Essentials of
Pediatric Radiology

Essentials of Pediatric Radiology

Edward M. Burton, M.D.

*Associate Professor of Radiology and Pediatrics and
Chief of Pediatric Radiology
Medical College of Georgia
Augusta, Georgia*

Alan S. Brody, M.D.

*Associate Professor of Radiology and Pediatrics
Children's Hospital Medical Center
Cincinnati, Ohio*

1999
THIEME
New York • Stuttgart

Thieme New York
333 Seventh Avenue
New York, NY 10001

Editorial Director: Avé McCracken
Executive Editor: Jane Pennington, Ph.D.
Assistant Editor: Jinnie Kim
Developmental Editor: Kathleen P. Lyons
Director, Production & Manufacturing: Maxine Langweil
Production Editor: Pam Ritzer
Marketing Director: Phyllis Gold
Sales Manager: David Bertelsen
Chief Financial Officer: Seth F. Fishman
President: Brian D. Scanlan
Cover Designer: José Fonfrias
Cover Illustration: Robert Finkbeiner
Compositor: The Publisher's Resource Development Group
Printer: The Maple-Vail Book Manufacturing Group

Cover illustration of hands, Robert Finkbeiner, Medical Illustrator, Department of Radiology, Medical College of Georgia, Augusta, GA.

Library of Congress Cataloging-in-Publication Data
Burton, Edward M.
    Essentials of pediatric radiology / Edward M. Burton and Alan S.
  Brody.
      p.   cm.
    Includes bibliographical references and index.
    ISBN 0-86577-802-7. — ISBN 3-13-115681-3
    1. Pediatric radiology.   I. Brody, Alan S.   II. Title.
    [DNLM: 1. Diagnostic Imaging—in infancy and childhood.
  2. Diagnostic Imaging—methods.   3. Pediatrics.   WN 240B974e   1999]
  RJ51.R3B87   1999
  618.92'00757—dc21
  DNLM/DC
  for Library of Congress   98-34484
                                                                  CIP

Important note: Medical knowledge is ever-changing. As new research and clinical experience broaden our knowledge, changes in treatment and drug therapy may be required. The authors and editors of the material herein have consulted sources believed to be reliable in their efforts to provide information that is complete and in accord with the standards accepted at the time of publication. However, in view of the possibility of human error by the authors, editors, or publisher of the work herein, or changes in medical knowledge, neither the authors, editors, publisher, nor any other party who has been involved in the preparation of this work, warrants that the information contained herein is in every respect accurate or complete, and they are not responsible for any errors or omissions or for the results obtained from use of such information. Readers are encouraged to confirm the information contained herein with other sources. For example, readers are advised to check the product information sheet included in the package of each drug they plan to administer to be certain that the information contained in this publication is accurate and that changes have not been made in the recommended dose or in the contraindications for administration. This recommendation is of particular importance in connection with new or infrequently used drugs.

Some of the product names, patents, and registered designs referred to in this book are in fact registered trademarks or proprietary names even though specific reference to this fact is not always made in the text. Therefore, the appearance of a name without designation as proprietary is not to be construed as a representation by the publisher that it is in the public domain.

Printed in the United States of America
Printer: The Maple-Vail Book Manufacturing Group

5 4 3 2 1
TNY ISBN 0-86577-802-7
GTV ISBN 3-13-115681-3

To Adam, Mathew, and Scott, who don't understand why Daddy spends so much time doing letters; and especially to Marsha, who does.

Alan S. Brody

To Paula, Adam, and Laura whose love, support, and encouragement helped guide me through the circuitous journey of my career.

Edward M. Burton

CONTENTS

FOREWORD

Two well-known pediatric radiologists have combined their clinical experience as well as reviewed the literature to produce a practical and concise approach to pediatric radiology. The differing styles of the two authors complement each other. They begin with an excellent section on "how to" perform imaging in pediatric patients. This "Quick Start" section will be especially helpful to pediatric radiology residents and fellows. The outline form used throughout the book makes it extremely easy to look up material. The authors thoroughly cover the traditional organ systems: nervous, musculoskeletal, cardiovascular, respiratory, and genitourinary. There is an additional section on conditions with multisystem involvement, such as child abuse, phakomatoses, leukemia, cystic fibrosis, sickle cell disease, histiocytosis, and AIDS. The clinical pathways or guidelines for appropriate imaging are presented in multiple, easy to read diagrams. The two appendices on routine projections and pediatric nuclear imaging are also presented in the same precise, easy to find style presented throughout this textbook. *Essentials of Pediatric Radiology* should become the *Harriet Lane* of pediatric radiology.

Joanna Seibert, M.D.
Arkansas Children's Hospital
University of Arkansas for Medical Sciences
Little Rock, Arkansas

FOREWORD

At a recent Morning Report on the pediatric services of a large area academic medical center here in North Carolina, a 14-month old child was presented who had a 5-month history of failure to thrive. The story was that of a malnourished infant who had episodes of watery diarrhea, oral thrush, and at presentation, high fever and Herpes simplex gingivostomatitis. The complete blood count showed an anemia consistent with a chronic disease, a normal urinalysis, and serum electrolytes with a profoundly low potassium and moderately low bicarbonate. The logical diagnosis appeared to be either a primary or a secondary immunodeficiency, perhaps related to AIDS . . . logical at least until an extensive, 8-day, in-hospital evaluation failed to demonstrate any immunologic abnormalities whatsoever. Attention then focused on this child's history of diarrhea, which appeared to be clinically consistent with a secretory diarrhea. A serum vasoactive intestinal peptide level was markedly elevated. A contrast CT scan of the abdomen demonstrated a suprarenal mass with calcifications. Once a stage I ganglioneuroblastoma was removed, the child thrived.

The point of this clinical story was not missed by those attending the Morning Report session. The key to early diagnosis often, and certainly in this case, is found in an appropriately chosen radiologic evaluation. In fact, the pediatric radiologist who attends these Morning Reports, in jest, suggested that a fair percentage of the time, one might forget about attempting a complex, speculative differential diagnosis and just do a total body CT scan. While the latter approach is of dubious merit, even a plain film of the abdomen taken much earlier in the case illustrated would have provided the tip-off, as the tumor-related calcifications were readily visible with simple radiographs.

So what does all this have to do with this book? *Essentials of Pediatric Radiology* will provide excellent guidance, not just to the fellows in pediatric radiology, but also to pediatric medical residents who care for children with enigmatic and complex problems. Pediatric radiology, like radiology in general, is an organized and systematic discipline. The codified nature of the discipline is reflected in the quality of *Essentials of Pediatric Radiology,* which presents lucid insights into all of radiology as applied to children. The telegraphic style of the presentation allows for a comprehensive yet concise review of the field with an emphasis on what is unique about children. The presentation of this work lends itself to the use of algorithms, which are illustrated in Chapter 9. Although algorithms are not the "cup of tea" of many and are sometimes variously described as the "cookbooks" of medicine or the "crutch" of those bereft of intellect, they are profoundly useful teaching instruments; and if thought of as such, they do indeed add great insight and clarity to difficult clinical problems, and simple ones as well.

Essentials of Pediatric Radiology will obviously find a comfortable spot on the library shelves of radiologists in training and of many staff radiologists as well. There is also much to be learned in this work by medical students who rotate on to pediatric services and by pediatric medical attendings as well. While parts of this book, particularly the technological aspects of the discipline, are not necessarily appropriate for reading by a wider audience beyond radiologists, a good bit of the work is. It is rich in its provision of descriptions of what studies to order and under what circumstances. It tells us of the pitfalls to be avoided when requesting specific studies. In fact, Chapter 1, subtitled "Approach to Image Acquisition and Interpretation" should be on the reading list of all those who care for children. This chapter provides a concise overview about the core of pediatric radiology relevant to each of us.

Get a "head start" with the "quick start" features of Chapter 1. Better yet, don't stop there. Run the whole race.

James A. Stockman III, M.D.
President, The American Board of Pediatrics
Chapel Hill, North Carolina

PREFACE

A patient, surrounded by a group of medical students and their attending physician, became alarmed by the young neophytes. The patient asked, "Are they all students?" The attending physician replied, "In medicine, we are always students."

As physicians, we have incorporated this philosophy in our careers and wish to share what we have learned from our training and experience with others interested in the medical care of children. As pediatricians and pediatric radiologists, we have been well served by always thinking of the child as well as the image of the child. This book furnishes the necessary data that radiology trainees must have in their quest for board certification and that practicing pediatricians and radiologists will find useful to enhance their knowledge of pediatric radiology.

This book was written for all those who use imaging in the care of children. The practice of pediatric imaging requires special knowledge and understanding of children and the diseases that affect them. We designed this book to provide a concise source of information that addresses all aspects of pediatric imaging.

The text consists of three parts. The Quick Start chapter provides an overview of imaging in children. We describe many common childhood diseases, the techniques used to image them, and their imaging appearance. Quick Start provides numerous tips and suggestions for practicing radiologists to obtain quality, focused studies on children that will provide better service to their clinical colleagues.

The majority of the book is a series of chapters arranged according to organ system. The text and illustrations provide extensive information regarding pediatrics and its imaging. In addition, entities that encompass multiple systems, such as sickle cell disease and AIDS, are included in a separate chapter.

In the final chapter, we present a series of clinical pathways that allow us to share our approach to the evaluation of a number of common problems that children may have. Although there are many ways to successfully care for each problem, we offer approaches that we have found useful.

The appropriate imaging of children is a cooperative venture that requires the participation of the clinician and the radiologist. As physicians and lifelong students who happen to be pediatricians or radiologists, we can learn from each other. The fruit of our collaboration will be the health and well-being of children.

Edward M. Burton, M.D.
Alan S. Brody, M.D.

ACKNOWLEDGMENTS

I can acknowledge only a few of the teachers who helped me to learn and to grow. Without them this book would not exist. Steve Shelov first showed me how much joy teaching adds to the practice of medicine. Hideyo Minagi taught me that good radiologists are first good doctors. Charles Gooding and Bob Brasch introduced me to pediatric radiology. Scott Dunbar always remembered that we were entrusted with the well-being of a child. Don Kirks brought all of modern imaging to the care of children. Drs. Dunbar and Kirks, two very different men, were alike in their dedication to those that they taught. Jerry Kuhn supported me and encouraged me to continue to grow as I began clinical practice. Janet Strife keeps me pointed in the right direction. Finally, my thanks to the children and their parents who have always been the best teachers.

Alan S. Brody, M.D.

As I teach third-year medical students aspects of pediatric radiology, I usually ask them which field of medicine they plan to enter. Then I ask them why they have made that specific choice. Often, they are undecided or unsure. I recall that, at a similar time in my medical training, I found myself inspired to become a pediatrician by one of my teachers. Gerold Schiebler was my role model and first mentor. During my early career as a clinician, my interest in radiology was encouraged by my friend, Bill Bloom. Fortunately, Robert Woolfitt enlisted me in his training program and enabled me to become a radiologist. To combine my careers of pediatrics and radiology seemed appropriate; the fellowship program in pediatric radiology at Children's Hospital Medical Center in Cincinnati provided an extraordinary faculty. Scott Dunbar was a superb teacher and forthright leader. I am indebted to Rich Towbin, Bill Ball, Janet Strife, Diane Babcock, Kim Han, Alan Oestreich, and Robert Kaufman for their teaching and friendship. Don Kirks joined the faculty in the middle of my training and encouraged me to be an academic pediatric radiologist, for which I am grateful. In Memphis, Barry Gerald provided amiable leadership, support, and friendship. During my first days at LeBonheur Children's Medical Center, Barry advised me to publish. When my career detoured and seemed to bottom out, Eugene Binet and the Medical College of Georgia provided an opportunity to resurrect my medical life. At MCG, I am grateful for the support and friendship of my colleagues in radiology and pediatrics. Specifically, I thank Gisela Mercado-Deane, Bill Kanto, and Charlie Howell. Finally, I wish to thank my co-author Alan Brody for many years of friendship and my medical editor, Laura Burton, who has lived my medical career by my side.

It has taken me a long time to understand that Gerold Schiebler's message to me is that teaching others is rewarding and satisfying in ways we often don't recognize initially. Just as our teachers touch our lives and guide us, we bequeath direction to our students.

Edward M. Burton, M.D.

INTRODUCTION

Radiology is a two-part discipline. The first part involves perception of an image and recognition of normal and abnormal findings. Accurate interpretation requires that the image be properly obtained. Chapter One includes basic information as well as helpful tips to get you "up and running" and to help you develop a logical, systematic approach to image interpretation in pediatric radiology.

The second part of radiology involves applying your knowledge or database of medicine to correlate the imaging findings with pathophysiology. The information to augment your database of pediatrics will be found in subsequent chapters arranged according to systems. The "quick start" icon will be found in various chapters to reinforce imaging acquisition or interpretation. The "quick start" icon in chapters 2 through 8 refers the reader to the appropriate section within the Quick Start chapter.

Finally, the last chapter presents a series of algorithms or imaging pathways that will assist you in utilizing radiologic imaging appropriately to diagnose common pediatric problems.

Now, let's get going!

Essentials of
Pediatric Radiology

CHAPTER ONE QUICK START

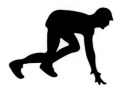

APPROACH TO IMAGE ACQUISITION AND INTERPRETATION

I. **RADIOGRAPHY (TECHNIQUE: APPENDIX 1)**
  A. **Approach to lateral chest radiograph interpretation [Figs. 1-1 and 1-2]**
    1. Most clinicians and radiology residents prefer the frontal chest radiograph to the lateral because they are more familiar with the frontal view.
    2. However, cardiac size, middle lobe, and lower lobe abnormalities may be easier to interpret on the lateral view.
       a. If you have a two-view chest series, look at the lateral view first. Do not ignore the lateral view!
    3. Evaluate
       a. Tracheal air column: note focal or diffuse narrowing and deviation. Identify the inferior vena cava and posterior cardiac border, which should be close to one another **[Fig. 4-42]**
       b. As your eye tracks down along the spine, the lung parenchyma should become darker
       c. If lung parenchyma becomes lighter in appearance, it usually indicates an airspace process in a lower lobe or pleural effusion **[Fig. 1-3; see also Fig. 5-30]**
          • Pleural effusion first collects in the posterior sulcus, best seen on lateral view on upright film

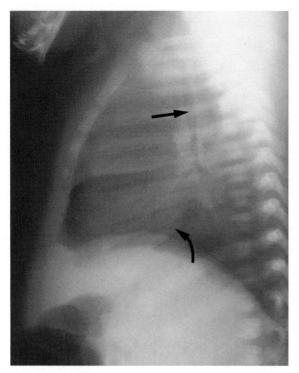

Fig. 1-1 Lateral chest radiograph: Normal newborn. Note segmented sternum, shape of hemidiaphragms, position of posterior cardiac border (curved arrow), tracheal air column (straight arrow), well-expanded and aerated lungs.

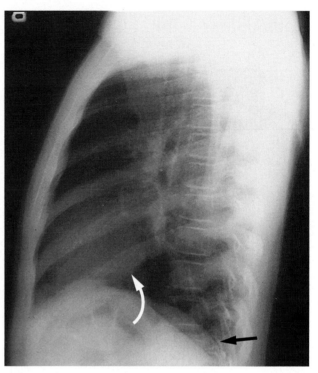

Fig. 1-2 Lateral chest radiograph: Normal child. Note posterior cardiac border (curved arrow) and normal posterior sulcus (straight arrow). As your eye follows the vertebral column inferiorly, lung parenchyma becomes "darker as you go down." This is normal. Notice normal vertebral bodies.

PITFALL

• Underinflation accentuates heart size, vessels appear enlarged, indistinct (simulates congestive heart failure)

    d. The air-filled lung should extend to where the ribs curve posteriorly on the lateral view and laterally on frontal view
- If a soft-tissue density is between air-filled lung and rib, it is pleural effusion or thickening

    e. Identifying the hemidiaphragms
- On upright lateral image, air in gastric fundus or splenic flexure of colon should be below left hemidiaphragm
- Right hemidiaphragm extends to anterior chest
- Left hemidiaphragm usually does not extend to anterior chest

B. **Approach to PA or AP (frontal) chest radiograph interpretation [Figs. 1-4 and 1-5; see also Fig. 5-1]**

  1. Adequate exposure

    a. Visualize vertebral bodies through cardiac shadow, disc spaces, central pulmonary vessels
- Overexposed (too dark)
- Underexposed (too light)

  2. Adequate inspiration
- Six anterior ribs or nine posterior ribs above diaphragm

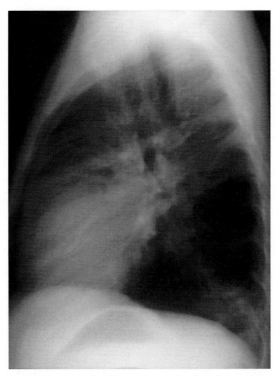

Fig. 1-3 Lateral chest radiograph: Opacity overlies lower thoracic spine. Note that lung overlying vertebral column becomes whiter inferiorly than superiorly. This is abnormal, indicating lower lobe opacity. Left hemidiaphragm identified by proximity to stomach bubble. Lower lobe opacity.

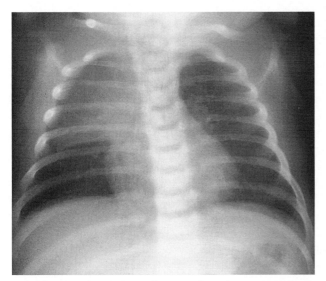

Fig. 1-4 AP chest radiograph: Normal newborn. Note prominent thymic "sail" to right of midline. Cardiac size is normal, lungs are well-expanded and aerated. Pulmonary vessels are normal.

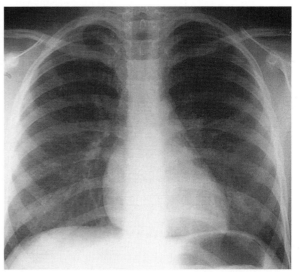

Fig. 1-5 PA chest radiograph: Normal child. Note symmetric pulmonary blood flow, normal cardiac size and shape, well-aerated lungs.

▶TIP
Look for increased
linear density
overlying pedicles
along spine;
descending aorta
usually identified
by this finding,
especially in
infants and small
children

3. Outside-in approach: If you look at heart and lungs first, especially if abnormal, you may ignore soft tissue, upper abdomen, rib, shoulder, or clavicle lesion. Beware the second abnormality!

4. Evaluate
   a. Placement of tubes and lines (endotracheal, thoracostomy, or feeding tube, central catheters, ventriculoperitoneal tubes, etc.) **[Figs. 5-4, 5-5, 5-10, 5-16 through 5-18]**
   b. Soft tissues for edema, calcification
   c. Ribs for patient rotation, asymmetry, anomaly **[Figs. 3-9 and 3-19]**, fracture **[Figs. 3-14 and 8-3],** periosteal reaction, and evidence of prior surgery
   d. Spine for unusual shape or segmentation anomalies
   e. Clavicles for position (lordosis or rotation), fracture, or periosteal reaction
   f. Humeri for unusual shape (previous trauma or neuromotor dysfunction)
   g. Chest and abdomen for surgical clips, gastrostomy tubes, or distention
   h. Hemidiaphragms for symmetry
   i. Mediastinum and hila for shape and calcification **[Figs. 5-51, 5-53, 5-57; see also Figs. 2-126 and 8-9]**
   j. Cardiac size and shape
      • Transverse diameter in children can be up to 60% of thoracic diameter
      • Due to overlying thymus, aortic knob usually not seen in infants
      • Identify expected tracheal deviation due to adjacent aortic knob
         Left aortic arch deviates trachea to right
         Right aortic arch deviates trachea to left **[Fig. 5-19]**
         On expiratory radiograph, trachea deviates to side opposite aortic arch

5. Lung parenchyma
   a. Normality of parenchyma identified by perception of vascular markings. As patient improves from focal or diffuse parenchymal disease, you will be able to perceive the margins of pulmonary vessels more clearly.
      • Conversely, as focal or diffuse parenchymal disease occurs or worsens, your ability to perceive the edge of vessels will decrease.
   b. Asymmetry of pulmonary blood flow, hyperlucency, shift of midline structures **[Fig. 1-6; see also Figs. 4-2 and 4-16]**
      • Due to decrease in overlying soft tissues
         Poland syndrome (absence of pectoralis muscle)
         Resection of upper limb
      • Decreased pulmonary blood flow
         Due to unilateral vascular obstruction
         – Pulmonary artery obstruction
         – Thromboembolic disease
         Reflex vasoconstriction
         – Bronchial obstruction or air trapping
      • Increased pulmonary blood flow
         Unilateral pulmonary artery shunt **[Fig. 4-17]**

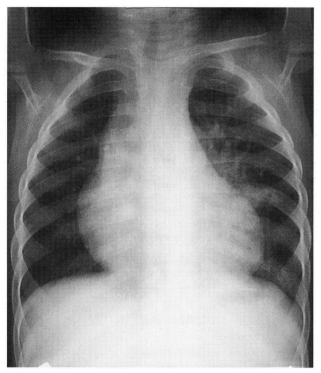

Fig. 1-6 PA chest radiograph: Pulmonary blood flow is decreased on right and increased on left. Asymmetric pulmonary blood flow.

- Pulmonary hyperinflation **[Figs. 5-33, 5-43 through 5-45]**
  Unilateral air trapping (foreign body aspiration, extrinsic bronchial obstruction)
  Emphysema, congenital or acquired
- Extra air in thorax
  Pneumothorax, pneumomediastinum
- Shift of midline
  Obliquity of patient position
  - Note ribs, medial clavicle
  - If right ribs longer than left ribs on AP film, patient is rotated to right
  - If left ribs longer than right ribs on AP film, patient is rotated to left
  - Right medial clavicle further from middle of spine than left medial clavicle = right rotation
  - Left medial clavicle further from middle of spine than right medial clavicle = left rotation
  - Chest asymmetry (scoliosis)
  Less volume on one side (atelectasis, pulmonary hypoplasia, agenesis) **[Figs. 5-20 and 5-26]**

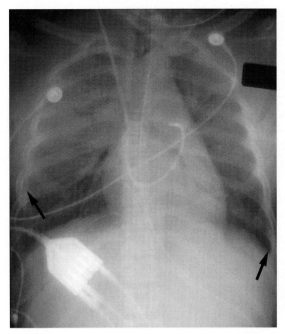

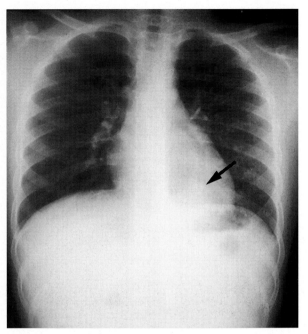

Fig. 1-7 PA chest radiograph: Diffuse airspace opacity with multiple air bronchograms, indicated as gray lucencies that branch and taper. Also note bilateral pleural effusion (arrows).

Fig. 1-8 PA chest radiograph: Opacity seen through cardiac shadow on left (arrow). Left lower lobe retrocardiac airspace opacity.

Increased volume on one side (pleural effusion, lobar emphysema, diaphragmatic hernia, cystic adenomatoid malformation, mass) **[Figs. 5-5, 5-24, 5-25, and 5-59]**

Increased pressure on one side (tension pneumothorax, air trapping due to partial bronchial obstruction or foreign body aspiration) **[Fig. 5-12]**

c. Look for air bronchograms (especially *through* the heart for left retrocardiac airspace opacity, a commonly missed area of atelectasis/pneumonitis) **[Figs. 1-7 and 1-8]**

  ● Branching lucencies in periphery or peripheral to right and left main bronchi

d. Alveolar or airspace opacities identified by homogeneous opacity, cloudlike appearance, air bronchograms **[Figs. 1-8 through 1-10; see also Figs. 5-27, 5-29, 5-30, 5-34, 5-35, 5-46, 5-47, 4-4 and 4-37]**

  ● Alveolar or airspace opacities include alveolar edema, pneumonitis, atelectasis, pulmonary contusion, or hemorrhage

e. Interstitial or airway opacities identified by lacelike, linear, reticular, or fine or coarse nodular opacities; often look like "chicken wire, doughnuts, or bagels" **[Figs. 1-11 and 1-12; see also Figs. 5-7, 5-8, 5-31, 5-32, and 5-37 through 5-40]**

  ● Interstitial or airway opacities include bronchiolitis, reactive airway disease,\bronchopulmonary dysplasia, interstitial edema, cystic fibrosis, chronic aspiration, fibrosis

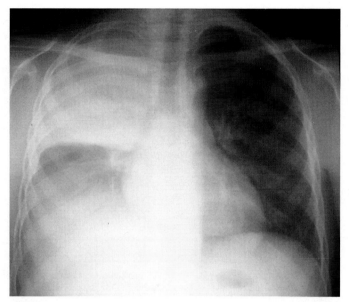

Fig. 1-9 PA chest radiograph: Airspace opacities in right upper and lower lobes. The right middle lobe is uninvolved.

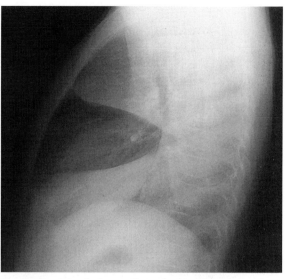

Fig. 1-10 Lateral chest radiograph: Same patient as Figure 1-9. Airspace opacities in right upper and lower lobes. The right middle lobe is uninvolved.

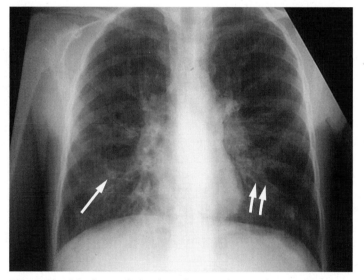

Fig. 1-11 PA chest radiograph: Pulmonary hyperinflation, manifested by flattened hemidiaphragms. Note numerous "doughnuts" or "bagels," indicating bronchial wall thickening (arrow) seen end-on. Also note "tram-tracks" (double arrow) indicating bronchial wall thickening seen along long axis. Interstitial opacities.

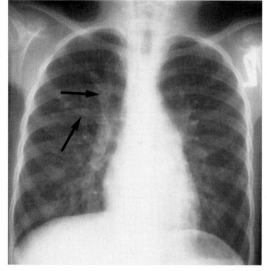

Fig. 1-12 PA chest radiograph: Pulmonary hyperinflation, manifested by flattened hemidiaphragms. Note numerous "doughnuts" or "bagels," indicating bronchial wall thickening (arrows) seen end-on. Interstitial opacities.

6. Air leaks:
   a. Pulmonary interstitial emphysema (PIE) **[Fig. 1-13; see also Figs. 5-3 and 5-14]**
      - More lucent, somewhat broader than air bronchograms
      - Round or rodlike, unlike air bronchograms, which branch like a tree

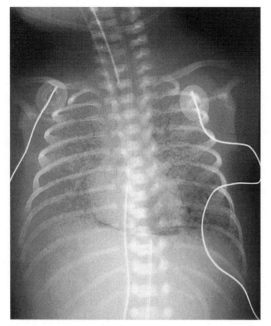

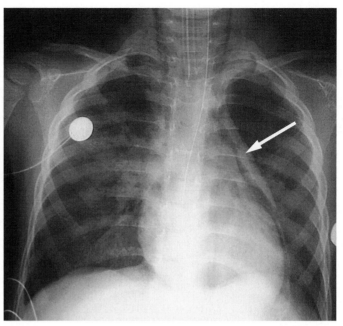

Fig. 1-13 PA chest radiograph: Dark, round lucencies (pulmonary interstitial emphysema, PIE) seen best in left lower lobe. These do not branch and are darker than air bronchograms, which can be seen in left upper and right upper lobes. Also note curvilinear lucency at base of heart (pneumomediastinum).

Fig. 1-14 PA chest radiograph: Near drowning. Mixed interstitial opacities in right perihilar area and airspace opacities in left retrocardiac area and right lower lobe. The oblique soft tissue density separated from the left cardiac border is the thymus (arrow). Air density is between heart and thymus. Also note air extending into soft tissues of the neck. Pneumomediastinum (uplifted thymus).

b. Pneumomediastinum (PMD) **[Figs. 1-13 through 1-16; see also Fig. 5-14]**
   - Identified by uplifted thymus (do not mistake left lobe of thymus in PMD for the left pulmonary artery)
   - Lucency outlines complete extent of diaphragmatic surface of both hemidiaphragms (continuous diaphragm sign)
   - Often associated with subcutaneous air dissecting into axilla or neck (unusual in newborn, common in child or adult)

c. Pneumopericardium (PCD) **[Fig. 5-15]**
   - Air almost completely encircles heart, extending to level of aorta/pulmonary artery (looks like "ring around the 'cor'lar'")

d. Pneumothorax (PTX) **[Figs. 1-17 and 1-18; see also Figs. 5-11 and 5-12]**
   - In supine patient, hemithorax more lucent, normal thin dark (Mach) line around heart too broad, air in costophrenic angle produces "deep sulcus sign"
   - Tension PTX produces midline shift away from lucency, widens rib interspaces, displaces hemidiaphragm downward
   - Clinically, heart may be displaced and small, indicating hypotension due to decreased venous return and reduced cardiac output

7. The opaque hemithorax:
   a. Opaque hemithorax with midline shift toward opacity = atelectasis
      - Do not put chest tube into this opaque hemithorax, or into opposite more lucent hemithorax **[Fig. 1-19; see also Fig. 4-30]**

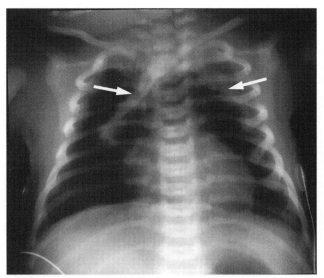

Fig. 1-15 AP chest radiograph: Newborn with respiratory distress. Note oblique soft tissue structures separated from cardiac border bilaterally. These structures are the lobes of the thymus (arrows) uplifted by air. Pneumomediastinum (uplifted thymus).

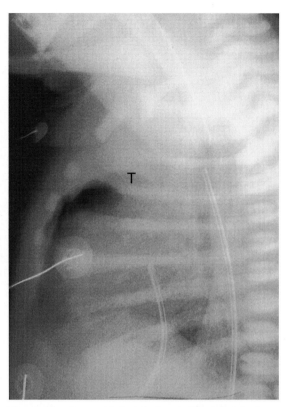

Fig. 1-16 Cross-table lateral chest radiograph: Newborn with respiratory distress. Note air anteriorly uplifting thymus (T). Pneumomediastinum.

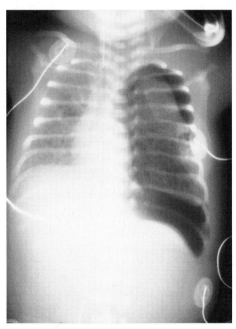

Fig. 1-17 AP chest radiograph: Lucent air collection in left hemithorax, depressed left hemidiaphragm, displaced heart and mediastinum to right. Note left lung fails to collapse due to stiffness or noncompliance and small cardiac size, indicating decreased venous return, or hypovolemia, and poor cardiac output. Tension pneumothorax.

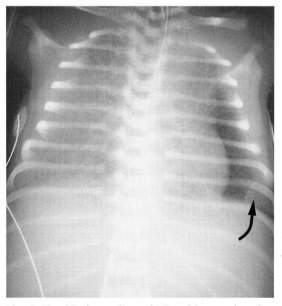

Fig. 1-18 AP chest radiograph: Broad lucency lateral to left cardiac border. Note small area of opaque lung at left costophrenic angle (curved arrow). Anterior pneumothorax.

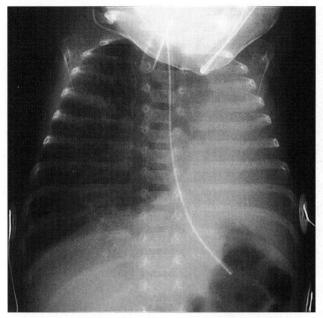

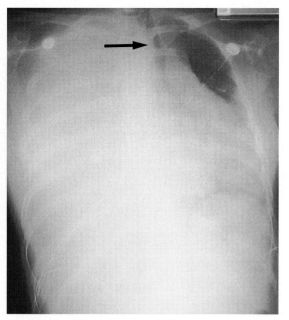

Fig. 1–19 AP chest radiograph: Complete opacity of left hemithorax with shift of heart and mediastinum to left. Left lung atelectasis.

Fig. 1–20 PA chest radiograph: Complete opacification of right hemithorax with displacement of trachea (arrow) to left, indicating increased volume in right hemithorax. Large right pleural effusion.

      b. Opaque hemithorax with midline shift = pleural effusion or mass **[Fig. 1-20]**

      c. Opaque hemithorax with no midline shift = pulmonary consolidation, unilateral pulmonary edema **[Fig. 1-21]**
- Often hazy, rather than opaque

C. **The Abdomen**
   1. Exposure
      a. Satisfactory exposure enables discrimination of properitoneal fat line, fat around inferior edge of liver
- If fat identifying liver edge absent, consider ascites or hemoperitoneum
   2. Positioning
      a. Patient should be straight
      b. Include lung bases to pubic symphysis
      c. Collimate side-to-side to abdominal wall
   3. Bowel gas pattern **[Fig. 1-22]**
      a. In older child, few small bowel air-filled loops normal
- Fecal material in colon common
      b. In infant, multiple small and large bowel air-filled loops common
      c. Focally dilated gas-filled bowel may indicate either obstruction or inflammatory disease
      d. In the newborn, you cannot discriminate between dilated large and small bowel. The newborn colon has no haustra and the small bowel has no valvulae conniventes.

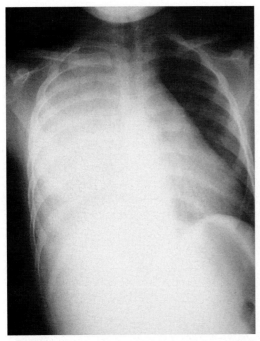

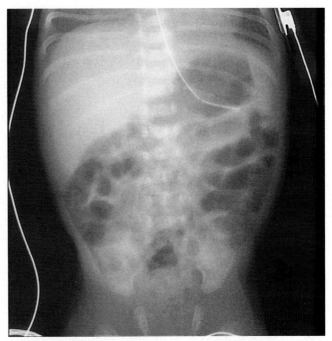

Fig. 1-21 PA chest radiograph: Complete opacification of right hemithorax with air bronchograms in right upper lobe and right lower lobe behind heart. No mediastinal shift. Right lung consolidation.

Fig. 1-22 AP abdomen radiograph: Normal newborn. Gas is distributed throughout bowel. All visualized loops have approximately equal caliber.

4. Pneumatosis **[Figs. 6-31 and 6-32]**
    a. Air in the wall of the bowel appears as a smooth (linear) or bubbly (mottled) pattern
    b. Smooth pattern is thought to be sub**S**erosal air
        - Pneumatosis parallels air in lumen of bowel
        - If involved bowel collapsed or if wall thickened, curvilinear pneumatosis produces geometric pattern (sine wave, circle)
    c. Mottled pattern is sub**M**ucosal air
        - Mottled pneumatosis can be confused with air mixed with fecal material.
    d. In the newborn, either pattern is a hallmark of necrotizing enterocolitis
        - Look for branching pattern of air in liver (portal venous air)
            Portal venous air peripheral (portal flow drives air outward)
            Biliary air central (bile flow drives air toward common bile duct)
5. Free air **[Figs. 1-23 and 1-24]**
    a. In the supine patient, air around the falciform ligament appears as a vertical or oblique line in the right upper quadrant
        If the radiograph is suspicious for free air, obtain an upright or left lateral decubitus (LLD) film
        - Upright film: Image obtained AP; air-fluid levels horizontal
            On upright film, look under diaphragm
            Upright film most sensitive projection in older child
            LLD in older child used if child unable to stand

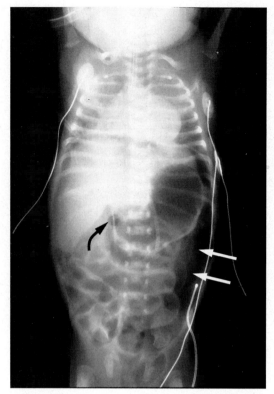

Fig. 1-23 AP chest/abdomen radiograph: "Football" sign. Note free air along left side of abdomen, air outlining bowel wall (arrows), air outlining falciform ligament (curved arrow). Hemidiaphragms are elevated. Pneumoperitoneum.

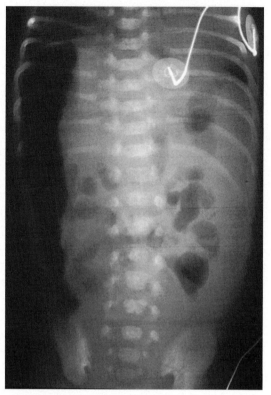

Fig. 1-24 LLD abdomen radiograph: Air overlying right lobe of liver. Pneumoperitoneum.

- LLD: patient placed left side down, film and cassette placed vertically behind patient's back, X-ray tube in front of patient's abdomen.
  - Image should resemble AP film, but air-fluid levels are vertical and intraluminal air predominates in right side of abdomen
  - Free air identified over right lateral liver edge usually
  - In premies and newborn, use LLD
  - NOTE: infant should be placed in LLD position for 5 to 10 minutes prior to X-ray exposure to allow gas to rise to nondependent position
- Cross-table lateral reported as more sensitive, but difficult to discriminate free air from air in distended loop of bowel. In general, LLD preferred

b. In the presence of a pneumothorax or pneumomediastinum, free peritoneal air may have dissected from chest

c. In the newborn with hyaline membrane disease and pulmonary interstitial emphysema but not pneumothorax or pneumomediastinum, free peritoneal air should be considered of abdominal origin (perforation)
  - Cross-table lateral radiograph of the abdomen with an air/fluid level in the peritoneum indicates air from visceral perforation rather than air dissected from the chest.

6. Small bowel obstruction **[Fig. 1-25; see also Figs. 6-17, 6-18, and 6-21]**
   a. Dilated air-filled loops of proximal bowel with paucity or absence of gas in distal bowel or colon/rectum
      • Few dilated loops indicates proximal bowel obstruction
      • Many dilated loops indicates distal bowel obstruction
   b. Obstruction of small bowel filled primarily with fluid and small amount of air indicated by "string of pearls" sign
      • Appearance resembles pearl necklace; produced by bubbles of air floating in fluid in multiple loops of bowel
7. Ascites **[Fig. 1-26; see also Fig. 7-47]**
   a. Loops of bowel float on top of peritoneal fluid
      • Bowel is centrally positioned and displaced from flanks
      • Loops often separated from each other by fluid
   b. Early sign of ascites is loss of fat plane at inferior liver margin
      • Indicates fluid in Morison's pouch (hepatorenal fossa)
      • Seen in older children; unusual in infants
8. Abdominal mass **[Fig. 1-27; see also Figs. 6-26 and 7-32]**
   a. Look for displacement of bowel loops around mass or air within mass (intussusception)
   b. Masses arising from pelvis displace bowel superiorly
   c. Midline pelvic masses suggest bladder distention or bladder outlet or vaginal obstruction (posterior urethral valves in newborn male, hydrometrocolpos in newborn female)
   d. Lateral pelvic mass extending into abdomen suggests ovarian origin in female

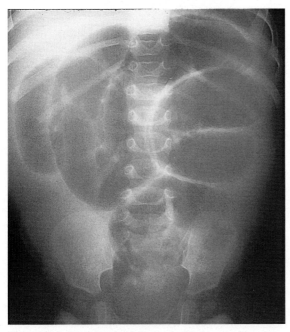

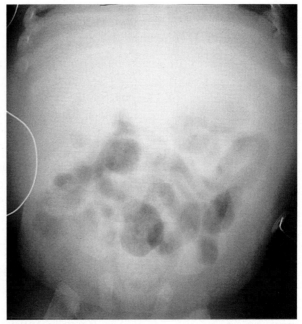

Fig. 1-25 AP abdomen radiograph: Numerous dilated air-filled loops of small bowel with paucity of gas in colon. Small bowel obstruction.

Fig. 1-26 AP abdomen radiograph: Newborn with ascites. Note centrally placed loops of bowel and abdominal protuberance.

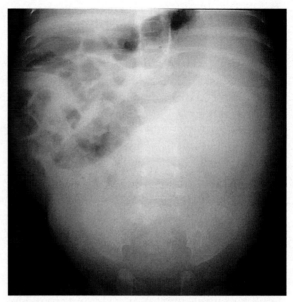

Fig. 1-27 AP abdomen radiograph: Newborn with abdominal mass. Note displacement of bowel superiorly and toward the right by large noncalcified soft-tissue mass that fills the left side of abdomen and lower abdominal and pelvic areas.

9. Calcification **[Fig. 6-64]**
   a. Within mass suggests germ cell tumor, neuroblastoma, adrenal tumor or hemorrhage
   b. Linear or geometric pattern suggests meconium or barium peritonitis
   c. Rounded calcification suggests gallstones, renal or ureteral calculi, appendicolith, ingested radiopaque pills (iron, other heavy metals, Pepto-Bismol, etc.)

D. **The Skull**
1. Lateral skull evaluation **[Figs. 1-28 and 1-29]**
   a. Coronal, lambdoid, and squamosal sutures seen in normals
   b. Normal sutures <2 mm in width
      ● Sutures >2 mm suggest increased intracranial pressure or diastasis (infiltration by tumor, underossification of skull, or diastatic fracture) **[Figs. 2-90 and 2-91]**
   c. Overlapping sutures may be present in newborn, due to molding during delivery
   d. Fracture identified as lucent line(s) that do not correspond to normal sutures **[Fig. 1-30]**
      ● Plain film more sensitive than CT
         If CT obtained along axis of fracture, fracture line may not be identified
   e. Depressed skull fracture represented as focal increased calvarial density (unexpected area of sclerosis) **[Fig. 1-31]**

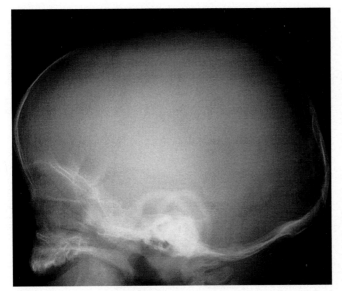

Fig. 1-28 Lateral skull radiograph: Normal 4-month-old infant. Note relationship between size of face and capacity of calvaria.

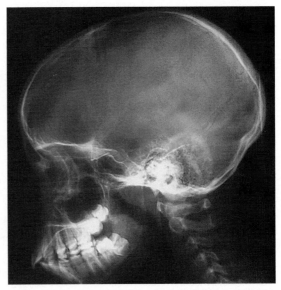

Fig. 1-29 Lateral skull radiograph: Normal 11-year-old child. Note relationship between size of face and capacity of calvaria.

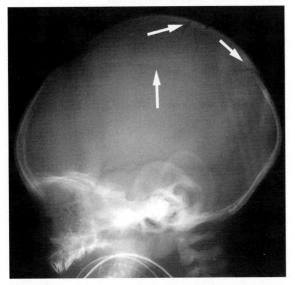

Fig. 1-30 Lateral skull radiograph: Child abuse. Comminuted parietal fractures (arrows). Skull fracture.

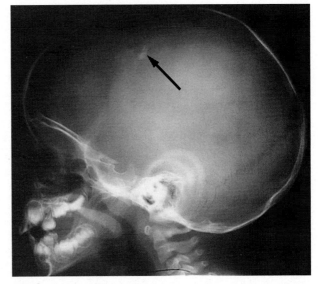

Fig. 1-31 Lateral skull radiograph: Focal area of sclerosis (arrow) posterior to level of coronal suture. Depressed skull fracture.

2. AP skull evaluation **[Fig. 1-32]**
   a. Sagittal suture unfused and <2 mm in width
   b. Orbits rounded and symmetric
      • Two orbits should be separated in distance by transverse diameter of one orbit
      • Abnormal interorbital distance suggests hypertelorism/hypotelorism

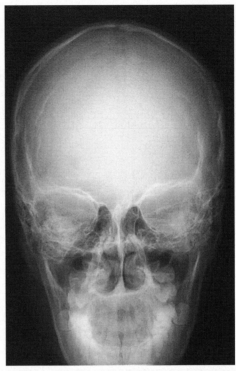

Fig. 1-32 AP skull radiograph: Normal 11-year-old child. Note symmetry of orbits, well-aerated paranasal sinuses.

3. Sinus radiographs
   a. AP or Caldwell + Waters + lateral to include adenoids
   b. High incidence of false negatives and positives
   c. Sinusitis is difficult diagnosis both clinically and radiographically
      • Soft tissue in sinuses on radiograph present in >50% of asymptomatic children <1 year of age, common through school age
4. Craniofacial ratio
   a. Number of faces that can fit within area of calvarium on lateral skull radiograph:
      • Newborn, 3–4 : 1; Premature, may be 5 : 1
      • By age 6 years, 2–2.5 : 1
      • Adult = 1.5 : 1
5. Synostosis patterns **[Figs. 1-33 and 1-34; see also Fig. 2-87]**
   a. Dolichocephaly or scaphocephaly (elongated from front-to-back)—sagittal (most common, 55%)
   b. Trigonocephaly (triangular)—metopic
   c. Brachycephaly (high over frontal part of skull)—bilateral coronal (second most common, 12%)
   d. Plagiocephaly (lopsided)—unilateral coronal (harlequin eye)
   e. Turricephaly or acrocephaly (tower skull, high over parietal part of skull)—all sutures
   f. Kleeblattschädel—cloverleaf skull

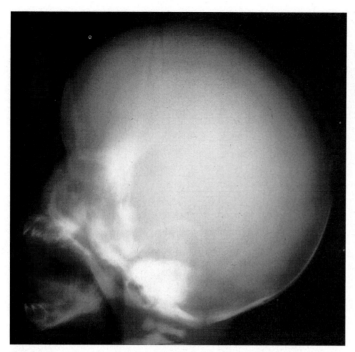

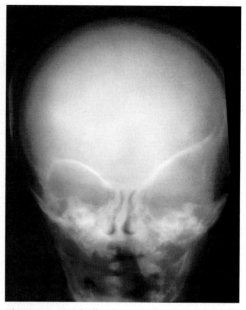

Fig. 1-34 AP skull radiograph: Normal right orbit, elevated and irregular left supraorbital ridge (Harlequin eye). Unilateral coronal synostosis.

Fig. 1-33 Lateral skull radiograph: Protuberant frontal calvarium due to bilateral coronal synostosis.

6. Increased intracranial pressure
   a. Sutures should not be more than 2 mm apart
   b. Excessive digital markings on calvarium

E. **The Spine**
1. Look at lateral image first **[Fig. 1-35]**
   a. Lines drawn along anterior vertebral body, posterior vertebral body, and spinolaminar line (normal sclerotic line at base of lamina) should be smooth along spinal axis.
      • Interruption or step-off indicates subluxation
2. Vertebral body shape
   a. Rectangular with smoothly contoured superior and inferior endplates
   b. Decreased vertebral body height = platyspondyly (diffusely oval, flat, or pear-shaped, usually congenital) **[Fig. 1-36; see also Figs. 3-5 and 3-7]**, compression (usually post-traumatic) **[Fig. 8-2]**, or vertebra plana (focal nearly complete loss of height, i.e., Langerhans' cell histiocytosis, osteomyelitis)
   c. Increased vertebral body height in lumbar spine indicates neuromotor dysfunction, patient not ambulatory
      • Confirm by gracile long bones, scoliosis, hip subluxation, ventriculo-peritoneal shunt
   d. Segmentation abnormalities **[Fig. 1-37]**
      • Butterfly vertebra
         Defect or waist in central portion of vertebral body
      • Hemivertebra
         Absence of lateral, ventral, or dorsal portion of vertebral body

PITFALL

• Note: Apparent anterior malalignment of vertebral bodies at C2–C3 (occasionally at C3–C4) with normal spinolaminar line indicates pseudosubluxation, a normal variant in children

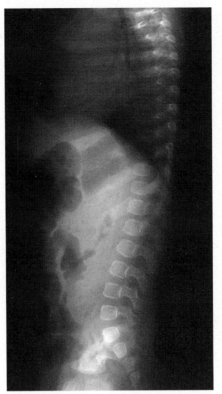

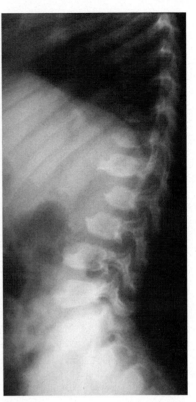

Fig. 1-35 Lateral thoracolumbar spine radiograph: Note size and shape of vertebral bodies, regular disc spaces. Normal spine.

Fig. 1-36 Lateral thoracolumbar spine radiograph: Patient with mucopolysaccaride disease. Flattened vertebral bodies with central and inferior beaking. Platyspondyly.

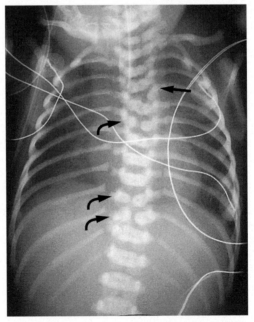

Fig. 1-37 AP spine radiograph: Hemivertebra (arrow), multiple butterfly vertebrae (curved arrows). Vertebral segmentation abnormality (VATER).

- Block vertebra

  Fusion of two (or more) adjacent vertebral bodies, no intervening disc space

  Height of block vertebra equals height of two normal adjacent vertebral bodies + intervening disc space

3. Scoliosis: Described by convexity of curve (right = dextroscoliosis, left = levoscoliosis)

F. **Long bones**

1. Detail film-screen combination recommended for best resolution
2. At least two views at right angles necessary
   a. Additional coned-down views may be needed for suspicious areas
3. Child abuse evaluation
   a. Individual long bone radiographs recommended
   b. Coned-down view of any suspicious areas may be needed
   c. Babygram is not adequate and should be discouraged
4. Age of appearance of ossification centers
   a. First molar = 33–34 wks gestation
   b. Second molar = 36 wks gestation
   c. Humeral head = 37 wks gestation – 4 months post-term
   d. Femoral head = 2 wks–7 months after birth in females, 3 wks–7 months in males
5. Fractures
   a. Evaluate
      - Orientation of fracture plane (transverse, oblique, spiral)
      - Angulation

        Specify direction of angle apex or convexity
      - Distracted or overriding
      - Displacement

        Specify relationship of proximal and distal fragments
      - Open (compound) or closed
      - Number of fragments (simple, comminuted)
      - Stage of healing **[Fig. 3-70]**
   b. Buckle fracture **[Fig. 3-67]**
      - Note smooth continuous cortical margin of long bones, metacarpals, metatarsals, phalanges
      - Abrupt angulation of cortical margin suggests buckle fracture

        Most common in distal radius
   c. Multi-bone unit fractures (Ring structures)
      - Just as a ring cannot be broken at only one point, a fracture in a multi-bone unit (jaw, pelvis, forearm, lower leg) often comprises a second fracture or dislocation
   d. Metaphyseal-epiphyseal fractures **[Figs. 3-57 through 3-65]**
      - Salter classification I–V:

        I = through physis

        II = metaphysis and physis

        III = physis and epiphysis

        IV = metaphysis, physis, and epiphysis

        V = occult injury of physis resulting in physeal growth disturbance

▶TIP
There will be a dislocation at a joint, angulated fracture of both bones, or angulated fracture of one bone and plastic bowing fracture of other bone [Fig. 3-68]. You *must* image the joints at both ends of an angulated forearm or lower leg fracture.

6. Patterns of bone loss or addition **[Figs. 3-47, 3-49 through 3-55]**
   a. Focal, circumscribed, well-defined or marginated
   b. Diffuse, poorly-defined or marginated
   c. Sclerotic, lytic, expansile, permeative, motheaten
7. Periosteal new bone formation **[Figs. 1-38 through 1-43; see also Figs. 3-34, 3-47, and 8-11]**
   a. *Smooth* (benign), *laminar* (often malignant, esp. Ewing's), *interrupted* (often malignant, esp. osteosarcoma; but osteomyelitis can produce Codman's triangle)

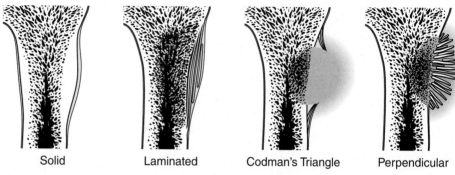

Solid   Laminated   Codman's Triangle   Perpendicular

Fig. 1-38 Periosteal patterns: Thin or thick solid periosteal reaction indicates nonaggressive pathologic process. Multiple layers of periosteum develop a laminated pattern as a reaction to an underlying pathologic process. This pattern implies a more aggressive lesion than the solid pattern. Codman's triangle denotes an aggressive lesion that has broken through the periosteum into the surrounding soft tissues. A perpendicular, or sunburst, pattern reveals a very aggressive underlying lesion.

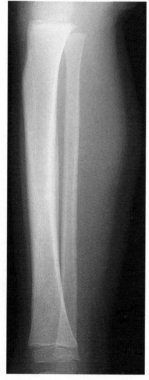

Fig. 1-39 Lateral lower leg radiograph: Smooth periosteal reaction along shaft of tibia.

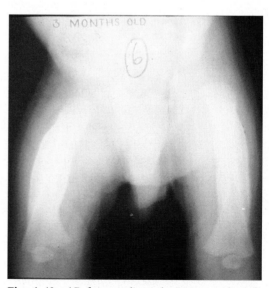

Fig. 1-40 AP femur radiograph: Patient with Caffey's disease. Thickening of cortex and periosteal new bone formation along shaft of femurs. Smooth periosteal reaction.

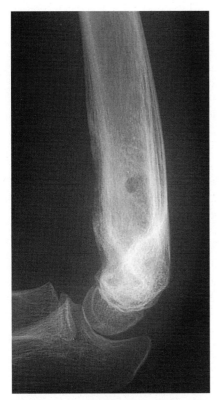

Fig. 1-41 Lateral humerus radiograph: Laminated periosteal reaction in a 9-year-old child with Ewing's sarcoma.

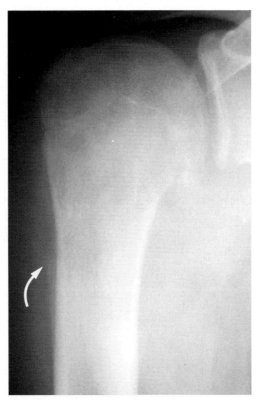

Fig. 1-42 AP humerus radiograph: Patient with osteosarcoma. Disrupted periosteal reaction (curved arrow) associated with poorly marginated motheaten pattern in proximal humeral metaphysis. Codman's triangle.

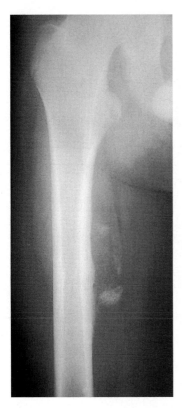

Fig. 1-43 AP femur radiograph: Soft-tissue calcification, disrupted periosteal new bone formation, and soft tissue ossification. Osteosarcoma, disrupted periosteal reaction.

      b. Focal (trauma, neoplasm, or infection)

      c. Diffuse (physiologic in 2–6 month old, metabolic, congenital infection, i.e., syphilis, toxic, i.e., prostaglandin)

   8. Abnormal shape

      a. Overtubulated = too thin or gracile **[Fig. 1-44]**

         Ex: Neuromotor dysfunction, osteogenesis imperfecta

      b. Undertubulated = too thick, Erlenmeyer flask-like **[Fig. 1-45]**

         Ex: Gaucher's disease, osteochondromatosis (diaphyseal aclasia)

G. **The Joints**

   1. Knee

      a. Lateral view first **[Fig. 1-46; see also Fig. 3-42]**

      b. Suprapatellar bursa located between pre-femoral fat posterior and triangular fat deep to the quadriceps tendon anterior. Suprapatellar bursa runs obliquely, less than 1 cm in width in all ages.

   2. Ankle

      a. Lateral view first

      b. First collection of effusion is anterior to talus. Fat anterior to talus is displaced by fluid/soft tissue density, producing "teardrop" appearance **[Fig. 3-38].**

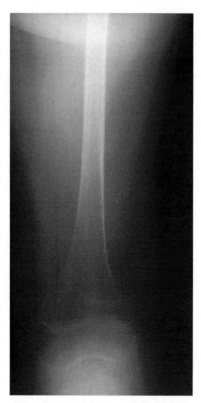

Fig. 1-44 AP femur radiograph: Patient with muscular dystrophy. Marked osteopenia (femoral condyle is barely seen), overtubulation of shaft (too narrow).

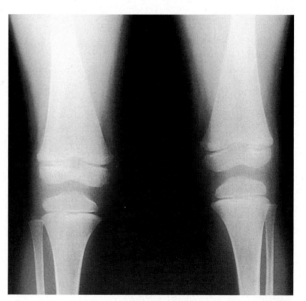

Fig. 1-45 AP knee radiograph: Patient with Gaucher's disease. Undertubulation (shaft too thick) of diaphysis and mild sclerosis.

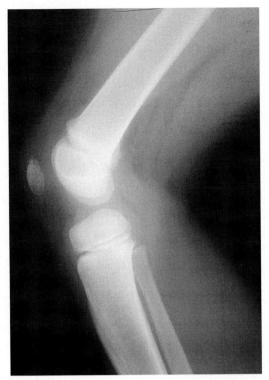

Fig. 1-46 Lateral knee radiograph: Normal growth plates, patella, and suprapatellar bursa.

   c. Only 2 to 3 cc joint fluid required to produce the "teardrop"

   d. Posterior ankle joint requires approximately 8 cc joint fluid to visualize distended capsule

3. Wrist

   a. Distal radius and ulna are nearly parallel

   b. In lateral view, line through ulna intersects triquetrum, most dorsal carpal bone (abnormal in Galeazzi fracture-dislocation)

   c. Fracture of carpal navicular may be subtle

     ● Specific positioning and oblique views may be necessary in appropriate clinical setting

4. Shoulder

   a. Note relationship of humeral head to glenoid fossa

   b. Shape (round) and density of humeral head

   c. Proximal humeral physis may resemble a fracture

     ● Be careful not to overcall

     ● Clinical evaluation or radiograph of opposite shoulder may be useful

5. Hip

   a. Note relationship of femoral head to acetabulum

   b. Shape (round) and density of femoral head **[Fig. 3-22]**

     ● Femoral heads should be equal in size and shape

   c. Medial joint space between acetabulum and most medial part of femoral head bilaterally should be symmetric (<2 mm difference)

6. Elbow **[Figs. 1-47 and 1-48; see also Fig. 3-68]**
   a. CRITOE/2,3,4,8,9,10. Capitellum, Radial head, Internal epicondyle, Trochlea, Olecranon, External epicondyle/Usual year of ossification.
   b. Internal epicondyle can occasionally precede Radial head; if Trochlea present but not Internal epicondyle, this indicates fracture of Internal epicondyle with entrapment (requires open reduction)
   c. Posterior fat pad sign
      • Always abnormal; indicates water, blood, pus, or cells in joint or synovial thickening
      • Traumatic joint effusion in child most commonly due to supracondylar fracture, which may be subtle
         For occult supracondylar fracture, immobilize and re-image in 10 to 14 days
   d. Anterior fat pad sign
      • Normally seen anterior to trochlear notch on lateral view
         If elevated or distorted, indicates joint fluid, etc.
   e. Radiocapitellar line
      • Line drawn through long axis of proximal shaft of radius should intersect capitellum in every plane (abnormal in Monteggia fracture-dislocation and occasionally in nursemaid's elbow)
   f. Anterior humeral line
      • Line drawn along anterior cortex of distal humerus should intersect middle 1/3 of capitellum
      • Line intersecting anterior 1/3 of capitellum indicates posterior displacement of capitellum (frequently seen in supracondylar fracture)

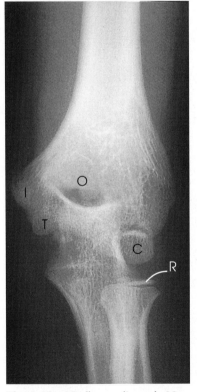

Fig. 1-47 AP elbow radiograph: Normal elbow ossification centers. Capitellum (C), radial head (R), internal epicondyle (I), trochlea (T), olecranon (O). External epicondyle not ossified in this patient.

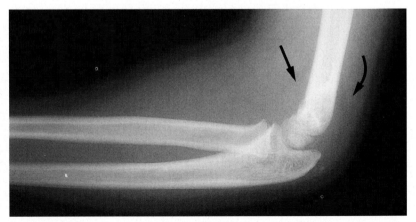

Fig. 1-48 Lateral elbow radiograph: Uplifted anterior fat pad (arrow); posterior fat pad (curved arrow). Elbow effusion.

H. **Hand**
1. Three views recommended (AP, lateral, oblique)
2. Note soft tissues
    a. Soft tissue swelling over dorsum, palmar, or local area may indicate underlying fracture.
3. Periosteal reaction along shaft of phalanges seen in sickle cell disease, child abuse, juvenile rheumatoid arthritis, leukemia, previous trauma
4. Cortex along phalanges and metacarpals should be smooth line
    a. Note abrupt angulation of buckle fracture
5. Metacarpals **[Fig. 3–18]**
    a. First metacarpal/thumb hypoplasia/dysplasia suggests radial ray dysplasia (i.e., Fanconi anemia, VATER, Holt-Oram syndrome)
    b. Straight edge along the heads of 3rd, 4th, 5th metacarpals should intersect all three metacarpal heads
        ● Short 4th or 5th metacarpal may indicate dysplasia, i.e., Turner's syndrome, pseudohypoparathyroidism
    c. In assessing bone age, compare metacarpal and phalangeal epiphyses with standard (Greulich and Pyle). Do not use carpal bones to assess bone age, except in young infant who may lack metacarpal/phalangeal epiphyses.

I. **Foot**
1. Normal hindfoot
    a. Angle between talus and calcaneus approximately 30°
    b. In AP and lateral views, talus points toward first metatarsal
    c. In AP view, calcaneus points toward fourth metatarsal
2. Hindfoot varus **[Fig. 3-20]**
    a. Talus, calcaneus nearly parallel in AP, lateral views
    b. Talus points toward second metatarsal
3. Hindfoot valgus **[Fig. 3-21]**
    a. Talo-calcaneal angle obtuse in AP, lateral views
    b. Talus points medial to first metatarsal

II. **FLUOROSCOPY**
A. **Airway [Figs. 1-49 through 1-51]:**
1. Performed in child with hoarseness, stridor, or cough, in conjunction with esophagogram/UGI
2. Place child in AP position
    a. Observe vocal cord movement for symmetry, abduction, and adduction
    b. Observe subglottic air column for narrowing, asymmetry, intraluminal soft tissue **[Figs. 2-94 and 2-95]**
3. Place child in right lateral position
    a. Observe airway for backward bowing of epiglottis or fluttering of aryepiglottic folds (laryngomalacia) and tracheal caliber change (tracheomalacia) or deviation
    b. Laryngomalacia noisier on quiet breathing
    c. Tracheomalacia noisier with crying

▶TIP
If epiglottitis considered, obtain lateral neck radiograph
Do not manipulate child **[Fig. 2-93]**

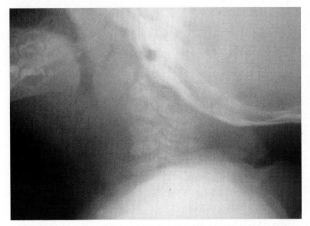

Fig. 1-49 Lateral airway radiograph: Taken in expiration. Apparent prevertebral soft tissue thickening and buckling of tracheal air column. Pharyngeal buckling.

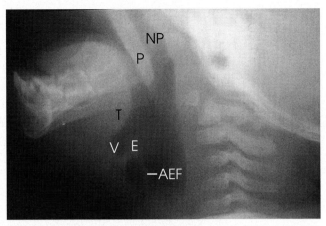

Fig. 1-50 Lateral airway radiograph: Same patient as Figure 1-49, moments later. Taken in inspiration. Normal prevertebral soft tissues. Nasopharyngeal air column (NP), palate (P), tongue (T), vallecula (V), epiglottis (E), aryepiglottic folds (AEF). Normal airway.

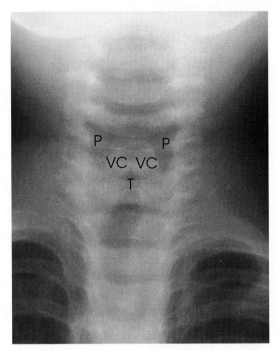

Fig. 1-51 AP airway radiograph: Pyriform sinus (P), vocal cords (VC), subglottic trachea (T). Normal airway.

B. **UGI, Esophagography**
  1. Key elements
    a. Be patient
      ● When performing any fluoroscopic study on a child, the radiologist must be patient
        Most children are apprehensive when placed on the fluoroscopic table

Teamwork between the parent or caregiver, technologist, and radiologist will help ensure a well-done study with a minimum of trauma to the child or parent.

b. Swallowing function if enteric tube is not used **[Fig. 1-52]**
- Observe multiple swallows in all infants
  Infant with developmental delay, former premies most likely to have swallowing dysfunction
- Swallowing dysfunction, intermittent aspiration may cause "bronchitis" in otherwise normal young infants
  Chest radiograph shows "dirty" chest appearance of perihilar bronchial wall thickening (peribronchial cuffing)
  "Silent" aspiration = tracheal aspiration without coughing

c. Course and caliber of esophagus **[Figs. 6-2 through 6-6]**
- Aortic arch and left atrium often seen as normal indentations
- Anterior indentation with soft tissue structure interposed between esophagus and trachea = pulmonary artery sling **[Fig. 4-31]**
- Posterior vascular indentation = subclavian artery **[Figs. 4-22 and 4-26]**
  If aorta on left (identify aorta on AP fluoro) = left aorta + aberrant right subclavian artery (normal variant)
  If aorta on right (identify aorta on AP fluoro) = right aorta + left subclavian artery or double aortic arch (vascular ring)
- H-type tracheoesophageal fistula (TEF)
  May be difficult to identify

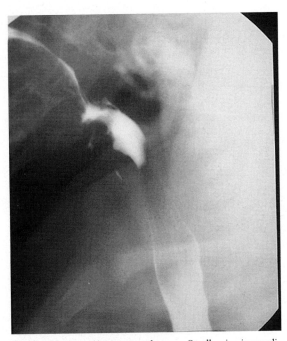

Fig. 1-52 Lateral barium esophagram: Swallowing incoordination. Note barium penetrating vocal cords (linear oblique contrast posterior to base of tongue), contrast in trachea (linear vertical contrast inferior to vocal cord contrast).

- Need straight lateral projection to separate esophagus from trachea
- Use of feeding tube to ensure distention recommended

  Placement of feeding tube important to distinguish laryngeal aspiration from TEF

  Occasionally repeat study necessary to diagnose

d. Gastric size, shape, and emptying **[Figs. 6-7 and 6-10]**
- Duration of gastric emptying variable in normal infants and children
- Elongation of pylorus and "string sign" = pyloric stenosis

e. Course of duodenum, duodeno-jejunal junction (DJJ) **[Figs. 1-53 through 1-55; see also Figs. 6-15, 6-21 through 6-25]**

f. Gastroesophageal reflux (GER)
- All babies spit up!

  Evaluation for GER is performed to identify or exclude gastric or bowel obstruction or malrotation, esophageal obstruction or vascular anomaly indenting the esophagus, swallowing dysfunction

  – Reflux of gastric acid may cause laryngospasm, hoarseness, incomplete laryngeal closure during swallowing, aspiration

g. Be patient

2. Technique

a. NPO × 3–4 hours for infant, 6–8 hours for older child

b. Child positioning and restraint
- Premature infants require warmth of heat lamps or equivalent device while in fluoro suite
- In infant less than 6 months of age, use a restraining device such as an Octagon board
- In older child or if a restraining device is unavailable, hold the child's legs at the knees to prevent motion and ensure proper positioning
- The technologist, nurse, or family member should hold the upper extremities extended and out of the field-of-view
- Place child in right lateral position

▶TIP

The position of the ligament of Treitz (duodeno-jejunal junction) must be identified regardless of whether the study requested is esophagography or UGI.

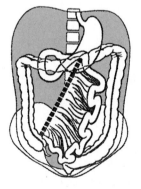 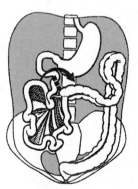 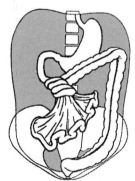

Fig. 1-53 GI rotation-malrotation: Normal small and large bowel position occurs early in gestation and involves 270 degree counterclockwise rotation each of DJJ and ceco-colic loop. This rotation places the DJJ to left of spine and at level of duodenal bulb and cecum in right lower quadrant. The wide small bowel mesentery between DJJ and distal small bowel anchors the small bowel and prevents twisting (image on left). Central image shows abnormal position of DJJ and cecum (malrotation) and shortened mesentery, which allows twisting to occur. Image on right shows midgut volvulus.

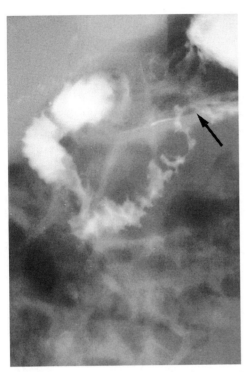

Fig. 1-54 AP UGI series: Contrast in duodenal "C" loop. Arrow at normal DJJ.

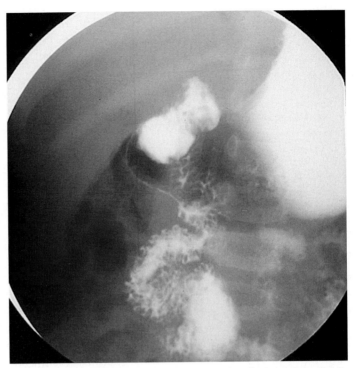

Fig. 1-55 AP UGI series: Contrast column coiling downward along right side of spine. Malrotation.

c. If a feeding tube is not used, the technologist or family member should feed the child by bottle or syringe
- Use nipple and bottle infant is used to, if possible
- Mother is usually the best feeder

d. Observe swallowing while the child is in the right lateral position
- Note sucking, swallowing coordination, nasopharyngeal reflux, vocal cord penetration or tracheal aspiration

e. Observe esophagus for stricture, indentation, fistula, and peristalsis

f. With child in right lateral position, fill the stomach partially until emptying into the duodenum is identified

g. When contrast enters the second portion of the duodenum, place child supine to identify the DJJ
- The child must be straight AP to accurately identify DJJ
  DJJ position verified to exclude or confirm malrotation
  – Normal position of DJJ is to left of spine and at level of bulb/pylorus

h. Obtain AP esophagram

i. Allow enough time for the child to drink the barium solution with or without additional water (or Kool-Aid) to distend the gastric fundus to evaluate for GE reflux
- Augment barium with water or Kool-Aid; most children will agree to ridding their mouth of the barium taste by drinking Kool-Aid, which distends the stomach, improving the likelihood of diagnosing GE reflux

- Additional water can be given to clear the barium from the esophagus prior to GER evaluation

j. Evaluate for GER
- Evaluate for GER at intermittent intervals for approximately 3 minutes (q15 seconds)

C. **Diagnostic contrast enema [Figs. 6-19, 6-28, 6-39 through 6-43]:**

1. Performed to identify causes of lower GI bleeding (i.e., polyps), small bowel obstruction (i.e., intussusception or distal bowel atresia), complications of inflammatory disease (i.e., post-necrotizing enterocolitis strictures), and to evaluate functional abnormality (i.e., Hirschsprung's), colonic anomaly (i.e., imperforate anus before complete repair)

   Evaluation for malrotation: UGI preferred

   a. Barium or water soluble contrast (gastrograffin diluted 4 : 1 or 15% Hypaque)
   b. Mucosal detail depicted with barium is better than that shown by water soluble contrast
   c. In the setting of Hirschsprung's disease, barium can harden and remain in the colon as a barium ball
   d. Water soluble contrast material can soften meconium plugs and can be used to treat meconium ileus
   e. Attention to fluid and electrolyte balance is necessary if hypertonic water soluble contrast is used in small infants
   f. Administration of barium into the GI tract can interfere with subsequent CT scans of the abdomen or with nuclear studies of the GU or GI systems, such as a Meckel scan
   g. If an abdominal CT scan is contemplated, a barium swallow or UGI series should follow the CT scan, rather than vice versa.

2. Technique

   a. Place soft rubber catheter into anus and secure with tape to buttocks
   b. Place child in right lateral position in same fashion as used for UGI
      - In prematures and infants less than 3 months of age, careful injection by hand can be used

        If bag drainage used, begin with bag 1 foot above table top
   c. Observe caliber of rectum compared to that of sigmoid. Normally, rectum is larger than sigmoid (in Hirschsprung's, rectum typically is smaller than sigmoid) **[Figs. 1-56 through 1-59]**
   d. Fill colon to the cecum, noting strictures, filling defects, and cecal position, and attempt to reflux ileocecal valve
   e. To reduce radiation exposure, camera spot images preferred over multiple static overhead films
   f. Rectal balloon? Do not use in infants or in children with possible Hirschsprung's disease

3. Air contrast barium enema (BE)

   a. It is usually difficult for children younger than teenage to hold air and barium long enough to obtain a good quality study.

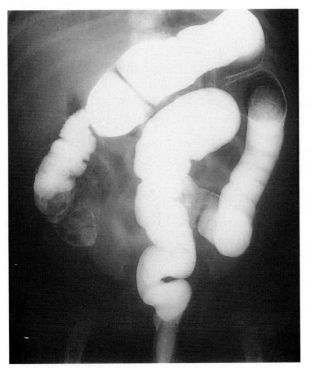

Fig. 1-56 AP BE: Normal newborn study.

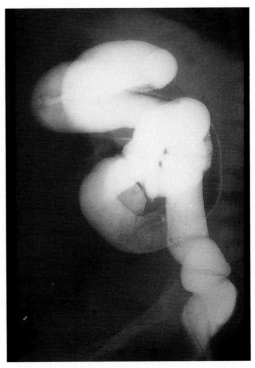

Fig. 1-57 Lateral BE: Normal newborn study.

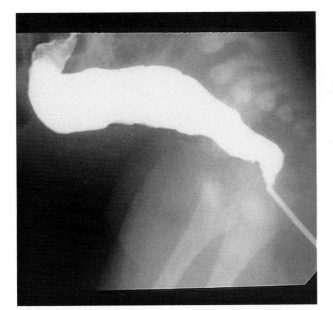

Fig. 1-58 Lateral view from barium enema: Narrowing of rectum compared to sigmoid (abnormal recto-sigmoid ratio), spiculation in rectum due to unrestrained muscular contractions. Hirschsprung's disease.

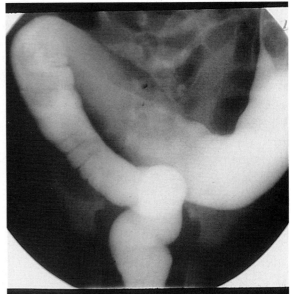

Fig. 1-59 AP view from contrast enema: Caliber of distal sigmoid is smaller than that of proximal sigmoid. Note caliber change. Hirschsprung's disease.

      b. In teenager, perform double contrast air and BE in same fashion as in adult.

      c. To identify polyps in young children, use very thin, dilute barium. You can visualize polyps more easily through the dilute contrast than through standard barium contrast [**Fig. 6-43**]

D. **Reduction of intussusception [Figs. 1-60 and 1-61]**

    1. Do not perform or attempt reduction without surgical back-up.

    2. Absolute contraindications to reduction:

      a. Clinical signs of peritonitis

      b. Pneumoperitoneum

    3. Duration of symptoms (>48 hours) or small bowel obstruction (SBO) indicates decreased rate of successful reduction

    4. "Dissection" sign (barium in interstices of intussusceptum) is associated with unsuccessful hydrostatic reduction

    5. Type of contrast: barium, water-soluble, or air?

      a. Barium

        • Risk of perforation and intraperitoneal barium untenable

        • Barium has no advantage over water-soluble, but has increased risk of morbidity if perforation occurs

      b. Air

        • Use Shiels device

        • Maintain pressure <120 mm Hg

        • Seal using rubber washer and tape plug

          Washer against anus pulled tightly to anus with overlying tape on buttocks to seal

          Foley with balloon can be used

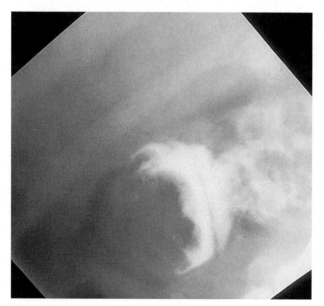

Fig. 1-60 Contrast enema: Soft tissue mass composed of invaginated bowel within colon contrast column. Small amount of contrast in interstices of intussusceptum. Intussusception.

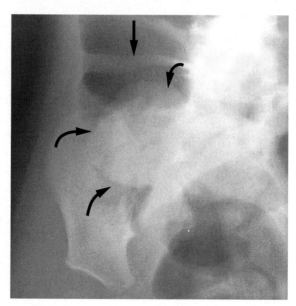

Fig. 1-61 Air reduction of intussusception: Air in ascending colon (arrow) outlines soft tissue mass (curved arrows) composed of loops of bowel at ileocecal valve.

c. Water soluble contrast
- Cystoconray™, 15% Hypaque™

  Both slightly hyperosmolar (400 to 600 mOsm/l)
  Undiluted Gastrograffin™ or Hypaque™ approximately
  2000 mOsm/l (very hyperosmolar, and not recommended)
- Seal buttocks similarly to air reduction
- Bag approximately 3 ft above table top

d. Air reduction in setting of SBO may be confusing due to proximal and distal intraluminal air

e. Water-soluble recommended for infant <6 months of age
- These patients are more likely to perforate during reduction
- If perforation occurs, sigmoid is most common location

f. Rule of "Threes": 3 tries of 3 minutes each with the bag 3 ft above the table

g. Sedation? An IV should be placed prior to BE. After two attempts with near-complete reduction, sedation is a reasonable adjunct
- Appropriate dose of IV morphine (0.2 mg/kg) or fentanyl (1 μg/kg) may be given prior to the third attempt
- The intussusceptum should have been advanced nearly to the ileocecal valve, suggesting a third attempt with sedation may be successful

h. 14% will reduce spontaneously between time of BE and surgery

i. Recurrence rate is 10% postradiologic reduction and 5% postoperative reduction

j. Reduction defined as complete elimination of intussusceptum through ileocecal valve and free reflux into distal small intestine for ileocolic intussusception, or elimination of small bowel (SB) intussusception with reflux into proximal SB

6. Intussusception: pneumatic reduction
   a. Success rate = 81%
   b. Recurrence in 11%
   c. Bowel perforation in 2.8%
   - Including tension pneumoperitoneum
   d. Predictors of bowel perforation
   - Young age of patient (<6 months)
   - Long duration of symptoms (>2 days)
   e. Predictors of failure
   - Ileoileocolic intussusception (27%)
   - Long duration of symptoms (>2 days)
   - Following failed hydrostatic reduction
   f. If successful, technique is faster than hydrostatic and less messy
   g. Incomplete reduction may be difficult to assess due to air both proximal and distal to intussusceptum

7. Intussusception: hydrostatic reduction
   a. Success rate = 75%
   b. Recurrence in 10%
   c. Bowel perforation in 0.7%

    d. Most important: seal of buttocks to maintain pressure and liquid in colon. Use tape unsparingly to bind buttocks or Foley catheter with balloon carefully distended in rectum to obstruct anus

E. **Contrast enema reduction of meconium ileus uncomplicated by bowel atresia, perforation, or volvulus [Fig. 1-62; see also Fig. 6-20]:**
   1. Technique
     a. Place soft rubber catheter into rectum and securely tape buttocks together
     b. Carefully administer hypertonic Hypaque (20 to 30%) with/without mucomyst 1% by hand injection.
     c. Hypaque/mucomyst solution made by diluting equal quantity 2% mucomyst with 40 to 45% Hypaque
     d. Caliber of entire colon and variable amount of small bowel is reduced up to level of most proximal obstruction (obvious caliber change at this site)
     e. More than one reduction attempt may be necessary
     f. Successful reduction occurs when contrast enters large caliber small bowel
     g. Perform in conjunction with pediatric surgeon, who can manage complications and fluid/electrolytes.

F. **Contrast enema for Hirschsprung's [Figs. 1-58 and 1-59; see also Figs. 6-39 and 6-40]**
   1. Technique
     a. No preparation of colon necessary

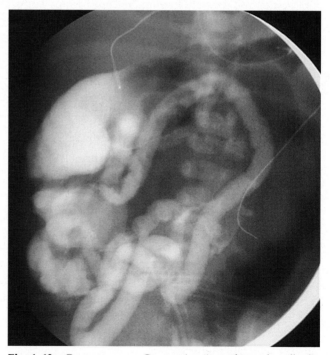

Fig. 1-62 Contrast enema: Contrast in microcolon and small caliber small bowel, with retrograde filling of dilated loop in right upper quadrant. Meconium ileus with hydrostatic reduction.

b. Rectal manipulation including rectal examination or rectal temperature shortly before contrast enema can make diagnosis more difficult by decompressing distended colon

c. In young infant, a small amount of air injected through the tubing may enable the diagnosis before positive contrast enters the rectum

d. With child in right lateral position, slowly administer contrast, noting caliber of rectum compared to that of sigmoid

e. Normally, rectum is larger than sigmoid (in Hirschsprung's, rectum typically is smaller than sigmoid)

f. Identify transition between narrowed distal aganglionic segment and dilated proximal, normal colon

G. **Voiding cystourethrography**

1. Technique

   a. Wash the external genitalia with antiseptic solution

   b. In male, squirt 2% viscous xylocaine into penile meatus to locally anesthetize urethra
      - Catheterization will then be less painful

   c. Catheterize the urethra with catheter of appropriate size (5 Fr. feeding tube in newborn and young infant or girl less than 2 to 4 years, 8 Fr. feeding tube in older child, 10–12 Fr. rubber catheter in teenager)

   d. Under fluoroscopic guidance, fill bladder with iodinated contrast, such as Cystoconray, from a bottle approximately 3 ft above the table level

   e. Place child in right and left oblique position to observe each vesicoureteral junction in early and late bladder filling

   f. If reflux occurs, document images of renal collecting system, ureter, and possible bladder diverticula (camera or digital devices produce less radiation exposure to patient than spot film) **[Figs. 7-5 through 7-10]**

   g. Observe size, shape and capacity of the bladder, dome of bladder for irregularities, and presence of filling defects (mass or ureterocele) or sinus tract (urachal remnant)

   h. Do not remove catheter from urethra prematurely
      - The child may protest he/she must void, but the contrast will continue to fill the bladder
      - Urgency can be predicted when contrast backs up in tubing

   i. In the oblique or lateral position, a boy voids into a urinal

   j. While on the fluoro table, older girls can void into a bedpan or onto towels

   k. As child voids, observe caliber of urethra, noting dilatation of posterior urethra, caliber change, and completeness of voiding

   l. Bladder capacity

Age (yrs.)	Approximate bladder volume (cc)
0–1	30–150
1–3	100–300
3–8	100–450
>8	150–600

▶TIP
Young infants will not have developed a transition zone. The diagnosis can and should be suggested on the basis of an abnormal rectosigmoid ratio alone. While contrast enema remains a useful test, suction biopsy provides definitive diagnosis. Suction biopsy is safe and easily performed in experienced hands, and should be performed if the diagnosis is strongly suspected clinically.

III. ULTRASONOGRAPHY

A. General rules for sonographers:

1. Darken room sufficiently to visualize monitor without increasing the power, which makes the image diffusely echogenic
2. Use a transducer and field-of-view (penetration) appropriate for size of patient and anatomy evaluated
    a. For example, a 3.5 mHz transducer may be appropriate for an adult, but is inappropriate for an infant
    b. Use the highest frequency transducer available to enhance image resolution while still penetrating the area of interest
    c. The higher the frequency of the transducer, the greater the sensitivity, but the shallower the tissue penetration
    d. In general, a 7 mHz transducer is recommended for infants and small children; a 4 to 5 mHz transducer is recommended for older children
    e. Using a large field-of-view or inappropriate penetration produces images that are minified and difficult to interpret. In the small child or infant, 8 to 10 cm penetration will suffice

B. Renal ultrasonography [Figs. 1-63 through 1-65]

1. Measure both kidneys for longest longitudinal length
2. Compare renal length with patient age or gestation in prematures
    a. Premie age in weeks (over 26 weeks) = length in mm (e.g., 28 week gestation = 28 mm length)

Patient age vs.	Renal length (cm)	Patient age vs.	Renal length (cm)
Term	4.0–6.0	5 yr.	6.3–9.0
6 mo.	4.7–6.8	8 yr.	7.1–9.8
1 yr.	5.6–7.8	12 yr.	8.0–10.7
3 yr.	5.8–8.4	15 yr.	8.8–11.6

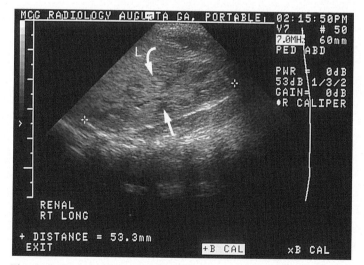

Fig. 1-63 Renal US: Newborn. Renal cortex (curved arrow) of same echogenic density (number of white dots on black background) as liver (L). Note prominent *normal* hypoechoic (fewer white dots on black background) medullary pyramids (straight arrow). Normal kidney US, newborn.

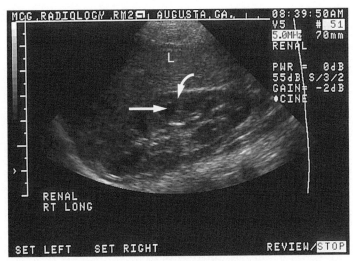

Fig. 1-64   Renal US: 2-year-old. Renal cortex (curved arrow) less echogenic density (fewer number of white dots on black background) than liver (L). Note prominent *normal* hypoechoic medullary pyramids (straight arrow) that look like "helmets." Normal kidney US, infant-young child.

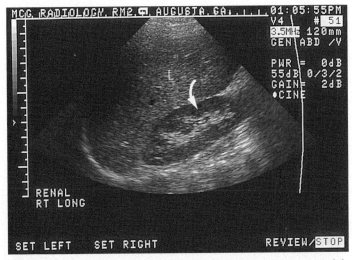

Fig. 1-65   Renal US: 8-year-old. Central renal sinus echogenic. Medullary pyramids less prominent than in Figures 1-63 or 1-64. Renal cortex (curved arrow) less echogenic density than liver (L). Normal kidney US, older child.

3. If one renal fossa lacks a kidney, document this finding
    a. Look for ectopic kidney in pelvis, if no history of nephrectomy
    b. If medial portion of kidney extends toward spine, carefully look for connection across midline (horseshoe kidney)
        • Place transducer in epigastrium in transverse plane
        • Using *gentle* sustained pressure with transducer, push downward and caudad to move overlying bowel away to visualize midline

4. Renal cortical echogenicity, compared to liver or spleen **[Figs. 7-17, 7-18, 7-21, and 7-50]**
    a. Cortical-medullary differentiation should be present at all ages
    b. Renal > liver/spleen in premature
    c. Renal ≥ liver/spleen in newborn
    d. Renal = liver/spleen at 6 to 12 months of age
    e. Renal ≤ liver/spleen over 12 months of age
5. Medullary pyramids **[Figs. 7-19 and 7-20]**
    a. Prominent in infants, children
    b. Hypoechoic, "helmet-shaped"
    c. Peripherally, bright echo of arcuate vessel identifies cortico-medullary junction
    d. Do not confuse with cyst or dilated calyx **[Figs. 7-22, 7-23, and 7-50]**
6. Urinary bladder
    a. Identify in all renal ultrasound studies
    b. Bladder wall thickness evaluated: should be ≤3 mm in distended state and ≤5 mm in collapsed state
7. If hydronephrosis found, evaluate ureter
    a. If distal ureter larger than proximal, consider ureterovesical junction (UVJ) stenosis or vesico-ureteral reflux

C. **Gallbladder ultrasonography**
1. Echogenic material within gallbladder **[Fig. 1-66]**
    a. Stones shadow
    b. Sludge may be focal (tumefactive sludge) or layered and does not shadow
2. Wall thickening
    a. Wall should be ≤3 mm thick
3. Size
    a. In newborn, >15 mm in length

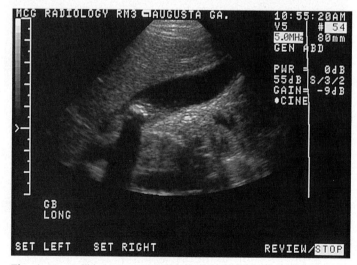

Fig. 1-66 Gallbladder US: Highly echogenic gall stone with posterior acoustic shadowing. Note non-shadowing sludge adjacent to gallstone within gallbladder. Gallstone (cholelithiasis).

　　　b. In older child, < length of right kidney
　　　　　● If longer, consider hydrops
　　4. Bile duct dilatation **[Fig. 6-57]**
D. **The pylorus [Fig. 1-67; see also Fig. 6-11]**
　　1. Finding the pylorus
　　　a. Place a 5 to 7 mHz linear transducer over the right upper quadrant of the abdomen in the transverse plane
　　　b. Use a short field-of-view (3 to 6 cm)
　　　c. If the child has hypertrophic pyloric stenosis (HPS), you may see a "bull's-eye appearing structure" immediately. Lucky you!
　　　d. If not seen, and a search is required, identify the gall bladder in the transverse plane. The pyloric channel should be seen to the left of the gall bladder.
　　　e. To facilitate your search, have the infant drink a clear solution of sugar water or Pedialyte, turn the infant toward the right and place the transducer over the right upper quadrant. You may need to stoop to get below the patient
　　　f. If the child does not have HPS, you will see fluid distending the pylorus as it enters the duodenum
　　　g. Align the transducer along the long axis of the pyloric channel
　　　h. If you see thickening of the pyloric muscle, compare it with the muscular wall of the gastric antrum
　　　i. Measure from the outer margin of the hypoechoic wall to the outer margin of the linear hyperechoic mucosa; this is the wall thickness
　　　j. Along the long axis of the pylorus, measure from the margin of the mucosa and the antrum to the most distal portion of the hypoechoic wall in the pyloric channel; this is the pyloric length

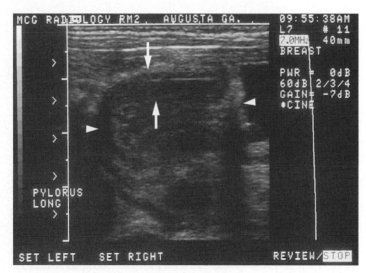

Fig. 1-67 Pyloric US: Along long axis of pyloric channel. Wall thickness measured between arrows. Pyloric channel length measured between arrowheads. Hypertrophic pyloric stenosis (HPS).

E. **The appendix [Figs. 1-68 and 1-69; see also Fig. 6-35]**
  1. Finding the appendix
      a. Place a 5 to 7 mHz linear transducer over the right lower quadrant of the abdomen in the transverse plane.
      b. Use a short field-of-view (4–8 cm).
      c. There are two ways to find the appendix:
          • The slower and more frustrating method is to find the right colon and travel down to the cecum

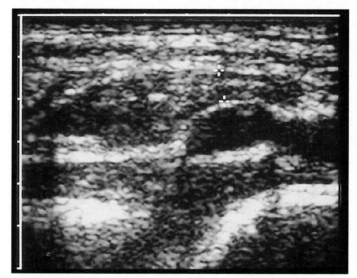

Fig. 1-68   Appendix US: Along long axis of appendix. Measurement between electronic cursors from wall to wall. Normal ≤6 mm. Normal appendix.

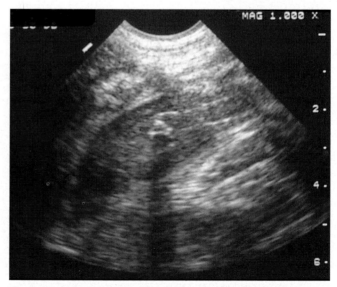

Fig. 1-69   Appendix US: Along long axis of appendix. Thickening of appendiceal wall and widening of lumen bounded by echogenic mucosa. Note appendicolith with posterior acoustic shadowing. Acute appendicitis.

- The faster way is to find the right iliac artery and vein by color Doppler in the transverse plane. The appendix will be just superficial to these vessels and, usually, just beneath the sharply echogenic peritoneum

  Limitation: retrocecal appendix or appendix in unusual location

2. In a patient with peritoneal signs, place the transducer gently on the abdomen. Slowly but with constant pressure, push downward while visualizing the appendix.
3. Once you identify it, you can use color Doppler to check hypervascularity.
4. When you are sure you have visualized the appendix, tell the patient you will be lifting the transducer rapidly. You can then confirm rebound tenderness precisely related to the appendix.

F. **Vascular imaging [Figs. 6-51 and 7-26]**
   1. Abdominal aorta in infant
      a. Can best be visualized from left coronal approach
      b. Often the left renal artery and, sometimes the right renal artery, can easily be discerned at its origin with left coronal approach
      c. Anterior approach may be defeated by gas in GI tract
   2. Mediastinal veins
      a. Can be visualized with 5 to 10 mHz linear or sector transducer from a supraclavicular approach
      b. Turn the patient's head away from the side of interest: be patient
      c. This is often a difficult and time-consuming study

G. **Spine ultrasound in the newborn [Fig. 1-70; see also Figs. 2-120 through 2-122]**
   1. Performed in infants with imperforate anus or hemangioma, fatty skin lesion, or tuft of hair in the back
   2. Place infant in prone position
   3. A rolled towel can be put under the infant's abdomen to reduce lumbar lordosis

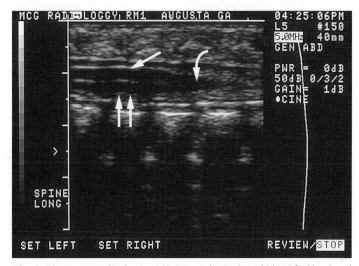

Fig. 1-70 Longitudinal spine US: Normal spinal cord identified by dorsal (single arrow), central, and ventral (double arrow) linear echoes. Normal conus medullaris is triangular in shape (curved arrow). Normal spine US.

4. Use a linear 5–7 mHz transducer with a short field-of-view (3 to 6 cm) longitudinally over the spine

5. The spine is hypoechoic with three linear echogenic landmarks
   - The most dorsal and ventral landmarks outline the cord; the central linear echo is the median longitudinal sulcus or central canal.

6. The conus is the triangular hypoechoic structure identifying the end of the cord. Normally, its most caudal extent is at L3 in the newborn.
   - To identify the level of the conus, place the transducer such that the conus is in the center of the linear field-of-view.
   - Using the hand that is not holding the transducer, feel for the twelfth rib and identify the spinous processes that correspond to the level of the conus.
   - Alternatively, you can tape a paper clip or other metallic object over the sonographic level of the conus and obtain a confirmatory radiograph.

H. **Hip Ultrasound [Figs. 1-71 and 1-72]**
   1. Place infant with one side down or supine
   2. To improve likelihood of cooperation, allow mother to feed infant from bottle
   3. Use linear/annular transducer with 5 to 10 mHz frequency
   4. Coronal projection **[Figs. 3-23 through 3-28]**
      a. Hip should be in the neutral position

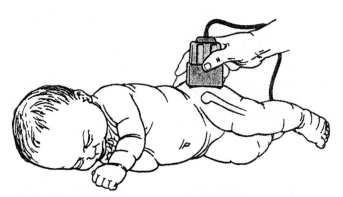

Fig. 1-71 Technique of coronal hip ultrasound.

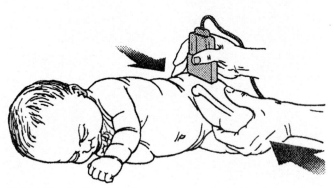

Fig. 1-72 Technique of transverse hip ultrasound without and with stress.

b. Place transducer over hip in coronal position

c. Find the femoral head and move the transducer to show the largest diameter

d. Rotate the transducer, cranial end posterior, to produce a straight line appearance of the supraacetabular ilium

e. Move transducer anterior and posterior to demonstrate the largest diameter of the femoral head and the echogenic triangle of the acetabular labrum

f. A normal hip can be made to appear abnormal, but an abnomal hip cannot be made to appear normal

g. Obtaining standard image and recognizing normal appearance is key

5. Transverse projection **[Figs. 3-29 through 3-32]**

a. Hip should be flexed to 90 degrees

b. Place transducer over the femoral head, along the axis of the flexed femur perpendicular to long axis of hip

c. Normal "U-view" is formed by the femoral head located between the symmetrically positioned posterior rim of acetabulum and ossified femoral shaft

d. If the femoral head is laterally displaced, the acetabular rim and the femoral shaft will be at different levels, and the symmetry of the "U" view will be lost

6. Transverse projection with stress applied

a. With transducer in transverse projection and with patient's hip flexed, gently push knee posterior, attempting to posteriorly displace femoral head from acetabulum

b. Note movement of femoral head relative to posterior acetabulum

7. Graf classification of hip dysplasia

a. Classification system for hip ultrasound allows identification of hip dysplasia and guides therapy

b. Angle measurements and anatomic terms have made a basically simple system appear very complex

c. With experience, most hips are classified by appearance with angle measurements used only for confirmation or confusing cases

d. Type 1. Normal

e. Type 2. Normally located femoral head, abnormally formed acetabulum

f. Type 3. Displaced femoral head, laterally located in abnormal acetabulum

g. Type 4. Femoral head displaced superolateral to the acetabulum

IV. **COMPUTED TOMOGRAPHY**

A. **Head CT**

1. Posterior fossa at 5 mm thick sections

2. Supratentorial compartment at 5 to 10 mm sections, depending on patient age, head size

a. Newborn, infants, microcephalics at 5 mm

3. Evaluation of acute trauma, unexplained seizure, increased intracranial pressure, etc.
   a. Perform first without IV contrast to exclude hemorrhage or calcification
   b. Obtaining a contrast-enhanced brain CT *only* may obscure findings of hemorrhage or calcification
4. If necessary, a contrast-enhanced brain CT can be performed after the noncontrast study is completed
   a. Contrast-enhanced brain CT
      - Following noncontrast CT to evaluate tumor, vascular malformation, complications of meningitis and/or abscess, possible dural sinus thrombosis
5. Position child's head straight in head-holder to avoid obliquity
6. Rubber inserts are placed on each side of the head, and the forehead can be taped to hold the head in the proper position

B. **Sinus CT**
1. Direct coronals, if possible
2. Axials can exclude gross abnormalities, if patient cannot be positioned for direct coronal
   a. IV contrast usually unnecessary, unless cavernous sinus thrombosis or intracranial complication suspected clinically or on noncontrast CT (NCCT)

C. **Body CT**
1. General
   a. Current CT scans generate images at 1 scan/second
   b. Typical 30–50 slice examination of the chest, abdomen, or pelvis completed in less than one minute
   c. Consequently, the requirement for sedation has been reduced substantially
   d. Images can be manipulated by computer and reformatted into innumerable planes *after* the patient has left the CT suite!
   e. IV contrast is necessary for most CT studies of the body in children **[Figs. 1-73 and 1-74]**
      - IV contrast-enhanced CT enables identifying and discriminating solid organ lesions which have different degrees of enhancement than normal parenchyma, depicting normal and abnormal vascularity, and distinguishing blood vessels from adenopathy. **[Figs. 6-44, 6-48, 6-49, 6-52, 6-53; see also Figs. 7-11, 7-30, 7-31, 7-34, and 7-38]**
      - Parents should be told beforehand that IV contrast may be necessary so they will not become upset when an IV is started in their child.
   f. CT scan of chest, abdomen, or pelvis does not usually require a separate noncontrast examination, unless calcification is suspected
   g. Most patients undergoing a CT of the chest, abdomen, or pelvis receive nonionic IV contrast material (1.5 to 2 cc/kg)
      - Nonionic contrast produces less nausea and overall warm feeling than ionic contrast

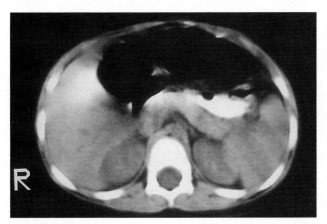

Fig. 1-73 Axial abdominal CT: Poor quality study without intravenous contrast precludes visualizing splenic laceration. Spleen laceration CT without IV contrast.

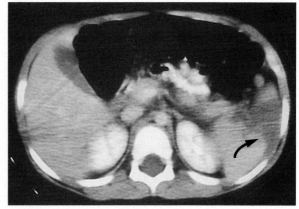

Fig. 1-74 Axial abdominal CT: Same patient as Figure 1-73. Addition of intravenous contrast easily allows visualization of splenic fracture (curved arrow). Spleen laceration CT with IV contrast.

    h. Oral contrast is usually administered 1 to 3 hours before the study to opacify the GI tract, except in the acutely injured patient
- Children who have sustained acute abdominal trauma may also be head-injured and often are nauseated; use no oral contrast in these patients

    i. Begin scan at end of the bolus of IV contrast

    j. IV contrast provides vessel identification in the mediastinum, abdomen, and pelvis

    k. Imaging in the vascular phase allows discrimination of subtle hepatic, splenic, or renal abnormalities, as well as mediastinal, retroperitoneal, and pelvic adenopathy

2. Sedation for CT

    a. Necessity reduced by faster CT scanners

    b. Patient motion can still degrade the image and defeat the imager

    c. Most children over the age of 4 will not require sedation, except those who are mentally retarded, immature, or anxious

    d. Parents in the scanning room with their child
- Parental tactile contact assuages the child's (and parents') apprehension
- The parent is a member of the team whose goal is to obtain a motion-free study as quickly as possible.

3. Body CT for childhood trauma **[Figs. 6-47, 6-61, and 6-62]**

    a. Performed after head CT in the multiply injured patient

    b. Patient is positioned properly on scanning table

    c. "Topogram"(Siemens) or "scoutview" (GE) is obtained

    d. Upper and lower limits of the scan are set

    e. Appropriate field-of-view chosen

    f. Scanner programmed to automatically increment the table

g. IV contrast should be administered by hand bolus (1.5 to 2 ml/kg) in small children or power injector in older child

h. Helical scan begun after entire bolus injected

i. Scans are performed with 5 to 10 mm slice thickness and 5 to 10 mm contiguous sections

j. If renal injury identified, obtain delayed CT through kidneys in approximately 5 minutes to exclude contrast extravasation
  - If "delayed" renal scan obtained too early, contrast extravasation, if present, may be missed **[Figs. 7-13 through 7-16, and 7-44]**

4. Filming

a. Window of 250-350 and Center of 45-60 (W250-350, C45-60)

b. Portions of the lungs imaged should be filmed at W800-1500, C-500

c. The scan should be viewed with bone settings on the monitor (especially in the pelvis, if included), and filmed at that setting (W1500-2000, C300), if abnormal.

d. View abdomen with lung settings to find subtle free air

V. MAGNETIC RESONANCE IMAGING

A. General

1. MRI depends upon

a. Strong magnetic field

b. Presence of mobile protons (most commonly found as hydrogen ions in water)

c. Inherent tissue characteristics exposed to a changing electro-magnetic environment

d. Powerful computers to interpret signal intensity and produce an image

2. Very basic concepts

a. Within a strong magnetic field, protons in a volume of tissue align themselves along the axis of the magnetic field and precess (or wobble) around this axis at a fixed frequency

b. If the aligned hydrogen nuclei are subjected to a radiofrequency (RF) pulse of the same frequency as the precessional frequency, the protons flip to a higher energy level

c. When the RF pulse is turned off, the protons return to their steady-state, and produce a small, but detectable signal that is sampled by a receiving coil in the magnet itself or in a coil around the body part imaged

d. Multiple repetitions are necessary to produce sufficient signal to create a diagnostic image

e. Currently, several sequences (different scans) are performed to complete a study

f. The most common sequences are referred to as T1-weighted (short TR, short TE), T2-weighted (long TR, long TE), and gradient-echo (variable flip angle $< 90°$)

g. Repetition time (TR) refers to the interval (in msec) between successive gradient impulses. Echo time (TE) refers to the time following each gradient impulse that the signal is listened for and detected

h. T1- and T2-weighting refers to spin–echo techniques, in which protons are flipped 90° (perpendicular to the magnetic field)
i. Short TR/short TE sequences usually 400–800 msec/12–30 msec
j. Long TR/long TE sequences usually 1800–9000 msec/60–120 msec
k. Because MRI is exquisitely responsive to water content, images are sensitive, but not specific
  • For example, within the marrow cavity of a long bone, hyperintensity can be a feature of a bone bruise (marrow edema) or marrow infiltration by inflammatory cells or tumor [Fig. 3–36]
l. An accompanying radiograph and clinical information are useful to yield the most useful information derived from musculoskeletal MRI
m. MRI can depict a lesion or abnormality in virtually any plane without altering the patient's position
3. Technical parameters for magnetic resonance imaging (Table 1)
4. MRI tissue characteristics [Figs. 1–75 through 1–79] (Table 2)

Table 1–1. Technical Parameters for Magnetic Resonance Imaging

Goal	Coil Size	FOV	Matrix	NSA	Slice Thick.	Skip	TR	TE
Inc. Resolution	—	⇓	⇑	—	⇓	—	—	—
Inc. S/N	⇓	⇑	⇓	⇑	⇑	⇑	⇑	⇓
Dec. Time	—	—	⇓	⇓	—	—	⇓	—
Inc. ROI	⇑	⇑	—	—	⇑	⇑	⇑	⇓
Dec. Alias	⇓	⇑	—	—	—	—	—	—

Key: Coil = radiofrequency coil size; FOV = Field-of-view; Matrix = Phase-encoding acquisition matrix; NSA = number of signals averaged; Skip = interval between slices; TR = repetition time; TE = echo time; Inc = increased; Dec = decreased; ⇑ = increased; ⇓ = decreased; — = no change; S/N = signal-to-noise; ROI = region of interest size; Alias = aliasing artifact

Table 1–2. MRI Tissue Characteristics

Tissue	T1	T2	Short TR/TE	Long TR/TE
Fat	Short	Medium	Very bright	± Gray/dark
Fibrous	Long	Very short	Dark	Very dark
Solid organ	Medium	Short	Medium	Dark
Fresh blood in brain	Long	Short	Dark	Dark
Old blood in brain	Short	Very long	Very bright	Very bright
Flow	Long	Short	Dark	Dark
Colloid	Short		Bright	
Edema	Long	Long	Dark	Bright
Most neoplasms	Long	Long	Dark	Bright
Inflammation	Long	Long	Dark	Bright

Note nonspecific nature of MR signal in various types of pathophysiology!!!
Key: T1 = T1 relaxation time; T2 = T2 relaxation time

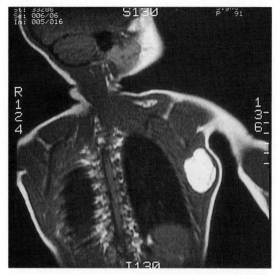

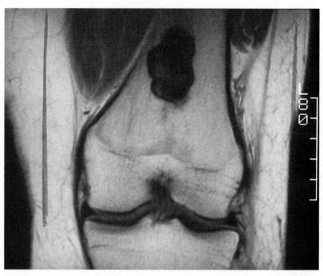

Fig. 1-75 Coronal T1-weighted MRI: Well-demarcated hyperintense mass in left chest wall. Lipoma.

Fig. 1-76 Coronal T1-weighted MRI: Lobulated hypointense lesion in distal femur. Fibrous lesion, nonossifying fibroma.

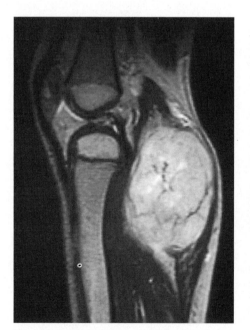

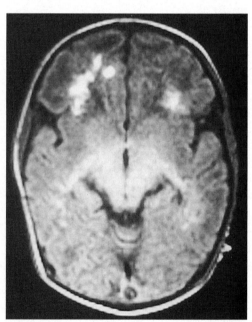

Fig. 1-77 Sagittal T2-weighted MRI: Lobulated, hyperintense mass within gastrocnemius. Rhabdomyosarcoma.

Fig. 1-78 Axial T1-weighted brain MRI: High intensity lesions in deep white matter adjacent to frontal horns. Hyperintensity is due to methemoglobin in hemorrhagic infarctions.

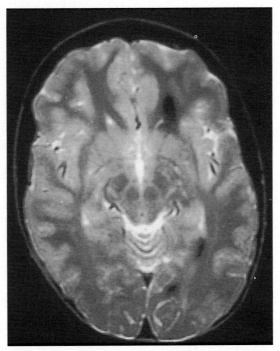

Fig. 1-79 Axial T2-weighted brain MRI: Several hypo-intense lesions in left hemisphere. These represent hemo-siderin from previous intracranial hemorrhage.

5. Intracranial hemorrhage on MRI
   a. Appearances on short TR/TE and long TR/TE images **(Table 3)**
B. **Tips for acquiring MRI studies in children**
   1. Most children less than 8 years of age require sedation
      a. Before sedating the patient, place an MR-compatible pulse oximeter on the child's finger or toe before placing the child in the scan room
         • Obtain baseline oxygen saturation; allow child to adjust to monitor

Table 1-3. Intracranial Hemorrhage on MRI: Appearances on Short TR/TE and Long TR/TE Images

	Center	Periphery		Adjacent Rim of Brain	Nearby White Matter
Acute	Hb/IRBC $-/\downarrow\downarrow$	$-/-$		$-/-$	Edema $-/\uparrow\uparrow$
Subacute	$-/\downarrow$	Mhb IRBC $\uparrow/\downarrow\downarrow\rightarrow\rightarrow$	Dilute Mhb IRBC $\uparrow/\uparrow\uparrow$	Hemosiderin $-/\downarrow\downarrow$	Edema $-/\uparrow\uparrow$
Chronic	Dilute Mhb $\uparrow\uparrow/\uparrow\uparrow$	Dilute Mhb LRBC $\uparrow\uparrow/\uparrow\uparrow$		Hemosiderin $-/\downarrow\downarrow$	$-/-$

Key: Hb = hemoglobin; IRBC = intact RBC; — = no change; $\uparrow$ = increased; $\downarrow$ = decreased; Mhb = methemoglobin; LRBC = lysed RBC; short TR/TE/long TR/TE

2. If intravenous sedation is necessary or IV contrast required, an IV should be established before placing the child in the scanner
   a. An IV drip should be maintained on a "keep open" basis so that the child and table do not have be manipulated when contrast is administered.
   b. Table or patient movement may interfere with sedation and prematurely terminate the study
   c. Inject the contrast into the tubing as close to the patient as possible without moving the patient
3. If the study requires EKG gating, place the leads on the child's chest before placing the child in the scan room
4. For the first scan, which is usually a localizer, use a large enough field-of-view and coil to completely cover the area of interest
   a. For example, to image an osteosarcoma of the distal femur, do not use a knee coil to image entire femur
     • The small knee coil will not visualize a skip lesion involving the proximal femur
     • Small coil provides high resolution over small area, but limits field-of-view
   b. To identify long length of tumor extent, or skip lesion, larger coil may be necessary

C. **Protocols for body MRI**
1. Standard protocols are only a starting point for the study
2. Altering sequences, area of interest, etc. may be necessary depending on findings
3. The child's short attention span and limited cooperation, and time constraints of sedation dictate efficiency of imaging.
   a. Get the most information in the shortest time possible!
4. Use a fast T2-weighted series (most often in the axial plane) after a localizing sequence to image the area of interest and identify signal abnormality
   a. Subsequently, additional sequences will be determined by imaging findings and/or need for IV contrast.
   b. If IV contrast used, obtain T1-weighted sequence prior to IV contrast, and T1-weighted sequence(s) after IV contrast.

D. **Cardiac MRI**
1. For intracardiac or great vessel anomaly
   a. Sequence #2 is EKG-gated thin section (3 to 4 mm) axial T1-weighted
   b. Then oblique coronal/sagittal T1-weighted sequence along axis of aortic arch for aortic coarctation
   c. 3D workstation valuable to depict reformats

VI. **NUCLEAR IMAGING (TECHNIQUE: SEE APPENDIX 2)**
A. **Bone scan [Fig. 1-80; see also Fig. 3-35]**
1. Metaphyses normally hot
2. Sharp straight border between physis and metadiaphysis is normal
3. If focal abnormality on bone radiograph, obtain coned-down nuclear image for specific area of interest
4. To differentiate cellulitis and osteomyelitis, images are obtained immediately and after 1.5 to 2 hours

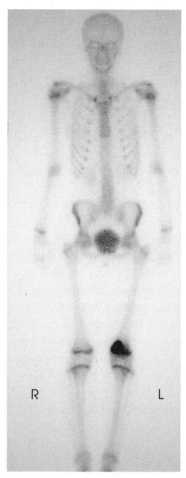

R   L

Fig. 1-80 ⁹⁹ᵐTechnetium bone scan: Normal metaphyses are sharply delineated, rectangular; abnormal metaphyseal uptake in distal left femur. Osteosarcoma, left distal femur.

5. Total body image alone unsatisfactory
6. For back pain:
   a. If SPECT available use it if planar bone scan is normal

B. **Hepatobiliary scan (HIDA scan)**
   1. For conjugated hyperbilirubinemia and suspected biliary atresia (BA) or choledochal cyst
   2. Following five days pretreatment with phenobarbital for BA
   3. Obtain delayed images up to 24 hours postinjection to identify small bowel excretion or filling of cyst

C. **Renal nuclear imaging**
   1. GFR, excretion, obstruction uropathy **[Fig. 7-12]**
      a. ⁹⁹ᵐTc-DTPA, MAG₃
      b. Place a catheter in the urinary bladder beforehand.
         • In the child with vesicoureteral reflux, isotope in the undrained bladder may reflux back into the kidney and interfere with evaluation of excretion.

    2. Pyelonephritis, renal scarring, cortical tagging to identify pelvic kidney **[Figs. 1-81 and 1-82]**
        a. ^{99m}Tc-DMSA, glucoheptonate

VII. **SEDATION**
  A. **First, do no harm!**
    1. It is possible to perform good quality CT or MRI without sedation in young children.
    2. Parental support and tactile contact between parent and child may obviate need for sedation.
    3. Sedation requires institutional commitment from anesthesiology and nursing.
        a. Guidelines–institutional policy for radiologic sedation should be reviewed by anesthesiology department
        b. Nursing support mandatory
    4. Sedation in outpatient setting without appropriate monitoring, nursing support, and emergency backup is risky.
  B. **If sedation required, patient monitoring is key**
    1. Prior to sedating the patient, obtain a medical history, focusing on drug allergy, underlying medical problems, and current medications.
    2. In children with upper airway obstruction who manifest stridor, snoring, or wheezing or who have cardiac disease, obtain oxygen saturation with oximetry prior to considering sedation. These types of patients are at risk for desaturation due to sedation.
  C. **Heart rate monitoring and pulse oximetry is mandatory in all patients**
  D. **Drugs**
    1. In children less than 18 to 24 months, oral chloral hydrate is first choice
        a. 40 to 60 mg/kg in infants $<$ 6 months of age

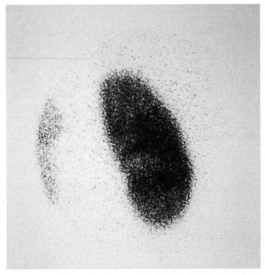

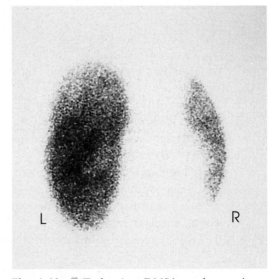

Fig. 1-81 ^{99m}Technetium-DMSA renal scan: Normal cortical uptake throughout right kidney. Contralateral kidney incompletely visualized on oblique pin-hole image.

Fig. 1-82 ^{99m}Technetium-DMSA renal scan: Acute pyelonephritis. Decreased cortical uptake in upper pole of left kidney.

b. 80 to 100 mg/kg in children 6 to 24 months
- Maximum chloral hydrate 1500 to 2000 mg

c. Chloral hydrate sedation in children over 2 years of age often unsuccessful

2. Sodium pentobarbital 3 to 5 mg/kg IV in children over age 2
3. Rate of successful sedation studies approximately 95%
- Patients who are difficult to sedate or are sedation failures often have a seizure disorder, mental retardation, or marked anxiety

4. Don't push the drugs to excess to sedate a patient who doesn't respond to the usual drug dosage

a. Such a patient may require anesthesia

E. **The worst scenario is to obtain a great study on a patient who has been brain-injured during sedation**

1. Document oxygen saturation, heart rate during study
2. Evaluate patient at end of study and monitor after study until alert
3. Do not discharge patient who is still sedated

Abbreviations

AP	Anteroposterior
CT	Computed tomography
CHF	Congestive heart failure
DJJ	Duodeno-jejunal junction
DMSA	Dimercaptosuccinate
DTPA	Diethylenetriamine pentaacetic acid
GE	Gastroesophageal
HPS	Hypertrophic pyloric stenosis
IV	Intravenous
MAG_3	Mercaptoacetyl triglycine
mHz	Megahertz (frequency in millions of cycles/sec)
MRI	Magnetic resonance imaging
PA	Posteroanterior
PCD	Pneumopericardium
PIE	Pulmonary interstitial emphysema
PMD	Pneumomediastinum
PTX	Pneumothorax
Tc	Technetium (radioactive isotope)
TE	Echo time in MRI
TR	Repetition time in MRI
UGI	Upper gastrointestinal series
UVJ	Uretero-vesical junction

CHAPTER TWO   PEDIATRIC CENTRAL NERVOUS SYSTEM

I. **ANOMALIES [Table 2-1, p. 71]**
   A. **The Chiari malformations**
   - Simply put, the posterior fossa is too small for its contents
   - In all three types, cerebellar tonsils are displaced below foramen magnum
   - In Chiari II (also called Arnold-Chiari), cerebellum is also displaced upward through tentorial hiatus; tectum is kinked or "beaked," obstructing aqueduct of Sylvius and producing hydrocephalus associated with spina bifida
   - In Chiari III, a cervico-occipital encephalocele is also present
     1. Chiari I malformation **[Fig. 2-1]**

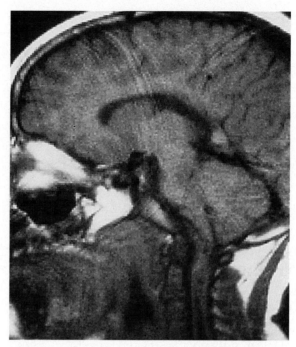

Fig. 2-1 Sagittal T1-weighted MRI: Cerebellar tonsils below level of foramen magnum. Note syrinx in lower cervical cord. Chiari I malformation.

   a. Downward displacement of cerebellar tonsils and inferior cerebellum below cranio-vertebral junction
   - Normal position of cerebellar tonsils below foramen magnum: ≤6 mm in first decade, ≤5 mm in second to third decades, ≤4 mm in fourth to eighth decades
   b. Medulla normal
   c. Associated with obstructive hydrocephalus, syringomyelia, syringobulbia
   d. Symptoms
   - Can simulate multiple sclerosis
   - Brain stem, cranial nerve dysfunction
   e. No spinal dysraphism
2. Chiari II malformation **[Figs. 2-2 and 2-3; see also Fig. 2-68]**
   a. Posterior fossa too small for its contents
   b. Large foramen magnum
   c. Downward displacement of cerebellar tonsils, inferior cerebellum, lower pons, medulla, fourth ventricle below cranio-vertebral junction
   d. Upward displacement of cerebellum ("towering cerebellum")
   e. Myelomeningocele
   f. Radiographic findings
   - Craniolacuna (disappears after 6 months, regardless of hydrocephalus) **[Fig. 2-90]**

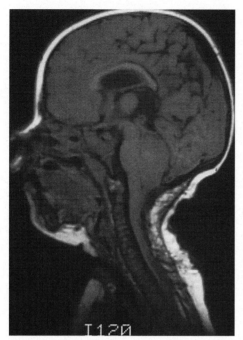

Fig. 2-2 Sagittal T1-weighted MRI: Cerebellar tonsils extend caudad to C2-3 level, dysplastic occipital lobe, elongation of fourth ventricle. Note enlarged massa intermedia. Chiari II malformation.

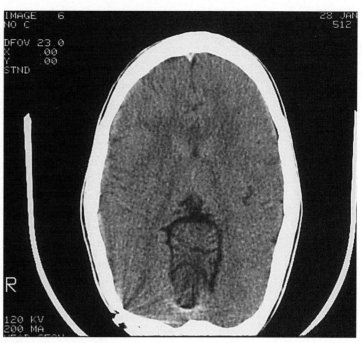

Fig. 2-3 Axial brain CT: Cerebellar vermis protrudes through tentorium ("towering cerebellum"). Chiari II malformation.

- Lückenschädel
- Myelodysplasia
- Enlarged foramen magnum

   g. Computed tomography (CT) and/or magnetic resonance imaging (MRI) findings
- Petrous scalloping
- Falx and tentorial hypoplasia
- Interdigitation in interhemispheric fissure
- Hydrocephalus
- Cerebellum displaced upward
- Wide tentorial incisura
- Mesencephalic beaking
- Anterior, inferior beaking of lateral ventricles
- Large massa intermedia
- Elongated fourth ventricle

  3. Chiari III malformation
    a. Downward displacement of medulla, fourth ventricle, cerebellum below cranio-vertebral junction
    b. Occipital/high cervical encephalomeningocele

B. Absence of corpus callosum (ACC) [Figs. 2-4 and 2-5]
  1. Primary embryonic agenesis or dysgenesis secondary to in utero inflammation or vascular insult
  2. Partial or complete

3. Isolated anomaly or part of complex anomaly
4. Separation of lateral ventricles by Probst bundles
    a. In ACC, cingulate gyrus extends inferiorly and separates anterior horns
5. Sharply angled frontal horns *concave upwards*
    a. Normal frontal horn is convex upwards
6. No septum pellucidum
7. Dilated occipital horns (colpocephaly)
    a. Looks like a "keyhole"
8. Associations
    a. Holoprosencephaly
    b. Chiari II malformation
    c. Dandy-Walker cyst
    d. Septo-optic dysplasia
    e. Midline lipoma
    f. Midline arachnoid cyst
    g. Encephalocele
    h. Gray matter heterotopia
    i. Aicardi's syndrome
        • Predominantly females, ACC, arachnoid cysts, butterfly vertebra

C. **Posterior fossa malformations**
    • These lesions comprise hypoplasia of the cerebellum, encystment of the fourth ventricle, enlargement of the cisterna magna, or arachnoid cyst
    • If a lesion does not exactly fit into one of the following categories, it should be described anatomically.

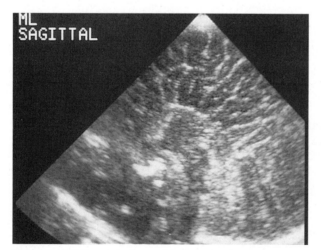

Fig. 2-4 Midline sagittal cranial US: Gyri radiate toward midportion of brain ("sunray appearance"). Absence of corpus callosum.

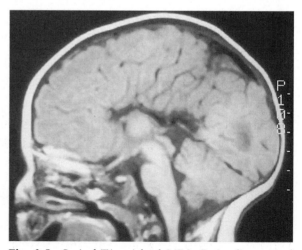

Fig. 2-5 Sagittal T1-weighted MRI: Gyri radiate toward mid-portion of brain, identical to Fig. 2-4. Absence of corpus callosum.

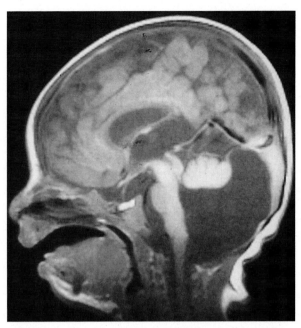

Fig. 2-6 Sagittal T1-weighted MRI: Absence of inferior vermis, cystic enlargement of fourth ventricle elevating straight sinus. Dandy Walker cyst.

1. Dandy-Walker cyst (DWC) **[Fig. 2-6]**
   a. Cystic dilatation of fourth ventricle
   b. Atresia of foramen of Magendie
   c. Vermian dysgenesis
   d. Huge posterior fossa cyst communicating with fourth ventricle
   e. Small cerebellar remnant
   f. Large posterior fossa
   g. Occiput thinned, ballooned
   h. Torcula above lambdoid suture ("Torcular-lambdoid inversion") on lateral skull X-ray
   i. Radiographic findings
      - High transverse sinus
      - Head size may be enlarged
   j. Associated anomalies
      - Agenesis of corpus callosum
      - Encephalocele
      - Holoprosencephaly
2. Dandy-Walker variant
   a. Partial vermian agenesis without torcular elevation
   b. Posterior evagination of tela choroidea of IV ventricle
   c. Some cases described as DW variant may represent vermian or cerebellar hypoplasia
3. Vermian or cerebellar hypoplasia
   a. Inferior lobules hypoplastic

      b. Cerebellar peduncles, pons, brain stem may be small

      c. Fourth ventricle, basal cisterns, vallecula, cisterna magna prominent

      d. Anatomic signs + cerebellar and brain stem dysfunction = Joubert's syndrome

  4. Retrocerebellar arachnoid cyst

      a. Also called Blake's pouch cyst **[Fig. 2-7]**

      b. No cerebellar dysgenesis

      c. Mass effect on cerebellum, displaced anteriorly

      d. Cyst may extend through tentorium

D. **Holoprosencephaly**

- Holoprosencephaly subdivided into complete absence of falx, midline separation of hemispheres or ventricles (alobar), partial (formation of falx) separation of hemispheres and ventricles (semilobar), or mild fusion of hemispheres in frontal lobes (lobar).

    Severity of mental or developmental deficiency coincides with severity of midline fusion (holoprosencephaly)

- Familial risk of holoprosencephaly (5 to 15%)
- Association of holoprosencephaly with trisomy 13, 18

  1. Alobar **[Fig. 2-8]**

      a. Facial malformation, hypotelorism

      b. Microcephaly

      c. Minimal cortex

      d. No falx

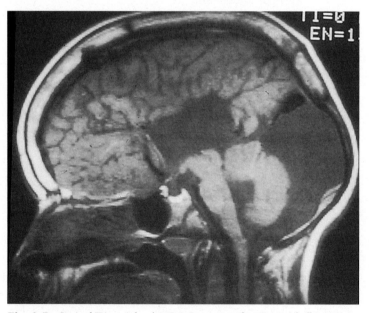

Fig. 2-7 Sagittal T1-weighted MRI: Presence of entire cerebellar vermis. Enlarged cisterna magna, thin occipital calvarium. Also note absence of corpus callosum. Mega cisterna magna (Blake's pouch cyst).

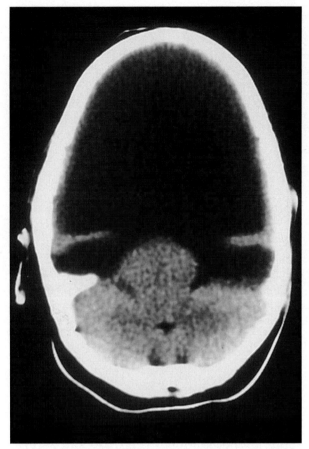

Fig. 2-8 Axial brain CT: Monoventricle, absence of midline structures. Alobar holoprosencephaly.

    e. Hemispheres fused at midline
    f. No olfactory bulbs/tracts
    g. Large monoventricular cavity
    h. Fused thalami
2. Semilobar
    a. Intermediate form
    b. Microcephaly
    c. Single ventricle
    d. Rudimentary occipital lobes, falx, interhemispheric fissure
3. Lobar
    a. Normal size brain
    b. Two hemispheres except rostrally
    c. Fused frontal horns
    d. Variable formation of corpus callosum, olfactory lobes
    e. Variable extent of thalamic fusion and facial deformity
    f. Absent septum pellucidum

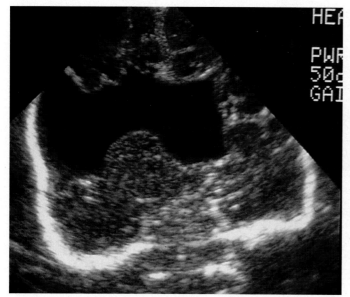

Fig. 2-9 Coronal cranial US: Square appearance of frontal horns of lateral ventricles, absence of septum pellucidum. Note gap between right temporal lobe and right frontal lobe, communication with lateral ventricle. Schizencephaly and absence of septum pellucidum.

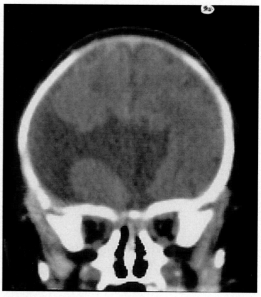

Fig. 2-10 Direct coronal brain CT: Same patient as Figure 2-9. Absence of septum pellucidum, schizencephaly involving right hemisphere. Note optic nerve hypoplasia. Compare diameter of optic nerve with diameter of extraocular muscles. Diameter of optic nerve should equal that of extraocular muscles. Septo-optic dysplasia.

E. **Septo-optic dysplasia (SOD) [Figs. 2-9 and 2-10]**
1. Described by De Morsier (1956)
2. Agenesis of septum pellucidum and hypoplasia of optic nerves
3. Females (80%)
4. Hypopituitarism
5. Hypotonia
6. Blindness
7. Squared frontal horns
8. Flattened roof and pointed floor of lateral ventricles
9. Dilatation of suprasellar and chiasmatic cisterns
10. Enlarged optic recess
11. Association with in utero infection, esp. cytomegalovirus (CMV)
12. Association with migrational disorders, esp. schizencephaly
13. Isolated absence of septum pellucidum may be found in otherwise normal people during neuroimaging for trauma, etc.

F. **Arachnoid cyst [Fig. 2-11]**
1. Size depends on flow dynamics into and out of cyst
   a. Small: rapid flow into and out of cyst
   b. Large: very slow efflux of cerebrospinal fluid (CSF) from cyst
   c. Medium: intermediate
2. Dilated, expanded CSF space (aberration in formation of subarachnoid space), or intraarachnoid cyst (splitting and duplication of arachnoid membrane)

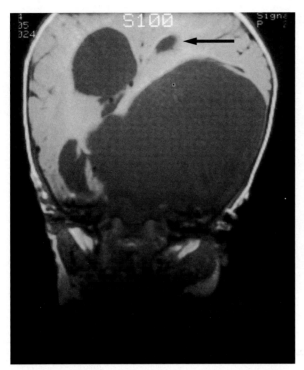

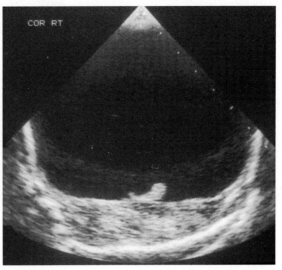

Fig. 2-11 Coronal T1-weighted MRI: Cystic structure displaces midline to right, markedly narrows left lateral ventricle (arrow). Arachnoid cyst.

Fig. 2-12 Coronal cranial US: Fluid-filled structure above level of tentorium with absence of cortical mantle. Note preservation of posterior fossa. Hydranencephaly.

a. Middle cranial fossa	50 to 66%
b. Suprasellar, quadrigeminal region	10%
c. Posterior fossa or frontal	5%

G. **Aqueductal stenosis**
 1. Two-thirds of cases of congenital hydrocephalus
 2. Seen in one-third of cases of Chiari II malformation

H. **Hydranencephaly [Fig. 2-12]**
 1. Occlusion of supraclinoid carotid arteries in third through sixth fetal months
 2. Hemispheres replaced by membranous sac of leptomeninges overlying glial layer that is remnant of cortex and white matter
 3. Posterior fossa, brain stem preserved; islands of temporal, frontal, or occipital lobes fed by posterior circulation
 4. Thalami are unfused
 5. Falx present
 6. Differential diagnosis (DDx):
    a. Alobar holoprosencephaly (no falx, fused thalami)
    b. Severe hydrocephalus
    c. Porencephaly
    d. Cystic encephalomalacia

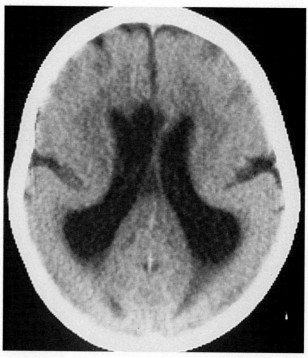

Fig. 2-13 Axial brain CT: Smooth surface of brain with infolding at Sylvian fissures. Note unusual white matter distribution. No interdigitating subcortical white matter; this white matter looks like a sergeant's "chevron." Lack of interdigitating white matter is a clue to presence of a migrational disorder. Lissencephaly.

I. **Migrational disorders**

    1. Lissencephaly or agyria (smooth brain) **[Fig. 2-13]**

        a. Normal brain has six layers

        b. Agyria-pachygyria complex: usually four layers

- Molecular layer, outer cellular layer, cell-sparse layer, inner cellular layer with disorganized neurons
- Cell-sparse gliotic layer with impaired migration distally
- Agyria: smooth surface, may coexist with pachygyria
- Pachygyria: broad, flat gyri, lack of sulcation, focal or diffuse
- Retardation, seizures, hypotonia
- CT/MRI: smooth brain, thickened cortex, shallow Sylvian fissures
- Associated gray matter heterotopia

        c. Type I lissencephaly: microcephaly

- Miller-Dieker (lissencephaly, ACC, micrognathia, short arm 17)
- Norman-Roberts (Miller-Dieker without chromosomal abnormality)
- Neu-Laxova (icthyosis, short limbs, perinatal death)

        d. Type II lissencephaly: macrocephaly

- Walker-Warburg (lissencephaly, hydrocephalus, retinal dysplasia, vermian hypoplasia with/without Dandy-Walker cyst)

- Cerebroocularmuscular syndrome (COMS): Walker-Warburg + congenital muscular dystrophy
  - HARD + E: Hydrocephalus, Agyria, Retinal Dysplasia, Encephalocele
  e. Type III lissencephaly: isolated lissencephaly with cerebrocerebellar lissencephaly
2. Polymicrogyria
   a. Numerous small gyri, cortex thickened, excessively convoluted
   b. Diffuse or focal, often in insular region in patient with abnormal sylvian fissure
   c. Polymicrogyria lines the cleft seen in schizencephaly
   d. Enlarged anomalous cortical veins
   e. White matter interdigitations follow convolutions
   f. Associations
      - Zellweger's cerebrohepatorenal syndrome
      - CMV
      - Cortical dysplasia
3. Schizencephaly **[Figs. 2-14 and 2-15]**
   a. Full thickness clefts lined with gray matter
   b. Pial-ependymal seam
   c. In utero vascular event
   d. May be associated with absent septum pellucidum (SOD), ACC
   e. Type I (Closed lip)
      - May be neurologically normal or seizures/spasticity

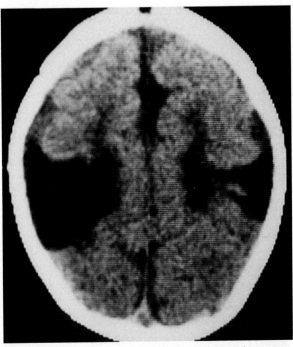

Fig. 2-14 Axial brain CT: Gap between gyri with communication to lateral ventricle bilaterally. Bilateral open-lipped schizencephaly.

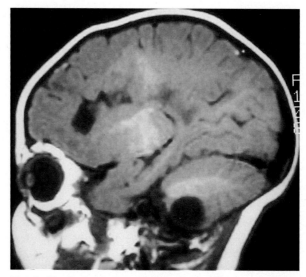

Fig. 2-15 Parasagittal T1-weighted MRI: Thin gap in frontal lobe, communication with frontal horn of lateral ventricle. Closed-lip schizencephaly. Incidentally noted posterior fossa arachnoid cyst and thickened gyri in frontal lobe indicating polymicrogyria or pachygyria.

- Fused cleft; unilateral or bilateral; at or near pre- or postcentral sulcus
  f. Type II (Open lip)
  - Retardation, seizures, hypotonia
  - Unfused cleft filled with CSF; lined by polymicrogyria
  - May be associated with hydrocephalus
  e. DDx: Porencephaly
  - Occurs after brain is formed, destructive or encephaloclastic, lined by white matter
4. Heterotopia **[Fig. 2-16]**
  a. Isolated or associated with other migrational disorders

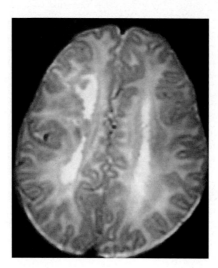

Fig. 2-16 Axial T2-weighted MRI: Several small nodules projecting into lateral ventricles (gray matter heterotopia), disorganized gyral pattern in right frontal lobe (pachygyria).

   b. Neurons in abnormal locations due to migration arrest
   c. Subependymal to cortex in location
   d. May simulate subependymal tubers of tuberous sclerosis
   e. Band heterotopia
      • In patients with heterotopic gray matter, continuous band of neurons in white matter between ventricles and cortex
      • Cortex–white matter band–heterotopic gray matter band–deep white matter
5. Hemimegalencephaly
   a. Focal or diffuse
   b. Enlarged cortical neurons
   c. Intractable seizures, hemiplegia, developmental delay
   d. Polymicrogyria, lissencephaly, heterotopia associated
   e. Distorted thickened cortex and ipsilateral ventricular dilatation
   f. Decreased myelination
J. **Phakomatoses**
   1. Tuberous sclerosis (TS) **[Figs. 2-17 through 2-19]**
      a. Autosomal dominant, variable penetrance
      b. Definitive diagnosis
         • Cortical tubers or subependymal nodules
         • Multiple renal angiomyolipomas and/or cysts
         • Cardiac rhabdomyomas
         • Adenoma sebaceum or subungual fibromas
         • Subependymal giant cell tumors
      c. Presumptive diagnosis (presence of two of the following)
         • Hypopigmented macule ("ash-leaf spot")
         • Shagreen patch

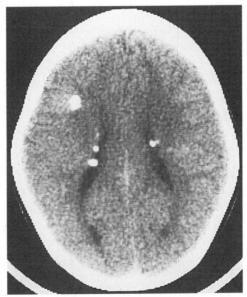

Fig. 2-17 Axial brain CT: Calcified subependymal nodules projecting into lateral ventricles, calcified parenchymal tuber in frontal lobe with associated cortical dysplasia. Tuberous sclerosis.

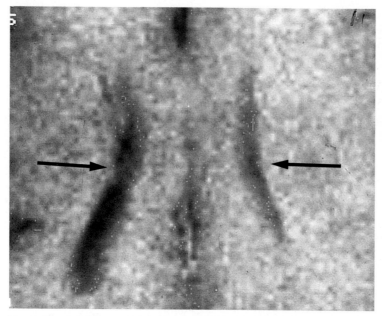

Fig. 2-18 Axial T1-weighted MRI: Several subependymal nodules project into both lateral ventricles (arrows). These are either heterotopic gray matter or tubers. Tuberous sclerosis.

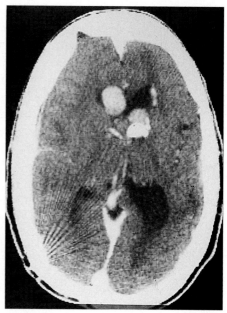

Fig. 2-19 Axial brain CT: Two enhancing tumors at the foramina of Monro in patient with tuberous sclerosis. Subependymal giant cell astrocytoma.

- Infantile spasms (hypsarrhythmia on electroencephalogram)
- Single retinal hamartoma
- Multiple renal cysts
- Cardiac rhabdomyoma
- First-degree relative with TS

d. Skin lesions   90%
e. Brain hamartomas   90%
f. Retinal hamartomas   50%
g. Renal hamartomas   50 to 80%
h. Variability of neurologic symptoms from none to disabled
i. Other signs
  - Lymphangiomyomatosis
  - Osteosclerosis; cysts in small bones of hand or foot
j. Subependymal nodules
  - Same CT density as brain, except when calcified
  - T1: isointense to hyperintense; T2: hypo- to isointense
k. Giant cell tumors
  - Usually at foramen of Monro
  - Slow growing, calcified, enhance on CT and MRI
  - T1: Hypo- to isointense; T2: hyperintense
l. Increased incidence of meningiomas, astrocytomas
m. Cortical tubers
  - Cortical and subcortical sclerosis or dysplasia
  - Gray and white matter; neural and glial giant cells
  - Diminished and disordered myelination, gliosis

- CT: hypodense to calcified
- T1: Hypo- to isointense; T2: hyperintense (gliosis)
2. Neurofibromatosis: NF-1 **[Figs. 2-20 through 2-22]**
   a. Autosomal dominant, variable penetrance
   b. NF-1 (von Recklinghausen, peripheral)
   c. One out of 2000–3000 live births
   d. Long arm chromosome 17
   e. Presence of two or more of following:
      - ≥6 cafe au lait spots, > 5 mm before, > 15 mm after puberty
      - ≥2 neurofibromas **[Fig. 8-5]**
      - ≥1 plexiform neurofibroma
      - Axillary or inguinal freckling
      - ≥2 iris hamartomas (Lisch nodules)

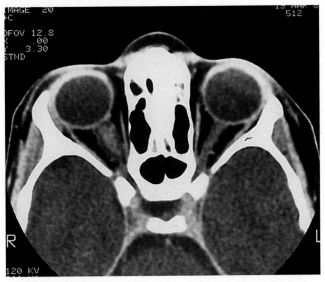

Fig. 2-20   Axial brain CT: Enhancement along course of right optic nerve in patient with neurofibromatosis-1. Optic glioma.

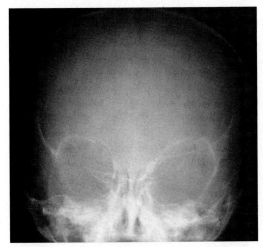

Fig. 2-21   AP skull radiograph: Absence of left lesser wing of sphenoid produces "empty orbit sign." Neurofibromatosis, sphenoid dysplasia.

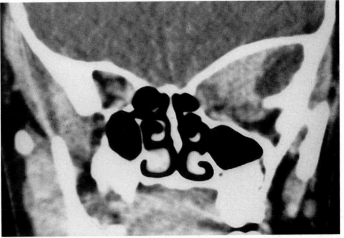

Fig. 2-22   Direct coronal orbital CT: Same patient as Figure 2-21. Widened left orbit, elevated supraorbital ridge; CT correlate of "empty orbit sign." Neurofibromatosis, sphenoid dysplasia.

- • ≥1 bone lesions (sphenoid dysplasia, pseudoarthrosis, etc.)
- • First-degree relative with NF-1
  f. Hamartomas
  g. Optic nerve glioma (15 to 40%)
- • Low grade pilocytoma astrocytoma
  h. Parenchymal gliomas (10%)
- • Astrocytomas
  i. Malignant nerve sheath tumors (MNST)
- • 50% occur in patients with NF-1
- • Incidence of MNST in patients with NF-1 ≥5%
  j. Sphenoid dysplasia (pulsating exophthalmos)
  k. Lambdoid defect
  l. Dural ectasia of internal auditory canal, neural foramina
  m. Lateral meningocele
  n. Kyphoscoliosis
- • Short segment thoracic scoliosis (NF-1 or Marfan's)
3. Neurofibromatosis: NF-2
  a. Autosomal dominant, variable penetrance
  b. NF-2 (bilateral acoustic, central) **[Fig. 8-7]**
  c. Deletions on chromosome 22
  d. Presence of one of following:
- • Bilateral VIII nerve schwannomas
- • First-degree relative with NF-2 + single VIII nerve mass
- • Any two of following: schwannoma, neurofibroma, meningioma, glioma (ependymoma), juvenile posterior subcapsular lens opacity
4. Sturge-Weber syndrome **[Fig. 2-23]**
  a. Encephalotrigeminal angiomatosis
  b. Port-wine stain in cranial nerve V1 distribution + leptomeningeal angiomatosis

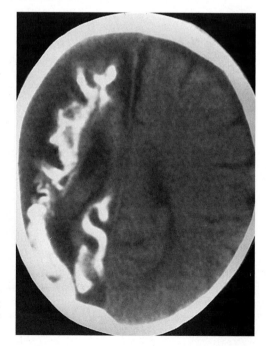

Fig. 2-23 Axial brain CT: Extensive gyral calcification and right hemisphere atrophy. Sturge Weber syndrome.

   c. Facial or leptomeningeal angioma unilateral or bilateral (25%)

   d. Choroidal angioma: congenital glaucoma (buphthalmos)

   e. Usually occipital

   f. Seizures in >90%; retardation; hemiplegia

   g. Hemiatrophy; Davidoff-Dyke-Masson

   h. Abnormal venous drainage ⇒ progressive dystrophic gyral calcification

   i. CT: Gyral calcification in dystrophic cortex

   j. MRI: Atrophy, enhanced shows ischemic cortex

Table 2-1. CNS Development Overview

Week	Normal	Anomalies
Primary Inductive Process		
2	Neural plate	Anencephaly
3	Neural tube	Dysraphia
		Cephalocele
		Meningomyelocele
		Chiari malformation
4	Formation of:	
	Prosencephalon	
	Metencephalon	
	Rhombencephalon	
5	Formation of:	Holoprosencephaly
	Telencephalon	Facial anomalies
	Diencephalon	
6	Commissural plate	Dysgenesis-corpus callosum
Cell Proliferation		
3–6	Proliferation of undifferentiated cells in primitive ependymal zone	Cerebellar hypoplasia; Dandy-Walker cyst
		Phakomatoses
	⇓	
	Neuroblasts	
Ventriculocisternal Development		
7–8	Choroid plexus perforation of fourth ventricle; Subarachnoid space	Anencephaly
		Arachnoid cyst
		Communicating hydrocephalus
		Acqueductal stenosis
		Non-communicating hydrocephalus
Neural Migration		
6–7	Mantle zone (primitive basal ganglia); Secondary migration of neuroblasts	Hydranencephaly
		Schizencephaly
	⇓	Heterotopia
	Cortical plate	Hemimegalencephaly
	(Primitive gray matter)	
20	Primary sulci	Lissencephaly
		Pachygyria
		Polymicrogyria
24–40	Secondary sulci	
36–60	Tertiary sulci	

From Mori K. Anomalies of the Central Nervous System. Neuroradiology and Neurosurgery. New York: Thieme-Stratton, Inc., 1985:20

II. MYELINATION AND WHITE MATTER ABNORMALITIES

A. Imaging of myelination
1. By MRI
2. Myelination of white matter (WM) indicated by high signal in WM (deep and subcortical) on T1-weighted images and low signal in WM on T2-weighted images
   a. Myelination is orderly sequence related to age [**Table 2-2 and Figs. 2-24 through 2-27**]

B. Formation of myelin
1. Formed by oligodendrocytes
2. Myelin sheath surrounds nerve process (axon)
3. Myelination occurs when the processes that are ensheathed become functional
4. Myelin rich in lipids (70 to 80%)
5. Lipids account for high signal on T1WI and low signal on T2WI. Lipids in myelin include:
   a. Cholesterol
   b. Galactolipids, which include cerebroside and sulfatide
   c. Phospholipids, which include various phosphoglycerides, sphingo-myelin, and plasmalogen

C. Myelin destruction and abnormal myelin formation result from:
1. Inflammatory, infectious, toxic or autoimmune disorders
2. Metabolic disorders that affect lysosomes, peroxisomes, or mitochondria

Table 2-2. Myelination Sequence Check List

T1WI at 1.5T	Age at Which Hyperintense WM seen on T1WI
Inferior and superior cerebellar peduncles	Birth
Dorsal pons, ventro-lateral thalamus partially myelinated	Birth
Optic tracts and radiations	2 Mo
Cerebellar WM	3 Mo
Splenium of corpus callosum	4 Mo
Genu of corpus callosum	6 Mo
Anterior limb of internal capsule	2–3 Mo
Deep frontal WM	3–6 Mo
Adult pattern	8 Mo

T2WI at 1.5T	Age at Which Hypointense WM seen on T2WI
Cerebellar WM	3–5 Mo
Splenium of corpus callosum	6 Mo
Genu of corpus callosum	8 Mo
Anterior limb of internal capsule	11 Mo
Frontal WM	11–14 Mo
Peripheral and subcortical WM (Adult pattern)	18 Mo

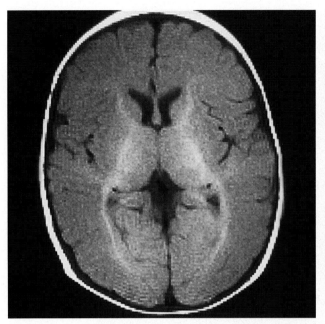

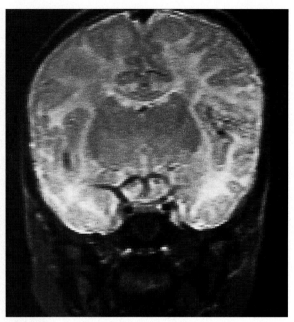

Fig. 2-24 Axial T1-weighted MRI: 3-month-old infant. Normal T1-weighted myelination pattern of white matter.

Fig. 2-25 Coronal T2-weighted MRI: 3-month-old infant. Normal T2-weighted myelination pattern of white matter.

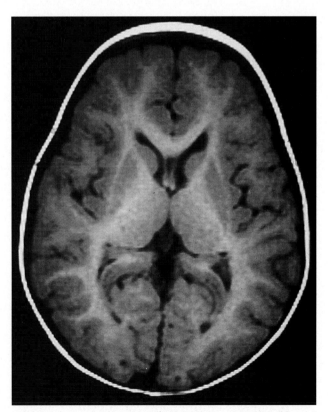

Fig. 2-26 Axial T1-weighted MRI: 1-year-old infant. Normal T1-weighted myelination pattern of white matter for child >8 months of age.

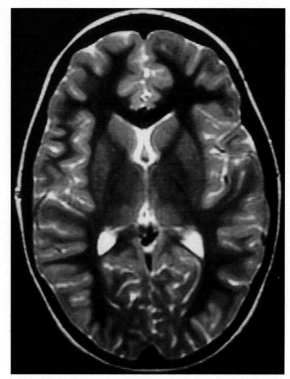

Fig. 2-27 Axial T2-weighted MRI: 2-year-old child. Normal T2-weighted myelination pattern of white matter for child >2 years of age.

D. **Demyelination (or myelinoclastic)**
   1. Myelin sheath originally normal, but damaged by toxic metabolites
   2. Pattern of demyelination lacks symmetry, lesions sharply demarcated, irregularly involves subcortical arcuate fibers; usually spares cerebellar WM
   3. Includes subacute sclerosing panencephalitis (SSPE), progressive multifocal leukoencephalopathy, human immunodeficiency virus (HIV) demyelination, multiple sclerosis (MS), postinfectious, and chemotherapy-radiotherapy-induced demyelination
E. **Dysmyelination**
   1. Intrinsic abnormality results in abnormal formation or destruction of essential components of myelin
   2. Newest myelin is peripheral
   3. Therefore, myelin affected in dysmyelinating disease is central
   4. Pattern of myelination symmetric, diffuse margins, involves cerebellar WM; spares subcortical WM
   5. Dysmyelination present in both lysosomal and peroxisomal disorders
F. **Peroxisomes are cytoplasmic organelles that contain enzymes necessary for oxidation of very long chain (24-26) fatty acids, oxidation of dicarboxylic acids, and synthesis of plasmalogen and phospholipids, components of myelin. Central nervous system (CNS) effects of peroxisomal diseases include:**
   1. Migrational disorders with dysmyelination, delayed myelination or demyelination (includes Zellweger, neonatal adrenoleukodystrophy)

Fig. 2-28 Axial brain CT: Hypodense white matter predominantly in posterior hemispheres with focal contrast enhancement. Adrenoleukodystrophy.

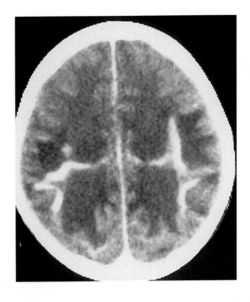

2. Symmetrical dysmyelination or demyelination
3. Cranial or peripheral neuropathy
4. Peroxisomal diseases include:
    a. Zellweger's syndrome (cerebro-hepato-renal syndrome)
        - Liver dysfunction, cataracts, seizures, migrational disorders, delayed myelination and possible demyelination, cortical renal cysts, stippled calcification of patella and greater trochanter, triradiate cartilage of hips, retardation, hypotonia
    b. X-linked adrenoleukodystrophy **[Fig. 2-28]**
        - Onset usually age 5 to 7 years in boys
        - Accumulation of very long chain fatty acids
        - May be preceded by adrenal insufficiency precipitated by intercurrent infection
        - Regression and behavior disturbance
        - Peritrigonal WM lesions first; extends through splenium of corpus callosum
        - Early occipital involvement
        - Extends anteriorly; atypical cases asymmetric, unilateral, or unusual distribution
        - WM-3 affected zones
            Central zone of gliosis, sometimes with cavitation or calcification
            Intermediate zone of inflammation + demyelination, which enhances with contrast
            Peripheral zone of demyelination without inflammation. Involves central WM, posterior, splenium of corpus callosum (CC)

G. **Lysosomes are cytoplasmic organelles that maintain normal function of the cell by removing worn out cytoplasmic structures (products of metabolism) or phagocytosed material, such as bacteria**
    1. Lysosomal storage disorders occur when enzyme defects in lysosome function result in material trapped in storage granules, interfering with cell function
    2. Lysosomal storage disorders produce disturbed turnover of myelin

> ►TIP
> Delayed myelination + migrational disorders = peroxisomal diseases

3. Involves myelin of deep WM
   a. Large, confluent symmetric deep WM involvement with sparing of subcortical U-fibers
      - No migrational disorder
4. Lysosomal disorders: autosomal recessive
   a. Classified by abnormal material stored in lysosomes
5. Lysosomal storage diseases include:
   a. Sphingolipidoses, such as:
      - Gangliosidoses
         GM1 Gangliosidosis–resembles Hurler syndrome
         Retardation, spasticity
         Demyelination and gliosis of WM
      - Fabry's disease
         Skin rash (angiokeratoma corporis), autonomic dysfunction, sensory neuropathy
         Multifocal small infarcts
         Includes demyelination
      - Metachromatic leukodystrophy
         Deficiency of arylsulfatase A
         Sulfatide accumulates in neural cells
         Classified by age at time of onset
         - Neonatal—rapid downhill course
         - Infantile—presents at 1 to 4 years of age with polyneuropathy, ataxia, retardation, speech deterioration, incoordination (Most common form, late infantile—1 to 2 years of age)
         - Juvenile—presents with dementia, behavior disorders, progressing to spastic quadriparesis
         Peripheral neuropathy
         Progressive WM loss
         - CT or MR:
            Symmetric WM abnormality in centrum semiovale, including cerebellum, peripheral WM spared
            Diffuse, spares U-fibers
            Bilateral, symmetric with both demyelinated and delayed myelination
      - Globoid cell leukodystrophy (Krabbe's disease)
         Cerebroside accumulates in lysosomes of histiocytes
         Age at presentation 1 to 6 months
         Psychomotor regression, hypertonia, fever, opisthotonus, seizures, hyperirritability, feeding problems
         Extensive demyelination with sparing of subcortical fibers
         High density on CT in thalamus, basal ganglia, and caudate
         Progressive high signal in deep WM
         Progressive atrophy, death by 2 years of age
      - Niemann-Pick disease
         Hepatosplenomegaly, lymphadenopathy
   b. Mucopolysaccharidoses
      - Hunter's and Hurler's syndromes, etc.

- Atrophy with prominence of perivascular (Virchow-Robin) spaces
    c. Others
        - Cystinosis
        - Pompe's glycogen storage disease
            Involves heart, tongue + gliosis
        - Wolman's disease
            Type of sudanophilic leukodystrophy
            Hepatosplenomegaly, adrenal calcification
        - Canavan disease
            Spongy degeneration
            Autosomal recessive in Jewish infants
            Onset in first 6 months of life
            Elevated levels of N-acetylaspartic acid
            Apathy, hypotonia, megalencephaly
            Subcortical U-fibers involved preferentially
            Occipital lobes more than frontal and parietal lobes
            Globus pallidus severely affected
        - Ceroid lipofuscinosis
            Marked cerebral and cerebellar atrophy; myoclonus, ataxia, retardation, visual loss

H. **Dysmyelinating leukodystrophies without defined enzyme defect**
    1. Alexander's leukodystrophy
        a. Psychomotor retardation, megalencephaly, hydrocephalus, seizures, spasticity
        b. CT
            - Hypodense frontal lobes with enhancement between frontal horn and WM
        c. MRI
            - Bilateral frontal lobe T1 and T2 prolongation
            - Extends posteriorly to parietal lobes and internal capsule (genu involved late)
    2. Cockayne's syndrome
        a. Late infancy; dwarfism, deafness, cataracts, optic atrophy, mental deficiency
        b. Autosomal recessive
        c. Thickened leptomeninges
        d. Extensive calcification, esp. basal ganglia, and vessel walls

I. **Mitochondria are cell membrane organelles that provide energy for the cell via adenosine 5'-triphosphatase (ATP)**
    1. Mitochondrial dysfunction includes:
        a. Defects of substrate transport across mitochondrial membrane
            - Carnitine deficiency
        b. Defects of respiratory chain
            - Hypoxic-ischemic encephalopathy
            - Carbon monoxide intoxication
            - Cyanide intoxication
        c. Defects of oxidative phosphorylation
            - Various aminoacidopathies

2. Distribution of mitochondrial disorders
   a. Deep gray matter involvement and peripheral WM involvement + abnormal muscles
   b. Involves caudate, putamen, periaqueductal gray; cortex less common, demyelination unusual
3. Clinical features
   a. Seizures, muscle weakness, mental deterioration, sensorineural hearing loss, ophthalmoplegia, retinitis pigmentosa, peripheral neuropathy, symmetric or asymmetric CNS deficits
   b. Endocrine effect including growth hormone deficiency, short stature, hypoparathyroidism, hypothyroidism
   c. Anemia, myocardopathy; hepatopathy
4. Leigh's disease
   a. Neonatal and adult forms
   b. Hypotonia, psychomotor deterioration, brain stem and basal ganglia dysfunction, including ataxia, ophthalmoplegia, dystonia, swallowing difficulties, nystagmus, developmental delay, failure to thrive (FTT)
   c. CT
      • Decreased density in basal ganglia (putamen), dorsal brain stem, cerebellum
   d. MRI
      • Increased signal in caudate, putamen, periaqueductal gray matter, cerebellum, midbrain, medulla, thalami, frontal and insular cortex, dorsal pons on T2WI + demyelination (unusual)
5. MERRF (Myoclonus, Epilepsy, Ragged Red Fibers)
   a. Myoclonus, epilepsy, ragged red fibers + lactic acidosis, profound ataxia
   b. Cortical and WM atrophy, including deep WM
6. MELAS (Mitochondrial Encephalopathy with Lactic Acidosis and Strokelike episodes)
   a. Myopathy, encephalopathy, lactic acidosis, nausea, vomiting, strokelike events with hemianopsia and hemiplegia
   b. Usually second decade of life
   c. Involves cortex and subcortical WM; abnormal signal in putamen on T2WI
7. Kearns-Sayre syndrome
   a. External ophthalmoplegia, retinitis pigmentosa, heart block, endocrine dysfunction, ataxia, myopathy
   b. Involves subcortical WM, globus pallidus, thalami, dorsal brain stem, substantia nigra, cerebellar WM
   c. Periventricular WM spared
8. Menkes disease (trichopoliodystrophy)
   a. Coarse, sparse, kinky hair
   b. Seizures, hypothermia, hypotonia
   c. X-linked recessive

d. Impaired intestinal absorption of copper

e. Primary disease a mitochondrial enzyme defect

f. Cerebral arteries thin walled, tortuous with splits in intima

g. Metaphyseal spurring, diaphyseal periostitis

h. Wormian bones

i. Large bladder diverticula

j. Large subdural collections

k. Rapid progression of atrophy

l. Short T1 in cortex early in disease (bright on T1WI)

9. Alpers syndrome (progressive cerebral poliodystrophy)

a. Intractable seizures, myoclonus

b. Involves cerebral gray matter and liver

c. Cortical atrophy, especially occipital

d. Decreased WM volume + delayed myelination

10. MELAS, MERRF, Kearns-Sayre in older patients

11. Leigh's, Menkes, Alpers in infants or young children

J. **Other mitochondrial disorders**

1. Amino/organic acidopathies

a. Toxic metabolites produce damage in perivenous spaces

b. Retarded myelination or hypomyelination

c. Irregular, mottled demyelination, spotty distribution

d. Subcortical U-fibers are not spared

2. Maple syrup urine disease

a. Onset shortly after birth, vomiting, FTT, seizures, decreasing consciousness

b. Cerebral edema; if survival, then atrophy

c. At 3 to 8 weeks of age, deep cerebellar WM, dorsal brain stem, cerebral peduncles, posterior limb of internal capsule (PLIC) show spongiform change

d. Myelination delayed

3. Phenylketonuria (PKU)

a. Deficiency of phenylalanine hydroxylase; toxic buildup of phenylpyruvic and phenylacetic acids

b. Migrational disorders, delayed and defective myelination, especially in deep cerebral WM

4. Nonketotic hyperglycinemia

a. Apnea and hypotonia shortly after birth

b. Seizures, myoclonus, severe developmental delay

c. Partial and complete agenesis of corpus callosum

d. Defective myelination and demyelination

5. Methylmalonic and propionic acidemia

a. Both present with ketoacidosis

b. Spastic quadriparesis, retardation early onset

6. Galactosemia

a. Vomiting in newborn, increased intracranial pressure, cataracts, jaundice, hepatosplenomegaly, hypoglycemia

b. Extensive cerebral WM edema

7. Hyperammonemia defects, which include urea cycle abnormalities
   a. Present with seizures, ataxia, coma
   b. WM edema and gliosis
   c. Includes citrullinemia, argininosuccinic aciduria (both autosomal recessive), and X-linked ornithine carbamyl transferase, which presents with strokelike episodes
      • Imaging shows gray and white matter "infarcts"

8. Organic acidurias
   a. Glutamic aciduria Type I
      • Results in hyperammonemia and metabolic acidosis
   b. Delayed and defective myelination
      • Degeneration and low density on CT in lentiform and caudate nuclei
      • Frontotemporal atrophy with widening of Sylvian fissure
   c. Glutamic aciduria Type II
      • Neonatal hypoglycemia, renal cysts
   d. Cystinuria
      • Life-threatening renal failure
      • Crystals in choroid plexus, necrosis of internal capsule
   e. Homocystinuria
      • Presents at 6 to 9 months of age with cerebro-occlusive disease, seizures, retardation

9. Carnitine deficiency
   a. Carnitine necessary for long chain fatty acid oxidation, peroxisomal fatty acid oxidation, branched chain amino acid metabolism, mitochondrial membrane stabilization
   b. Carnitine deficiency primary or secondary to organic acidurias, hemodialysis or renal failure
   c. Mitochondrial cytopathy with encephalopathy, cardiomyopathy
   d. Presents with hepatic encephalopathy, Reye-like encephalopathy, hypoglycemia, heart failure

10. Fatty acid enzyme defects
    a. Include medium chain acyl CoA dehydrogenase (MCAD), most common type
    b. Present with metabolic decompensation, hypoketotic hypoglycemia, carnitine deficiency, acidosis

K. **Destructive leukodystrophies**
   1. Periventricular leukomalacia (PVL)
      a. See section on hypoxia
   2. Trauma
      a. Irradiation with/or without intrathecal methotrexate
      b. Mineralizing microangiopathy
         • Patchy or diffuse deep WM involvement
         • Calcification on CT

▶TIP
Urea cycle defects and metabolic defects producing metabolic acidosis/hypoglycemia induce diffuse global insult that simulates hypoxic-ischemic encephalopathy by neuroimaging.

L. **Primary defect unknown**
   1. Pelizaeus-Merzbacher
      a. First decade of life; X-linked recessive
      b. Pendular nystagmus, cerebellar ataxia, intermittent shaking of head, choreoathetoid movement, psychomotor retardation
      c. Arrested myelination, not dysmyelination
         • Therefore, WM is not bright because myelin is simply not formed
         • Slow, progressive atrophy

M. **Infectious or inflammatory causes of demyelination**
   1. Secondary to ischemia associated with bacterial meningitis, encephalitis-induced necrosis
   2. Progressive multifocal leukoencephalopathy (PML)
      a. Papovavirus in immunocompromised, autoimmunodeficiency syndrome (AIDS)
         • MRI
            Focal lesions-confluent areas on hyperintense white matter on T2WI
   3. Subacute sclerosing panencephalitis (SSPE)
      a. Defective measles virus
      b. Clinical features: mental deterioration, behavior problems, seizures
      c. Posterior cerebral demyelination (occipital)
      d. Spares subcortical fibers
         • Similar distribution in adrenoleukodystrophy
      e. Also involves cortical gray matter, brain stem
         • Congenital cytomegalovirus (CMV)
            Hypodensity in white matter
         • Multiple sclerosis (MS)
            Hyperintense cerebral and cerebellar white matter and brain stem on T2WI
   4. Acute disseminated encephalomyelitis (ADEM)
      a. Two to four weeks after vaccination or viral illness
      b. Autoimmune
      c. Clinical: abrupt onset, confusion, cranial nerve palsies, seizures
         • CT
            Patchy, hypodense white matter; nodular or gyriform enhancement
         • MRI
            Patchy high signal in hemispheric WM, asymmetric, often involves gray-white junctions
            May involve gray matter
   5. Congenital cytomegalovirus (CMV)
      a. Associated with migrational disorders
      b. WM distribution may mimic ADEM
   6. Multiple sclerosis (MS) **[Figs. 2-29 and 2-30]**
      a. Demyelinating disease
      b. Female predominance in those rare children with MS
      c. Chronic, relapsing course

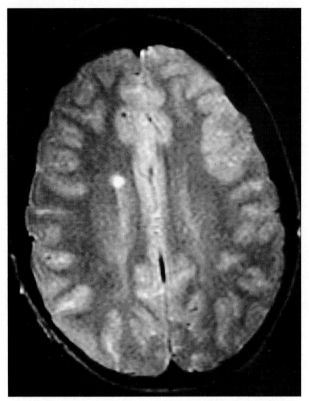

Fig. 2-29 Axial T2-weighted MRI: 14-year-old girl. Focal hyperintense lesions in deep white matter. Multiple sclerosis.

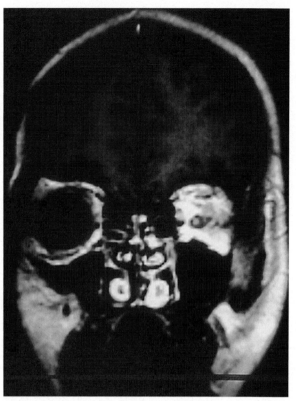

Fig. 2-30 Coronal gadolinium-enhanced T1-weighted MRI: Same patient as Figure 2-29. Enhancement in left optic nerve, indicating optic neuritis. Multiple sclerosis.

    d. Presenting symptoms: sensory (26%), optic neuritis (14%), diplopia (11%)

    e. Elevated IgG in CSF

    f. MRI

       • Asymmetric, focal lesions of hyperintensity on T2WI in deep white matter or spinal cord

       • Usually spares subcortical white matter

       • Gadolinium enhancement in lesions of acute demyelination

       • Lesions may be large enough to be confused with neoplasia

N. **Differentiating features of some white matter disorders**

    1. Megalencephaly: Alexander or Canavan disease

    2. Calcification of basal ganglia: Krabbe's disease, Cockayne's syndrome

    3. Adrenoleukodystrophy—occipital involvement, then frontal

    4. Alexander—frontal involvement first, then posterior

    5. Pelizaeus-Merzbacher—persistently infantile pattern of myelination

    6. Migrational disorders + WM abnormality: peroxisomal disorders, CMV, PKU

    7. Preferential subcortical WM involvement: Canavan disease

III. **HYPOXIA AND THE DEVELOPING BRAIN**
   A. **Incidence of intracranial hemorrhage inversely related to birthweight (Table 2-3)**

Table 2-3. Incidence of Intracranial Pathology as a
Function of Birthweight

Birth Weight (g)	Intracranial Hemorrhage
<750	60%
750–999	50%
1000–1249	38%
1250–1499	22%
1500–1749	7%
1750–1999	5%
2000–2250	6%
>2250	5%

From: Sims ME, Halterman G, Jasani N, Vachon L, Wu PYK. Indications for routine cranial ultrasound scanning in the nursery. *J Clin Ultrasound* 1986;14:443–447.

   B. **Germinal matrix/intraventricular/parenchymal hemorrhage [Figs. 2-31 through 2-37; see also Fig. 2-72]**
   1. Highly vascular germinal matrix is zone of neuroblast formation and migration
   2. Germinal matrix lines ventricular system, including caudothalamic groove, most common site of hemorrhage
   3. Germinal matrix involutes after 34 weeks gestation
      a. Germinal matrix hemorrhage usually prior to 34 weeks gestation
   4. Hemorrhage occurs because of fragile vascular bed, lack of cerebrovascular autoregulation, fluctuating arterial and venous pressures resulting from patent ductus arteriosus (PDA), hypoxia, ventilatory support, other perinatal stressors

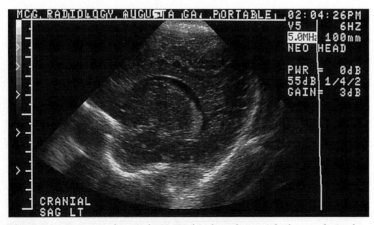

Fig. 2-31 Parasagittal cranial US: Within lateral ventricle, hyperechoic choroid plexus tapers anteriorly and terminates at the level of the caudo-thalamic groove (arrow). Normal parasagittal newborn cranial US.

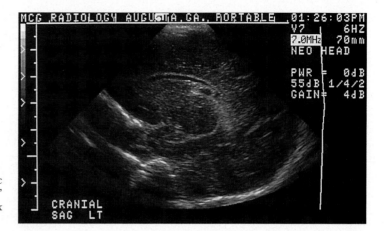

Fig. 2-32 Parasagittal cranial US: Hypoechoic "cyst" (arrow) in caudo-thalamic groove. The "cyst" is a hyperacute or resolving grade I germinal matrix hemorrhage (GMH).

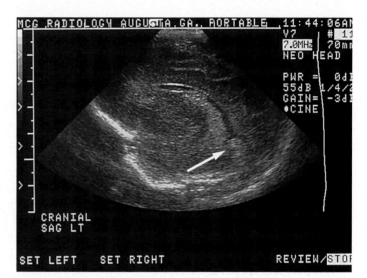

Fig. 2-33 Parasagittal cranial US: Hyperechoic choroid plexus becomes "thicker" at level of caudo-thalamic groove. The area of thickness actually represents germinal matrix hemorrhage (GMH). Note low-level echoes within normal size lateral ventricle and small hyperechoic clot (arrow) in posterior horn of lateral ventricle. Grade II GMH.

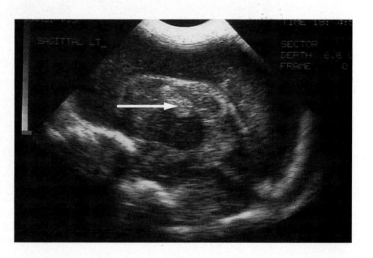

Fig. 2-34 Left parasagittal cranial US: "Cast clot" within lateral ventricle. Note extension of germinal matrix hemorrhage (GMH) (arrow) into lateral ventricle. Grade III GMH.

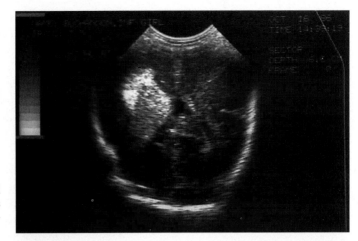

Fig. 2-35 Coronal cranial US: Clot fills right lateral ventricle; echogenic lesion in right frontal lobe indicates parenchymal hemorrhage or infarction. Grade IV germinal matrix hemorrhage.

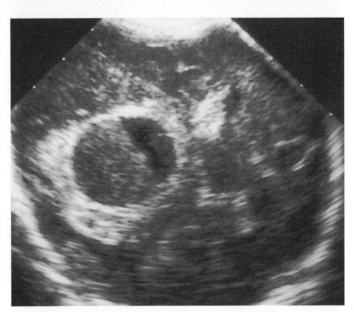

Fig. 2-36 Coronal cranial US: Fluid-fluid level in acute parenchymal hemorrhage.

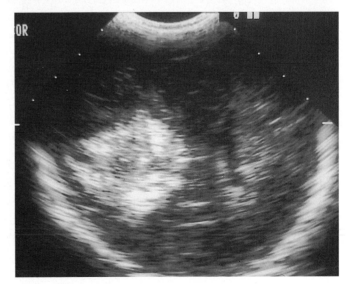

Fig. 2-37 Coronal cranial US: Same patient as Figure 2-36, 24 hours later. Conversion of hypoechoic sonographic pattern of acute hemorrhage to more typical echogenic parenchymal hemorrhage.

5. Germinal matrix hemorrhage grades I–IV
    a. I: Confined to subependymal matrix, normal ventricular size
    b. II: Intraventricular hemorrhage (IVH) without ventricular dilatation
    c. III: IVH with ventricular dilatation
    d. IV: Grade III + parenchymal hemorrhage
6. Prognosis usually good for grades I and II; worst for grade IV
7. Subependymal hemorrhage (SEH) usually resolves completely or small residual "cyst" indicates evidence of prior germinal matrix hemorrhage
8. Intraventricular hemorrhage indicated by clot, fluid-fluid level, or intermediate-level echoes in ventricle
    a. Several days after IVH, ependymal thickening noted by ultrasound
    b. Posthemorrhagic hydrocephalus occurs in about 75% grade III–IV
        • Arrested hydrocephalus in 75%
        • 10% will require ventricular shunt
9. Likelihood of neurologic sequelae increases with severity of hemorrhage
10. Parenchymal hemorrhage [Fig. 1-78]
    a. Occurs as periventricular venous hemorrhagic infarction, periventricular leukomalacia, or isolated parenchymal hemorrhage

C. **Periventricular hemorrhagic infarction**
1. Usually in prematures following or associated with Grade III hemorrhage
2. 80% of cases associated with large intraventricular hemorrhage
3. Incorporates large area of WM; dense, homogeneous on ultrasound
4. Probably secondary to periventricular venous congestion
5. High morbidity (80–100%) and mortality (37% if localized, 81% if extensive)

D. **PVL [Figs. 2-38 through 2-40]**
1. Manifestation of partial asphyxia in prematures and some term newborns
2. Characterized by focal necrosis of periventricular WM dorsal and lateral to external angles of ventricle
3. Most common sites are trigone and adjacent to frontal horn
4. Hemorrhage into areas of PVL may be microscopic to massive: its incidence varies inversely with gestational age
5. Varied degree of severity from cystic cavities to diminished myelin with dilated lateral ventricles
6. Only 28% of periventricular WM lesions detected by ultrasound
7. Spastic diplegia and intellectual deficit correlated with PVL
8. Pathogenesis is systemic hypotension and impaired cerebral blood flow (arterial border zone)
    a. Usually in prematures; can occur in term newborn
9. Higher incidence in smaller premies; postulated that less severe insult necessary in smallest of premies; conversely, more severe insult required in larger infants to produce PVL
10. On MRI, characterized by decreased WM volume and hyperintensity in older infant or child, without peritrigonal myelinated layer of WM
11. PVL in premature less than 26 weeks gestation only manifested by decrease in WM volume

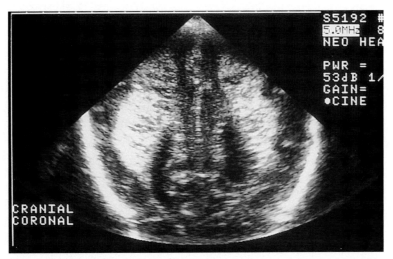

Fig. 2-38 Coronal cranial US: Extensive hyperechogenic lesion in deep white matter bilaterally. Periventricular leukomalacia (PVL), acute.

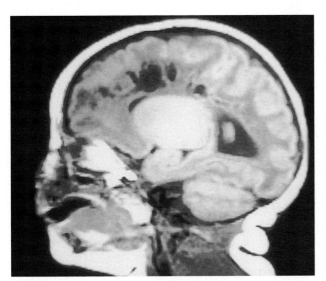

Fig. 2-39 Parasagittal T1-weighted MRI: Numerous cysts or cavitations in deep white matter. Periventricular leukomalacia (PVL), subacute.

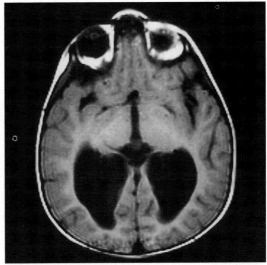

Fig. 2-40 Axial T1-weighted MRI: Ventricular widening, narrowed periventricular white matter, and approximation of gyri to lateral ventricle. Periventricular leukomalacia (PVL), chronic.

12. PVL in premature more than 26 weeks gestation manifested by decrease in WM volume and hyperintensity in WM due to gliosis
13. On ultrasound, characterized by hyperechogenic and coarse pattern of WM in neonate
    a. Difficult distinction between normal "peritrigonal blush," which has a paintbrush effect at trigone

E. **Isolated parenchymal hemorrhage**
1. Occurs primarily in term infants
2. Associated with birth trauma, congenital bleeding diathesis, such as hemophilia, or due to anticoagulants, used in extracorporeal membrane oxygenation (ECMO)

F. **Cerebral edema [Figs. 2-41 and 2-42]**
1. Occurs in term newborns due to perinatal asphyxia, low cardiac output states, shock (fetomaternal or twin-twin transfusion, placental abruption), metabolic catastrophe (organic acidemias, urea cycle enzyme defects)

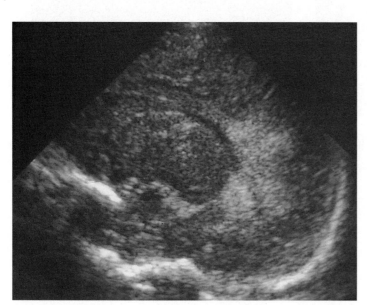

Fig. 2-41 Parasagittal cranial US: Monotonous echogenic pattern throughout cortex and white matter, lack of differentiation between gray and white matter; narrowed lateral ventricles. Cerebral edema.

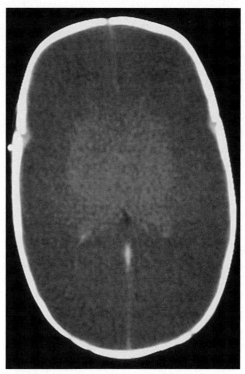

Fig. 2-42 Axial brain CT: Marked, diffuse hypodensity throughout hemispheres, contrasted with central structures. Note hyperdensity in interhemispheric fissure indicating slow or absent blood flow, subarachnoid hemorrhage, or polycythemia. Cerebral edema.

2. Difficult radiographic diagnosis by CT
   a. Diffuse loss of gray-white differentiation
3. Note gray-white differentiation on ultrasound
   a. Normal: Periphery of hemisphere less echogenic than deep structures
   b. Cerebral edema: Monotonous pattern with no differentiation between gray and white matter
   c. By MRI, T1-weighted images may be more useful than T2-weighted images to detect cerebral edema

G. **Hypoxic–ischemic encephalopathy (HIE)**
   1. Pathophysiology
      a. Neurons susceptible to oxygen and glucose deprivation directly or to injury from excitatory amino acids such as glutamate
      b. Excitatory amino acids function at N-methyl-D-aspartate (NMDA) receptor sites
      c. Excessive release or impaired uptake of excitatory amino acids from intersynaptic cleft results in excess excitatory amino acids at receptor sites
      d. Excess excitatory amino acids causes depolarization of cell membranes, calcium influx into cells, free radical formation, mitochondrial dysfunction, depletion of energy stores and cell death
      e. Proposed causes of brain injury include HIE, hypoglycemia, status epilepticus
      f. Areas susceptible to HIE in newborn are those with active myelination and those with high levels of NMDA receptor sites
   2. Patterns of injury
      a. Selective neuronal necrosis of cortex involves hippocampus, deep gray matter
      b. Leukomalacia of deep and subcortical WM
      c. Focal or generalized infarction
   3. Ischemic injury in first trimester causes congenital malformations
   4. Ischemic injury in third trimester causes PVL
      a. 24–26 weeks at time of hypoxic insult:
         • Ventricular widening with loss of deep WM, minimal or absent gliosis
         • Limited response to neural tissue injury
         • Liquefaction necrosis of deep WM, sloughing of brain into ventricle
         • Imaging displays ventriculomegaly, thin WM, no T2 prolongation by MRI
         • Large ventricles at birth with decreased WM volume = intrauterine damage before 27 to 28 weeks
      b. 28–36 weeks at time of hypoxic insult:
         • Deep WM gliosis
         • Cortex and subcortical WM spared
         • Damaged deep WM, reflected by bright areas on T2WI
         • Enlargement of ventricles, irregular border

▶TIPS
• BE CAREFUL: If nursery room light excessive, technologist may increase gain on ultrasound machine
• Excess gain will render entire scan spuriously echogenic, simulating cerebral edema
• Internal control: Compare temporal lobe with deep structures of basal ganglia and thalamus
• The temporal lobe should be less echogenic

c. With ongoing PVL:
- Early, gyri at short distance from ventricular wall
- Four weeks later, gyri closer to ventricles with ventricular enlargement, indicating necrosis and absorption
- Six weeks later, chronic PVL, loss of WM, apposition of gyri to ventricle

d. 36 weeks at time of hypoxic insult:
- Deep WM gliosis; mild subcortical WM gliosis

e. Term at time of hypoxic insult:
- Parasagittal cortical watershed, deep and subcortical WM gliosis

f. Post-term at time of hypoxic insult:
- Cortex and subcortical WM, relative sparing of deep WM

5. In prematures, the "watershed" is between deep perforating vessels (ventriculofugal) and medullary arteries from cortex inward (ventriculopedal) = deep periventricular WM (at trigone and frontal horn of lateral ventricle). As central perforators develop, the "watershed" moves outward with gestational age in third trimester. At and shortly after term, "watershed" is peripheral in cortical and subcortical regions.

6. Clinical signs of perinatal asphyxia
   a. Low scalp and cord pH, low Apgar score, depressed fetal heart rate, meconium stained amniotic fluid, neurologic deterioration shortly after birth
   b. Hyperalert initially or lethargic, poor suck, apnea, abnormal tone and movement
   c. Seizures in first day of life, death rate 11% term, 60% premies
   d. 25% of survivors have sequelae such as retardation, cerebral palsy, epilepsy

7. Partial vs. total (profound) asphyxia
   a. Severity determined by degree and duration of hypoxia and hypotension

8. Partial asphyxia
   a. Hypotension, cerebral edema, hypoperfusion affect the "watershed"; brain stem, thalami, basal ganglia relatively perfused
   b. Term with partial asphyxia:
      - Poor differentiation between involved cortex and unmyelinated subcortical WM giving appearance of discontinuous cortex
      - T2WI: should see discrete dark signal in cortex
      - Cortex and WM look isointense (loss of gyral pattern)
      - Acute event may be difficult to see on MRI
   c. Chronic effects of partial asphyxia:
      - Atrophy, shrunken gyri, ulegyria (base of gyri shrunken, gyrus looks like a mushroom)
      - Extension of hyperintensity from central to subcortical areas and shrunken gyri

9. Total asphyxia
   a. Complete absence of cerebral blood flow

   b. Brain stem, thalami, basal ganglia are areas of highest metabolic requirement typically affected by absent blood flow

   c. Thalami, basal ganglia, hippocampi, dorsal brain stem consistently affected by absent blood flow in both premies in third trimester and term newborns
- Perirolandic cortex spared in premies, but affected in term newborns

   d. Volume of affected brain related to severity and duration of insult
- >25 minutes cardiorespiratory arrest affects entire brain

   e. In term infants, abnormal signal in basal ganglia, thalami, lenticular nuclei, hippocampi, corticospinal tracts, relative cortical sparing (except perirolandic cortex involved)

   f. Older patients with cardiac arrest-basal ganglia, cortex, lentiform nuclei involved

10. Imaging of presumed perinatal asphyxia

   a. CT in acute perinatal and postnatal asphyxia
- Basal ganglia (BG) hypodensity
- Subtle finding in newborns in whom basal ganglia may be isodense to deep WM

        "Normal" hyperdense basal ganglia in asphyxiated newborn may actually represent petechial hemorrhage into BG **[Fig. 2-43]**
- Cerebral edema **[Fig. 2-58]**

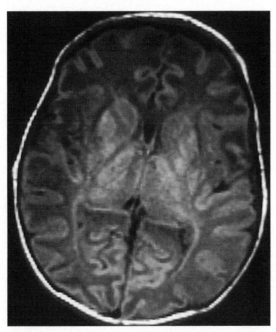

Fig. 2-43 Axial T1-weighted MRI: Asphyxiated newborn 10 days old. High signal in basal ganglia, thalami most likely reflecting petechial hemorrhage. Perinatal asphyxia, hypoxic-ischemic encephalopathy.

Loss of gray-white differentiation

Diffuse hypodensity

Relative hyperdensity in dural sinuses reflects slow flow or no flow

- DDx: Polycythemia or hyperflow from arteriovenous malformation (AVM)

- Focal infarct in "watershed"

Cortical infarct in term; PVL poorly depicted by CT

b. MRI in perinatal and postnatal asphyxia

- Distinguishing normal from abnormal in first days of life:

Posterior limb of internal capsule (PLIC) *hyperintense* in normal term newborn on T1WI

In asphyxia, PLIC is *hypointense* on T1WI

Pre- and post-central gyri in term newborn:

- Normal newborn—gyri bright on T1 and dark on T2 seen along length of gyrus

- Asphyxia—deep portion of gyrus only bright on T1 and dark on T2

- First 2 to 3 days after perinatal asphyxia:

Low signal on T1WI, high signal T2WI in involved areas

Term, profound asphyxia—ventrolateral thalami, lentiform nuclei, posterior mesencephalon, hippocampi, corticospinal tracts to perirolandic cortex

Partial asphyxia—vascular boundary zones ("watershed")

- Four to five days after injury:

T1 shortening, which lasts 4 to 10 weeks

T2 hypointensity appears in first month, lasts 2 to 3 months

- With time, areas of T1 and T2 shortening change to T1 and T2 lengthening (hypointense on T1, hyperintense on T2).

- MR >1 year postinjury—atrophy or T2 prolongation

c. Profound postnatal asphyxia **[Fig. 2-44]:**

- Areas affected include corpus striatum, anterior frontal, parieto-occipital cortex with perirolandic and thalamic sparing.

- MR weeks to months later—atrophy or T2 prolongation

d. MR in first 10 days after birth to assess asphyxial injury:

- T1 hyperintensity seen as early as 3 days postpartum; T2 shortening (hypointensity) seen after 6 to 7 days postpartum.

- Study requires support, warming of sick newborn

e. Prognostic value of early MRI:

- Normal MRI at 24 to 72 hours predicts good outcome

- Extensive brain edema with loss of cortical ribbon, ventrolateral thalamic injury—poor outcome

f. MRI more useful weeks to months after perinatal asphyxia

- Normal large water content of neonatal brain can preclude conspicuity of lesions

g. Myelination delay: seen in premies and term newborns with perinatal asphyxia **(Table 2-4)**

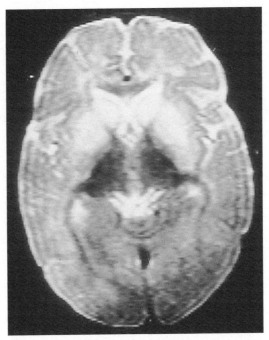

Fig. 2-44 Axial T2-weighted MRI: Hyperintensity in caudate nuclei, basal ganglia in suffocated 6-month-old infant. Postnatal asphyxia, hypoxic-ischemic encephalopathy.

Table 2-4. Indications for MRI in Neonatal Neuro-Imaging

Asphyxia/CNS injury
   Severity
   PVL on ultrasound
   Delayed development

Delayed myelination syndromes
   Bronchopulmonary dysplasia
   Progressive hydrocephalus
   Infant of a diabetic mother

Hemorrhage ≥3 days

Birth trauma
   Skull fracture on plain film/CT
   Subdural/epidural collections
   Suspected venous sinus thrombosis

Complex hydrocephalus
   Intraventricular cysts
   Arachnoid cysts

CNS malformations

Further evaluation of abnormal ultrasound scan

IV. **INFLAMMATION**
   A. **Prenatal infections. TORCH = Toxoplasmosis, Others (AIDS), Rubella, Cytomegalovirus (CMV), and Herpes simplex**
      1. Toxoplasmosis
         a. Second most common in utero infection
         b. 1:1000–8000 pregnancies in U.S.
         c. Congenital infection in 17%, 25%, 65% of infected pregnancies in first, second, third trimesters, respectively
         d. 50% of infected newborns have CNS injury
         e. Severity worst in first trimester, decreases during gestation
         f. Multifocal involvement; no migrational disorder
         g. Periventricular and multifocal calcifications
         h. Hydrocephalus, microcephaly
      2. AIDS
         a. HIV infects T4 helper cells
         b. Secondary infection with *Pneumocystis carinii* **[Fig. 8-20],** CMV, *Candida, Herpes simplex* (HS)
         c. Congenital via infected mother (78%) or acquired from infected blood products
         d. 30% of infected mothers have congenitally infected offspring
         e. Pediatric CNS disease more likely due to direct HIV encephalitis than opportunistic infections (unlike adults)
         f. HIV perivascular cytopathy tends to affect basal ganglia, pons, white matter
         g. Clinical features: failure to thrive, progressive spastic quadriplegia, dementia
         h. CT or MRI
            • Cerebral atrophy (89%)
            • Basal ganglia calcification (34%)
            • Demyelination, delayed or deficient myelination
      3. Rubella
         a. Rare since immunization for rubella
         b. Clinical features: cataracts, glaucoma, chorioretinitis, hepatosplenomegaly, patent ductus arteriosus, microcephaly, microscopic CNS calcification
      4. CMV **[Fig. 2-45; see also Fig. 2-73]**
         a. Most common in utero infection
         b. 5% of pregnant women excrete CMV
            • Offspring of 40% infected with CMV
         c. 1% of all newborns have evidence of CMV exposure
            • 1 to 5% of these have CMV disease
            • 20% of diseased infants have retardation or deafness
         d. Clinical features: hepatosplenomegaly, jaundice, thrombocytopenia, deafness, chorioretinitis
         e. CNS: microcephaly, periventricular calcification, seizures, migrational disorders, cerebellar hypoplasia, subependymal cysts in occipital horns, linear echogenic pattern in thalami seen on ultrasound

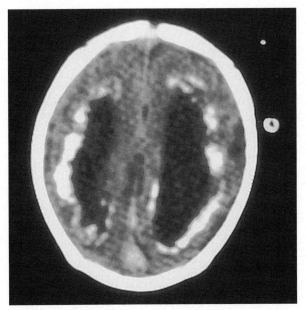

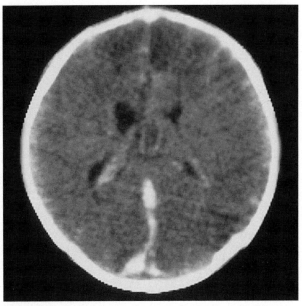

Fig. 2-45 Axial brain CT: Periventricular calcification in patient with microcephaly. Congenital cytomegalovirus (CMV) encephalopathy.

Fig. 2-46 Axial brain CT: Infant with group B streptococcal meningitis. Filling defect in straight sinus, multifocal cortical hypodense lesions. Meningitis; dural sinus thrombosis and cortical venous infarction.

- Infection in 1st–2nd trimesters = frequent CNS injury
  - Early infection ⇒ migrational disorders
  - Late infection ⇒ porencephaly

B. **Perinatal infections**
  1. HS
     a. 75% of HS infections due to Type II (genital)
     b. Via direct contact of eyes, skin, mucous membranes with cervix or vaginal lesions
     c. *Diffuse* brain involvement
        - Acquired herpes in older children or adults focal (frontal and temporal lobes)
     d. Treated with acyclovir
  2. Enterovirus
     a. Encephalitis, myocarditis
C. **Neonatal meningitis [Fig. 2-46]**
  1. Most common is Group B *streptococcus*
     a. Also *Escherichia coli, Listeria monocytogenes*
  2. Sepsis in 1.5/1,000 births; meningitis in 20%
  3. Diffuse exudate + ventriculitis
  4. Early complications
     a. Infarction, venous sinus thrombosis common
     b. Subdural effusions uncommon in first week of life
     c. Effusions with gram negatives after first week of life
  5. Late complications
     a. Atrophy
     b. Dystrophic calcification (4–5 weeks ofter onset)

  c. Ventriculomegaly
   • Obstructive hydrocephalus due to inflammation at aqueduct, fourth ventricle, or arachnoid granulations, or atrophy and necrosis with ex vacuo dilatation
  d. Ventriculitis
   • May form loculations, seal off portions of infected ventricle, predispose to shunt malfunction or dependency
  e. Cystic encephalomalacia
   • Due to neuronal necrosis, direct or ischemic

D. **Cerebral abscess [Fig. 2-47]**
 1. Complication of meningitis, but may occur without it
 2. Citrobacter, Proteus, Pseudomonas, Serratia, S. aureus
 3. Usually large, hemispheric, lack defined capsule
 4. CT: pre-contrast, wall tends to be hyperdense
 5. MRI: hyperintense wall on T1WI = abscess

E. **Fungal infection**
 1. Candidiasis
  a. CNS involved in two-thirds of cases of systemic candida infections

F. **Infections in infants, children**
 1. Bacterial meningitis
  a. Purulent leptomeningeal exudate
  b. *N. meningitidis, H. influenzae, S. pneumoniae*
  c. Thromboses of cortical veins, dural sinuses

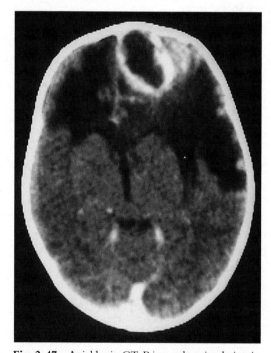

Fig. 2-47 Axial brain CT: Ring-enhancing lesion in left frontal lobe. Note extensive white matter edema in left hemisphere extending across midline through corpus callosum into right frontal lobe. Cerebral abscess, vasogenic edema.

  d. Overwhelming infection associated with marked brain swelling, low-flow state
   • CT: diffusely hypodense supratentorial compartment, middle cerebral artery hyperdense, "reversal sign"
  e. Sequelae: hydrocephalus or atrophy
2. Cerebral abscess
  a. Associated with cyanotic heart disease, otitis media, mastoiditis, sinusitis (especially frontal or sphenoid)
3. HS encephalitis
  a. HS Type I: from oropharynx via salivary contact to sensory nerve fibers
  b. Localized to frontal and temporal lobes, usually unilateral
  c. Treated with acyclovir
4. Demyelinating disorders
  a. See section on myelin and white matter abnormalities
5. Tuberculosis **[Fig. 2-48]**
  a. Basilar meningitis
   • Also sarcoid and fungal meningitis
  b. Perivascular inflammation; frequent thromboses
  c. Tuberculomas can occur anywhere in brain
6. Lyme disease
  a. *Borrelia burgdorferi*
  b. Multifocal white matter involvement
   • Also thalami, basal ganglia

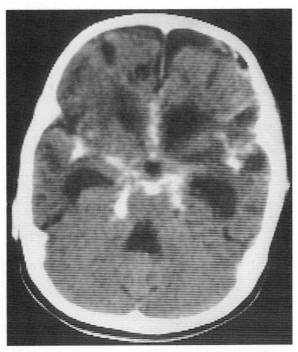

Fig. 2-48 Axial brain CT: Ventricular widening. Beaded appearance of anterior, middle, and posterior cerebral vessels, right hemisphere parenchymal hypodensity. Basilar meningitis; tuberculosis.

7. Cysticercosis
   a. Pork tapeworm (*Taenia solium*)
   b. Mexico, Central or South America
   c. Lesions spread from CSF spaces to ventricles
   d. CT
      - Chronological changes
         Initially parenchymal edema
         Small enhancing lesions without edema
         Cysts enlarge, with ring enhancement
         Eccentric nodule on cyst wall
         Calcification of cyst wall

V. **TUMORS**
   - Brain tumors: second most common pediatric neoplasm, after leukemia
   A. **Supratentorial**
      - More common in children <1 year of age and after second decade of life
      - Neuroepithelial tumors (astrocytoma, ependymoma, primitive neuro-ectodermal tumors [PNET], malformations (dermoid, epidermoid, hamartoma), developmental cysts, germ cell, meningeal, nerve sheath tumors, metastases in decreasing order of incidence
      1. Gliomas **[Fig. 2-49]**
         a. Include astrocytoma, oligodendroglioma, ependymoma
         b. Histologic grading from 1 to 4
            - Glioblastoma multiforme = 4

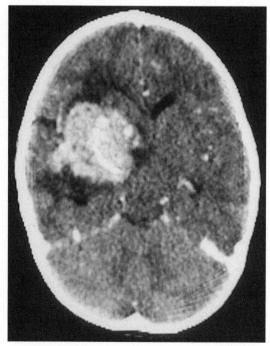

Fig. 2-49 Axial brain CT: Vasogenic edema surrounding enhancing mass in right basal ganglia and thalamus. Note areas of calcification within mass. Astrocytoma.

c. Imaging may not correlate with grading
d. Hemispheric astrocytoma
  - 30% of supratentorial tumors
  - Clinical signs of increased intracranial pressure and focal deficits; seizures from temporal lobe lesions
  - Hypointense on T1WI, hyperintense on T2WI
  - Variable enhancement
  - Variable tumor necrosis, cyst formation, hemorrhage, and surrounding edema
e. Ependymoma
  - 6% of gliomas; 40% occur in supratentorial area
  - Located in or near ventricle
  - Cysts and calcification common
f. Oligodendroglioma
  - 1% of pediatric brain tumors
      Male and adolescent predominance
  - Well-circumscribed, solid, variable contrast enhancement
  - Calcification common (50% on CT)
g. Chiasmatic and hypothalamic astrocytoma
  - Cannot be differentiated by imaging
  - Bulky, frequent invasion of sella, third ventricle, posterior fossa
  - Hydrocephalus common
  - Hypointense on T1WI, hyperintense on T2WI
  - Marked enhancement
2. Choroid plexus tumors **[Fig. 2-50]**
    a. 40 to 50% in first decade

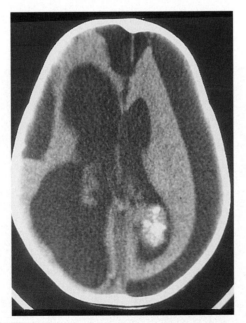

Fig. 2-50 Axial T1-weighted MRI: Hyperintense mass in left choroid plexus with associated ventriculomegaly and extra-axial fluid collection. Choroid plexus papilloma.

b. In children, most in lateral ventricle, especially atrium
  – In adults, more common in fourth ventricle
c. Cysts, hemorrhage, and calcification common

3. PNET
  a. See below

4. Ganglioglioma and gangliocytoma [**Fig. 2-51**]
  a. Mature ganglion cells mixed with glial tissue
  b. Benign, slow-growing
  c. Usually peripheral in hemisphere
  d. Most common in temporal, occipital lobes
  e. Present with focal deficits or seizures
  f. Well circumscribed mass with minimal, if any, edema
  g. Hypointense on T1WI, inhomogeneous
  h. Hyperintense on T2WI
  i. Variable enhancement
  j. Cysts and calcification (35% on CT) common

5. Meningioma
  a. 4% of pediatric brain tumors
  b. More common in second decade
  c. Associated with neurofibromatosis, prior irradiation
  d. Usually more aggressive than adult meningiomas
  e. Childhood meningioma more commonly cystic, intraventricular, equal gender incidence
  f. Calcification, hyperostosis occasional, seen on CT
  g. Iso- to hypointense on T1WI, hyperintense on T2WI
  h. Marked enhancement

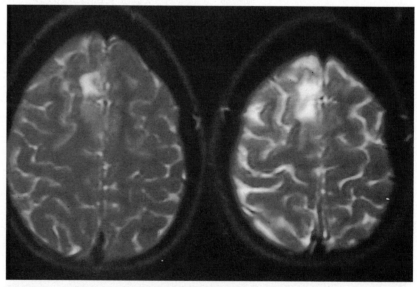

Fig. 2-51 Axial T2-weighted MRI: Focal hyperintense right frontal cortical lesion without surrounding vasogenic edema. Ganglioglioma.

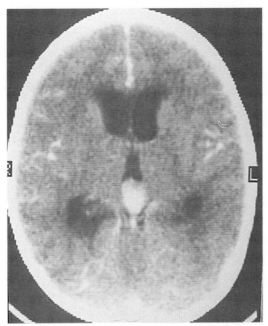

Fig. 2-52 Axial brain CT: Enhancing mass in pineal gland with associated ventriculomegaly. Pineoblastoma.

B. **Pineal region masses [Fig. 2-52]**
1. 8% of pediatric brain tumors; half are germ cell tumors
2. Usually present with hydrocephalus due to aqueduct compression
   a. Parinaud's sign: paralysis of upward conjugate gaze due to compression of superior colliculus
   b. Argyll-Robertson pupil: intact accommodation in absence of light reflex due to involvement of Edinger-Westphal nucleus
   c. Also, precocious puberty and diabetes insipidus
3. Enlargement of pineal >1 cm should be considered tumor
4. Smooth, anterior margin projects into third ventricle
5. Pineal calcification of any size by CT in child <6 years of age is not physiologic and should be considered tumor
6. Germ cell tumors
   a. Germinoma
      • Pineal germinoma almost always in males
      • Suprasellar germinoma in both genders
      • Hypointense on T1WI, hyperintense on T2WI
      • Marked enhancement
      • Parenchymal invasion, CSF spread common
   b. Teratoma
      • Pineal teratoma almost always in males
      • Inhomogeneous mass with cyst, calcification, cartilage, hair, fat
   c. Pineocytoma and pineoblastoma
      • 20% of pineal region tumors

- CT
  - 25 to 50% calcify
  - Iso- or hyperdense, with enhancement
- MRI
  - Hypo- to isointense on T1WI, iso- or minimally hyperintense on T2WI
  - Homogeneous enhancement
- Pineocytoma: calcified, cystic, benign
- Pineoblastoma: associated with bilateral retinoblastoma ("trilateral retinoblastoma")
  - Considered a PNET

C. **Sellar and suprasellar tumors**
1. 25% of pediatric brain tumors are parasellar in location
2. Includes craniopharyngioma, optic pathway and hypothalamic glioma, Rathke's cleft cyst, hypothalamic hamartoma, germinoma, lipoma, epidermoid, dermoid, pituitary tumors
3. Craniopharyngioma **[Fig. 2-53]**
   a. More than half of pediatric sellar tumors
   b. Peak age ranges of 6–12 years and 4th–5th decades
   c. Presents with headache, visual field cut (bitemporal hemianopsia), diplopia, growth retardation
   d. Suprasellar (75%), extending into sella (21%), third ventricle, posterior fossa, hemisphere
   e. Difficult to resect because tumor becomes adherent to neural structures
   f. Calcification in 75 to 90%
   g. Cyst variable in signal due to cholesterol, keratin, protein content
   h. 15% entirely solid
4. Optic pathway astrocytoma **[Fig. 2-54]**
   a. Most common intracranial neoplasm in NF-1
   b. 50% of children, 75% of adults with optic nerve astrocytoma do not have NF-1
   c. Expansion of optic nerve or chiasm
   d. CT
      - Iso- or hypodense, variable enhancement
      - Cyst, calcification, hemorrhage unusual except after irradiation
   e. MRI
      - Hypointense on T1WI, hyperintense on T2WI
      - Marked enhancement
5. Hypothalamic and chiasmatic astrocytoma
   a. Similar appearance to each other
   b. "Diencephalic syndrome": emaciation, hyperactivity
6. Germinoma
   a. Suprasellar germinoma most common germ cell tumor in this location
   b. Germinoma more common in suprasellar region than pineal
   c. Most common presentation is diabetes insipidus
      - Also visual field defect, pituitary dysfunction

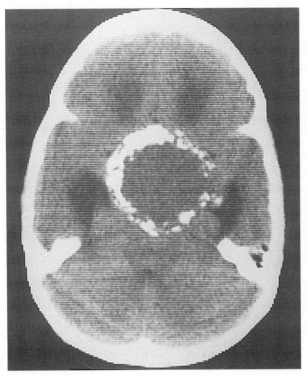

Fig. 2-53 Axial brain CT: Large midline mass with central cyst and peripheral calcification. Note associated ventriculomegaly. Craniopharyngioma.

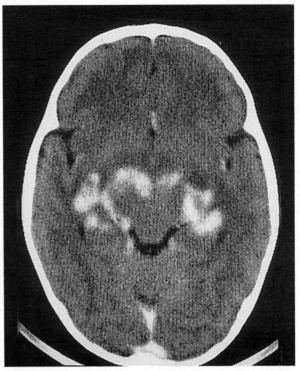

Fig. 2-54 Axial brain CT: Lesion enhances along optic pathway bilaterally, involves optic chiasm and extends to lateral geniculate body. Optic pathway glioma.

    d. Iso- to hyperdense on CT

    e. Usually no calcification or cysts

    f. Hypointense on T1WI, only minimally hyperintense on T2WI

    g. Markedly and homogeneously enhances on CT or MRI

  7. Pituitary adenoma

    a. 30% of sellar and parasellar masses in children

    b. Presents with delayed puberty, galactorrhea, gigantism, hypercortisolism

    c. Macroadenomas usually hormonally inactive

    d. Microadenomas usually functional

    e. CT

      • Image in coronal plane, 1 to 3 mm sections

      • Precontrast images may show calcification

      • Postcontrast images obtained quickly after bolus (differential enhancement: normal pituitary enhances more rapidly than hypodense microadenoma)

    f. MRI

      • Thin sections

      • Sensitivity increased 10 to 30% with contrast and rapid postbolus imaging

  8. Rathke's cleft cyst

    a. Benign

    b. Iso- or hyperdense on CT

      c. No calcification or enhancement

      d. Mucoid material or cholesterol in cyst

      e. May be hyperintense on T1WI, iso- or hypointense on T2WI

  9. Hypothalamic hamartoma

      a. Presents with precocious puberty, laughing fits (gelastic seizures)

      b. Isodense to brain on CT, without calcification or enhancement

      c. Isointense to gray matter on T1WI; hyperintense on T2WI, no enhancement

 10. Langerhans' cell histiocytosis

      a. Not a neoplasm but part of differential diagnosis

      b. Presents with diabetes insipidus

      c. Appears as thickened infundibulum

      d. Isodense on CT; isointense on T1WI, minimally hyperintense on T2WI

      e. Associated with absence of posterior bright spot of neurohypophysis
- DDx includes germinoma, sarcoid, and tuberculosis

 11. Epidermoid and dermoid

      a. 4% of parasellar tumors in childhood

      b. Imaging characteristics: see infratentorial lesions

D. Infratentorial

- More common than supratentorial tumors between ages 1–10
- Glioma, ependymoma, PNET (including medulloblastoma and primary cerebral neuroblastoma), choroid plexus tumors, metastases, skull base lesions (including rhabdomyosarcoma and chordoma) in decreasing order of incidence

  1. Brain stem glioma **[Fig. 2-55]**

      a. 10 to 20% of solid childhood CNS tumors

      b. Peak incidence age 5 to 6 years

      c. Cranial nerve involvement common

      d. Pons involved in 40 to 60%, medulla in 20–25%, midbrain in 15–20%

      e. Produces alteration in size, shape of brain stem; may be exophytic

      f. CT
- Homogeneous; iso- or hypodense
- Calcification in <10%
- Cyst or necrosis unusual
- Hemorrhage and contrast enhancement unusual

      g. MRI
- Sagittal images key to define cephalocaudal extent
- T1WI: usually hypointense; enhancement variable
- T2WI: homogeneous, hyperintense

      h. DDx
- ADEM

     Systemic signs, symptoms

     Also enlarges brain stem, hyperintense on T2WI
- Demyelinating diseases

     Follow WM tracts

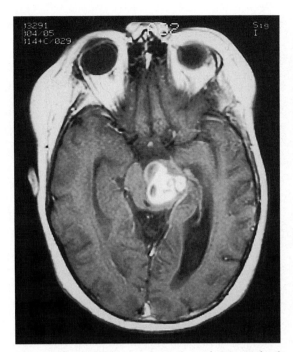

Fig. 2-55 Gadolinium-enhanced axial T1-weighted MRI: Multilobulated mass in cerebral peduncle with deviation of aqueduct of Sylvius and associated ventriculomegaly. Brain stem glioma.

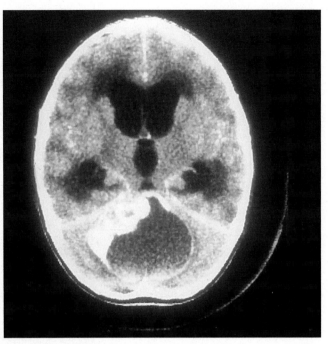

Fig. 2-56 Axial brain CT: Midline ring-enhancing cystic mass with enhancing mural nodule. Note ventriculomegaly and periventricular hypodensity indicating transependymal flow and acute obstructive hydrocephalus. Cerebellar cystic astrocytoma.

- Vascular malformation
  Old and new hemorrhage (hemosiderin)
  Serpiginous signal voids
2. Cerebellar astrocytoma **[Fig. 2-56]**
   a. 80% hemispheric, 20% vermis; 80% cystic, 20% solid
   b. Peak age range: 5 to 13 years
   c. Clinical presentation: hydrocephalus due to fourth ventricle obstruction
   d. Usually low-grade; most common type is juvenile pilocytic astrocytoma
      - Pilocytic astrocytoma also occurs in optic pathway, hypothalamus, midbrain, cerebral hemisphere
   e. CT
      - Solid component iso- or hypodense
      - Cyst hypodense
      - Calcification unusual
      - Variable contrast enhancement
   f. MRI
      - Cyst hyperintense to CSF on T1WI (due to protein in cyst)
      - Cyst wall irregular if mural nodule present
      - Solid component or nodule iso- or hypointense on T1WI
      - Tumor and cyst hyperintense on T2WI
      - Tumor and cyst wall enhance

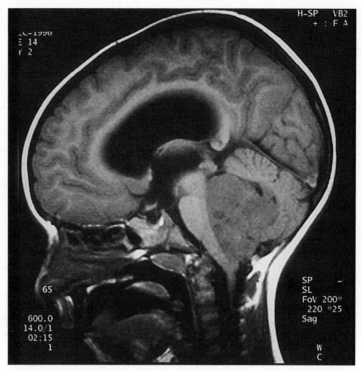

Fig. 2-57 Midline sagittal T1-weighted MRI: Heterogeneous hypodense mass distorts cerebellum, fourth ventricle, and pons, with associated ventricular obstruction. Primitive neuroectodermal tumor (PNET), medulloblastoma.

    g. Postsurgery
        • Lack of enhancement within 48 hours = complete removal
  3. PNET ("small blue cell tumors") **[Fig. 2-57; see also Fig. 2-128]**
    a. Includes medulloblastoma, pineoblastoma, ependymoblastoma, cerebral neuroblastoma
    b. Also noncerebral neuroblastoma, Ewing's sarcoma
    c. Peak incidence infratentorial PNET: 5–8 years
    d. Male predominance 2–3 : 1
    e. Most common origin inferior vermis
    f. Clinical presentation: hydrocephalus due to fourth ventricle obstruction
    g. Spreads by direct extension or CSF dissemination
        • Systemic metastases or via ventriculoperitoneal shunt
    h. 90% midline; lateral or hemispheric more common in older patients
    i. CT
        • Calcification, hemorrhage unusual
        • 50%: Homogeneous, hyperdense
           May be iso- or hypodense
           Homogeneous enhancement

- 50%: Heterogeneous with small areas of necrosis
      Inhomogeneous enhancement
  j. MRI
     - Homogeneous on T1WI and T2WI
     - Hypointense on T1WI; hyperintense on T2WI
     - Prominent central vessels (signal voids)
     - Enhancement inhomogeneous, variable
  k. Tends to recur, spread by meningeal metastases
     - 10 to 40% have leptomeningeal disease at diagnosis
4. Ependymoma
  a. Age range, 6 months to 18 years; peak at 3 to 5 years
  b. Usually related to ventricle (fourth, lateral, third)
  c. Majority in children in posterior fossa
     - Majority in adults supratentorial
  d. Clinical presentation: hydrocephalus due to fourth ventricle obstruction
  e. Heterogeneous; calcification, necrosis common
  f. CT
     - Calcification in 60%
     - Inhomogeneous; hypo-, iso-, or hyperdense
     - Variable enhancement
  g. MRI
     - Intraventricular relationship best seen on sagittal T1WI
     - Hypo-, iso-, or hyperintense on T1WI
     - Inhomogeneous on T1WI and T2WI
     - Signal void from calcification or vascularity
     - Variable, inhomogeneous enhancement
  h. Local recurrence or leptomeningeal spread
5. Choroid plexus tumors
  a. More common in supratentorial compartment
  b. Male predominance
  c. Arise from tela choroidea adjacent to inferior medullary velum of fourth ventricle
  d. Calcification common (20 to 25%)
  e. Homogeneous enhancement on CT or MRI
6. Schwannoma
  a. Bilateral acoustic schwannoma in NF-2
  b. Isodense on CT; isointense on T1WI, hyperintense on T2WI
  c. Marked contrast enhancement on MRI
7. Dermoid, epidermoid
  a. Classified as developmental malformations
  b. Approximately 1% of all brain neoplasms
  c. Dermoids more common than epidermoids in children
  d. Both occur in spinal canal, usually associated with dysraphism or dermal sinus
  e. Present as meningitis from infected dermal sinus tracking into dermoid or chemical meningitis from rupture into CSF space
  f. Epidermoid: cyst lined by keratinizing squamous epithelium
     - Usually off-midline

- Periphery of posterior fossa, cerebellopontine or prepontine cistern, or craniocervical junction
- Hypodense cyst without wall enhancement on CT
- Iso- to hyperintense on T1WI; hyperintense on T2WI

g. Dermoid: cyst lined by squamous epithelium + hair, sebaceous or sweat glands, and connective tissue
- Midline
- Heterogeneous on CT and MRI

8. Hemangioblastoma
   a. Looks like cystic astrocytoma, but occurs in older age group
      - Peak ages, 12 to 70 years; rare under 12 years of age
   b. Highly vascular tumor, associated with von Hippel-Lindau (VHL)
      - VHL: autosomal dominance; retinal or spinal hemangioblastoma, renal cell carcinoma, pheochromocytoma, pancreatic carcinoma, liver, renal cysts
   c. Cystic mass with mural nodule
      - Cyst hyperdense on CT, hyperintense on T1WI
      - Mural nodule markedly enhances on CT, MRI

E. **Metastatic**
   1. CNS metastases rare in children
   2. Most common are leukemia, lymphoma, neuroblastoma
      a. Meningeal enhancement uncommon in leukemia, even with CSF leukemia
   3. Dural, epidural metastases **[see Fig. 7-33]**
      a. Hypointense on T1WI, hyperintense on T2WI
      b. Marked enhancement

VI. **TRAUMA**
- Head trauma accounts for 50% of deaths in age group 1 to 14 years

A. **Birth trauma**
   1. Molding
      a. Due to passage through birth canal
      b. Resolves in 4 to 6 weeks
   2. Caput succedaneum
      a. Subcutaneous bleeding not confined by calvarial sutures
      b. May be source of significant blood loss at birth
   3. Cephalohematoma (subgaleal hematoma)
      a. 2 to 5% of deliveries
      b. Bounded by sutures
      c. Bleeding into subperiosteum
      d. Chronic: may present as firm, calcified mass deforming skull
   4. Intracranial hemorrhage
      a. Subdural hematoma
         - May be spontaneous or related to difficult delivery through birth canal
            Extraction devices
            Forceps

b. Subarachnoid hemorrhage
  - May be seen in otherwise normal vaginal delivery or associated with birth trauma
  - Usually of little clinical significance
5. Infarction
   a. Usually spontaneous; involves middle cerebral artery, L > R
   b. May be associated with protein C or S deficiency, polycythemia, hypoxic-ischemic encephalopathy
   c. Involves watershed areas
      - Between anterior and middle cerebral and middle and posterior cerebral arteries in term
      - Between central perforating arteries and peripheral gyral arteries in premies and some term neonates (periventricular leukomalacia)
   d. Cause of neonatal seizures, hemiparesis

B. **Skull fractures [Figs. 1-30 and 1-31]**
   1. Fracture alone does not predict significant intracranial insult
   2. Radiograph better study than CT to identify skull fracture
      a. CT may not identify fracture in same plane as CT slice
      b. CT obtained without intravenous (IV) contrast to distinguish intracranial injury
   3. Neurologic evaluation is best indicator of significant intracranial injury
      a. Glasgow Coma Scale of ≤14 = risk for intracranial sequelae
      b. Altered level of consciousness, seizures, focal neurologic deficits correlate with intracranial injury
   4. Linear parietal fracture usually due to accidental fall
   5. Dense margin of fracture indicates depressed fragment
      a. Surgical elevation for depression >5 mm
   6. Multiple, comminuted, or diastatic fractures or those that cross sutures associated with more severe trauma than linear
      a. Due to severe accidental or nonaccidental trauma
   7. Leptomeningeal cyst (growing fracture) **[Fig. 2-91]**
      a. Children <4 years of age
      b. Diastatic fracture
      c. Indicates dural tear

C. **Parenchymal injury**
   1. Concussion
      a. Loss of consciousness, nausea, vomiting
      b. CT usually normal
   2. Contusion
      a. 16% of pediatric head trauma
      b. Focal brain swelling with or without hemorrhage
      c. Coup-contrecoup mechanism
      d. Swelling usually increases for first 2–4 days
      e. May heal without consequence or with atrophy, gliosis, scarring
      f. May become seizure focus
      g. CT
         - Hypodense area of edema, hyperdense hemorrhage, or mixture

h. MRI
- Useful to detect small contusions inconspicuous on CT, additional areas of injury

3. Diffuse brain swelling [Figs. 2-41, 2-42, and Fig. 2-58]
   a. More common in children than adults
   b. Possible mechanisms:
      - Axonal injury (acceleration-deceleration)
      - Cortical necrosis (hypotension)
      - Hypoxic-ischemic injury
   c. CT
      - Diffuse hypodensity, slitlike ventricles, sulcal effacement, narrowed basal cisterns
        Especially ambient and quadrigeminal cisterns
      - Hypodense brain stem in setting of diffuse supratentorial edema suggests posterior cerebral artery ischemia
      - "Dense cerebellar sign": hypodense supratentorial contents with relatively hyperdense cerebellum
      - "Reversal sign": relatively hyperdense white matter compared to gray matter [Fig. 2-58]
        Indicates global insult, usually hypoxic-ischemic encephalopathy [Fig. 8-1]
        – DDx: Severe trauma, child abuse, meningoencephalitis, near-sudden infant death syndrome (SIDS), drowning

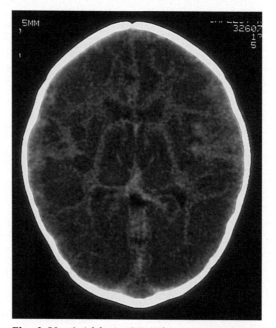

Fig. 2-58 Axial brain CT: White matter is hyperdense compared to gray matter, a "reversal" from the usual and expected pattern. Also note hypodense thalami and basal ganglia. Hypoxic-ischemic encephalopathy, "reversal" sign.

4. Shearing injuries
   a. At corpus callosum, gray-white junctions
   b. Best seen on MRI as hemorrhagic foci
5. Parenchymal hematoma
   a. CT
      - Hyperdense mass of blood with surrounding hypodense zone of edema
   b. MRI
      - Signal intensity varies with evolution of brain hematoma

D. Extra-axial hemorrhage
   1. Epidural hematoma **[Fig. 2-59]**
      a. Clinical presentation may be delayed
      b. No loss of consciousness at time of injury in 57% of children, 85% of infants
      c. Lucid interval >24 hours in >30%
      d. Either arterial (middle meningeal artery) or venous (dural sinus) injury in children
      e. Skull fracture absent in 32 to 60% of children
      f. CT
         - Biconvex, adjacent to inner table of skull
         - Does not cross sutures
         - Homogeneous, hyperdense, or mixed density

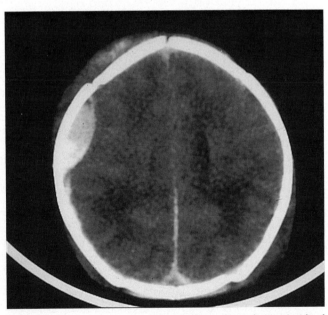

Fig. 2-59 Axial brain CT: Elliptical hyperdense lesion (epidural hematoma) adjacent to right hemisphere with mass effect, hyperdense subarachnoid hemorrhage in posterior interhemispheric fissure, and cephalohematoma.

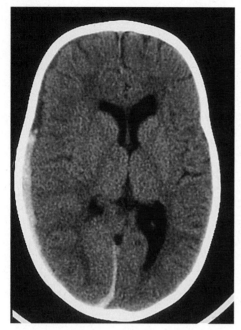

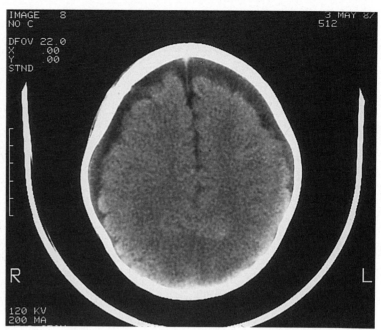

Fig. 2-60 Axial brain CT: Hyperdensity with hematocrit level along right hemisphere extending into interhemispheric fissure. Notice mass effect upon adjacent sulci compared with opposite hemisphere. Subdural hematoma, acute.

Fig. 2-61 Axial brain CT: Child abuse. Hypodense fluid collection in subdural space bilaterally. Subdural hematoma, chronic.

2. Subdural hematoma (SDH) **[Figs. 2-60 and 2-61]**
   a. Acute, subacute, and chronic
   b. Subacute, chronic due to prior trauma
   c. In <2 years of age, consider child abuse
   d. Increased incidence in children with cerebral atrophy, ventricular shunts
   e. Clinical signs
      - Acute: signs of increased intracranial pressure, bulging fontanelle, seizures, altered mental status, focal neurologic signs
      - Subacute, chronic: anemia, macrocephaly, boxlike appearance of calvaria
   f. CT
      - Crescent-shaped fluid/blood collection along inner table
      - Can cross sutures
      - Convexity and posterior interhemispheric SDH in child abuse
   g. MRI
      - Evolution of blood breakdown products but no hemosiderin
   h. DDx of chronic SDH: benign subdural effusion of infancy
      - 3 months to 2 years of age
      - Head circumference upper limits of normal-enlarged, but head growth along same percentile
      - Enlarged subdural and subarachnoid spaces
      - Otherwise normal growth, development
3. Subarachnoid hemorrhage
   a. Occurs in head trauma, rupture of aneurysm or AVM

b. CT
- Hyperdensity in subarachnoid spaces, sulci, cisterns
- DDx: Slow or no flow in dural sinuses, arteries, veins (brain death, severe increased intracranial pressure, thrombosis), polycythemia, marked hypodensity of supratentorial compartment (cerebral edema)

E. Child abuse [Figs. 2-61 and 2-62; see also Figs. 1-30, 3-69, 3-70, 6-7, 6-15, 6-62, 8-1 through 8-3]
1. Head trauma is leading cause of death in child abuse
2. 10% of all injured children <5 years of age in emergency rooms are victims of some form of abuse
3. 70% of head trauma due to child abuse have concurrent skeletal injuries (ribs, long bones)
4. John Caffey: pediatric radiologist first reported in 1946 association of long bone fractures and subdural hematomas
5. Fred Silverman: described skeletal findings of child abuse in 1953
6. Caffey: "Whiplash-shaken infant syndrome" in 1972
7. Duhaime (1992): shaking + impact of head involved in mechanism of injury
8. Other possible mechanisms include strangulation, suffocation
9. Radiographic findings
   a. Long bone fractures in non-ambulatory infant, corner-bucket handle metaphyseal fractures due to jerking/twisting of extremity, multiple or bilateral skull fractures, or skull fractures that cross sutures
10. CT
    a. Subdural hematomas of varied duration
       - Often bilateral SDH
       - Interhemispheric SDH
    b. Diffuse cerebral edema most common parenchymal lesion [Fig. 2-62]
       - "Reversal sign" or "dense cerebellar sign"

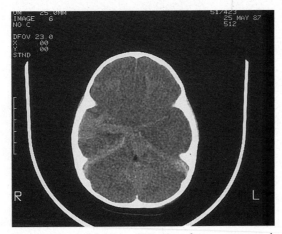

Fig. 2-62 Axial brain CT: Hypodense cortex and patchy, relatively hyperdense white matter. Note hypodensity of cerebellar hemispheres. Hypoxic-ischemic encephalopathy, "reversal" sign, child abuse.

11. MRI

    a. Useful when index of suspicion high, CT findings "normal" or unclear, and to further characterize abnormal CT

VII. **VASCULAR DISEASE AND ISCHEMIA**

  A. **Perinatal stroke [Fig. 2-63]**

    1. Recognized cause of seizure in newborn

      a. Seizures occur 8 to 72 hours after birth

      b. Often unassociated with perinatal asphyxia or obstetric abnormalities

    2. Causes of infarction include: hypoxic-ischemic encephalopathy, protein C or S deficiency, placental emboli, polycythemia, injury to carotid vessels, meningitis

    3. Usually involves middle cerebral artery, left more often than right

  B. **Vascular malformation**

    • Symptoms vary from asymptomatic to headache to massive hemorrhage

    1. AVM **[Fig. 2-64]**

      a. Nidus fed by cerebral or dural arteries, drained by deep or superficial veins

      b. Risk of hemorrhage 3 to 4%/year

      c. Presents in neonates with congestive heart failure (CHF), macrocrania or hydrocephalus

        • Vein of Galen malformation usually fed by anterior and posterior circulation

          Radiograph: cardiomegaly, pulmonary venous congestion, dilated upper mediastinum from enlarged superior vena cava

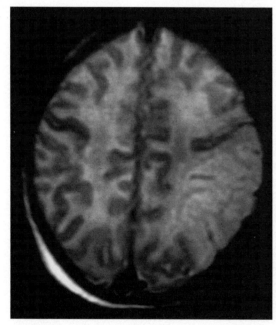

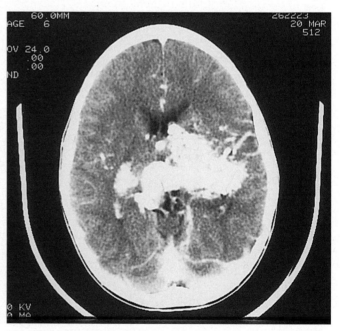

Fig. 2-63 Axial T2-weighted MRI: Newborn with focal seizures. Loss of cortical ribbon in left parietal lobe. Note poor distinction between gray and white matter in affected area. Neonatal stroke.

Fig. 2-64 Axial brain CT: Irregular and extensive enhancing vascular lesion in left frontal cortex, basal ganglia, midline and right hemisphere. Arteriovenous malformation (AVM).

d. Older children: spontaneous hemorrhage, stroke, progressive deficit from shunting of blood from cortex, or seizures

e. Most supratentorial: parietal, occipital, thalamic, basal ganglia, frontal in descending order

f. Multifocal AVMs:
- Wyburn-Mason syndrome: unilateral or bilateral facial nevi, retinal vascular malformation, multiple cerebral AVM

g. CT or MRI
- Serpiginous arteries with large draining vein(s)

2. Cavernous angioma **[Fig. 1-79]**

a. Familial inheritance if multiple angiomas present

b. Increased incidence of cavernous angiomas in children receiving craniospinal irradiation for leukemia
- Usually 6–12 months after radiotherapy completed

c. Symptoms: seizures, acute hemorrhage, sudden neurologic deficits

d. CT: ring or punctate calcified lesions

e. MRI: small lesions hypointense on T2WI indicating hemosiderin, solitary lobulated mass heterogeneous on T1WI and T2WI with acute and/or chronic hemorrhage

3. Venous angioma

a. Usually asymptomatic

b. Small enhancing lesion on CT or signal void on MRI

c. Prominent stellate vessels drain into cortical veins

4. Capillary telangiectasia

a. Usually asymptomatic in children

b. In adults can present with seizures or hemorrhage

c. Association: Weber-Osler-Rendu syndrome (pulmonary AVMs)

C. **Aneurysm**

1. Congenital defects in arterial wall in 75 to 80%, posttraumatic in 15 to 20%, mycotic in 5 to 10%

2. Associated with aortic coarctation and autosomal dominant polycystic kidney disease

a. Arterial ectasia in patients with Menkes' syndrome and neurofibromatosis

D. **Stroke in children [Figs. 2-65 and 2-66]**

1. Idiopathic in 20 to 50%; ischemic in 55%, hemorrhagic in 45%

2. Known causes include:

a. Cardiac disease
- Cyanotic congenital heart disease
- Emboli from dysrhythmia, cardiac tumor, prosthetic valve

b. Hypercoagulability
- Protein C or S deficiency
- Antithrombin III deficiency
- Hyperviscosity (polycythemia)

c. Cerebrovascular malformations and aneurysms

d. Moya-moya ("puff of smoke")
- Progressive carotid artery occlusion with lenticulostriate collaterals

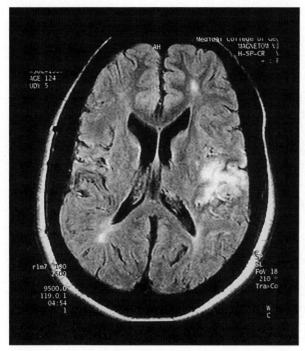

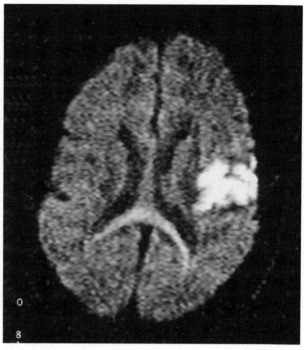

Fig. 2-65 Axial TRIM MRI (9500/119): Patient with sickle cell anemia. Hyperintense lesion in left frontal white matter, right peritrigonal white matter, and left parietal lobe involving gray and white matter. Cerebral ischemia/infarction.

Fig. 2-66 Axial diffusion-weighted echoplanar MRI: Same patient as Figure 2-65. Hyperintensity in area of left parietal ischemia, but not in white matter lesions seen in Figure 2-65. Acute cortical stroke.

- Found in sickle cell disease, neurofibromatosis, postradiation, arteritis
- MRI: Cortical ischemia + signal voids in basal ganglia representing moya-moya collaterals
- Angiography: stenosis of carotid, anterior and middle cerebral arteries; multiple serpiginous collaterals from lenticulostriate and thalamoperforators, that look like a "puff of smoke"

e. Metabolic abnormalities
- Homocystinuria

  Arterial and venous cerebrovascular disease from intimal fibrosis

  Multiple infarcts common
- Dyslipoproteinemia and premature atherosclerotic disease
- Fabry's disease

  Enzyme deficiency of β galactosidase A

  Angiokeratomas of skin, cataracts, peripheral neuropathy

  Lipids accumulate in endothelium, producing thrombosis
- Mitochondrial cytopathy

  MELAS

f. Meningitis and/or septicemia
- Due to pyogenic bacterial or mycobacterial meningitis

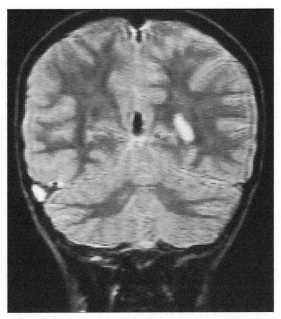

Fig. 2-67 Coronal T2-weighted MRI: Hyperintensity in right sigmoid sinus. Right sigmoid sinus thrombosis.

- Due to hemolytic-uremic syndrome (associated with *E. coli* infection)
  g. Arteritis
  - Secondary to meningitis or encephalitis, systemic lupus erythematosus (SLE), juvenile rheumatoid arthritis (JRA)
  h. Trauma
  - Carotid or vertebral artery dissection
    Also due to Marfan's, Ehlers-Danlos
  i. Sickle cell disease (SCD) **[Figs. 2-65 and 2-66]**
  - 6 to 20% of children with stroke have SCD; 0.7% of children with SCD have stroke
  - Ischemic and hemorrhagic infarcts
  - Occurs in hemoglobin SS and SC, rarely in AS

E. **Venous infarction**
  1. Thrombosis of cortical veins or dural sinuses **[Fig. 2-67; see also Fig. 2-46]**
  2. Due to meningitis, mastoiditis, cholesteatoma, trauma, dehydration (especially hypernatremic), hypercoagulable states
  3. Infarction crosses arterial boundaries
  4. CT: "delta" sign of central thrombosis with surrounding dural sinus enhancement
  5. MRI: absence of expected signal void and/or hyperintense signal from dural sinus

VIII. **HYDROCEPHALUS**

A. **Obstructive [Fig. 2-68; see also Fig. 2-71]**

1. Level of obstruction

    a. Posterior third ventricle/aqueduct

      - Aqueductal stenosis
      - Aqueductal obstruction

        Supratentorial or infratentorial neoplasm

        Kinking of aqueduct in Chiari II malformation

      - Tectal lesion
      - On MRI, note normal signal void in aqueduct indicating flow

        If signal in aqueduct present, flow may be turbulent or absent

        Cine-MR (sagittal CSF flow during cardiac cycle) can depict

          flow presence or absence

    b. Fourth ventricle

      - DWC
      - Infratentorial mass or neoplasm

    c. Basal cisterns

      - Basilar meningitis

        Tuberculous or other granulomatous lesion

      - Intracranial hemorrhage
      - Central herniation

    d. Arachnoid granulations

      - Pyogenic meningitis
      - Intracranial hemorrhage

    e. Impaired venous absorption

      - Narrowed jugular foramen

        Achondroplasia **[Fig. 2-69]**

        – Obstruction also at foramen magnum

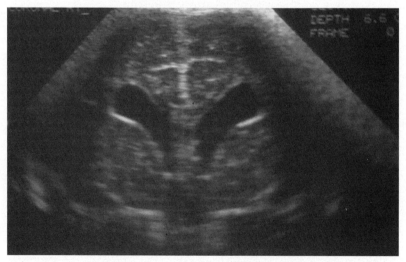

Fig. 2-68 Coronal cranial US: Mild ventriculomegaly. Note smooth ventricular wall. Chiari II malformation, non-communicating hydrocephalus.

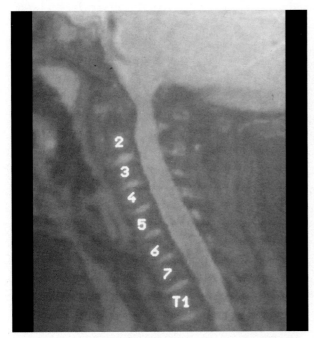

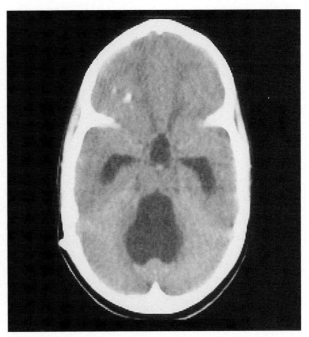

Fig. 2-69 Midline sagittal MRI: Patient with achondroplasia. Note markedly narrowed foramen magnum indenting CSF around spinal cord. Communicating hydrocephalus.

Fig. 2-70 Axial brain CT: Mild dilatation of temporal horns of lateral ventricles and third ventricle, but disproportionate dilatation of fourth ventricle. Entrapped fourth ventricle.

  f. Entrapped lateral or fourth ventricle **[Fig. 2-70]**
   • Dilated segment of ventricular system enlarged out of proportion to remainder of system
    Usually in patients with ventricular shunts and loculations or septations
     – Indicates prior ventricular hemorrhage or ventriculitis with synechia formation

B. **Nonobstructive**
  1. Ex vacuo ventriculomegaly
   a. Parenchymal volume loss
    • Diffuse
     Cystic encephalomalacia
     – Postglobal insult
      Asphyxia
      Meningitis/encephalitis
     Metabolic catastrophe
     – Degenerative disorders
     – Dysmyelination or demyelination
     Congenital malformations
     – Lissencephaly
     – Holoprosencephaly

- Focal
  Congenital malformations
    - Pachygyria
    - Schizencephaly
    - Hemimegalencephaly
        Encephalomalacia (encephaloclastic porencephaly)
        Postinfarction or traumatic
- Deep white matter
  Periventricular leukomalacia
    - Hypoxic–ischemic
  Demyelination
  Postinfarction

C. **Sonographic patterns of ventriculomegaly**
  1. Smooth **[Fig. 2-71]**
     a. Typical appearance for obstructive hydrocephalus, without hemorrhage
     b. Look for signs of Chiari malformation and for fourth ventricle (Dandy–Walker malformation, aqueductal stenosis)
  2. Thickened but smooth **[Fig. 2-72]**
     a. Usually indicates IVH several days after event
        - Previous scans, if available, will have demonstrated IVH
  3. Thickened and irregular or beaded **[Fig. 2-73]**
     a. Look carefully for evidence of hyperechogenic foci in thalami or basal ganglia
     b. This appearance suggests periventricular calcifications and intrauterine infection (cytomegalovirus or toxoplasmosis)
     c. CT is recommended to confirm intracranial calcifications

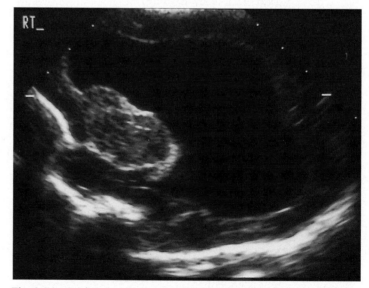

Fig. 2-71 Right parasagittal cranial US: Moderate ventriculomegaly, without ependymal thickening or irregularity. Hydrocephalus; smooth ventriculomegaly.

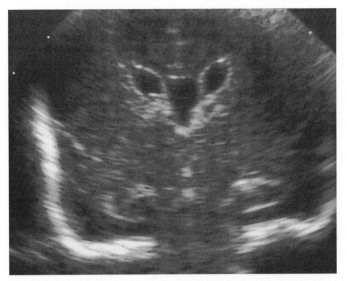

Fig. 2-72 Coronal cranial US: Smooth thickening of ependyma of frontal and temporal horns of lateral ventricles secondary to intraventricular hemorrhage. Thick, smooth ventriculomegaly.

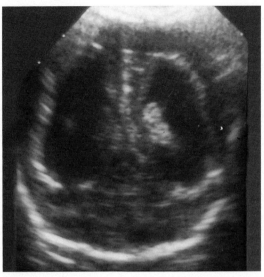

Fig. 2-73 Coronal cranial US: Irregularly beaded, thickened ependyma of enlarged lateral ventricles in patient with congenital cytomegalovirus encephalitis. CT showed periventricular calcification. Thick, irregular ventriculomegaly.

IX. **INTRACRANIAL CALCIFICATIONS**
- NOTE: In order to simplify the approach to the differential diagnosis of intracranial calcification in children, we have chosen to use the mnemonic **VICTIMS:**

V	Vascular
I	Infection/Inflammation
C	Congenital
T	Tumor, Trauma, Toxic
I	Idiopathic
M	Metabolic
S	Syndrome

This mnemonic is an aid in constructing a differential diagnosis for a variety of clinical and radiologic situations, in addition to intracranial calcifications.

A. **Basal ganglia [Fig. 2-74]**
1. Vascular
2. Inflammatory
   a. Congenital rubella (usually microscopic)
   b. SLE
   c. AIDS
      - Calcification bilateral, symmetric; involves putamen and outer portion of globus pallidus
   d. Subacute necrotizing encephalomyelopathy (Leigh's disease)
   e. Measles, pertussis, coxsackie B

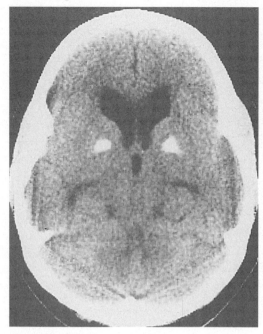

Fig. 2-74 Axial brain CT: Patient with systemic lupus erythematosus (SLE). Symmetric basal ganglia calcification and mild ventriculomegaly.

3. Congenital
4. Tumor, trauma, toxic
   a. Hypoxic–ischemic brain injury
   b. Carbon monoxide
   c. Cyanide
   d. Hydrogen sulfide
   e. Radiotherapy
5. Idiopathic
   a. Physiologic (> age 40)
      • Considered "physiologic" in asymptomatic adults over 40 years of age; every child less than 20 years of age with basal ganglia calcification reported in several studies had an underlying abnormality
   b. Fahr's disease (idiopathic familial cerebrovascular ferrocalcinosis)
      • Manifested by progressive mental deterioration and growth delay
6. Metabolic
   a. Hypoparathyroidism
   b. Pseudo-hypoparathyroidism
   c. Disorders of calcium metabolism
      • Vitamin D intoxication
      • Phenytoin (Dilantin) and/or phenobarbital
   d. Carnitine deficiency
   e. Lactic acidemia and mitochondrial myopathy
   f. Krabbe's disease (globoid cell leukodystrophy)
   g. Carbonic anhydrase II deficiency (marble brain disease)

7. Syndromes
   a. Kearns-Sayre syndrome
      - Progressive external ophthalmoplegia, retinitis pigmentosa, and heart block
      - Microcephaly, short stature, muscular weakness
   b. Down's syndrome
   c. Cockayne's syndrome
      - Autosomal recessive dwarfism characterized by senile facies, sensorineural hearing loss, abnormal retinal pigmentation, cerebellar dysfunction, and microcephaly
   d. Cerebro-oculo-facio-skeletal (COFS) syndrome
      - Cataracts, microcephaly, kyphosis, joint immobility
   e. Oculodento osseous dysplasia (ODOD)
      - Microphthalmia, skeletal dysplasia with sclerosis, enamel hypoplasia, and digital malformation
   f. Marinesco-Sjögren syndrome
      - Autosomal recessive spinocerebellar degeneration manifested by progressive ataxia, nystagmus, weakness, and cataracts

B. **Thalamus [Fig. 2-75; see also Fig. 2-49]**
   1. Hypoxic-ischemic brain injury
   2. Gliomas
   3. Meningitis
      a. Mycobacteria

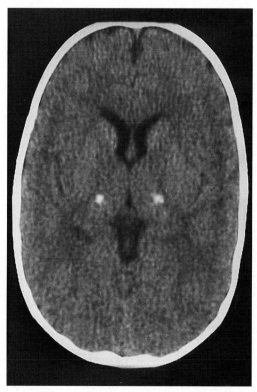

Fig. 2-75   Axial brain CT: History of perinatal asphyxia. Symmetric thalamic calcification.

    4. Carbonic anhydrase II deficiency (marble brain disease)
       a. Osteopetrosis, renal tubular acidosis, and intracranial calcification
       b. Extremely dense calcifications in basal ganglia, thalami, and cerebral cortex
    5. Krabbe's disease (globoid cell leukodystrophy)

C. Pineal gland
    1. Physiologic (> age 6)
       a. 3% of normal children ages 6 to 8 years, 10% in ages 9 to 12 years, 20% in ages 13 to 16 years, 40% in ages 17 to 20 years
       b. The youngest normal child with pineal calcification = 6 years of age
       c. NOTE: Pineal calcification in child <6 even without a mass should be considered pineal tumor until proved otherwise
    2. Pineoblastoma
    3. Pineocytoma
    4. Germinoma
    5. Teratoma

D. Sellar-parasellar
    1. Craniopharyngioma **[Fig. 2-52]**
       a. Calcifies in 70 to 90%; conglomerate or rim-like calcification
    2. Dermoid/epidermoid

E. Ventricular
    1. Choroid plexus papilloma/carcinoma
    2. Meningioma
    3. Ependymoma
       a. Calcifies in 30%
    4. CMV
       a. Choroid plexus calcification
    5. Toxoplasmosis
       a. Choroid plexus calcification
    6. Physiologic: Choroid plexus (> age 1 year)
       a. Physiologic choroid plexus calcification increases with age; found in 0.2 to 0.4% of asymptomatic patients in first decade of life, in 15 to 25% in second decade
    7. Neurofibromatosis (choroid plexus)
       a. Neurofibromatosis is the most common cause of extensive choroid plexus calcification
    8. Sturge-Weber syndrome (choroid plexus hemangioma)

F. Subependymal/periventricular
    1. Tuberous sclerosis
    2. Linear sebaceous nevus syndrome (of Jadassohn)
    3. CMV **[Fig. 2-45]**
       a. Subependymal calcification
    4. Toxoplasmosis
       a. 32% have calcification on plain film; calcifications variable in size and number
       b. Involves cerebral cortex, caudate nucleus, choroid plexus, and periventricular foci
       c. Cortical calcification resembles a "snowflake" pattern

5. Herpesvirus
   a. Radiographically visible calcifications as early as 17 days after neonatal onset
   b. Calcifications described as periventricular, punctate, nodular, or gyriform
   c. Acquired herpes encephalitis in older children; gyriform
6. Congenital rubella
   a. Microscopic calcification not visible radiographically

G. **Tentorium**
   1. Hypercalcemia
      a. Hypervitaminosis D
      b. Hyperparathyroidism
      c. Idiopathic hypercalcemia of infancy (Williams syndrome)
   2. Basal cell nevus syndrome (Gorlin-Goltz syndrome)
      a. Autosomal dominant syndrome
      b. Consists of multiple basal cell nevi, cysts of the jaw, and various tumors of the gastrointestinal (GI) and genitourinary (GU) systems; occasionally present at birth
      c. Occasional patients found with decreased responsiveness to parathyroid hormone
      d. Increased incidence of medulloblastoma and craniopharyngioma

H. **Falx**
   1. Hypercalcemia
      a. Hypervitaminosis D
      b. Hyperparathyroidism
      c. Idiopathic hypercalcemia of infancy (Williams syndrome)
   2. Basal cell nevus syndrome (Gorlin-Goltz syndrome)

I. **Parenchymal**
   1. AVM
      a. 40% have calcification; tubular or gyriform
   2. Sturge–Weber syndrome
      a. 25% bilateral; gyriform
   3. TS
      a. 94 to 97% of patients in several series; 80% of calcifications subependymal, located along the body of the lateral ventricle and/or the foramen of Monro
      b. 20 to 60% calcifications are noted in the cortex
      c. Subependymal and cortical calcifications thought to represent calcified tubers or heterotopic glial tissue
   4. Neurofibromatosis
   5. Linear sebaceous nevus syndrome (of Jadassohn)
   6. Gliomas
      a. Brain stem glioma may calcify after radiotherapy, rarely before
      b. Ganglioglioma
      c. Oligodendroglioma
      d. Astrocytoma
         • Cerebellar astrocytomas calcify in 15%
   7. PNET
      a. Medulloblastomas calcify in 5 to 10%

8. Chronic trauma
9. Encephalitis
   a. Measles
   b. Pertussis
   c. Coxsackie B
   d. Congenital rubella
   e. Herpes virus
10. Meningitis
    a. Bacterial
       - Gyriform
    b. Mycobacterial
       - Calcification not seen until at least 18 months after onset of disease; 1 to 6% of tuberculomas
11. Cysticercosis
12. Trichinosis
13. Echinococcosis
14. Paragonimiasis
15. Carbonic anhydrase II deficiency (marble brain disease)
16. Cockayne's syndrome
17. COFS syndrome
18. Lipoid proteinosis (Urbach-Wiethe disease)
    a. Hippocampi or amygdala

J. **Gray-white junctions [Fig. 2-76]**
   1. Radiotherapy
      a. CNS prophylaxis before 5 years and at least 2400 rads = higher incidence of dystrophic calcification

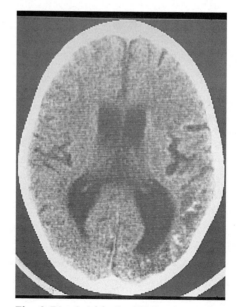

Fig. 2-76 Axial brain CT: Previous radiotherapy and intrathecal methotrexate. Note atrophy and gyriform calcification in left hemisphere.

2. Methotrexate
   a. Combination of chemotherapy and radiotherapy results in a much higher incidence of calcification than methotrexate used alone
3. Folate deficiency
   a. Celiac disease

K. **WM**
1. Adrenoleukodystrophy
2. Krabbe disease (globoid cell leukodystrophy)
3. Tuberous sclerosis
4. Marinesco-Sjögren syndrome
5. Hypoxic-ischemic insult in periventricular leukomalacia

L. **Midline locations**
1. Dermoid
2. Epidermoid
3. Lipoma

M. **Dura**
1. Chronic hematoma

X. **PEDIATRIC EAR AND TEMPORAL BONE**
A. **Normal anatomy**
1. External auditory canal derived from first branchial groove
2. Middle ear cavity derived from first pharyngeal pouch
3. Ossicles derived from first and second branchial arches
4. Stapes footplate derived from otic capsule
5. Inner ear derived from neuroectoderm
6. Vestibule: central portion of bony labyrinth; leads anterior into cochlea and posterior into semicircular canals
7. Semicircular canals (SCC): superior, lateral (or horizontal), posterior
   a. SCC are posterior and superior to cochlea
8. Cochlea has 2-1/2 to 2-3/4 turns
9. Geniculate ganglion located superior to cochlea and anterior to SCC
10. Internal auditory canal (IAC)
    a. Contains four cranial nerves: VII (facial), VIII (acoustic), VIII (superior and inferior vestibular)
    b. Since cochlea and geniculate ganglion are anterior to SCC, VII and acoustic nerve are anterior to superior and inferior vestibular nerves in IAC
    c. Since geniculate ganglion is superior to cochlea, VII is superior to acoustic N in anterior portion of IAC
11. Scutum: spur-shaped bony structure at top of tympanic membrane (on coronal CT)
12. Prussak's space: space between scutum and ossicles
    a. Pars flaccida cholesteatoma originates in Prussak's space and erodes scutum

B. **Congenital malformations**
1. External auditory canal atresia **[Fig. 2-77]**
   a. Incidence: 1:10,000 to 20,000

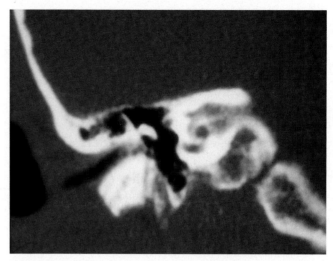

Fig. 2-77 Direct coronal temporal bone CT: External auditory canal atresia. Note ossicle fused to lateral bony wall.

    b. Membranous or bony atresia
    c. Associated ossicle abnormalities common
       • Malleus and incus fused to atresia plate most common
    d. Facial nerve canal often aberrant
    e. Inner ear abnormalities may coexist
  2. Inner ear anomalies
    a. Michel deformity
       • Aplasia of cochlea, vestibule, SCC
    b. Mondini deformity
       • Combined middle and apical coils of cochlea, forming single cavity above normal basal turn
       • Most common congenital cochlear anomaly
       • Associated with syndromes: CHARGE, DiGeorge, Klippel-Feil, Pendred syndromes
    c. Pseudo-Mondini deformity
       • Common cochlear chamber; absence of basal turn of cochlea
    d. Widened vestibular aqueduct
       • Vestibular aqueduct seen on axial CT posteromedial to posterior SCC
       • Compare diameter of vestibular aqueduct to posterior SCC
         Vestibular aqueduct diameter should = posterior SCC
         If vestibular aqueduct diameter > posterior SCC, vestibular aqueduct is widened
    e. IAC
       • Lined by dura
         Dural dehiscence may be associated with congenital cochlear anomaly
          – Dural dehiscence associated with recurrent pneumococcal meningitis
       • Widened by tumor (schwannoma, as in NF-2; hemangioma), dural ectasia in NF-1

C. **Inflammation**
  1. Otitis media
     a. Acute or chronic
     b. Clinical diagnosis
     c. Complications
        - Mastoiditis, cholesteatoma, dural sinus thrombosis, facial nerve palsy, meningitis, brain abscess
     d. CT or MRI
        - Fluid in middle ear cavity; often effusion in mastoid air cells
  2. Mastoiditis
     a. Acute mastoiditis
        - Persistent ear pain, mastoid tenderness, postauricular erythema
        - CT shows bone destruction (osteomyelitis)
        - "Coalescence" when destruction of bony septa separating air cells produces single or few large cavities
  3. Dural sinus thrombosis
     a. Transverse or sigmoid sinuses
     b. CT
        - Hyperdense sinus on non-contrast CT
        - "Delta" sign at sigmoid or transverse sinus with contrast enhancement
     c. MRI
        - Hyperintensity along course of sinus on T1WI
        - Distinguished from laminar signal showing slow flow in dural sinus (can also be seen in patients with mastoiditis)

D. **Tumor**
  1. Cholesteatoma **[Fig. 2-78]**
     a. Sac of squamous epithelium

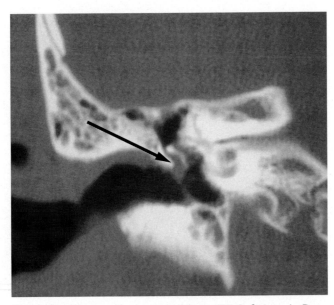

Fig. 2-78   Direct coronal temporal bone CT: Soft tissue in Prussak's space (arrow), interposed between ossicle and scutum. Note associated thickening of tympanic membrane. Cholesteatoma.

      b. 98% acquired; 2% congenital

      c. Congenital
- No prior history of inflammation
- Middle ear most common site; others are geniculate ganglion, cerebellopontine angle, petrous apex

      d. Acquired
- Due to recurrent or chronic otitis media
- Clinical hearing loss, chronic otorrhea
- From Prussak's space, erodes scutum (pars flaccida)

2. Fibrous dysplasia **[Fig. 2-79]**

      a. Temporal bone in 18% with skull involvement

      b. Amorphous thickening of bone that encroaches on external auditory canal, foramina

3. Langerhans' cell histiocytosis

      a. Lytic destruction of mastoid

4. Acoustic schwannoma

      a. NF-2
- Bilateral acoustic schwannoma in 90%

      b. NF-1
- Usually unilateral

      c. From vestibular nerve in IAC

      d. CT or MRI
- Postcontrast enhancement
- Enlarged IAC

5. Rhabdomyosarcoma

      a. Most common malignant tumor of ear and temporal bone

      b. Aggressive bone destruction

      c. Tends to recur, metastasize to lung, bone, invade meninges

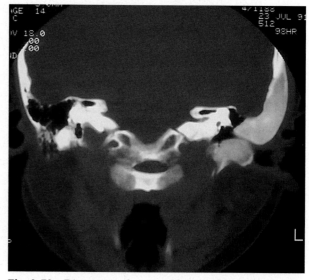

Fig. 2-79 Direct coronal temporal bone CT: Ground-glass appearance of expanded temporal bone with marked narrowing of left external auditory canal. Fibrous dysplasia.

6. Metastasis
   a. Due to leukemia or neuroblastoma

E. **Trauma**
   1. Temporal bone fracture **[Fig. 2-80]**
      a. Relationship to axis of petrous ridge
      b. Oblique
         - Most common: across external canal, extends medially and traverses tegmen above, eustachian tube, carotid canal below to foramen lacerum or sphenoid sinus; parallel to petrous ridge
         - Crosses middle ear and ossicular chain
         - Conductive hearing loss due to ossicular disruption
         - Facial nerve injury usually transient
      c. Longitudinal
         - Vertical course from temporal squamosa to external canal through geniculate ganglion; coronal plane
         - Crosses middle ear and ossicular chain
         - Conductive hearing loss due to ossicular disruption
         - Facial nerve injury usually transient
      d. Transverse
         - Perpendicular to axis of petrous ridge; parasagittal plane
         - Sensorineural deafness due to labyrinthine injury
         - Facial nerve transected
   2. CSF otorrhea
      a. Perilymph fistula secondary to surgery, trauma, or congenital inner ear anomaly
         - Dural dehiscense at IAC
         - Recurrent meningitis (usually pneumococcal), CSF otorrhea

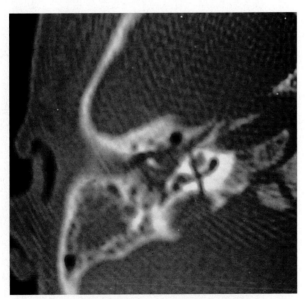

Fig. 2-80 Axial temporal bone CT: Fracture through cochlea, associated fluid in middle ear cavity. Temporal bone fracture.

XI. **THE PEDIATRIC ORBIT**

A. **Leukocoria (white retinal reflex)**
- Retinoblastoma
- Persistent hyperplastic primary vitreous (PHPV)
- Coats' disease
- Norrie's disease
- Retrolental fibroplasia
- Sclerosing endophthalmitis

1. Retinoblastoma **[Fig. 2-81]**
   a. Most common intraocular neoplasm in childhood
   b. 1:20,000 births
   c. 90% sporadic; 10% familial (autosomal dominant with 80% penetrance)
   d. Sporadic usually unilateral; familial usually bilateral
   e. Arises in retina, grows anterior into vitreous, posterior through optic nerve sheath
   f. Distant spread via hematogenous or CSF pathways
   g. 95% calcified; eye is normal in size to slightly enlarged
   h. Enhances on CT
      - Trilateral retinoblastoma = bilateral + pineoblastoma (or retinoblastoma involving vestigial photoreceptors in pineal)

2. Persistent hyperplastic primary vitreous (PHPV)
   a. Microphthalmia + leukocoria, without calcification

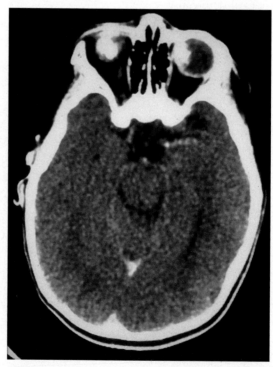

Fig. 2-81 Axial orbit CT: Markedly hyperdense, calcified masses in both globes. Bilateral retinoblastoma.

b. Arrest in maturation of eye

c. Hyaloid artery traverses globe from retina to lens, bisects globe

3. Coats' disease

   a. Vascular anomaly of the retina with telangiectasias, neovascularity

   b. Retinal detachment common; unilateral

   c. Globe normal in size; no calcification or enhancement of subretinal exudate

4. Norrie's disease

   a. Familial disorder; seizures, sensorineural hearing loss, cataracts, mental retardation

   b. Normal size eye at birth, decreases over time

5. Retrolental fibroplasia

   a. Vasoconstriction in retina produced by chronic exposure to high oxygen concentration in premature infants

   b. Neovascularity, hemorrhage, retinal detachment

   c. Eye normal in size-small

   d. Bilateral, often asymmetric

   e. Calcification rare

6. Sclerosing endophthalmitis (manifestation of visceral larva migrans)

   a. *Toxocara canis* in canine feces

   b. Usual age, 6 to 14 years

   c. Retinal detachment, occasional calcification

   d. No enhancement on CT

B. **Congenital malformations**

1. Coloboma

   a. Incomplete closure of posterior retina

   b. Concave anterior retina at or near insertion of optic nerve

   c. Associated with encephalocele, agenesis of corpus callosum

   d. Component of CHARGE syndrome

2. Optic atrophy

   a. Component of SOD (De Morsier's syndrome)

      • Absence of septum pellucidum

      • Hypopituitarism

      • Optic nerve hypoplasia

C. **Tumors**

1. Hemangioma **[Fig. 2-82]**

   a. Capillary hemangioma most common benign orbital mass in child <2 years of age

      • Adult hemangioma is cavernous

   b. Generally grows for first 6 months, static size between 6 to 18 months

   c. Preseptal or postseptal: no calcification

      • Preseptal: well-defined mass with intense contrast enhancement
        No bone destruction or erosion

      • Postseptal: intraconal, extraconal, or mixed
        May fill orbit or extend into extra-orbital spaces
        Intense contrast enhancement
        Smooth remodeling of bone; no destruction

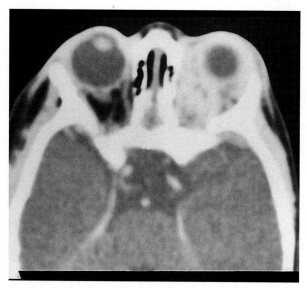

Fig. 2-82 Axial orbit CT: Extensive enhancement of vascular lesion involving intraconal and extraconal spaces throughout left orbit. Capillary hemangioma.

2. Varices
   a. Proptosis increases with crying, Valsalva
   b. May be pulsatile exophthalmos
   c. Venous malformation
3. Lymphangioma or lymphemangioma **[Fig. 2-83]**
   a. Lymphatic or mixed lymphatic/vascular malformation
   b. Heterogeneous; increase in size following hemorrhage or inflammation
   c. Margins poorly defined, infiltrates without respect to tissue planes
4. Dermoid **[Fig. 2-84]**
   a. Dermoid second most common tumor of orbit in child <10 years
   b. Dermoid: arises from epithelial rests
   c. Resembles cyst with higher attenuation material centrally
   d. Remodels bone
5. NF-1 **[Figs. 2-21 and 2-22]**
   a. Dysplasia of NF-1 includes absence of lesser wing of sphenoid: defect in posterior orbit, transmission of CSF pulsations, and "pulsating exophthalmos"
   b. Plexiform neurofibroma: infiltrating tumor extends along course of nerves; lesion irregular, sometimes bizarre in shape
      • Moderate enhancement on CT and MRI
6. Encephalocele **[Figs. 2-88 and 2-89]**
   a. Thin section sagittal or coronal CT or MRI shows bony defect
   b. Another cause of pulsating exophthalmos
7. Langerhans' cell histiocytosis
   a. Formerly histiocytosis X
   b. Smoothly marginated lytic defect in orbit + soft tissue mass
   c. Homogeneous on CT and MRI (on T1WI and T2WI)
   d. Enhancement on CT and MRI

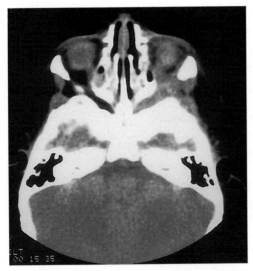

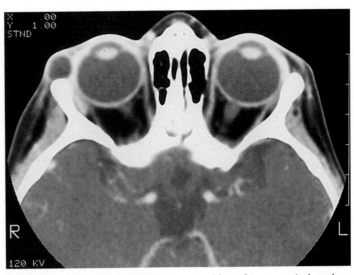

Fig. 2-83 Axial orbit CT: Heterogeneous lesion in posterior left orbit extends into infratemporal fossa and superior orbital fissure. Note punctate calcification in center of mass. Orbital lymphangioma.

Fig. 2-84 Axial orbit CT: Well-demarcated hypodense mass in lateral aspect of right orbit. Dermoid.

8. Rhabdomyosarcoma
   a. Most common malignant lesion of orbit in children
   b. Embryonal, alveolar, pleomorphic types
      • Embryonal most common in children
   c. Density on CT and intensity on MRI similar to muscle
      • Mild-moderate contrast enhancement on both
   d. Imaging cannot differentiate between sarcoma, lymphoma, small round cell tumors
   e. Aggressive lesion with bone destruction, infiltration, poor margination
9. Neuroblastoma **[Fig. 2-85]**
   a. Most common solid malignancy in childhood

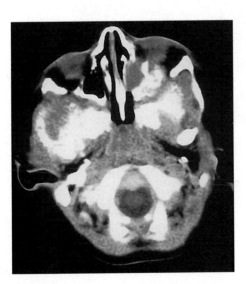

Fig. 2-85 Axial orbit CT: Infiltration and erosion of posterior left orbit, bony erosion of right temporal bone with associated soft tissue mass. Metastatic neuroblastoma.

      b. Orbital involvement due to metastases

      c. Involves orbital wall or roof adjacent to meningeal surface

      d. Bone destruction and infiltration, spiculation, with soft-tissue mass on both sides of orbit where involved

10. Lymphoma

      a. Painless proptosis

      b. Solid or infiltrating mass; rarely intraconal

      c. Homogeneous on CT and MRI with mild-moderate enhancement

11. Optic pathway glioma **[Fig. 2-20]**

      a. NF-1, often bilateral

      b. Fusiform or globular enlargement of optic nerve sheath

      c. Homogeneous on CT and MRI; no calcification unless prior radiotherapy

      d. Minimal-moderate enhancement on CT and MRI

D. **Inflammation**

  1. Optic neuritis **[Fig. 2-30]**

      a. Multiple sclerosis

      b. Viral

      c. Leukemic

  2. Orbital cellulitis **[Fig. 2-86]**

      a. Due to ethmoid sinusitis (infection extends through lamina papyracea to medial orbit), local infection, septicemia

      b. Preseptal: superficial to orbital septum (identified by drawing straight line from inner canthus to anterolateral orbital wall)

        • Imaging usually unnecessary

      c. Postseptal: Deep to orbital septum

        • Chemosis, proptosis, decreased range of motion, decreased acuity, diplopia

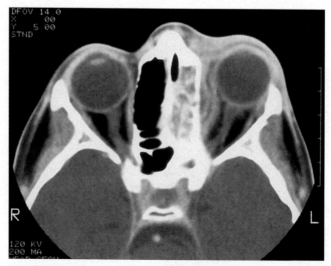

Fig. 2-86 Axial orbit CT: Soft tissue fills left ethmoid air cells. Preseptal and post-septal inflammation. Note subperiosteal elevation in medial left orbit as well as deviation and thickening of left medial rectus muscle. Preseptal and post-septal orbital cellulitis.

- Treat 24 hours with intravenous antibiotics. If improved, no imaging necessary
- If no improvement, orbital CT: Contrast enhancement useful to identify cavernous sinus thrombosis **[Fig. 2-108]**

XII. **PEDIATRIC SKULL AND FACE**

A. **Cranio-facial relationship [Figs. 1-28 and 1-29]**
  1. In newborn, 3 to 4:1
  2. Premie, may be 5:1
  3. By age 6, 2 to 2.5:1

B. **Microcephaly**
  1. Consider in utero insult, such as cytomegalovirus, toxoplasmosis, fetal alcohol syndrome
  2. Usually longitudinal growth and weight are affected but head size is unaffected in placental insufficiency and intrauterine growth retardation (IUGR)
  3. Postnatally, lack of brain growth due to neonatal asphyxia or infection is associated with lack of skull growth (secondary craniosynostosis)

C. **Macrocephaly**
  1. Hydrocephalus
    a. Chiari II, aqueductal stenosis, posthemorrhagic or meningitis
  2. Subdural collections
    a. Chronic hematoma and child abuse
    b. "Benign" subdural collection of infancy
  3. Megalencephaly
    a. Anatomic: familial, neurofibromatosis, achondroplasia
    b. Metabolic: mucopolysaccharidoses, Alexander's, Canavan's diseases
    c. Syndromes: Soto's (cerebral gigantism)
  4. Calvarial
    a. Osteopetrosis, anemias

D. **Synostosis [Fig. 2-87; see also Figs. 1-33 and 1-34]**
  1. Sutures: sagittal, metopic, paired coronal, paired lambdoid, paired squamosal

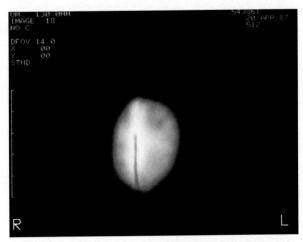

Fig. 2-87 Axial brain CT: Ridging and sclerosis along sagittal suture. Sagittal synostosis.

    2. Synostosis patterns
       a. Dolichocephaly or scaphocephaly—sagittal (most common 55%)
       b. Trigonocephaly—metopic
       c. Brachycephaly—bilateral coronal (2nd most common 12%)
       d. Plagiocephaly—unilateral coronal
       e. Turricephaly or acrocephaly—all sutures
       f. Kleebättschädel—cloverleaf skull
    3. Syndromes associated with synostosis
       a. Apert's = acrocephalosyndactyly
       b. Carpenter's = acrocephalopolysyndactyly
       c. Crouzon's = craniofacial dysostosis
    4. Secondary synostoses
       a. Metabolic
         • Treated rickets
         • Idiopathic hypercalcemia
         • Hyperthyroidism
         • Hurler's syndrome
       b. Dysplasias
         • Hypophosphatasia
         • Achondroplasia
         • Metaphyseal dysostosis
         • Rubinstein-Taybi syndrome
         • Down's syndrome
       c. Following ventricular shunting
       d. Associated with microcephaly
    5. Anomalies associated with synostosis
       a. Most frequent with coronal synostosis
       b. Cleft lip, palate
       c. Holoprosencephaly
       d. ACC
       e. Spina bifida, Chiari II malformation
       f. Congenital heart disease
       g. Hypogonadism
  E. Skull defects and abnormalities
    1. Cephaloceles **[Figs. 2-88 and 2-89]**
       a. Occipital most common in Western hemisphere
       b. Associated with midline defects (cleft palate, ACC, Dandy-Walker cyst)
       c. Nasal dermoid
       d. Median cleft face
    2. Epidermoid, dermoid (lucent with sclerotic rim)
    3. Craniolacuna **[Fig. 2-90]**
       a. Dysplasia associated with Chiari II malformation
       b. Resolves by 6 months of age whether shunted for hydrocephalus or not
    4. Neurofibromatosis **[Figs. 2-21 and 2-22]**
       a. Sphenoid wing dysplasia

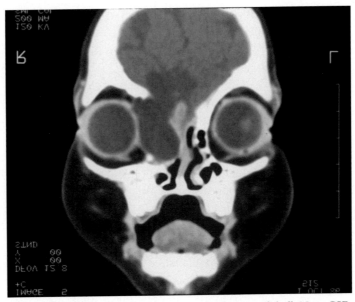

Fig. 2-88 Direct coronal CT: Defect in right base of skull. Note CSF-containing structure protruding into medial aspect of right orbit. Fronto-ethmoidal cephalocele.

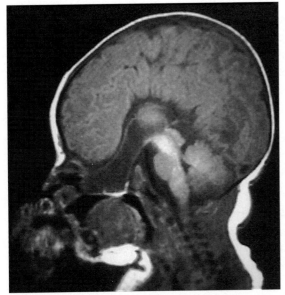

Fig. 2-89 Midline sagittal T1-weighted MRI: Patient with median cleft face syndrome. Third ventricle protrudes through defect in base of skull and cleft palate to abut the top of the tongue. Cephalocele.

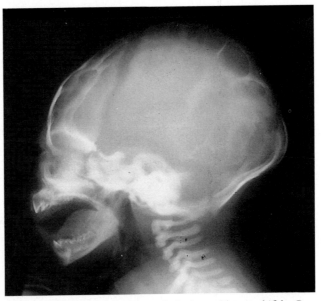

Fig. 2-90 Lateral skull radiograph: Patient with spina bifida. Cystic appearing calvaria, widening of squamosal and coronal sutures, microcephaly. Craniolacuna, sutural diastasis.

b. "Empty orbit sign"

c. Defect in lambdoid suture

d. Widening of optic foramen or internal auditory canal

5. Sturge-Weber syndrome

a. Davidoff-Dyke-Masson

- Hemiatrophy
- Unilateral calvarial thickening

6. Calvarial thickening

a. Dilantin effect

b. Sickle cell disease **[Fig. 8-14]**

c. Osteopetrosis

- Progressive obliteration of foramina

d. Healed rickets

e. Hypoparathyroidism

f. Fibrous dysplasia

- Ground-glass appearance
- Progressive obliteration of foramina

7. Wormian (intrasutural) bones

a. Normal variant

b. Osteogenesis imperfecta (OI)

c. hypothyroidism

d. Cleidocranial dysostosis

e. Hypophosphatasia

f. (NOTCH) + pyknodysostosis, rickets

8. Delayed sutural closure

a. Hypopituitarism (small sella)

b. Hypothyroidism (large sella)

9. Deficient calvarial mineralization (craniotabes)

a. Hypophosphatasia

b. Achondrogenesis

c. OI

F. **Skull fractures**

1. At birth

a. Linear, buckled, or depressed

b. Associated with cephalohematoma (does not cross sutures) or caput succadaneum (subgaleal, crosses sutures)

2. Leptomeningeal cyst **[Fig. 2-91]**

a. Associated with dural tear and underlying parenchymal injury

3. Child abuse **[Fig. 1-30]**

a. In children <2 years of age, more likely if fracture is multiple or complex, depressed, involves more than one bone, associated with intracranial injury

4. Accidental fractures more likely linear and parietal

5. Depressed fracture **[Fig. 1-31]**

a. Image with CT or tangential X-ray beam

b. On cross-table lateral, evaluate for pneumocephalus

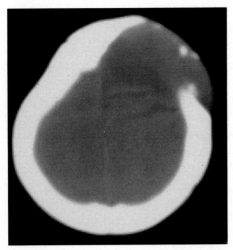

Fig. 2-91   Axial brain CT: Separation of calvarium by "cystic" lesion in patient with previous skull fracture. Leptomeningeal cyst ("growing fracture").

G. **Skull tumors**
  1. Benign
     a. Of 70 children with nontraumatic lump on head, 61% = dermoid, 9% = cephalohematoma, 7% eosinophilic granuloma, 4% = occult cephalocele
     b. Epidermoid, dermoid (lucent with sclerotic rim)
     c. Langerhans' cell histiocytosis (eosinophilic granuloma) **[Fig. 3-54]**
        • "Punched out" lesion with beveled edge
        • Greater involvement of inner table than outer table
     d. Hemangioma—radial appearance
     e. Chordoma (50% sacrum/coccyx, >50 yrs.; 35% skull base, 20 to 40 years; <15% vertebral, thoracic least common)
  2. Malignant
     a. Skull base tumors
        • Lymphoma
        • Nasopharyngeal carcinoma
        • Rhabdomyosarcoma
     b. Osteosarcoma
     c. Neuroblastoma (metastases to calvarium, base of skull, orbit, sutures) **[Fig. 7-33]**
H. **Skull and facial infections**
  1. Osteomyelitis
  2. Mastoiditis
     a. Association: dural sinus thrombosis
  3. Sinusitis
     a. "Potts' puffy tumor" (frontal sinusitis)
  4. Orbital cellulitis
     a. Association: cavernous sinus thrombosis

XIII. **HEAD AND NECK**
  A. **Congenital**
    1. Nasal inlet stenosis
    2. Normal diameter = 3 to 10 mm
    3. Holonasal stenosis
      a. <2 mm diameter
      b. Boys predominate, premies, maxillary hypoplasia, Apert syndrome
    4. Nasolacrimal mucocele
      a. Obstruction of nasolacrimal duct at level of inferior turbinate
      b. Association with chronic or recurrent dacryocystitis
    5. Choanal atresia **[Fig. 2-92]**
      a. 1:5000 births
      b. Bony atresia 90%, membranous atresia 10%
      c. Plate is 2 to 4 mm anterior to posterior edge of vomer
      d. Normal choanal diameter >3 mm; atresia <3 mm
      e. Lateral wall of choana is medially deviated
      f. Girls predominate; 75% bilateral; 80% have associated anomalies
      g. CHARGE syndrome: Colobomata, Heart disease, Atresia of choanae, Retarded growth/development, Genital anomalies, Ear anomalies
      h. Fetal alcohol syndrome
    6. Laryngomalacia
      a. Most common laryngeal anomaly
      b. "Aryepiglottic hypermobility or laxity"
      c. Inspiratory stridor on quiet breathing; disappears with crying
    7. Vocal cord paralysis
      a. Second most common laryngeal anomaly
      b. Inspiratory stridor most pronounced with crying
      c. Half without associated anomalies

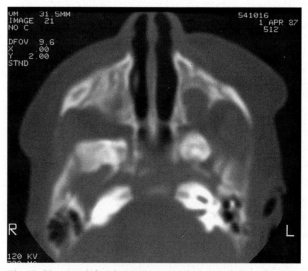

Fig. 2-92 Axial facial CT: Narrowed choana bilaterally with bony atresia plate. Choanal atresia.

     d. Associated anomalies: neurologic lesions (CNS, Werdnig-Hoffman, leukodystrophy), subglottic stenosis, hip dysplasia, cardiac, Down's syndrome

     e. Association with meningomyelocele (vocal cord paralysis may signal shunt malfunction)

     f. Postbirth trauma, surgery

  8. Midline defects: cleft palate, cephaloceles

     a. DDx of neonatal nasopharyngeal mass includes hamartoma, teratoma, dermoid, hemangioma, neuroblastoma, glioma, and encephalocele

     b. Presence of fat within a nasopharyngeal mass indicates either hamartoma, teratoma, or dermoid

       • Of these three rare fat-containing tumors, the hairy or teratoid polyp is most common

     c. Teratoma contains ectoderm, mesoderm, and endoderm

     d. The hairy polyp is a dermoid and has two germ layers, ectoderm and mesoderm

       • The hairy skin, of ectodermal origin, which covers the hairy polyp, is not indigenous to the nasopharynx; this finding distinguishes a hairy polyp from a hamartoma

B. Inflammation [Figs. 1-49 through 1-51]

  1. Cervical lymphadenitis

     a. Bacterial

       • Usually *S. aureus* or *S. pneumoniae*

     b. Granulomatous

       • Chronic granulomatous disease of childhood

     c. Toxoplasmosis

       • Exposure to cat or kitten

     d. Scrofula (mycobacterial)

     e. Cat-scratch disease

  2. Supraglottitis **[Fig. 2-93]**

     a. *H. influenzae;* 3 to 10 years of age

     b. Drooling; "tripod" body posture to maintain open airway (head held forward)

     c. Muffled voice, stridor, air hunger

     d. Swollen aryepiglottic folds; "thumb sign" of short, broad epiglottis

     e. 25% have subglottic involvement

     f. DDx: omega-shaped epiglottis, thermal injury, angioedema, epiglottic or aryepiglottic cyst, hemophilia

  3. Croup **[Fig. 2-94]**

     a. Viral; 1.5 to 3 years of age

     b. Hoarseness, inspiratory stridor

     c. Narrowing of subglottic trachea

     d. Loss of "shouldering" of trachea; as if the trachea were in a pencil sharpener

  4. Membranous croup **[Fig. 2-95]**

     a. Bacterial (*S. aureus, S. pneumoniae, C. diphtheria,* others)

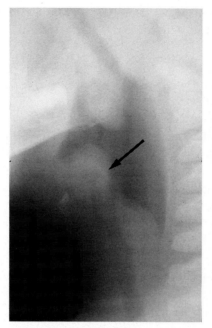

Fig. 2-93 Lateral airway radiograph: Short, thickened epiglottis, markedly thickened aryepiglottic folds (arrow). Acute epiglottitis.

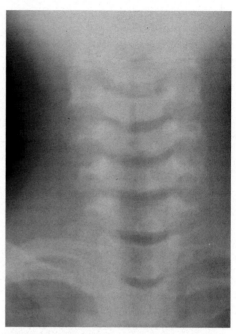

Fig. 2-94 AP airway radiograph: Circumferential narrowing of subglottic tracheal air column, as if the trachea has been placed in a pencil sharpener. Croup.

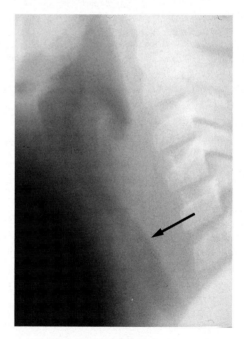

Fig. 2-95 Lateral airway radiograph: Narrowing of subglottic trachea. Note soft tissue within the tracheal air column (arrow). Membranous croup.

b. Signs, symptoms of viral croup + increased toxicity; less responsiveness to inhalation therapy

c. Most between 1–24 months of age; 20% > 4 years

d. Two-thirds have subglottic narrowing indistinguishable from viral croup; 1/3 have narrowing + membrane or mucosal irregularity

C. **Trauma**

1. Fibromatosis colli (congenital torticollis, wryneck) **[Figs. 2-96 and 2-97]**

   a. Asymmetric deformity of neck, flexion of head toward involved side, rotation of chin to opposite side

   b. Associated with birth trauma or forceps delivery

   c. Hemorrhage into sternocleidomastoid muscle can be identified by US, CT, or MRI

   d. Failure to resolve may cause facial asymmetry (flattening of face on ipsilateral side)

2. Subglottic stenosis

   a. Often postintubation

   b. Tracheal stenosis may be congenital; diffuse or segmental

3. Neonatal pharyngeal pseudo-diverticulum **[Fig. 2-98]**

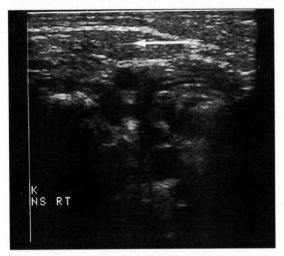

Fig. 2-96 Transverse neck US: Normal sonographic appearance of right sternocleidomastoid muscle (arrows). Note consistent diameter of muscle with sharp borders. Normal sternocleidomastoid muscle.

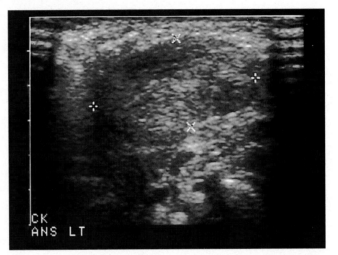

Fig. 2-97 Transverse neck US: Same patient as Figure 2-96. Rounded left sternocleidomastoid muscle contains echogenic hematoma (between electronic cursors). Fibromatosis colli.

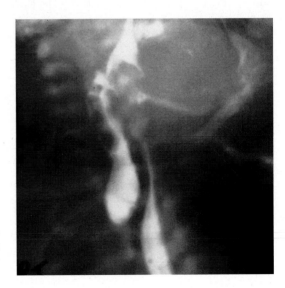

Fig. 2-98 AP esophagram: Traumatic intubation attempt at birth. Diverticulum extends from pharynx to mediastinum alongside barium esophageal column. Note narrowing of upper esophagus. Neonatal pharyngeal pseudodiverticulum.

a. Secondary to perinatal pharyngeal perforation
- Radiographic appearance can simulate esophageal atresia

b. Associated with pneumomediastinum

c. Conservative treatment, resolves in 2 to 3 weeks

D. **Tumors**

1. Benign nasopharyngeal masses

   a. Pseudomasses
   - Pharyngeal buckling

     Increased distance between hypopharynx and cervical spine seen on lateral radiograph in exhalation, during swallowing, or crying

     Due to elastic soft tissues of hypopharynx

     Children <2 years of age

     Disappears on full inspiration

   - Thymic herniation

     Thymus extends into lower neck on exhalation or crying: 2 months to 2.5 years of age

     Noisy breathing, apnea, cyanosis, suprasternal mass

   b. Cysts
   - Cystic hygroma

     Congenital malformation of lymph sacs; subset of lymphangioma

     Most common site is posterior triangle of neck and supraclavicular fossa

     30 to 50% present at birth with respiratory distress or mass

     Nonencapsulated; tend to infiltrate soft tissues in neck or chest

     Poorly circumscribed, multiloculated, low density mass on CT

     May rapidly enlarge due to hemorrhage or infection

     Associated with syndromes, such as Turner's, Noonan's, fetal alcohol, familial pterygium colli

   - Branchial cleft cyst **[Fig. 2-99]**

     20% of all neck masses in children

     90% arise from second branchial cleft, 8% from first branchial cleft, 2% from third branchial cleft

     Most common location is at anterior border of sternocleido mastoid muscle, lateral to carotid sheath

     May present as infected mass; can communicate with pharynx, pyriform sinus, or valleculae

     Fascial planes usually preserved, unless infection is present

     Unilocular with thin walls, unless infected

   - Ranula **[Fig. 2-100]**

     Retention cyst of salivary gland, usually sublingual

     Usually do not extend below hyoid

     Simple ranula is confined to floor of mouth

     Plunging ranula extends through mylohyoid

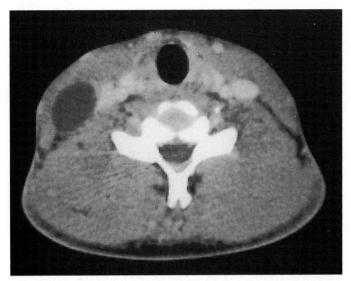

Fig. 2-99 Axial neck CT: Well-demarcated homogeneous hypodense mass medial to right sternocleidomastoid muscle and lateral to carotid sheath. Branchial cleft cyst.

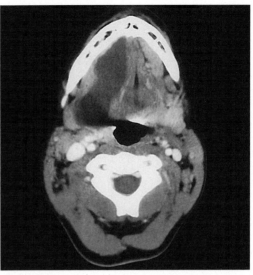

Fig. 2-100 Axial neck CT: Homogeneous hypodense lesion in floor of mouth, extends from posterior border of mandible. Ranula.

- Thyroglossal duct cyst **[Fig. 2-101]**
    Midline mass from base of tongue to mediastinum
    Can be off midline
    Can penetrate hyoid bone
    Most are at or just below hyoid
    Fistula to thyroid may promote recurrence
    US to determine if normal thyroid tissue present

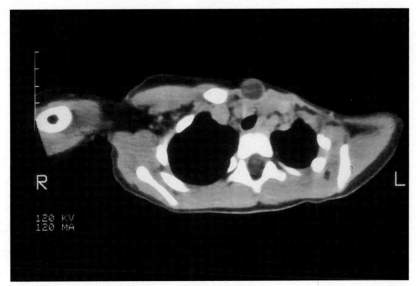

Fig. 2-101 Axial neck CT: Superficial hypodense lesion in midline with mildly thickened and enhancing rim. Thyroglossal duct cyst.

- Thymic cyst [**Fig. 2-102**]

    Thymus arises from third and fourth pharyngeal pouches

    Migrates caudally in neck to mediastinum

    Embryologic thymic remnant in neck accounts for cervical thymic cyst

    Diagnosis depends upon the finding of remnants of thymic tissue with characteristic Hassall corpuscles in the fibrous tissue wall

    Masses derived from the third pharyngeal pouch are usually adherent to the carotid sheath and pass downward lateral to the thyroid capsule and along the anterior border of the sternocleidomastoid muscle to the manubrium

    Thymic cysts may have an intimate relationship to the carotid sheath

c. Hemangioma [**Fig. 2-103**]

- Most common tumor of the head and neck in children
- Most common cause of subglottic soft tissue mass
- Posterolateral indentation on trachea
- Capillary
- Usually involutes by 5 to 6 years of age
- Very vascular, with areas of AV shunting, fibrosis, and hemorrhage

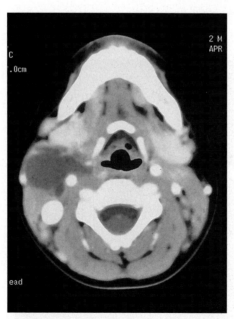

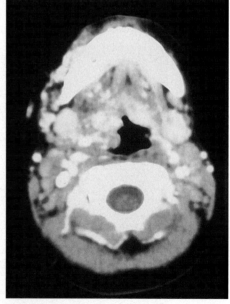

Fig. 2-102   Axial neck CT: Homogeneous hypodense lesion along anteromedial border of sternocleidomastoid muscle. Note extension of lesion between internal jugular vein and carotid artery, within carotid sheath. Thymic cyst.

Fig. 2-103   Axial neck CT: Marked enhancement of extensive vascular lesion that extends superficial to mandible, within floor of mouth, and into right parapharyngeal space. Hemangioma.

d. Juvenile angiofibroma **[Fig. 2-104]**
- Teenage males, epistaxis, nasal obstruction, 0.5% head/neck tumors
- Located in/around sphenopalatine foramen (SPF)
- Staging:
    I: Limited to posterior nares; IB into one or more sinuses
    IIA: Through SPF to medial pterygomaxillary fossa (PMF)
    IIB: Occupies PMF, displaces posterior wall of maxillary antrum, orbital extension
    IIC: Through PMF to infratemporal fossa or cheek
    III: Intracranial extension
- Highly vascular, grows through foramina, bright enhancement, T2 hyperintensity
- Ascending pharyngeal, internal maxillary arteries
- Anterior bowing of posterior wall of maxillary antrum, erosion of pterygoids, displacement of nasal septum, grows through foramina
e. Thyroid
- Goiter
- Cyst
- Adenoma
- Carcinoma
    Increased incidence in patients subjected to radiotherapy
- Inflammatory thyroiditis

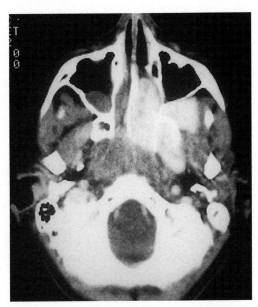

Fig. 2-104 Axial facial CT: Homogeneously-enhancing lesion in left posterior nasopharynx, infratemporal fossa, and parapharyngeal space. Note scalloping of both pterygoid plate and bony nasal wall and extension through sphenopalatine foramen. Juvenile angiofibroma.

- Lingual thyroid
    Usually removed because it is commonly dysfunctional
    Patient must be placed on thyroid replacement hormone
- US
    Solid vs. cystic mass
    Solitary vs. multiple thyroid lesions
- Nuclear study
    Solitary "cold" nodule
    − 20 to 30% malignant
      "Cold" nodule in multinodular gland
    − Approximately 5% malignant
      "Warm" or "hot" nodules usually functioning adenomas

f. Papillomatosis
- Papillomavirus type 6
    Subtype human papilloma virus (HPV)-6C associated with more extensive disease
- Of 532 patients with laryngeal papillomatosis, 5% involved trachea/proximal bronchi, <1% involved lung parenchyma
- Laryngeal papillomas at ages 6 months to 14 years of age
- Lung lesions 1 to 11 years later **[Fig. 5–42]**
    Lung lesion: round nodule, solid or cystic, thin or thick wall
    Slow growing, may be confluent, air/fluid levels when infected
    Papillomas destroy normal tissue
    Chronic restrictive lung disease
    Malignant transformation to squamous cell carcinoma
    Do not regress or disappear
    Aerial dissemination, following endoscopic removal

2. Malignant nasopharyngeal masses
a. Lymphoma **[Fig. 2–105]**
- Tend to be homogeneous in MR signal; no calcification
- In face, paranasal sinuses, and skull base, non-Hodgkin's lymphoma (NHL) is aggressive, erodes bone
- In NHL, 25 to 30% have involvement of Waldeyer's ring or cervical nodes
- Most common presentation of Hodgkin's is painless cervical lymphadenopathy (90%)
- In children < 10, NHL > Hodgkin's
- In all childhood lymphomas, Hodgkin's > NHL

b. Nasopharyngeal carcinoma **[Fig. 2–106]**
- Increased incidence in Asian adults, Alaskan adult natives
- Association with Ebstein Barr virus
- Nasal, eustachian tube obstruction; cranial nerve involvement common
- Aggressive, destructive, skull base involvement (may be sclerotic)
- Local and distant mets

c. Rhabdomyosarcoma
- Most common soft tissue sarcoma in children

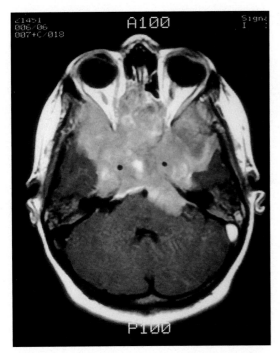

Fig. 2-105 Gadolinium-enhanced axial T1-weighted MRI: Extensive enhancing mass involves nasopharynx and base of skull; invades intracranial contents to level of cerebellopontine cistern. Nasopharyngeal lymphoma.

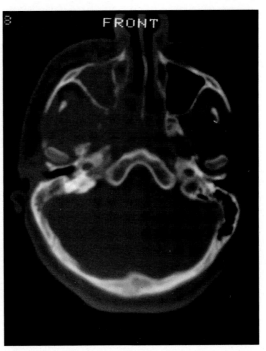

Fig. 2-106 Axial facial CT: Soft tissue mass destroys right pterygoid plate, fills nasopharynx, erodes wall of right maxillary sinus. Nasopharyngeal carcinoma. Note fluid within right mastoid air cells, indicating Eustachian tube obstruction.

- 40% occur in head and neck
- Orbit, nasopharynx, and middle ear most commonly affected
- Embryonal and botryoid types in head and neck; alveolar in extremities
- Aggressive, frequent bone erosion
- Cervical lymph node involvement in 12 to 50%

E. **Paranasal Sinuses [Fig. 1-32]**

1. Sinusitis **[Fig. 2-107]**
   a. May be difficult clinical diagnosis in children
   b. Signs, symptoms overlap with simple upper respiratory infection
   c. Purulent rhinorrhea
   d. Associated with cystic fibrosis, asthma, immune deficiencies, allergic rhinitis
   e. Imaging
      - Poor correlation between sinus radiographs and CT
      - Radiographs: 35% false-positive, 45% false-negative
      - Mucosal thickening >4 mm suggests acute sinusitis
      - CT

         Direct coronal 3 mm thickness

         Prone or supine position

         Evaluate ostiomeatal complex, look for polyps, mucosal thickening, air-fluid levels

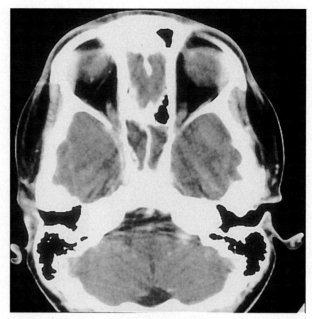

Fig. 2-107   Axial facial CT: Soft tissue or fluid in sphenoid sinus. Note enhancement and thickening of dura of right medial temporal lobe due to parameningeal inflammation. Sphenoid sinusitis.

   f. Complications
- Orbital cellulitis **[Fig. 2-86]**
- Cavernous sinus thrombosis **[Fig. 2-108]**
- Pott's puffy tumor: subgaleal abscess of forehead due to frontal sinusitis
- Cerebritis
- Parameningeal inflammation: due to sphenoid sinusitis
  - Enhancement of meninges on CT
  - Abnormal CSF

2. Fungal sinusitis
   a. Chronic sinusitis unresponsive to antibacterial therapy
   b. Hyperdensity on CT, hypointensity on MRI

3. Mucocele
   a. Accumulation of secretions in chronically obstructed sinus
   b. Frontal (60%), ethmoid (25%)
   c. Expansion of sinus filled with mucoid material: no air in sinus

4. Polyps
   a. Nasal polyps in 23% of patients with chronic rhinitis
   b. Polyp that exits sinus ostia to posterior nasal cavity = choanal polyp
   c. Most common from maxillary antrum = antrochoanal polyp
   d. Antrochoanal polyp
- Arises in maxillary sinus, through ostium into choana, to nasopharynx
- 3% of patients with nasal polyps have antrochoanal polyp

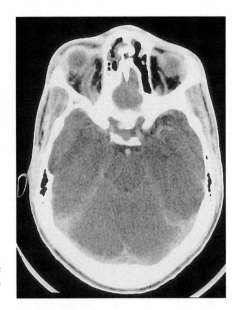

Fig. 2-108 Axial facial CT: Patient with sinusitis. "Tram-track" enhancement of right superior ophthalmic vein. Compare with contralateral normal superior ophthalmic vein. Cavernous sinus thrombosis.

- 71% are 10 to 39 years of age; male:female = 1.3:1
- 57% unilateral, 42% bilateral
- Expansion of opaque maxillary sinus; no bone destruction
- Positive sniff test at fluoro = air outlines nasopharyngeal component
- DDx: mucocele, inflammatory or allergic polyp, angiofibroma, carcinoma, lymphoma, rhabdomyosarcoma
  e. Polypoid rhinosinusitis
- Expansion of nasal cavity (can produce hypertelorism) or sinus, ethmoids predominate
- No nasopharyngeal component
- CONSIDER CYSTIC FIBROSIS

F. **Laryngeal and extrathoracic tracheal obstruction**
1. Laryngomalacia
2. Vocal cord paralysis
3. Supraglottitis
4. Croup and membranous croup
5. Subglottic stenosis
6. Neonatal pharyngeal pseudo-diverticulum
7. Hemangioma
8. Papillomatosis

XIV. **SPINE**
A. Vertebra
1. Vertebral development
a. Vertebra = body + posterior elements
b. Body is rectangular; height slightly < width **[Fig. 1-35]**
c. Vertebral body originates from dorsal and ventral ossification centers
d. Notochord in ventral portion of body atrophies, disappears
- Notochord enlarges in disc area to become nucleus pulposus

2. Vertebral malformations
   a. Agenesis of body from failure of both ossifications centers
   b. Hemivertebra: unilateral, dorsal, or ventral location **[Fig. 1–37]**
      - Congenital scoliosis with unilateral
      - Congenital kyphosis with dorsal
      - Ventral hemivertebra rare
   c. Coronal cleft
      - Vertical lucency seen on lateral view of spine on radiograph
      - Due to failure of fusion of anterior and posterior ossification centers
   d. Butterfly vertebra **[Fig. 1–37]**
      - Failure of fusion of lateral halves of vertebral body
   e. Block vertebra
      - Adjacent bodies fused
      - Height of two involved bodies = height of two normal adjacent vertebrae + interposed disc space
   f. Hypoplastic vertebra
   g. Platyspondyly **[Figs. 3–5, 3–7, and 3–36]**
      - Flattened vertebrae, variable degree of severity
      - Thanatophoric dysplasia: marked platyspondyly, "H" or "U" shape
      - Achondroplasia
      - Spondyloepiphyseal dysplasia
      - Mucopolysaccharidosis
      - Osteogenesis imperfecta
   h. Elongated vertebra
      - Neuromotor dysfunction: nonambulatory
   i. Posterior scalloping
      - Normal
      - Neurofibromatosis
      - Achondroplasia
      - Spinal cord tumor
   j. End plate deformity
      - SCD: infarcts
      - Schmorl's nodes: central disc herniation
      - Limbus vertebra (anterior disc herniation): irregular anterosuperior fragment of end plate sheared by anterior disc herniation
      - "Ring" apophysis: "ununited" fragments at anterosuperior and/or anteroinferior end plate separated from body by unossified cartilage; normal finding
   k. Beaking
      - Anteroinferior
        Normal
        Achondroplasia
        Hurler's syndrome
        Hypothyroidism

- Central
  Morquio's syndrome
3. Vertebral inflammation
  a. Osteomyelitis **[Figs. 2-109 through 2-111]**
     - Lumbar spine most common
     - Starts in disc space or end plate, typically involves two adjacent bodies
       Low grade osteomyelitis may involve only portion of body

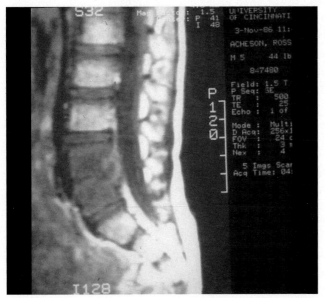

Fig. 2-109 Sagittal T1-weighted MRI: Hypointense L4 and L5 vertebral bodies with markedly narrowed intervening disc space. Discitis.

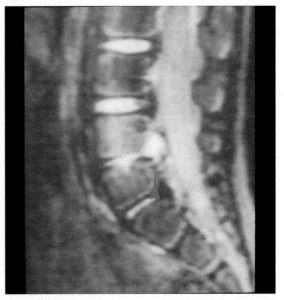

Fig. 2-110 Sagittal T2-weighted MRI: Same patient as Figure 2-109. Hyperintense L4 and L5 vertebral bodies with herniation of disc substance into L5 superior end plate and epidural disc herniation. Discitis.

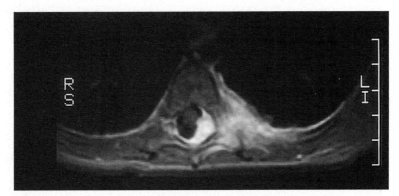

Fig. 2-111 Gadolinium-enhanced axial T1-weighted MRI with fat saturation: Enhancement in transverse process, pedicle, paravertebral soft tissues. Note inflammatory component within neural canal (epidural abscess) deviating spinal cord to right. Vertebral osteomyelitis with epidural abscess.

- *S. aureus* most common; cultures often show no growth
- Radiographs
    Narrowed disc space, irregular end plates
- Nuclear bone scan
    Increased uptake in two adjacent bodies
    Abnormal scan may precede radiographic abnormalities
    If planar bone scan normal, single photon emission computed tomography (SPECT) may show subtle abnormality of low grade osteomyelitis
- MRI
    Hypointense vertebral body, disc on T1WI
    Hyperintense vertebral body, disc on T2WI
    − Soft tissue mass, epidural abscess best seen after gadolinium enhancement

4. Vertebral tumors
- Note: "most common site" refers only to site within vertebral column

a. Osteoid osteoma
- Lumbar most common site; male predominance
- Central calcification surrounded by lytic area; reactive sclerosis around lesion
- Extremely hot on nuclear bone scan
- CT better than MRI to show diagnostic bone lesion

b. Osteoblastoma
- Cervical spine most common site
- Also called "giant osteoid osteoma"; >2 cm diameter
- Involves posterior elements
- Expansile, lytic lesion with sclerotic rim

c. Aneurysmal bone cyst (ABC)
- Two-thirds of ABC are secondary to primary bone tumor, such as giant cell tumor, nonossifying fibroma, fibrous dysplasia, osteoblastoma
- Expansile, lytic, vascular with areas of hemorrhage
- Cervical, thoracic spine most common sites
- CT
    Expansile, cystic
- MRI
    Heterogeneous signal on T1WI and T2WI
    Fluid-fluid or blood-fluid levels within cysts

d. Osteochondroma (exostosis)
- Cervical and thoracic spine most common sites
- Involves transverse or spinous processes
- Malignant degeneration in 1% of solitary and up to 25% of hereditary osteochondromatosis
- Cortex and marrow of lesion continuous with that of vertebra

e. Giant cell tumor
- Sacrum most common site
- Lytic, expansile, no calcified matrix
- Malignant degeneration in 10%

- CT

  Lytic lesion with nonsclerotic margin; no calcification

f. Osteosarcoma
  - Most common primary malignant bone tumor in childhood
  - Rarely involves vertebral column primarily, but metastases to spine common
  - Usually in second decade of life

g. Ewing's sarcoma **[Fig. 2-112]**
  - Second most common primary malignant bone tumor in childhood
  - Typically ages 5 to 15 years; male predominance
  - Primary or metastatic involvement of spine
  - Either lytic or sclerotic

h. Chordoma
  - Arises from notochord remnants
  - Clivus most common; sacrum next
  - Lytic with calcified soft tissue mass in 50%
  - Can cross disc space, mimicking osteomyelitis

i. Leukemia/lymphoma **[Fig. 8-8]**
  - Radiograph: osteopenia, lytic or sclerotic lesions, pathologic fracture

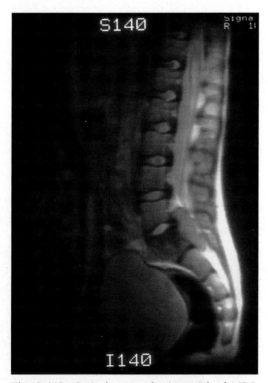

Fig. 2-112 Sagittal proton density-weighted MRI: Hypointense mass in S1 vertebral body with lobulated epidural soft tissue mass and small anterior presacral mass indenting urinary bladder. Ewing's sarcoma.

- Marrow infiltration alters fatty marrow signal in vertebrae
  Not identified by MRI in young children with red marrow
- Multifocal marrow involvement with epidural masses: THINK of non-Hodgkins' lymphoma
  DDx: histiocytosis, metastatic disease
  j. Hemangioma
  - Most common primary tumor of spine in all ages
  - Usually asymptomatic, found incidentally
  - Cavernous type of hemangioma
  - Vertically-oriented striated trabecular pattern on radiograph
  k. Langerhans' cell histiocytosis
  - Formerly called histiocytosis X (included Letterer-Siwe, Hand-Schüller-Christian, and eosinophilic granuloma)
  - Lytic lesion with/without soft tissue mass
  - Vertebra plana; disc spaces preserved
5. Vertebral trauma
  a. Cranio-cervical
  - Normal measurements in children
    Normal dens-basion distance 5 to 12 mm
    Anterior arch C1-dens: 2.5 mm in adults; 3 to 5 mm in children
    – Flexion-extension movement ≤2 mm
    C2–C3 pseudosubluxation
    – Line through spinolaminar line from C1 to C3 should pass within 1.5 mm of spinolaminar line of C2
    Dens-arch synchondrosis at base of dens **[Fig. 2-113]**
    – Dens should retain relationship with body of C2 on flexion, extension; it should not tip forward

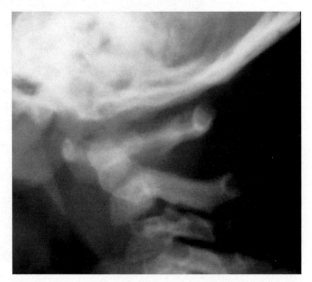

Fig. 2-113 Lateral coned-down cervical spine radiograph: Dens tipped forward relative to C2 vertebral body. Note widening at base of dens. Dens synchondrosis fracture.

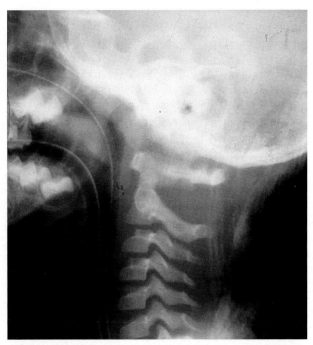

Fig. 2-114 Lateral cervical spine radiograph. Widening between base of skull and C1 and between C1 and C2. Note anterior displacement of clinoid relative to top of dens. Atlanto-occipital dislocation, atlanto-axial distraction.

- Upper cervical injuries in young child
  Head relatively heavy, supporting ligaments weak, facets small, more horizontal than in adult
  - Fulcrum at C2–C3
- Lower cervical injuries in older child (>6 years of age)
  Anatomy more like that of adult
  - Adult fulcrum at C5–C6
- Atlanto-occipital dislocation **[Fig. 2-114]**
  Dens-basion distance ≥14 mm
  Usually motor vehicle accidents; mortality and morbidity high
  Head usually displaced anterior to spine (if you drop a marble from the clivus, it should strike the top of the dens)
- C1 (atlas) fractures
  Hyperextension fracture through posterior synchondrosis
  - May be confused with normal unossified portions of posterior arch (smooth margins, wide unossified area)
  Jefferson, burst fracture through synchondroses
  - Lateral masses lateral to body of C2 on radiograph or CT
- C2 (axis) fractures
  Odontoid fractures
  - Often through dens synchondrosis; dens should not tip forward on body of C2

- Fracture through upper dens (Type I) uncommon

  Do not confuse with os terminale, an ossification center with oblique margins at tip of dens

  Os odontoideum

- Enlarged os terminale; may be associated with hypoplasia of posterior ring of C1

- Separation from body of C2 predisposes to instability (flexion/extension radiographs or fluoroscopy useful)

  Hangman's fracture

- Hyperextension fracture through posterior arch of C2

- Use spinolaminar line from C1 to C3 to determine malposition of spinolaminar point of C2

- Atlantoaxial instability **[Figs. 2-115 and 2-116]**

  Down's syndrome

- Also have increased incidence atlanto-occipital instability

- Special Olympics recommendations

  1) "Despite difficulties in obtaining good medical histories and physical and neurologic examinations . . ., it is clearly important that they receive these evaluations before participation in sports."

  2) "The Special Olympics does not plan to remove its requirement that all athletes with Down's syndrome receive radiographs of the cervical spine."

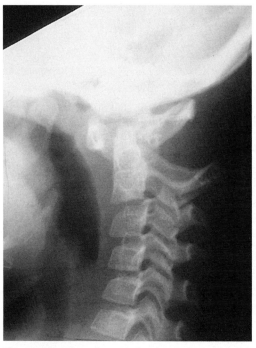

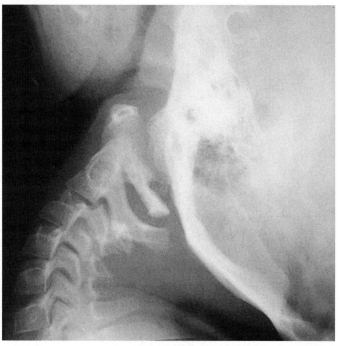

Fig. 2-115 Lateral cervical spine radiograph with flexion: Down's syndrome. Widening between posterior elements of C1 and C2 with anterior subluxation of C1 on C2. Atlanto-axial instability.

Fig. 2-116 Lateral cervical spine radiograph with extension: Same patient as Figure 2-115. Abnormal anterior movement of C1 relative to base of skull. Atlanto-occipital instability.

- Preoperative evaluation
  1) Preoperative neurologic assessment
  2) Children with Down's syndrome >2 years of age should have lateral neck radiographs in neutral, flexion, and extension positions
  3) Children with Down's syndrome and predental space >4.5 mm should have preoperative neurosurgical consultation
  4) Children with neurologic findings should have cervical stabilization before elective otolaryngologic procedures

Juvenile rheumatoid arthritis, ankylosing spondylitis, retropharyngeal inflammation allow transverse ligament laxity and widening of predental space

Hypoplastic odontoid
- Down's syndrome

  May also have hypoplastic posterior arch of C1, laxity of transverse ligament, all of which can compromise neural canal
- Morquio's syndrome

- Atlantoaxial rotary subluxation [Fig. 2–117]

  Secondary to trauma or pharyngeal inflammation

  Torticollis, spasm

  Offset of lateral mass of C1 relative to C2

  Predental space may be normal in mild rotation to widened with more severe rotation
  - Type I rotary fixation: with no anterior displacement
  - Type II rotary fixation: with 3 to 5 mm anterior displacement

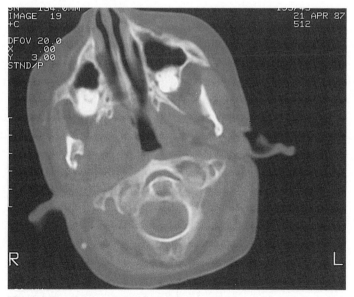

Fig. 2-117 Axial neck CT: Malalignment of C1 and C2. Note long axis between tip of nose and midline of C1 compared to axis of C2. Atlanto-axial rotary subluxation.

- Type III rotary fixation: with >5 mm anterior displacement
- Type IV rotary fixation: with posterior displacement
CT
- Line through transverse axis of C1 (through neuroforamina) should be parallel with similar line through body of C2
- Dens (should be midline) will also lie closer to one side of lateral mass of C1
- Lower cervical trauma
  Hyperflexion, hyperextension, distraction, compression, rotational injuries more common in older children
  Similar radiographic findings as in adults
- Obtaining cervical radiographs in children
  Obtain cross-table lateral rather than turning patient to true lateral
  Anteroposterior (AP), lateral in young children
  - Open mouth odontoid difficult due to lack of cooperation
    Can use reverse Water's for odontoid
  Add obliques, open mouth odontoid in older children
  Flexion-extension lateral views
  - Do not allow parent to flex child's neck in uncontrolled situation
  - Fluoroscopy excellent to protect child and obtain properly positioned views
    Place towel under child's head to reduce obliquity between head and level of shoulders
  - Coordinated movement of child by nurses, technologists, et al to protect child's neck

b. Thoracolumbar injuries **[Fig. 8-2]**
  - Usually hyperflexion injury
  - Vertebral compression + posterior ligament or posterior arch injury predisposes to instability
  - Burst fracture with retropulsion of fragments produces cord displacement and/or contusion
  - Chance fracture
    Lapbelt hyperflexion injury through lumbar spine
    Involves posterior elements, with or without vertebral compression fracture
    Associated with intra-abdominal injuries
    - Duodenum, pancreas, bowel, mesentery
  - Spondylolysis **[Fig. 2-118]**
    Fracture in pars interarticularis in lumbar spine
    Oblique lumber spine radiographs show "fractured neck" in Scottie dog
    Nuclear bone scan shows increase uptake in pars
    - But may be falsely negative; SPECT is most sensitive to diagnose

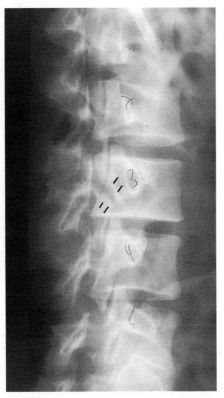

Fig. 2-118 Oblique lumbar spine radiograph: Abnormal pars interarticularis at L3. "Broken neck" in Scottie dog (outlined). Spondylolysis.

- Spondylolisthesis

  Slippage of upper body on lower body; usually lumbosacral

  Usually due to bilateral spondylolysis

  Grade I = upper body anterior <25% of AP diameter of lower body

  Grade II = 25 to 50% slip

  Grade III = 50 to 75% slip

  Grade IV = >75% slip

c. Calcifying discopathy
  - Disease of childhood; not associated with disc herniation
  - Systemic disease: fever, pain, elevated white blood cell, sedimentation rate
  - Cervical and thoracic spine involved
  - Disc height normal or increased
  - Spontaneous resolution of symptoms and calcification in cervical spine

d. Disc herniation
  - Anterior (see limbus vertebra)

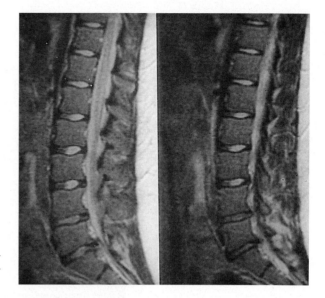

Fig. 2-119 Parasagittal T2-weighted MRI: L5–S1 disc herniation with disruption of hypointense posterior longitudinal ligament.

- Posterior **[Fig. 2-119]**

  Post-traumatic (vehicular, recreational) or spontaneous

  Teenagers

  Lumbar sites same as in adults (typically L4–L5 and L5–S1)

  e. Child abuse
  - Vertebral body compression and spinous process fractures **[Fig. 8-2]**

6. Scoliosis
   a. Lateral curvature of the spine >10 degrees
   b. Described by the location of curvature and direction of convexity
   c. Measurement
      - Find approximate center of curve
      - Identify vertebral body above and below this center farthest from horizontal
      - Draw line along superior endplate of vertebral body at beginning of curve and inferior endplate of vertebral body at end of curve; then draw perpendicular line to each of these lines
      - Angle between the two perpendiculars is angle of scoliosis
      - Accuracy is in the range of 5 degrees on repeat studies
   d. Types of scoliosis
      - Idiopathic scoliosis

        Infantile
        – M > F
        – Thoracic dextroscoliosis

          Usually resolves spontaneously
        – Thoracolumbar levoscoliosis

          Often progresses to severe scoliosis

        Juvenile
        – F > M
        – 4 to 9 years of age

- Thoracic dextroscoliosis
- Frequently progresses to severe scoliosis

Adolescent
- Most common type of scoliosis
- F ≫ M
- Thoracic dextroscoliosis most common, may be accompanied by thoracolumbar or lumbar levoscoliosis
- Isolated levoscoliosis rare in idiopathic adolescent scoliosis
- Likely inherited trait
- Increased incidence, M = F, in congenital heart disease
- Progression variable; depends on severity of curve, age, and rate of progression

- Congenital
  Structural abnormalities
  - Hemivertebrae
  - Vertebral body fusion
    Unilateral = vertebral or pedicle bar
  - Rib fusions
  Thoracic hypoplasia
  Frequently progresses
  Associated with congenital heart disease
- Neuromuscular
  Cerebral palsy
  Muscular dystrophy
  Myopathy
- Posttraumatic
  Radiation
  Postoperative
  Fracture
- Other causes
  NF-1
  - Short, acutely angulated curves common
  Marfan's syndrome
  DDx of short, segment thoracic scoliosis
  - NF-1, Marfan's syndrome
  Skeletal dysplasia

7. Kyphosis
   a. Increased convexity along posterior curvature of spine
   b. >40° in thoracic spine
   c. Causes
      - Scheuermann disease
        Most common cause of kyphosis
        Poorly understood abnormality of vertebral body endplate ossification
        M > F, preteen to teen
        Most commonly mid and lower thoracic spine

Endplate irregularity, disk space narrowing, vertebral body wedging
- Trauma
- Inflammation
- Neuromuscular disorders
  Osteopenia

B. **Spinal Cord**
  1. Development
     a. Cord formed from neuro-ectoderm; infolding of neural plate to form neural tube approximately 20 days gestation
     b. Neural tube separates from overlying ectoderm (skin) by 27 days
     c. Conus medullaris and filum terminale formed by 7 weeks
        - Normal level of conus medullaris is L3 or higher at birth, L2–3 disk space or higher by 3 months after birth

        - US of neonatal spinal column **[Fig. 1-70]**
             Use linear transducer in sagittal projection
             Spinal cord identified as hypoechoic linear structure with three echogenic lines (1 dorsal, 1 central, 1 ventral)
             Conus is acutely angled, triangular hypoechoic structure; once conus identified, feel for 12th rib to identify T12 spinous process.
             Count down along spinous processes to identify level of conus
             Normal variant
             – Ventriculus terminalis **[Fig. 2–120]**
                  Elliptical, focal widening of central canal just above level of conus
  2. Syrinx or syringohydromyelia
     a. Fluid in widened central canal
     b. Secondary to spinal cord tumor, trauma, ischemia, inflammation, or anomalies (Chiari I or II, lipomyelomeningocele, myelomeningocele, diastematomyelia)
     c. MRI
        - Sagittal T1WI and T2WI to define extent of syrinx
        - Axial T1WI to best show size and position of syrinx
        - If cause of syrinx is not apparent, contrast-enhanced T1WI necessary to exclude or identify underlying tumor or inflammation
  3. Spinal dysraphism
     a. Incomplete fusion of midline mesenchymal, bony, and neural structures
     b. Includes spina bifida and myeloschisis
        - Defect may be open or covered by skin
     c. Spina bifida
        - Incomplete fusion of bony spinal axis, anterior, posterior, or both
     d. Myeloschisis
        - Midline cleft of spinal cord
  4. Skin-covered spinal dysraphism **[Figs. 2-121 and 2-122]**
     a. Clinically, tuft of hair, hemangioma, skin thickening or dimple in midline of back, imperforate anus

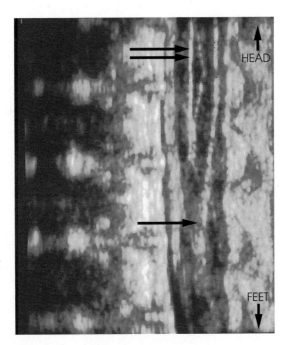

Fig. 2-120 Midline sagittal spine US: Focal widening of central canal (double arrow) just above level of conus medullaris (arrow), which is normal. Ventriculus terminalis, normal variant.

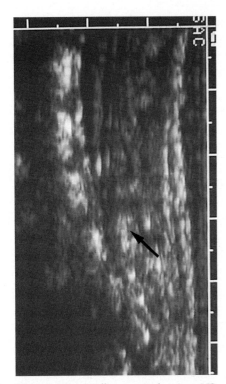

Fig. 2-121 Midline sagittal spine US (oriented in same plane as Figure 2-122): Newborn with small midline hemangioma over lower back. Spinal cord extends to L5 level. Cord intermixed with spinal lipoma (arrow). Tethered cord with lipomyelomeningocele.

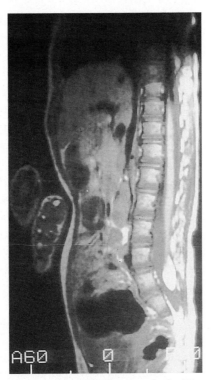

Fig. 2-122 Midline sagittal T1-weighted MRI: Same patient as Figure 2-121. Cord extends to L4–L5 level with hyperintense intraspinal lipoma attached to dorsal cord. Tethered cord with lipomyelomeningocele.

- Usually no neurologic abnormality at birth; neurogenic bowel, bladder dysfunction may be insidious, progressive. Because all infants are incontinent normally, patients with subtle findings above must be identified prior to loss of function. Neurogenic bowel, bladder is not reversible.

b. Radiographically, vertebral segmentation anomalies, sacral dysplasia

c. Image spinal column in newborn by US if a. or b. found

d. If spinal cord abnormal by US (low-lying conus or echogenic intraspinal lipoma), image spinal column by MRI

e. Spinal lipoma, lipomyelomeningocele
- Incomplete separation of cutaneous ectoderm from neuroectoderm
- 20 to 50% of skin-covered spinal dysraphism
- 50% have cutaneous stigmata
- Tethered cord (low-lying conus) common
- US
  - Low-lying conus; echogenic mass at dorsal border of spinal cord, nerve roots may be seen intermingling with fatty mass
  - US can be performed until posterior elements ossified, usually not later than 3 to 6 months of age
- MRI
  - Sagittal T1WI shows bright, fatty intraspinal mass
  - Axial T1WI best to identify associated hydromyelia

f. Meningocele
- Protrusion of meninges + CSF through anterior, posterior or lateral spinal defect
  - Anterior meningocele usually sacral
    - Part of Currarino triad (imperforate anus, sacral dysplasia with crescentic defect, anterior sacral meningocele)
  - Posterior meningocele usually lumbosacral
  - Lateral meningocele in thoracic spine
    - 85% have neurofibromatosis

g. Diastematomyelia **[Fig. 2–123]**
- Sagittal clefting of spinal cord into hemicords
  - One or two separate dural sacs
- Cleft divided by bone, cartilage or fibrous tissue if two dural sacs present
- Females involved in 90%
- Cutaneous stigmata and segmentation abnormalities at level of diastematomyelia; usually thoraco-lumbar
- Clinically, neurogenic bowel, bladder, orthopedic abnormalities
- Radiographs: segmentation abnormalities, bony bridge dividing cleft
- MRI
  - Sagittal imaging to determine cord tethering level
  - Axial T1WI and T2WI to identify hemicords and associated syrinx

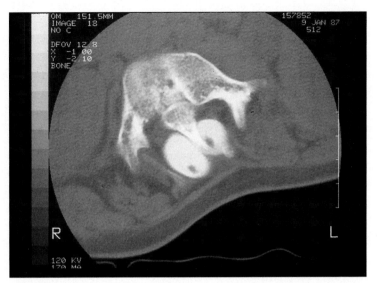

Fig. 2-123 CT myelogram: Two hemicords separated by bony bridge. Diastematomyelia.

       Hemicords reunite to terminate in single filum terminale in 90%

  h. Thick filum terminale
- Normal filum is ≤2 mm at L5–S1
- Cord tethered by thickened filum
- Filum thickened by lipoma in 30% of cases

5. Open spinal dysraphism
  a. Myelomeningocele
- Female predominance, 3:1
- Neural placode (spinal cord tissue) + nerve roots exposed to ambient environment through posterior spinal canal and skin defect
- Fetal US shows widened pedicles, defect; elevated α-fetoprotein level
- Associated with Chiari II malformation; nearly 100% develop ventriculomegaly

6. Neurenteric cyst
  a. Least common type of bronchopulmonary foregut malformation
  b. Communication between GI tract and spinal cord
  c. Vertebral segmentation abnormalities cephalad to defect
- Usually cervico-thoracic vertebral anomalies
  d. Entrapment of enteric lined cyst in neural canal
  e. Associated with thoracic or abdominal GI duplication cyst

7. Caudal regression syndrome
  a. Infants of diabetic mothers (16% of cases)
  b. Partial or complete dysgenesis of lumbosacral spine
  c. Associated with imperforate anus, renal anomalies, pulmonary hypoplasia
  d. Wedge-shaped or blunted conus

8. AVM
   a. Thoracic most common
   b. Clinically, subarachnoid hemorrhage
   c. MRI
      - Serpiginous signal voids represent abnormal vascular structures
9. Inflammation
   a. Epidural abscess
      - *S. aureus* most common; hematogenous spread
      - Thoracic and lumbar spine most common sites
      - Localized back pain, tenderness, fever
      - MRI modality of choice
         Abscess displaces thecal sac
         Signal of abscess different from adjacent CSF
         Gadolinium enhancement with fat suppression to discriminate
            vertebral involvement from fatty marrow
   b. ADEM
      - Postviral or vaccination immune-mediated process
      - Demyelinating inflammation of brain and spinal cord
      - MRI
         Patchy randomly distributed areas of signal hyperintensity on
            T2WI with variable gadolinium enhancement
         DDx: MS
   c. MS
      - Rare in children; occurs in teenagers; female predominance
      - Cervical cord most commonly affected
      - MRI
         Hyperintense lesions on T2WI; may involve ≥3 levels or en-
            tire cord
         Gadolinium enhancement variable, patchy
      - DDx: ADEM, transverse myelitis, infarct, neoplasm
10. Tumor
   a. Sacrococcygeal teratoma **[Fig. 2-124]**
      - Female > male; malignant elements more common in males
         Malignant elements in 10% at birth, 90% at 2 months of age
         Malignancy related to extent of glial tissue in teratoma
      - Composed of ectoderm, mesoderm, endoderm
      - Variable degree of intrapelvic/abdominal extension
         Cross-sectional imaging useful to define extent
   b. Astrocytoma **[Fig. 2-125]**
      - 50 to 60% of intramedullary tumors in children
      - 60% involve entire cord
      - Often contain cysts; secondary syringohydromyelia
      - MRI
         Focal or diffuse cord thickening
         Focal gadolinium enhancement
   c. Ependymoma
      - 20 to 30% of intramedullary tumors in children
      - Lumbosacral usually; may arise from filum terminale

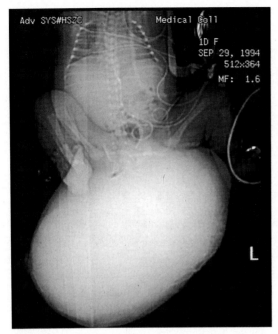

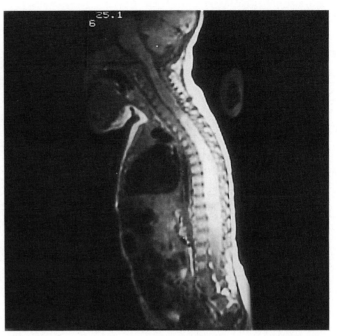

Fig. 2-124 Scoutview from CT: Huge soft tissue mass extends from pelvis and perineum. Sacrococcygeal teratoma.

Fig. 2-125 Gadolinium-enhanced sagittal T1-weighted MRI: Enhancement along long segment of cervical, thoracic, and lumbar cord with syrinx in upper cervical cord. Extensive spinal cord tumor.

- MRI
    May fill neural canal; intensity different than CSF on T1WI and T2WI
    Heterogeneous enhancement
  d. Hemangioblastoma
    - von Hippel-Lindau syndrome
    - Cervicomedullary and cervicothoracic most common sites
    - MRI
      Well demarcated; variable signal reflecting cysts, hemorrhage, signal voids from vascular supply
  e. Neuroblastoma **[Figs. 2-126 and 2-127]**
    - Extends into neural canal through neural foramina at one or multiple levels
    - MRI
      Longitudinal extent best seen on sagittal images
      Involvement into neural foramina best seen on axial images
  f. Neurofibroma
    - Plexiform neurofibroma diagnostic of neurofibromatosis
    - Extends into neural canal through neural foramina at one or multiple levels
  g. Metastasis **[Fig. 2-128]**
    - Most commonly due to drop metastases from intracranial neoplasms
    - Especially from PNETs (such as medulloblastoma or retinoblastoma), ependymoma, glioma
    - Also neuroblastoma, lymphoma, leukemia

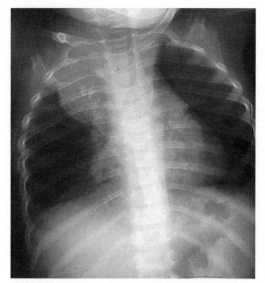

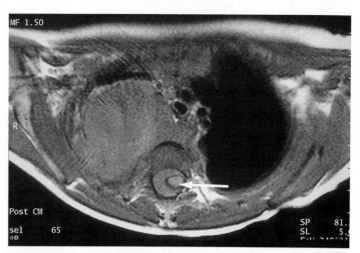

Fig. 2-126 PA chest radiograph: Calcified soft tissue mass in upper right thorax. Note deviation of trachea to left. Thoracic neuroblastoma.

Fig. 2-127 Gadolinium-enhanced axial T1-weighted MRI: Same patient as Figure 2-126. Soft tissue mass in posterior and middle mediastinum with extension across midline. Note deviation of trachea anterior and to left. The mass invades the neural canal and partially surrounds the spinal cord (arrow). Neuroblastoma with intraspinal component.

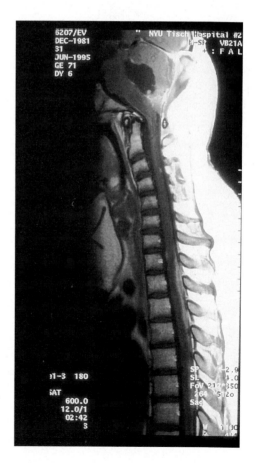

Fig. 2-128 Gadolinium-enhanced sagittal T1-weighted MRI: History of medulloblastoma resection. Enhancement along dorsal thoracic spinal canal, at C3 level, anterior border of pons and dorsal to medulla. Medulloblastoma with meningeal metastases.

- MRI
    Postgadolinium T1WI to identify drop mets
11. Trauma
    a. Spinal Cord Injury WithOut Radiographic Abnormality (SCIWORA)
        - Distraction, hyperextension or hyperflexion of vertebrae + ligamentous injury causing cord contusion, transection
        - Neurologic deficit immediate or delayed (up to 48 hours). Poor prognosis; worst in youngest patients

FURTHER READING

Anon. Atlantoaxial instability in Down syndrome: subject review. Pediatrics 1995;96:151–154.

Anon. National Heart, Lung, and Blood Institute report. Stroke Prevention Trial in Sickle Cell Anemia (STOP). Sept. 18, 1997.

Armington WG, Osborn AG, Cubberley DA, et al. Supratentorial ependymoma: CT appearance. Radiology 1985;157:367–372.

Ball WS Jr., ed. Pediatric Neuroradiology. Philadelphia: Lippincott-Raven; 1997.

Barkovich AJ. MR and CT evaluation of profound neonatal and infantile asphyxia. AJNR. 1992;13:959–972.

Barkovich AJ, Good WV, Koch TK, Berg BO. Mitochondrial disorders; analysis of their clinical and imaging characteristics. AJNR 1993;14:1119–1137.

Barkovich AJ, Naidich TP, ed. Pediatric neuroradiology. Neuroimag Clin N Amer 1994;4:201–455.

Barkovich AJ, Sargent SK. Profound asphyxia in the premature infant: imaging findings. AJNR 1995;16:1837–1846.

Barkovich AJ, Truwit CL. Brain damage from perinatal asphyxia: correlation of MR findings with gestational age. AJNR 1990;11:1087–1096.

Barkovich AJ, Westmark K, Partridge C, et al. Perinatal asphyxia: MR findings in the first 10 days. AJNR 1995;16:427–438.

Becker LE. Lysosomes, peroxisomes, and mitochondria: function and disorder. AJNR 1992;13:609–620.

Belman AL, Lantos G, Horoupian D, et al. AIDS: Calcification of the basal ganglia in infants and children. Neurol 1986;36:1192–1199.

Boesel CT, Paulson GW, Kosnik EJ, et al. Brain hamartomas and tumors associated with tuberous sclerosis. Neurosurg 1979;4:410–417.

Boltshauser E, Wilson J, Hoare RD. Sturge-Weber syndrome with bilateral intracranial calcification. J Neurol Neurosurg Psych 1976;39:429–435.

Brannan TS, Burger AA, Chaudhary MY. Bilateral basal ganglia calcifications visualized on CT scan. J Neurol Neurosurg Psych 1980;43:403–406.

Brunelle FOS, Harwood-Nash DCF, Fitz CR, Chuang SH. Intracranial vascular malformations in children: computed tomographic and angiographic evaluation. Radiology 1983;149:455–461.

Carli J, Perilongo G, Laverda AM, et al. Risk factors in long-term sequelae of central nervous system prophylaxis in successfully treated children with acute lymphocytic leukemia. Med Ped Oncol 1985;13:334–340.

Cavezudo JM, Vaquero J, Garcia-de-Sola R, et al. Computed tomography with craniopharyngiomas: a review. Surg Neurol 1981;15:422–427.

Couvreur J, Desmonts G. Congenital and maternal toxoplasmosis. A review of 300 congenital cases. Devel Med Child Neurol 1962;4:519–530.

Enzmann DR, Ranson B, Normal D, et al. Computed tomography of herpes simplex encephalitis. Radiology 1978;129:419–425.

Ferrari R, DiMauro S, Sherwood G, ed. L-Carnitine and Its Role in Medicine: From Function to Therapy. London: Academic Press; 1992; entire book.

Fielding JW, Hawkins RJ. Atlanto-axial rotary fixation. J Bone Joint Surg 1977;59:37–44.

Garrick R, Gomez MR, Houser OW. Demyelination of the brain in tuberous sclerosis. Mayo Clin Proc 1979;54:685–689.

Golden GS. Stroke syndromes in childhood. Neurol Clin N Amer 1985;3:59–75.

Harley EH, Collins MD. Neurologic sequelae secondary to atlantoaxial instability in Down syndrome: implications in otolaryngologic surgery. Arch Otolaryngol Head Neck Surg 1994;120:159–165.

Jacoby CG, Go RT, Beren RA. Cranial CT of neurofibromatosis. AJR 1980;135:553–557.

Kendall BE. Disorders of lysosomes, peroxisomes, and mitochondria. AJNR 1992; 13:621–653.

Ketonen L, Koskiniemi ML. Gyriform calcification after herpes simplex encephalitis. J Comput Assist Tomogr 1983;7:1070–1072.

Koller WC, Cochran JW, Klawans HL. Calcification of the basal ganglia: computerized tomography and clinical correlation. Neurol 1979;29:328–333.

Kumar R, Guinto FC, Jr., Madewell JE, et al. The vertebral body: radiographic configurations in various congenital and acquired disorders. RadioGraphics 1988;88:455–485.

Legge M, Sauerbrei E, Macdonald A. Intracranial tuberous sclerosis in infancy. Radiology 1984;153:667–668.

Levy SR, Abroms IF, Marshall PC, Rosquete EE. Seizures and cerebral infarction in the full-term newborn. Ann Neurol 1985;17:366–370.

Lorber J. Intracranial calcifications following tuberculous meningitis in children. Acta Radiol 1958;50:204–210.

Lorber J. The incidence and nature of intracranial calcification after tuberculous meningitis. Arch Dis Chld 1952;28:542–551.

Martin E, Barkovich AJ. Magnetic resonance imaging in perinatal asphyxia. Arch Dis Child 1995;72:F62–F70.

McArdle CB, Richardson CJ, Hayden CK, Nicholas DA, Crofford MJ, Amparo EG. Abnormalities of the neonatal brain: MR imaging. Radiology 1987;163:387–403.

McLaurin RL, Towbin RB. Tuberous sclerosis: diagnostic and surgical considerations. Ped Neurosci 1986;12:43–48.

Modic MT, Weinstein MA, Rothner AD, et al. Calcification of the choroid plexus visualized by computed tomography. Radiology 1980;135:369–372.

Murphy MJ. Clinical correlations of CT scan-detected calcifications of the basal ganglia. Ann Neurol 1979;6:507–511.

Mussbichler H. Radiologic study of intracranial calcifications in congenital toxoplasmosis. Acta Radiol 1968;7:369–379.

Noorbehesht B, Enzmann DR, Sullender W, et al. Neonatal herpes simplex encephalitis: correlation of clinical and CT findings. Radiology 1987;162:813–819.

Nordstrom DM, West SG, Andersen PA. Basal ganglia calcifications in central nervous system lupus erythematous. Arthrit Rheumat 1985;28:1412–1416.

Palmieri A, de Vecchio E, Pirolo R, et al. The current potential of neuroradiology in the diagnosis of tuberous sclerosis. Ital J Neurol Sci 1982;3:229–233.

Probst FP, Erasmie U, Nergadh A, et al. CT appearance of brain lesions in tuberous sclerosis and their morphological basis. Ann Radiol 1979;22:171–183.

Quencer RM. Intracranial CSF flow in pediatric hydrocephalus: evaluation with cine-MR imaging. AJNR 1992;13:601–608.

Simopoulous AP, Breslow A. Tuberous sclerosis in the newborn. Amer J Dis Child 1966;111:313–316.

Sims ME, Halterman G, Jasani N, Vachon L, Wu PYK. Indications for routine cranial ultrasound scanning in the nursery. J Clin Ultrasound 1986;14:443–447.

Truwit CL, Barkovich AJ, Koch TK, Ferriero DM. Cerebral palsy: MR findings in 40 patients. AJNR 1992;13:67–78.

Valk J, van der Knaap MS. Magnetic Resonance of Myelin, Myelination, and Myelin Disorders. Berlin: Springer-Verlag; 1989; entire book.

Volpe JJ. Current concepts of brain injury in the premature infant. AJR 1989;153:243–251.

Warkany J, Lemire RJ, Cohen MM. Mental Retardation and Congenital Malformations of the Central Nervous System. Chicago: YearBook Medical Publishers, Inc., 1981:341–346.

Wilkinson HA, Ferris EJ, Muggie AL, et al. Central nervous system tuberculosis: a persistent disease. J Neursurg 1971;34:15–22.

Zatz LM. Atypical choroid plexus calcifications associated with neurofibromatosis. Radiology 1968;91:1135–1139.

Zimmerman RA, Bilaniuk LT. Age-related incidence of pineal calcification detected by computed tomography. Radiology 1982;142:659–662.

I. **ANATOMY AND TERMINOLOGY**
   A. **Terminology [Fig. 3-1]**
      1. Long bones: epiphyses at both ends
      2. Short tubular bones: epiphysis at one end
      3. Round bones: wrists and ankles
      4. Epiphysis: ossification center bordered by articular cartilage
      5. Apophysis: ossification center not bordered by articular cartilage, usually at tendon insertions; also called traction epiphyses
      6. Physis: the growth center of tubular bones
         a. Beginning at the epiphysis, the physis consists of
            - Reserve zone
            - Proliferating zone
            - Hypertrophic zone, consisting of
               Zone of maturation
               Zone of degeneration
               Zone of provisional calcification
      7. Metaphysis: portion of long bone between the shaft and the physis
         a. The metaphysis bordering the physis contains:

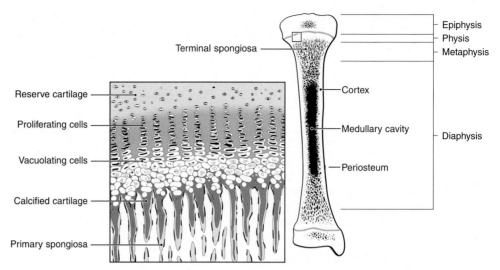

Fig. 3-1   Schematic indicates terminology of typical long bone organization.

- Zone of primary spongiosa
    Adjacent to physis, weakest part of the metaphysis and diaphysis
- Zone of secondary spongiosa
8. Diaphysis: the shaft of a tubular bone
9. Acromelic: bone shortening, most marked in the hands and feet
10. Rhizomelic: bone shortening, proximal greater than distal (femur and humerus)
11. Mesomelic: bone shortening, most marked in the forearms and lower legs (radius and ulna, tibia and fibula)

II. NORMAL DEVELOPMENT

A. Enchondral and intramembranous bone growth

1. Enchondral bone formation
    a. Governed by the physis and affected by disorders of cartilage
    b. Responsible for longitudinal growth of long bones and growth of the skull base
    c. Achondroplasia results in short, thick, long bones, as only enchondral growth is affected
2. Intramembranous bone formation
    a. Not affected by cartilage disorders
    b. Responsible for growth of flat bones
        - Pelvis
        - Cranial vault
    c. Transverse growth of long bones is by intramembranous ossification as bone is laid down by the periosteum (appositional bone)
    d. The majority of bone mass is formed via appositional bone
    e. Osteogenesis imperfecta (OI) results in long, thin bones due to defective intramembranous bone formation
3. Cartilaginous epiphyses initially have blood supply through the physis. These transphyseal vessels disappear by 18 months to 2 years of age. This change in blood supply explains the high incidence of epiphyseal osteomyelitis in infants, which becomes rare after age 2 years.

4. Sharpey's fibers attaching periosteum to bone are fewer and weaker in children than in adults, so periosteal elevation and periosteal new bone formation following trauma or infection occur more frequently in children.

B. **Marrow development**

1. Bone marrow is entirely hematopoietic at birth, progressing in a predictable fashion to mostly fat

2. Marrow conversion occurs first in the epiphyses, then the diaphyses, then the metaphyses

3. Bone marrow infiltration by tumor or infection is difficult to detect with magnetic resonance imaging (MRI) in red marrow **[Fig. 8-8]**

4. During progression from red to yellow marrow, patchy distribution can limit evaluation of bone marrow on MRI

C. **Skeletal maturation**

1. Newborn

   a. First molar appears at 33 weeks, second at 36 weeks

   b. Proximal humeral ossification center appears between 37 weeks post-conception and 4 months of age

2. Less than 1 year of age

   a. Maturation quite variable in first year; all radiographic methods are limited

   b. Sontag method

      • Radiograph one arm from shoulder to fingers and one leg from thigh to toes

      • Assume proximal femoral ossification center present

      • Compare number of ossified centers to standards

3. Over one year of age

   a. Greulich and Pyle standards

      • Anteroposterior (AP) radiograph of left hand and wrist compared to standards

         Approximately 60 well cared-for children in suburban Ohio had their hand and wrist radiographed serially during growth between 1931 and 1942

         The hand and wrist at the midpoint of skeletal maturation for all patients at each age was selected as standard

         Further studies showed that a typical population was less advanced at a given age than the study children. It is therefore necessary to calculate the expected bone age for a child's chronological age and compare the expected bone age with bone age standards.

      • Use Brush Foundation Table in Greulich and Pyle

      • Standards are dated and studies of current children and different ethnic groups are limited; however, this remains the system in use throughout the United States

      • Sontag and Greulich and Pyle standards continue to be useful especially for serial evaluation of children on growth hormone or other therapy

- Method

    Comment on abnormal bones
    - Cone epiphyses
    - Turner tufts
    - Bone density
    - Epiphyses markedly delayed vs. overall appearance suggests epiphyseal dysplasia, even if larger bone epiphyses normal

    Compare to standards of appropriate sex, without knowledge of patient age

    General tips
    - Distal bones are more useful than proximal
    - The wrist is extremely variable, so give it little weight in assessing bone age
    - In very young or nearly mature children, use appearance of ossification centers or fusion of physes
    - Width of epiphyses relative to the metaphyses is very useful
    - Epiphysis of the proximal phalanx of the thumb extends in ulnar direction past the metaphysis, then develops a "hook" as it conforms to the metaphysis. This characteristic distinguishes several standards.

III. **NORMAL VARIANTS FREQUENTLY CONFUSED WITH DISEASE**

A. **Nutrient foramina: lucencies extend through cortex with straight, parallel margins. They extend away from joint central to peripheral. In tibia may be seen as longitudinal central lucency**

B. **Scalloping of medial distal fibula: the distal fibular metaphysis often shows reciprocal shaping from the adjacent tibia. This finding can be confused with a buckle fracture or superficial bone destruction**

C. **Serpentine physes may appear as lucencies suggesting fractures**
    1. Proximal humerus
    2. Proximal tibia

D. **Distal femoral cortical irregularity [Fig. 3-2]**
    1. Posteromedial metaphysis
    2. May have an inferior bone spur suggesting a bone-forming neoplasm
        a. These may appear particularly striking in younger children who resume normal activity after serious illness
    3. Bone scan should not be necessary, but is usually negative

E. **Apophyses of the inferior pubic rami**
    1. These apophyses often ossify asymmetrically
    2. The appearance can suggest either a healing fracture or a bone tumor

F. **Physiological new bone formation**
    1. Occurs between 1 and 6 months of age
    2. Usually a single layer of new bone along diaphyses of long bones
    3. Usually bilaterally symmetrical
    4. Often affects only a portion of the circumference of the bone

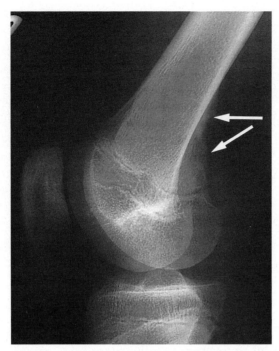

Fig. 3-2 Lateral knee radiograph: Distal femoral irregularity (arrows) along posterior cortex of femoral metaphysis.

G. **Dense metaphyseal bands**
　　1. Affect the zone of provisional calcification
　　2. Most commonly 2 to 6 years of age
　　3. Can simulate lead lines
　　4. Suspected lead ingestion requires biochemical evaluation
　　5. Biochemical evidence of lead ingestion without lead lines suggests recent rather than long-term ingestion
H. **Developing epiphysis may be irregular**
　　1. Acetabulum
　　2. Irregular ossification of medial distal femoral epiphysis
I. **Dorsal defect of patella**
　　1. Superolateral dorsal lucency in the patella
　　2. Frequent sclerotic margins
J. **Calcaneal apophysis**
　　1. Normally denser than adjacent bone
　　2. Frequently fragmented appearance
　　3. This normal appearance has been called Sever's disease (nondisease)
K. **Calcaneal pseudocyst [Fig. 3-3]**
　　1. Lack of trabeculae cause decreased bone density in the anterior calcaneus at its narrowest point
　　2. The margin may be slightly sclerotic
L. **Apophysis at base of fifth metatarsal (MT)**
　　1. A longitudinal physis separates this frequently flake-like apophysis from the shaft

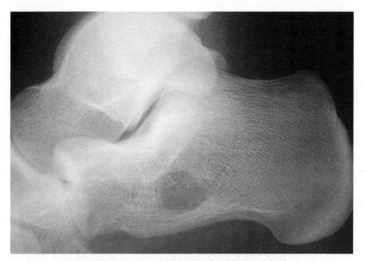

Fig. 3-3 Lateral ankle radiograph: Well-defined lucent appearance in region of calcaneus typical of calcaneal pseudocyst.

2. Especially on oblique views, this frequently appears displaced. Fractures in this area are almost always transverse; lack of overlying soft tissue swelling supports no focal trauma

IV. **BONE DYSPLASIAS: RADIOGRAPHIC ASSESSMENT**
   A. **Approach to bone dysplasia**
      1. Obtain a complete skeletal survey
      2. Evaluate the spine, the epiphyses, the metaphyses, the pelvis, and the chest for features of dysplasia syndromes
   B. **Spine**
      1. Vertebral bodies
         a. Small, oval or pear shaped
            - Spondyloepiphyseal dysplasia (infants)
            - Mucopolysaccharidoses
         b. Flattened
            - Thanatophoric dysplasia
            - Osteogenesis imperfecta
         c. Interpediculate distance does not increase caudally
            - Achondroplasia
            - Hypochondroplasia
         d. Scoliosis
            - Spondylometaphyseal dysplasia
   C. **Epiphyses**
      1. Small (compare hands with Greulich and Pyle standards)
         a. Spondlyoepiphyseal dysplasia
         b. Multiple epiphyseal dysplasia
         c. Hypothyroidism
   D. **Metaphyses**
      1. Flared and irregular
         a. Rickets
         b. Hypophosphatasia
         c. Metaphyseal chondrodysplasias

2. Flared and regular
   a. Achondroplasia

E. **Pelvis**
   1. Flat acetabular roofs
      a. Achondroplasia
      b. Ellis van Creveld
      c. Jeune syndrome
      d. Thanatophoric dysplasia
   2. Trident acetabular roofs (acetabular roof has sharp lateral points and broader central protrusion)
      a. Ellis van Creveld
      b. Jeune syndrome
      c. Thanatophoric dysplasia
   3. "Wine glass pelvis"
      a. Morquio's
   4. Small
      a. Campomelic dysplasia

F. **Chest**
   1. Short ribs
      a. Jeune syndrome
      b. Ellis van Creveld

G. **Limbs**
   1. Limb shortening
      a. Rhizomelic
         • Achondroplasia
         • Rhizomelic chondrodysplasia punctata
      b. Mesomelic
         • Osteochondromatosis (bayonet forearm)

H. **Hand**
   1. Radial ray anomalies
      a. Holt-Oram
      b. Fanconi anemia
      c. Thrombocytopenia-absent radius
   2. Carpal fusions
      a. Ellis van Creveld
   3. Turner tufts: tufts of distal phalanges as wide as base—strongly suggests Turner syndrome
   4. Cone epiphyses: physis V-shaped, with central portion of adjacent epiphysis projecting into the metaphysis
      a. Frequent normal variant when isolated, especially distal phalanx thumb or middle phalanx fifth digit
      b. Abnormal if seen in proximal phalanges
      c. Associations
         • Acrodysostosis
         • Achondroplasia
         • Multiple epiphyseal dysplasia
         • Spondyloepiphyseal dysplasia

- Pseudohypoparathyroidism
- Trichorhinophalangeal dysplasia

I. **Are there any associated abnormalities?**
1. Cardiac
2. Hematopoietic

J. **Were the abnormalities noted at birth, or later in life?**

V. **SPECIFIC BONE DYSPLASIAS**

A. **Osteochondrodysplasias affecting growth of tubular bones and spine (identifiable at birth)**
1. Achondroplasia **[Fig. 3-4]**
   a. Most common bony dysplasia
   b. Autosomal dominant
   c. Symmetrical shortening of long bones
   d. Metaphyseal flaring, frequent shallow V configuration
   e. Large brachycephalic cranium with small foramen magnum
      - Communicating hydrocephalus due to small foramen magnum or venous obstruction at jugular foramen **[Fig. 2-69]**
   f. Interpediculate distance does not increase caudally in lumbar spine
   g. Narrow sacrosciatic notch, flat acetabular roofs
2. Thanatophoric dysplasia **[Fig. 3-5]**
   a. Marked rhizomelic shortening of long bones
   b. "Telephone receiver" femurs

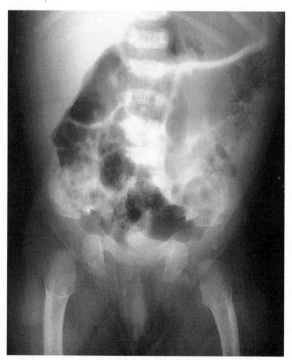 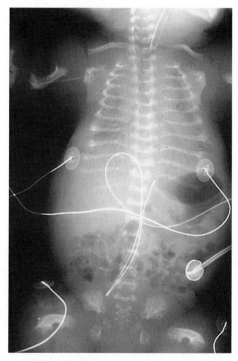

Fig. 3-4 AP radiograph of pelvis: Narrowed interpediculate distance (between pedicles), which should become progressively wider from L1 to L5, narrowed sacrosciatic notch, and abnormal proximal femora, which look like "ice cream scoops." Achondroplasia.

Fig. 3-5 AP babygram: Marked shortening of all bones, femur that resembles a "telephone receiver," and marked platyspondyly. Vertebral bodies look like an "H" or "U." Thanatophoric dysplasia.

    c. Flattening of vertebral bodies

    d. Small square iliac wings

3. Chondrodysplasia punctata **[Fig. 3-6]**

    a. Stippling likely results from in-utero insult

    b. Bone shortening and delayed appearance of ossification centers are seen later

    c. Rhizomelic form (autosomal recessive)

      • Rhizomelic shortening of extremities, especially humeri

      • Stippled calcifications of epiphyses and respiratory cartilage

      • Cleft vertebrae without stippling

      • Cataracts

    d. Conradi-Hünermann form (autosomal dominant)

      • More variable and less severe than recessive form

      • Stippling usually less marked than recessive form

4. Spondyloepiphyseal dysplasia congenita **[Figs. 3-7 and 3-8]**

    a. Infancy

      • Short limbs may be identified in utero

      • Retarded skeletal ossification

      • Abnormally small vertebral bodies, largest lower thorax, smallest cervical and sacral spine

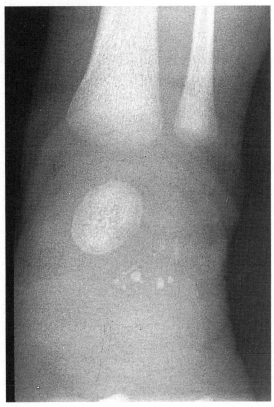

Fig. 3-6 AP ankle radiograph: Stippled ossification centers. Stippled epiphyses.

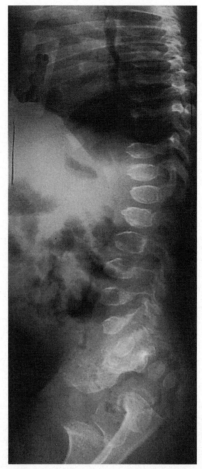

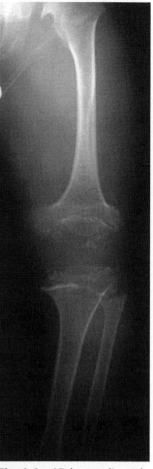

Fig. 3-7 Lateral thoracolumbar spine radiograph: Irregular platyspondyly with variable "beaking." Spondyloepiphyseal dysplasia.

Fig. 3-8 AP knee radiograph: Fragmentation of epiphyses, flaring of metaphyses. Spondyloepiphyseal dysplasia.

   b. Childhood
- Flattening, immaturity, and irregular ossification of vertebral bodies
- Odontoid hypoplasia
- Retarded pelvic and proximal femoral ossification
- Horizontal acetabular roofs
- Rhizomelic limb shortening
- Variable retarded and irregular epiphyseal metaphyseal ossification of long tubular bones

   c. Adult
- Severe spinal shortening, severe kyphoscoliosis
- Platyspondyly and irregular anterior endplates
- Marked coxa vara, high-riding femoral trochanter
- Normally located, deformed femoral head
- Relatively normal hands/feet

5. Asphyxiating thoracic dystrophy (Jeune syndrome) **[Figs. 3-9 and 3-10]**
   a. Short horizontal ribs

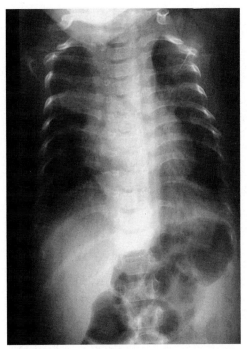

Fig. 3-9 AP chest radiograph: Short ribs, elongated chest compared to transverse chest diameter. Asphyxiating thoracic dystrophy (Jeune syndrome).

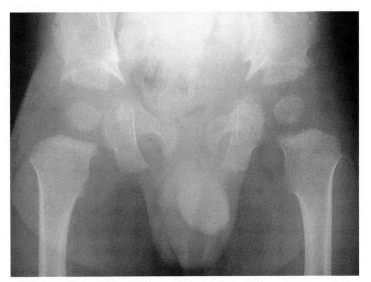

Fig. 3-10 AP pelvis radiograph: Trident pelvis. Differential diagnosis includes thanatophoric dysplasia, asphyxiating thoracic dystrophy, chondroectodermal dysplasia.

    b. Tubular thorax often with flaring of lowest ribs

    c. Flat acetabular roofs with medial and lateral, and rarely central, spikes

    d. "Bicycle handlebar" clavicles—the clavicles are long and convex upward

6. Chondroectodermal dysplasia (Ellis–van Creveld syndrome)

    a. Autosomal recessive

    b. At birth

      • Thorax similar to asphyxiating thoracic dystrophy

      • Trident pelvis

      • Shortening of tibia and fibula and the radius and ulna

      • Postaxial polydactyly of hands

      • Small exostosis from medial proximal tibia

    c. Later life

      • Pelvis becomes less abnormal over time

      • Fusion of carpals

      • Dental dysplasia

7. Cleidocranial dysplasia

    a. Delay in cranial ossification

    b. Hypoplastic clavicles, only rarely completely absent

    c. Delayed ossification of pubis and femoral necks with development of coxa vara

    d. Biconvex vertebral bodies persist into childhood

B. **Osteochondrodysplasias affecting growth of tubular bones and spine (identifiable in later life)**
1. Hypochondroplasia
    a. Underdiagnosed, findings frequently subtle
    b. Short stature with relatively long trunk and disproportionately short limbs
    c. Skull is normal, other findings suggest very mild achondroplasia
    d. Interpediculate distances decrease in lumbar spine less than in achondroplasia
    e. Lack of increasing interpediculate distance may be only abnormality
    f. Lordotic lumbosacral junction
2. Multiple epiphyseal dysplasia
    a. Identified after 2 years of age
    b. Small, dense, irregular epiphyses appear late
    c. Symmetrical, not universal involvement
    d. Tubular bones normal or slightly short
    e. Minimal spinal involvement
3. Metaphyseal chondrodysplasia **[Fig. 3-11]**
    a. Difficult to identify at birth or after skeletal maturity
    b. Best identified at young school age
    c. Flared and irregular metaphyses
    d. Schmid type most common
        • Coxa vara
        • Growth plate widening
        • Autosomal dominant
    e. McKusick type
        • Cartilage-hair hypoplasia

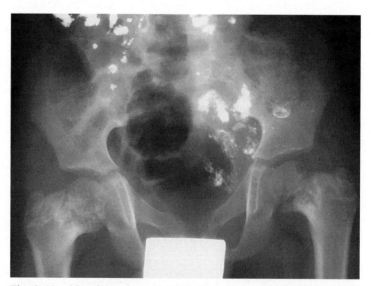

Fig. 3-11 AP pelvis radiograph: Widening of growth plate and irregularity of proximal femoral metaphyses. Metaphyseal chondrodysplasia.

- Sparse light hair, severe short-limbed dwarfism
- Autosomal recessive

   f. Jansen type
- Marked widening of physes that then fill in with irregular dense bone
- Lower extremities more affected than upper with genu varum
- Autosomal dominant

   g. Schwachman-Diamond type
- Short-limbed dwarfism
- Exocrine pancreatic insufficiency
- Cyclic neutropenia to pancytopenia

C. **Osteochondrodysplasias with disorganized development of cartilage and fibrous components of the skeleton**
   1. Osteochondromatosis or multiple hereditary exostoses **[Fig. 3-12]**
      a. Autosomal dominant
      b. Diaphyseal aclasia (lack of modeling) = dwarfism
      c. "Bayonet hand" in one-third due to ulnar shortening
      d. May cause pressure on nerves, vessels, spinal cord
      e. Bony masses protruding from bone at metaphysis, angled away from joint
      f. Cortex and medulla contiguous with normal bone
      g. Cartilage cap acts as growth center
      h. Most common at rapid growth areas (especially knees)
      i. Arise after birth and by 10 years of age
      j. Growth ceases with adjacent physis closure
      k. Malignant transformation (2% solitary, 15% multiple) extremely rare in childhood
      l. In most cases of multiple exostoses, more than one exostosis is seen on the radiograph that revealed the first exostosis
      m. If concern persists, normal AP of both knees excludes multiple hereditary exostoses
   2. Enchondromatosis (Ollier's disease) **[Fig. 3-13]**
      a. Sporadic inheritance
      b. Excessive hypertrophic cartilage from physis progresses into the medullary cavity at the metaphyses
      c. Multiple expansile, lucent lesions ± stippled central calcification
      d. Epiphyses frequently malformed
      e. One side of body more affected than the other
      f. Lesions heal after puberty, deformity may persist
      g. Malignant degeneration variably reported, from rare to 40%
      h. Other types described
- Acroform (hands and feet)
- Ray form
- Oligotropic (few, near joint)

   3. Maffucci syndrome
      a. Enchondromatosis associated with cavernous hemangiomas
      b. High incidence of malignancies

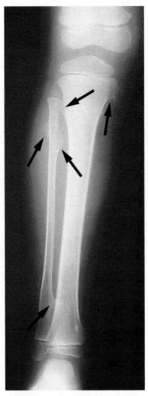

Fig. 3-12 AP lower extremity radiograph: Multiple exostoses (arrows). Osteochondromatosis.

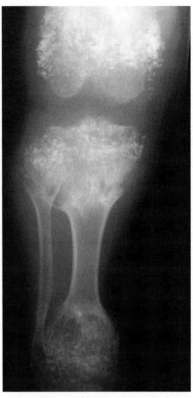

Fig. 3-13 AP lower extremity radiograph: Marked shortening of lower leg, abnormal chondroid material in widely flared metaphyses. Enchondromatosis.

4. Polyostotic fibrous dysplasia
   a. One-fourth of all patients with fibrous dysplasia have polyostotic disease
   b. 2 to 3% of these have McCune-Albright syndrome
      • Polyostotic fibrous dysplasia
      • Unilateral or markedly greater involvement on one side
      • Cafe-au-lait spots with irregular margins: "coast of Maine"
      • Precocious puberty
5. Neurofibromatosis
   a. Ribs: wavy contour, irregular sclerosis
   b. Extremities: pseudoarthroses at fracture sites
      • Occurs with 10% of fractures
      • Distal tibia most common site
   c. Bone dysplasia has a variable appearance
      • Mottled appearance and increased cortical thickness common
   d. Loose periosteum results in increased size and frequency of subperiosteal bleeds with trauma
      • Elevated periosteum then forms bone resulting in soft-tissue calcification
D. **Abnormalities of density of cortical diaphyseal structure and metaphyseal modeling**
   1. Osteogenesis imperfecta (OI) **[Fig. 3-14]**

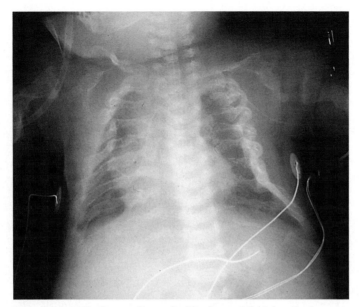

Fig. 3-14 AP chest radiograph: Newborn. Multiple rib fractures, deformity of both humeri due to previous fractures. Osteogenesis imperfecta.

a. Fractures, osteopenia and gracile bones, wormian bones
b. Type 1
  • Blue sclerae
  • Moderate osteopenia
  • Decreased fractures after puberty
c. Type 2
  • Lethal form
  • Extensive fractures at birth
  • Bones may be short and broad or gracile
  • Stillborn or neonatal demise
d. Type 3
  • Variable bony deformity
  • Moderate bony fragility
  • Normal sclerae
e. Type 4
  • Mild to moderate bony fragility
  • Normal sclerae
f. OI vs. child abuse
  • Sporadic type 4 mutation can present as child abuse. Definitive diagnosis is by fibroblast culture to evaluate collagen
  • This mutation is extremely rare; estimates suggest one case per century in an urban center
2. Osteopetrosis **[Figs. 3-15 and 3-16]**
  a. Congenital
    • Dense sclerosis of bones with poorly formed marrow cavity and poor modeling
    • Metaphyseal lucencies may suggest rickets
    • Bone within bone appearance, especially spine

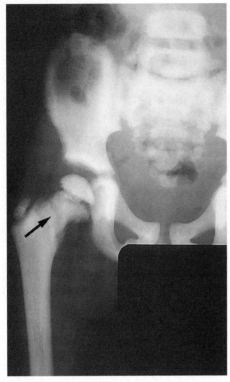

Fig. 3-15 AP pelvis radiograph: Diffusely sclerotic bone. Despite sclerosis, the bone is actually soft, indicated by intertrochanteric right hip fracture (arrow). Osteopetrosis.

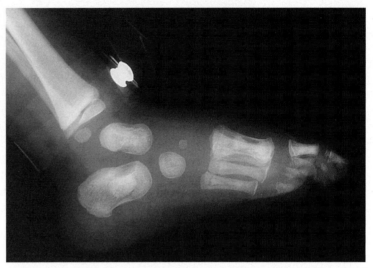

Fig. 3-16 Lateral foot radiograph: "Bone within bone" appearance of metatarsals, talus, and calcaneus. Osteopetrosis.

- Abnormal skull base may narrow foramina causing neurologic sequelae
- Bone is dense but fragile; frequent fractures as child grows
  b. Tarda
    - Often discovered incidentally
    - Milder findings, otherwise similar to congenital form
    - Tarda form may represent multiple different disorders with similar manifestations

E. **Limb reduction anomalies**
  1. Proximal focal femoral deficiency **[Fig. 3-17]**
    a. Type A: Femoral head within normal acetabulum, bony continuity between femoral shaft and head
    b. Type B: Femoral head within normal or dysplastic acetabulum, no bony continuity between shaft and head
    c. Type C: Femoral head absent or present as small ossicle, severely dysplastic acetabulum
    d. Type D: Absent femoral head and acetabulum
  2. Radial ray anomalies **[Fig. 3-18; see also Fig. 1–37]**
    a. VATER (Vertebral defects, Anal atresia, TracheoEsophageal fistula with esophageal atresia, and Radial and/or Renal anomalies) or VACTERL association (VATER + Cardiac + Limb anomalies)

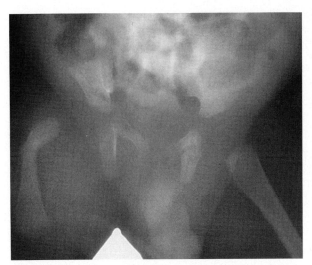

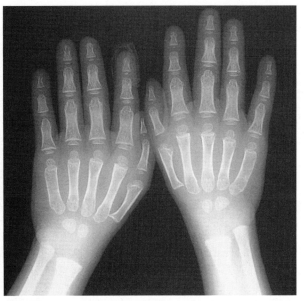

Fig. 3-17 AP pelvis radiograph: Hypoplastic, deformed proximal right femur. Femoral heads are not ossified. Shallow, dysplastic right acetabulum. Proximal focal femoral deficiency.

Fig. 3-18 AP hand radiograph: Patient with Fanconi anemia. Hypoplasia of first metacarpal and thumb. Radial ray anomaly.

    b. Thrombocytopenia absent radius (TAR) syndrome
- Thumb present
- Absent radius with radial angulation of hand on short upper arm
- Transient thrombocytopenia

    c. Holt-Oram syndrome
- Upper limb anomaly and congenital heart disease
- Thumb always abnormal, but not necessarily absent

    d. Amniotic band syndrome
- Exact cause uncertain
- Occurs in utero, no familial pattern
- Usually transverse unilateral or asymmetric soft tissue constricting bands
- May see bony amputation, syndactyly, distal deformity, or soft tissue calcification

F. **Congenital bowing deformities and pseudoarthroses**
  1. Campomelic dysplasia
    a. Bowed bones, usually proximal long bones
    b. Affects upper rather than lower extremities
    c. Enlarged and elongated skull
    d. Small scapulae
  2. Neurofibromatosis

G. **Mucopolysaccharidoses [Fig. 1–36]**
  1. Hunter/Hurler syndrome **[Fig. 3-19]**
    a. Enlarged skull, thick diploic space
    b. Mandible short, broad with missing condyles
    c. Persistence of infantile biconvexity of vertebrae
    d. Anterior, inferior beaking of vertebra at thoracolumbar junction

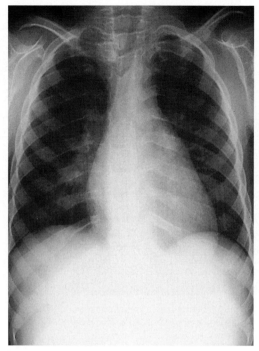

Fig. 3-19 PA chest radiograph: Broad ribs with medial narrowing ("oar-shaped ribs"). Hurler syndrome.

      e. Ribs paddle-shaped (broad anteriorly, narrow posteriorly)
      f. Lack of diaphyseal modeling
      g. Sloping ends of radius and ulna
      h. Pointing of proximal metacarpals
      i. Hurler: autosomal recessive, corneal opacities
      j. Hunter: X-linked recessive, no corneal clouding, less severe than Hurler's

  2. Morquio's
      a. Autosomal recessive
      b. Normal intelligence
      c. Platyspondyly, hooked vertebrae
      d. Odontoid hypoplastic, possible C1-C2 instability
      e. Flared iliac wings with narrow base ("wine-glass" configuration)
      f. Pointing of proximal metacarpals
      g. Genu valgum
      h. Failure of ossification of lateral proximal tibial epiphysis and metaphysis

VI. **THE PEDIATRIC ELBOW**
  A. **Order of appearance of ossification centers in elbow–CRITOE [Fig. 1-47]**
    1. Order is more consistent and important than age
      a. Capitellum: 2 years
      b. Radial head: 3 years

c. Internal epicondyle: 4 years

d. Trochlear: 8 years

e. Olecranon: 9 years

f. External epicondyle: 10 years

2. Absent ossification center in injured elbow may indicate displaced fracture.

a. Comparison radiograph of opposite elbow useful.

B. **Fat pads [Fig. 1-48]**

1. Anterior

a. Normally seen

b. Usually closely applied to the angle between humerus and ulna

c. When elevated by joint fluid or thickening, forms a thorn or sail appearance

2. Posterior

a. Seen only when displaced by joint space

b. Oblique lateral view can obscure fat pad

3. Positive posterior fat pad sign in elbow trauma should be treated as occult fracture

4. Synovial hypertrophy can cause positive posterior fat pad sign in absence of trauma

a. Juvenile rheumatoid arthritis (JRA)

b. Hemophilia

C. **Lines of the elbow**

1. Anterior humeral line

a. A line drawn along the anterior humeral cortex intersects the middle third of the capitellum

b. Abnormal in displaced supracondylar fractures

c. Capitellum displacement is posterior in 95%

2. Radiocapitellar line

a. A line drawn along the midline of the proximal radial shaft should intersect the capitellum on all views, including oblique radiographs

b. Abnormal in Monteggia fracture/dislocation and radial head dislocation

VII. **THE PEDIATRIC FOOT**

A. **Lateral talocalcaneal angle**

1. Normal = 25 to 50 degrees

2. Angle between midline of talus and inferior margin of calcaneus

3. AP angle dependent on technique and difficult to obtain reliably, so rely on lateral measurement

a. Decreased = hindfoot varus

b. Increased = hindfoot valgus

B. **Pes equinus**

1. Toe walking foot

2. Angle between the long axis of the tibia and the inferior margin of the calcaneus >90 degrees with dorsiflexion

C. **Pes calcaneus**

1. Angle between the long axis of the tibia and the inferior margin of the calcaneus <55 degrees

D. **Pes planus**
   1. Lines drawn along the inferior margin of the calcaneus and the inferior fifth metatarsal make an angle near 0 degrees

E. **Pes cavus**
   1. A line drawn along the inferior margin of the calcaneus and the inferior fifth metatarsal is <150 degrees

F. **Metatarsus adductus**
   1. Lateral calcaneal margin should parallel lateral margin of fifth metatarsal
   2. On AP view convex lateral angulation of the lateral margin of the calcaneus and the fifth metatarsal indicates metatarsus adductus

G. **Club foot (talipes equinovarus) [Fig. 3-20]**
   1. Congenital abnormality, etiology unknown; may be related to fetal positioning
   2. Components
      a. Equinus
      b. Metatarsus adductus
      c. Hindfoot varus

H. **Congenital vertical talus [Fig. 3-21]**
   1. Talocalcaneal angle >65 degrees
   2. True vertical talus distinguished from oblique talus by lateral maximal plantarflexion radiograph demonstrating the navicular anterior to dorsal margin of talus

I. **Tarsal coalition**
   1. Classically causes a stiff painful flat foot
   2. Usually an isolated abnormality
   3. 50% between calcaneus and navicular

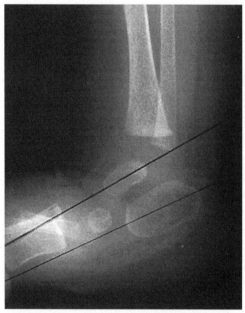

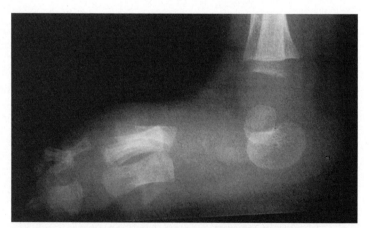

Fig. 3-20 Lateral ankle radiograph with forced dorsiflexion: Nearly parallel relationship between talus and calcaneus. Hindfoot varus, club foot.

Fig. 3-21 Lateral foot radiograph: Perpendicular relationship between talus and calcaneus. Hindfoot valgus, vertical talus.

4. 45% between talus and calcaneus
5. Can be bony or fibrous
6. Plain radiographs
   a. Calcaneonavicular coalition has elongated anterosuperior calcaneus on oblique radiographs
   b. In fibrous union see bony irregularity and decreased distance between calcaneus and navicular
   c. Talocalcaneal coalition shows a convex upward sclerotic line in the calcaneus below the middle talocalcaneal facet
7. Definitive diagnosis with computed tomography (CT), thin sections in axial and coronal plane

VIII. **DEVELOPMENTAL DYSPLASIA OF HIP (DDH)**
- This term is more accurate than congenital hip dislocation
- Dysplasia is frequently not present at birth
- Incidence of clinical DDH 1:1000
- Incidence of unstable exam in infants 1:100
  Therefore, only small percentage of unstable clinical exams have DDH
- Very rarely, may develop in initially normal children

A. **Clinical evaluation of the hip**
   1. Typical DDH occurs in otherwise normal infants
   2. Teratologic DDH is secondary to underlying neuromuscular disorder
   3. Hip ultrasound (US) approach discussed refers to typical DDH
   4. Barlow maneuver
      a. Flex and abduct hip while applying posterior pressure with the pelvis immobilized
      b. Causes unstable hip to dislocate
   5. Ortolani maneuver
      a. Flex and abduct hip while applying anterior pressure to femoral head
      b. Relocates dislocated mobile hip
      c. Useful primarily in infants age 1 to 2 months

B. **Imaging evaluation [Figs. 1–71 and 1–72]**
C. **Lines of the infant pelvis [Fig. 3–22]**
   1. Y-Y line of Hilgenreiner-horizontal line through triradiate cartilages
      a. Provides a baseline for comparison of acetabulae
   2. Perkin's line perpendicular to Y-Y line at lateral margin of acetabular roof
      b. The medial margin of the femoral neck should lie medial to Perkin's line
   3. Acetabular angle—angle between a line drawn along the acetabular roof and Y-Y line
   4. Shenton's line—curve drawn along the medial femoral neck and the lower margin of the superior pubic ramus
      a. Superior or lateral migration of the femur disrupts the continuity of this line
      b. Very sensitive for displacement in infants
      c. Less reliable in older children

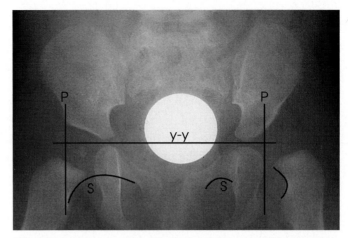

Fig. 3-22 AP pelvis radiograph: Shallow left acetabulum with oblique roof. Note sclerosis in supra-acetabular region of iliac wing (pseudo-acetabulum). Normal right femoral head has ossified; the abnormal left femoral head is not yet ossified. Lines of pelvis: Y-Y line of Hilgenreiner (Y-Y), Perkins line (P), Shenton's line (S). Note continuity of Shenton's line on right and discontinuity on left. Hip dysplasia.

D. **Hip US**
- Hip US accurately demonstrates the cartilaginous acetabulum, the labrum, and the femoral head
- Findings can be used to decide follow-up and treatment
- Examination has both static and dynamic components
  1. Static **[Figs. 3-23 through 3-28]**
     a. Coronal images with evaluation of morphology and measurement of angles
     b. Morphology distinguishes types
     c. Angle measurements distinguish subtypes, aid when morphology is intermediate between types
     d. Angle measurements
        - Baseline drawn along the straight line of the supraacetabular ilium
        - Alpha angle
          Angle between baseline and line drawn along bony acetabular roof **[Figs. 3-24 and 3-26]**
          Reflects acetabular formation
          Higher number indicates better formed acetabulum
          Most useful angle
        - Beta angle
          Angle between baseline and line drawn from promontory through labrum **[Figs. 3-24 and 3-26]**
          Reflects cartilage covering femoral head
          Lower number indicates better cartilage position
          Less useful than alpha angle
     e. Type 1 **[Fig. 3-24]**
        - Normal appearance

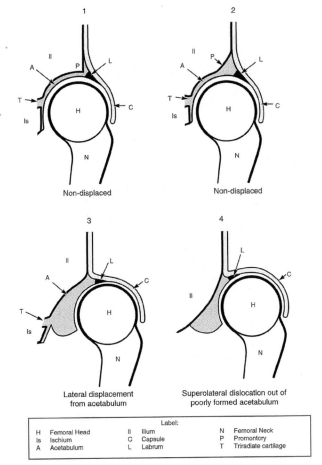

Non-displaced   Non-displaced

Lateral displacement
from acetabulum

Superolateral dislocation out of
poorly formed acetabulum

Label:					
H	Femoral Head	Il	Ilium	N	Femoral Neck
Is	Ischium	C	Capsule	P	Promontory
A	Acetabulum	L	Labrum	T	Triradiate cartilage

Fig. 3-23 Schematic of coronal hip US indicating Graf hip types.

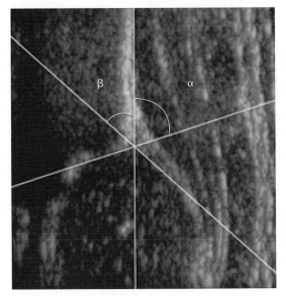

Fig. 3-24 Coronal hip US displayed in vertical orientation. Compare with Figure 3-23: Graf Type 1 hip. α angle = 71 degrees; β angle = 49 degrees.

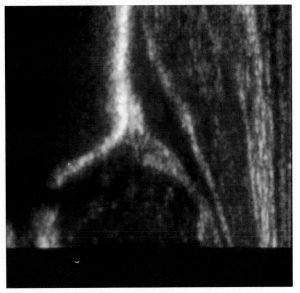

Fig. 3-25 Coronal hip US displayed in vertical orientation. Compare with Figure 3-23: Graf Type 2 hip.

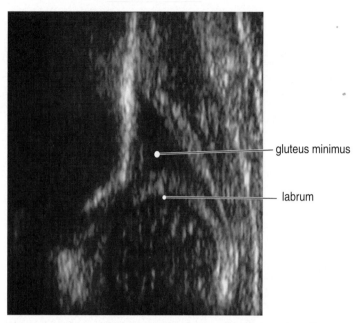

gluteus minimus

labrum

Fig. 3-26 Coronal hip US displayed in vertical orientation. Compare with Figure 3-23: Graf Type 3a hip. Note that the long axis of the iliac crest (vertical echogenic line) is medial to the midpoint of the femoral head. Larger white dot indicates gluteus minimus muscle; smaller white dot indicates tip of labrum.

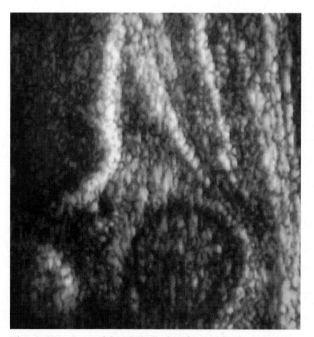

Fig. 3-27 Coronal hip US displayed in vertical orientation. Compare with Figure 3-23: Graf Type 3b hip.

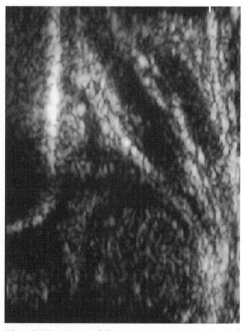

Fig. 3-28 Coronal hip US displayed in vertical orientation. Compare with Figure 3-23: Graf Type 4 hip.

- Angular promontory, acetabular depth ≥50% femoral head diameter, cartilage/labrum thin, covering femoral head
- α ≥60 degrees, β ≤55 degrees
- Dysplasia is very unlikely to develop in a child with type 1 morphology

f. Types 2A and 2B **[Fig. 3-25]**
- Rounded promontory, acetabular depth ≥50% femoral head diameter, cartilage/labrum thin or mildly thickened, covering >50% of femoral head
- α 50 to 59 degrees, β >55 degrees
- 2A: <3 months of age
  Frequently becomes normal on follow-up
  No treatment
  Repeat US in 6 weeks
  No further evaluation if type 1 on follow-up
- 2B: >3 months
  Progression possible if untreated
  Treat with abduction harness

g. Type 2C
- Morphology as 2A and B, but more severe rounding of promontory
- α 43 to 49 degrees, β 56 to 77 degrees
- Will likely progress if untreated
- Treat with reduction/abduction splint

h. Type 2D
- Identified best by dislocatablility on dynamic testing rather than specific morphology
- Usual features: rounded or flattened promontory, variable acetabular depth, cartilage/labrum elevated
- α 43 to 49 degrees, β 56 to 77 degrees
- Very likely to progress to complete dislocation
- Reduction/abduction splint until reduced followed by casting, or inpatient treatment

i. Type 3
- Abnormally located femoral head at rest, but still contiguous with acetabulum
- Shallow acetabulum with no well-defined promontory; broad short cartilage extends over medial portion of femoral head
- α <43 degrees, β >77 degrees
- 3A: Hypoechoic acetabular roof cartilage **[Fig. 3-26]**
- 3B: Hyperechoic acetabular roof cartilage **[Fig. 3-27]**
- Reduction/abduction splint until reduced followed by casting, or inpatient treatment

j. Type 4
- Dislocated hip **[Figs. 3-28 and 3-29]**
- Femoral head completely separate from minimally formed acetabulum; acetabular roof cartilage lies between femoral head and ilium

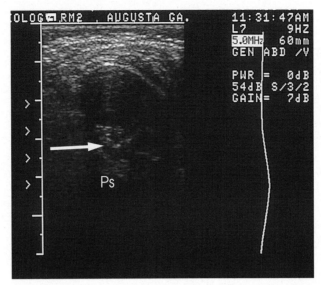

Fig. 3-29 Transverse hip US: Dislocated femoral head displaced from pseudoacetabulum (Ps) by echogenic fibrofatty material (arrow).

- Type 4 capsule forms an acute angle between the ilium and the femoral head, unlike all other types where capsule forms smooth line extending caudad from the ilium to cover femoral head
- Appearance of capsule best distinguishes type 4 from type 3
- α <43 degrees, β >77 degrees
- Inpatient treatment

2. Dynamic **[Figs. 3-30 through 3-32]**
   a. Transverse imaging while attempting to gently dislocate hip posteriorly with pressure on the knee and thigh
   b. Anterior traction can be used to attempt to relocate a dislocated hip
3. Combining static and dynamic examinations allows determination of hip type and planning of therapy

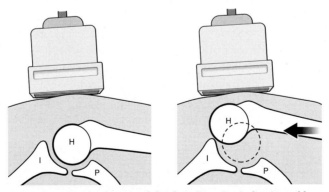

Fig. 3-30 Hip developmental dysplasia: Drawing indicating subluxation of femoral head overlying posterior lip of acetabulum during stress maneuver.

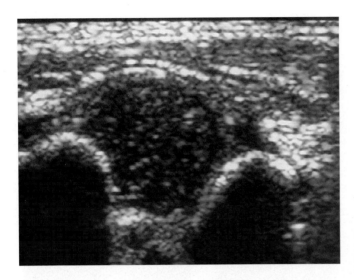

Fig. 3-31 Transverse hip US: At rest, the femoral head is normally located within the acetabulum, anterior to the posterior rim of the acetabulum. DDH.

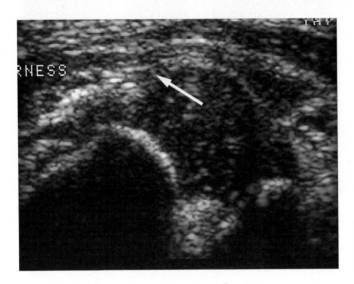

Fig. 3-32 Transverse hip US: Same patient as Figure 3-31, with stress applied. Femoral head has moved (arrow) laterally and posteriorly, and now partially overlies the posterior acetabular rim. DDH, subluxable hip.

IX. **INFECTION**

    A. **Pyogenic osteomyelitis**

        1. General

            a. Bacteria lodge in terminal capillaries of metaphyses, making metaphyses or metaphyseal equivalents the most common site of osteomyelitis

            b. Elevated sedimentation rate in almost all cases

        2. Imaging

            a. Radiographic changes **[Figs. 3-33 and 3-34]**

                • Deep soft tissue swelling may be seen several days after initial infection

                • Bone changes of focal demineralization may be seen as early as one week after infection. Periosteal new bone first seen 10 to 14 days after infection.

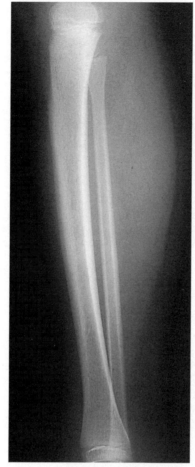

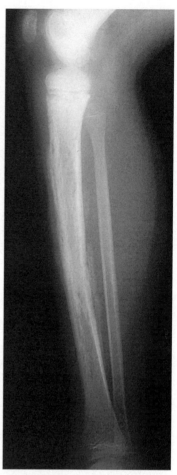

Fig. 3-33 Lateral lower leg radiograph: Deep soft-tissue swelling posterior to tibia. Early osteomyelitis.

Fig. 3-34 Lateral lower leg radiograph: Follow-up radiographic in same patient as in Figure 3-33. Motheaten appearance of tibia with disruption of periosteal reaction. Osteomyelitis.

- Lack of bone changes up to 3 weeks after infection does not exclude the diagnosis.
- Bone changes progress despite effective therapy

b. Radionuclide imaging **[Fig. 3-35]**
- Immediate (blood pool) and 2 hour images distinguish osteomyelitis from cellulitis
- Cellulitis shows diffuse increased activity on immediate (blood pool) images and increased activity in the soft tissues on delayed images.
- Hyperemia usually results in mild diffuse increased bone activity in cellulitis
- Osteomyelitis shows more focal increased activity in the bone on immediate images and localized increased bone activity with little soft-tissue activity on delayed images.
- Decreased activity in bone may indicate site of infarction due to increased intramedullary pressure due to infection

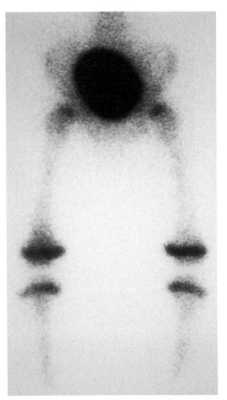

Fig. 3-35 Technetium-99m bone scan: Tri-angular area of uptake in distal femoral metaphysis. Osteomyelitis.

- Radionuclide imaging remains diagnostic at least 72 hours after effective antibiotic therapy is begun
  c. US imaging
    - Useful to demonstrate subperiosteal pus and site for biopsy/aspiration
  d. CT scanning
    - Best demonstrates devascularized isolated bone fragments (sequestra), which must be surgically removed
  e. MRI **[Fig. 3-36]**
    - As sensitive and specific as bone scanning
    - Normal marrow signal in older children virtually excludes osteomyelitis
    - MRI frequently identifies other causes of symptoms in patients who do not have osteomyelitis
3. Age-related features of osteomyelitis
  a. Infants
    - *Staphylococcus aureus (S. aureus)* most common, Group B *streptococcus* and gram negative organisms
    - Frequent multifocal disease with septic arthritis **[Fig. 3-37]**
      Often presents as fever without source
      Flat bones involved in 20%
  b. Older children
    - 90% *S. aureus*

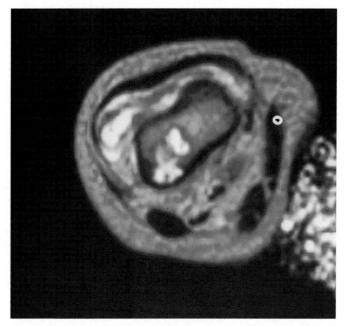

Fig. 3-36 Axial T2-weighted MRI through distal femur: Hyperintense lesion within medullary cavity and endosteal cortex with surrounding hyperintense edema. Neonatal osteomyelitis.

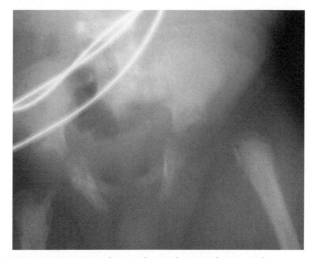

Fig. 3-37 AP pelvis radiograph: Newborn with sepsis. Marked displacement of left femur from acetabulum. Note irregularity of left acetabulum and demineralization of proximal femur. Neonatal osteomyelitis with septic hip dislocation.

- *Salmonella* increased in children with sickle cell anemia (but still less frequent than *S. aureus*)
- Long segment diaphyseal osteomyelitis in children with sickle cell anemia almost always caused by *Salmonella* **[Fig. 8-15]**
- It can be very difficult to differentiate osteomyelitis from bone infarction in sickle cell disease

4. Septic arthritis **[Fig. 3-38]**
  a. Secondary to bacteremia, not osteomyelitis

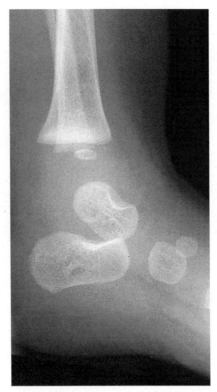

Fig. 3-38 Lateral ankle radiograph: Marked soft tissue swelling involving ankle joint with distortion of fat plane anterior to talus and tilting of talus on calcaneus. Septic arthritis.

   b. Infants—*S. aureus*

   c. Young children—*Haemophilus influenzae*

   d. Rare after first decade of life

   e. Hip—*S. aureus*

   f. Ultrasound most reliable indicator of effusion **[Figs. 3-39 and 3-40]**

   g. Transphyseal vessels present at birth disappear by 18 months to 2 years of age

   h. Epiphyseal bone changes with infection in children >2 years old suggest septic arthritis rather than osteomyelitis

   i. Bone scanning demonstrates increased activity on both sides of joint

   j. Increased activity differentiates septic arthritis from transient synovitis of the hip, but aspiration indicated if other clinical findings strongly suggest infection

B. **Tuberculosis**

   1. In long bones originates in epiphyses and rapidly extends to joints

   2. Isolated osteomyelitis extremely rare

   3. Dactylitis can occur in up to 10% of infants and young children with tuberculosis

   4. Bony expansion with soft tissue swelling classic

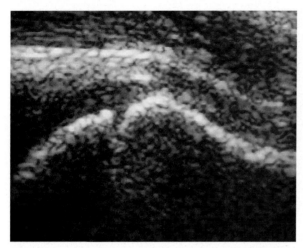

Fig. 3-39 US of hip joint: Soft tissues are closely approximated to hyperechogenic cortex of proximal femur. Normal hip US; no effusion present.

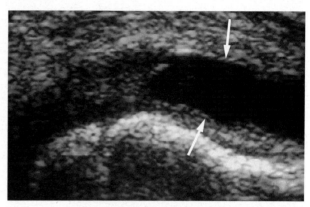

Fig. 3-40 US of hip joint: Soft tissues are displaced from hyperechogenic cortex of proximal femur by hypoechoic hip joint effusion (between arrows). Septic arthritis.

C. **Syphilis**
  1. Infantile
      a. Congenital syphilis is due to transplacental migration of spirochetes
      b. Blood-borne spirochetes most numerous during early infection, so congenital syphilis most likely due to maternal infection during pregnancy
      c. Bone changes probably require 6 weeks to appear and may therefore not be present at birth
      d. Multifocal metaphyseal lucencies frequently seen at birth
      e. "Sawtooth metaphysis" is not universal but is highly specific
      f. Wimberger sign later in infancy—destroyed areas of the medial tibial metaphysis **[Fig. 3-41]**
      g. Diffuse periostitis occurs after the first month
      h. These changes usually heal without sequelae
  2. Juvenile
      a. Diffuse or focal subperiosteal thickening of the cortex of the diaphyses
      b. Destructive lesions and periosteal reaction occur
  D. **Congenital infection**
  1. TORCH, especially cytomegalovirus and toxoplasmosis
  2. Longitudinal striation of metaphyses: "celery stalk" appearance
  3. Metaphyses irregular but not cupped
  4. Epiphyses irregular with frayed margins
  5. No periosteal new bone formation (as opposed to syphilis)
  6. Bone changes disappear by 6 months of age
X. **OTHER INFLAMMATORY CONDITIONS**
  A. **Toxic synovitis or transient synovitis of the hip**
  1. Development of noninfectious effusion
  2. Accompanied by pain and limp
  3. Children usually <10 years of age
  4. Ultrasound confirms fluid

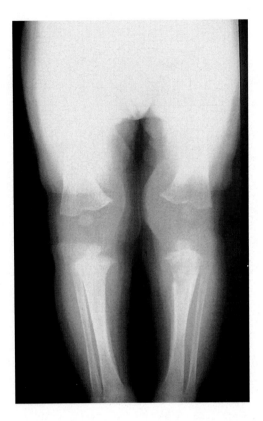

Fig. 3-41 AP lower extremities radiograph: Metaphyseal rarefaction; lytic lesion in proximal left tibia (Wimberger sign). Congenital syphilis.

5. Aspiration required to exclude septic arthritis
6. Nuclear medicine study usually normal; increased activity suggests septic arthritis

B. **JRA [Figs. 3-42 and 3-43]**
   1. Groups have different joint involvement, different clinical courses, and different immunogenetics
   2. Radial rather than ulnar drift of fingers
   3. 1 to 4% mortality
   4. Systemic
      a. 1/2 <5 years of age, M = F
      b. Spiking fevers 103 to 105°C
      c. 90% salmon rash
      d. 50% develop destructive polyarthritis
      e. Frequent growth retardation
   5. Polyarticular rheumatoid factor negative
      a. 1 to 3 years of age, M:F = 2:1
      b. Large and small joints
      c. Slowly progressive polyarticular inflammation
   6. Polyarticular rheumatoid factor positive
      a. Late school age to adolescence, F ≫ M
      b. Like adult rheumatoid arthritis (RA)
      c. Aggressive, destructive, polyarticular involvement
   7. Pauciarticular, early
      a. <5 years of age, F:M = 4:1

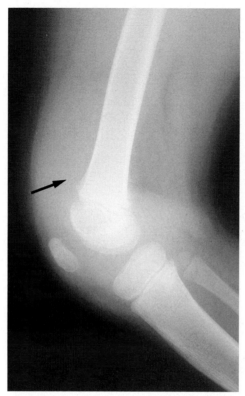

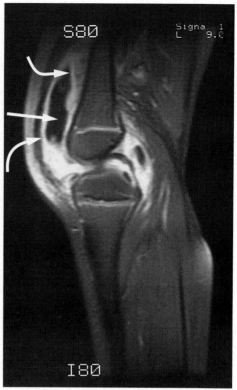

Fig. 3-42 Lateral knee radiograph: Fluid and/or soft tissue distends or thickens suprapatellar bursa (arrow). Prefemoral fat is obliterated. Soft tissue swelling also involves posterior portion of knee joint. JRA.

Fig. 3-43 Gadolinium-enhanced axial T1-weighted MRI: Same patient as in Figure 3-42. Non-enhancing fluid collection (arrow) and enhancing synovium/pannus (curved arrows). JRA. T1-weighted MRI with gadolinium enhancement can differentiate between soft tissue thickening or mass and fluid component or cyst.

      b. Large joints (knee, ankle, wrist, elbow); if small joints expect progression

      c. Develop limb length discrepancies

      d. 40% evolve to polyarticular course

    8. Pauciarticular, late

      a. >8 years of age

      b. M ≫ F

      c. Large weight bearing joints

      d. Probably a spondyloarthropathy

C. **Hemophilic arthropathy**

    1. Intraosseous hemorrhage

      a. Focal, well-defined lucent lesions within bone

    2. Changes due to intraarticular hemorrhage **[Fig. 3-44]**

      a. Chronic inflammation causes increased blood flow

      b. Epiphyses enlarge and fuse prematurely

      c. Cartilage destruction secondary to synovial overgrowth can be focal or diffuse

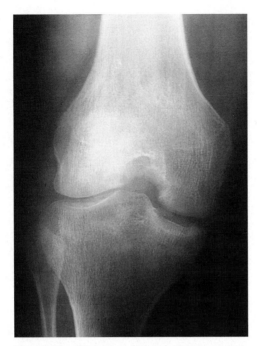

Fig. 3-44 AP knee radiograph: Square appearance of intercondylar notch. Differential diagnosis includes hemophilia and JRA.

XI. **BONE TUMORS**
  A. **Radiographic evaluation of bone tumors**
   - Aggressive vs. nonaggressive is more accurate than malignant vs. benign
     Osteomyelitis is an aggressive lesion that is not malignant
     Indolent malignancies can have a nonaggressive appearance
   - Evaluation of margin, periosteal reaction, and soft-tissue mass useful in determining aggressive vs. nonaggressive
   - Matrix and location are useful in suggesting cell-type-specific lesions
   - MRI provides a very useful evaluation of marrow involvement and soft-tissue extent, but
   - MRI appearance is far less specific than plain film appearance
   1. Margins
     a. Nonaggressive
       - Sclerotic **[Fig. 8-19]**
       - Sharply defined
     b. Aggressive
       - Ill-defined
       - Geographic
       - Motheaten **[Fig. 1-42]**
       - Permeative
   2. Periosteal new bone **[Fig. 1-38]**
     a. Nonaggressive **[Figs. 1-39 and 1-40]**
       - Thick, inseparable from underlying cortex
       - Thick wavy layer separate from underlying cortex

    b. Indeterminate
- Single thin layer
  Benign periosteal reaction of infancy is an important normal variant with this appearance

    c. Aggressive
- Several thin layers (onion skin) **[Fig. 1-41]**
- Thin layers increasing in number toward the lesion, but destroyed overlying the lesion (Codman triangle) **[Figs. 1-42 and 1-43]**
- Perpendicular to the cortical surface of bone (sunburst)

3. Soft-tissue mass, disruption of fat planes
    a. Aggressive **[Fig. 1-43]**

4. Matrix
    a. Osseous—cortical bone density
- Osteoma
- Osteoid osteoma
- Osteoblastoma
- Osteosarcoma
- Parosteal sarcoma

    b. Cartilage—snowflake, comma, speckled/stippled
- Osteochondroma
- Enchondroma
- Chondrosarcoma
- Chondroblastoma
- Chondromyxoid fibroma

    c. Fibrous—ground glass
- Fibrous dysplasia
- Bone cysts
- Fibroma, myxofibroma
- Nonossifying fibroma
- Fibrosarcoma

5. Location
    a. Epiphyseal
- Chondroblastoma

    b. Metaphyseal
- Infection
- Osteosarcoma

    c. Crossing the physis
- Giant cell

    d. Diaphyseal
- Ewing sarcoma

B. **Specific skeletal neoplasms**
1. Tumors of cartilage
    a. Osteochondroma
- Exophytic cartilaginous growths
  Improper modeling of growth plate persisting at metaphyseal periosteal surface produces bone growing outward from metaphysis
- Covered by cartilage cap; may have overlying bursa
- Continuous cortex with underlying bone

- Grows as long as growth plate is open
- More axial location, greater likelihood of malignant degeneration

b. Osteochondromatosis, or hereditary exostoses
  - See dysplasia section
c. Enchondroma
  - Anomalous rests of cartilage in endosteal cavity of metaphysis
  - Grows until growth plate of parent bone fuses
  - Well-defined lytic lesion in endosteal cortex of metaphysis or upper diaphysis
  - Stippled calcification may be seen in lytic lesion
  - More axial the location, greater likelihood of malignant degeneration
d. Chondrosarcoma
  - Malignant; chondroid matrix
  - Most arise from preexisting enchondromas or osteochondromas
  - Intramedullary type present as lytic destructive lesions ± stippled calcification
  - Extraosseous type does not destroy bone; shows proliferation of tumor attached to bone
  - Intramedullary more malignant than extraosseous type
e. Chondroblastoma **[Fig. 3-45]**
  - Benign; chondroblasts, nests of cartilage, giant cells
  - Adolescents
  - Lytic epiphyseal lesion; rarely locally aggressive with cortical breakthrough
  - Rarely metastasizes
f. Chondromyxoid fibroma
  - Benign; chondroblasts, myxomatous cartilage, fibrous tissue
  - Lytic; arises in lower metaphysis

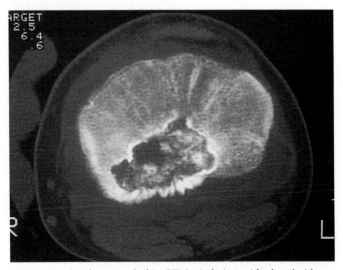

Fig. 3-45 Axial proximal tibia CT: Lytic lesion with chondroid matrix in epiphysis. Chondroblastoma.

- Dense sclerotic rim; may expand cortex
- Rarely degenerates to chondrosarcoma or fibrosarcoma
2. Tumors of osteoid origin
   a. Osteoma
      - Benign, localized overgrowth of bone.
      - Skull and paranasal sinuses
      - Consider Gardner's syndrome
   b. Osteoid osteoma **[Fig. 3-46]**
      - Lesion composed of connective tissue with a central nidus of osteoid tissue <1 cm in size
      - Lucent cortical lesion with marked surrounding sclerosis
      - If intracapsular, no sclerosis, associated with joint effusion
      - Presents with localized pain, classically relieved by aspirin
      - 90% <21 years old
      - Tibia and femur most common
   c. Osteoblastoma
      - >2 cm in size
      - Debate exists whether this is a large osteoid osteoma or a different lesion
      - Benign; metaphyseal; osteoid-producing lesion
      - Frequently have giant cells, vascular component
      - Vertebral column and sacrum, especially posterior elements
      - Lytic, destructive, expansile, tendency to recur if incompletely removed
   d. Osteosarcoma **[Figs. 3-47 and 3-48; see also Figs. 1-42 and 1-43]**
      - Most common primary malignancy of bone

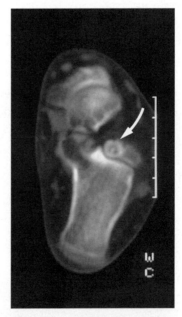

Fig. 3-46 Axial ankle CT: Target-like lesion (arrow) in talus. Note central nidus, adjacent sclerosis in calcaneus. Osteoid osteoma, talus.

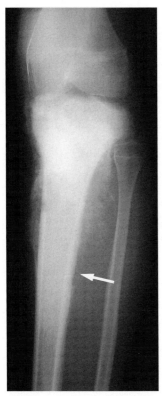

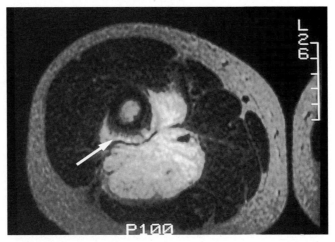

Fig. 3-47 AP knee radiograph: Sclerotic lesion of tibia with osteoid tumor new bone formation in soft tissues. Note disruption of periosteum (arrow). Osteosarcoma.

Fig. 3-48 Axial STIR MRI: Hyperintense abnormal signal in marrow and in soft tissues and muscle surrounding bone. Notice spiculated appearance of periosteum (arrow). Osteosarcoma.

- Central type is most common
- Pain and swelling are common, systemic illness is rare
- Most common about knee (70%), followed by proximal humerus
- 90% are metaphyseal, 10% diaphyseal
- Most common in second decade of life
- May occur in preexisting lesions such as fibrous dysplasia, giant cell tumor, and osteochondroma and following radiation
- Radiographic appearance: bone destruction mixed with sclerosis and tumor new bone formation
- 90% show tumor bone outside normal bone margin
- Rarely atypical appearance; entirely lytic or expansile bubbly lesion
- Aggressive periosteal reaction
- Metastases to lung frequent; may calcify, cavitate
- Skeletal metastases in 15% of patients involving flat bones such as ribs, skull, and vertebra
- Other types
  Parosteal or juxtacortical osteogenic sarcoma
  - Broad based extension of dense bone from cortex
  - Diaphyseal; most commonly distal femur

- Frond-like peripheral margin
- Less aggressive than central, older age group
- Parosteal sarcoma: central calcification
- Myositis ossificans: peripheral calcification

Telangiectatic
- Resembles aneurysmal bone cyst

Periosteal
- Rare
- Presents as cortical thickening

3. Giant cell tumor
   a. Tumor of osteoclasts
   b. >90% occur after physeal closure
   c. Lytic, sharply defined nonsclerotic margin
   d. Extends from metaphysis into epiphysis
   e. Locally aggressive, rarely metastatic
   f. High recurrence rate
   g. Knee, radius, ulna, sacrum

4. Fibrocystic and fibrous disease of bone
   a. Bone cyst **[Fig. 3-49]**
      - Metadiaphyseal
      - Lytic; smooth, slightly sclerotic border
      - Two-thirds to three-fourths in proximal humerus or femur
      - Two-thirds have pathologic fracture

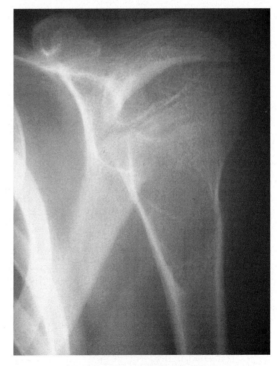

Fig. 3-49 AP shoulder radiograph: Lytic lesion of proximal humerus with pathologic fracture. Bony spicule within lytic lesion ("fallen fragment sign"). Unicameral bone cyst.

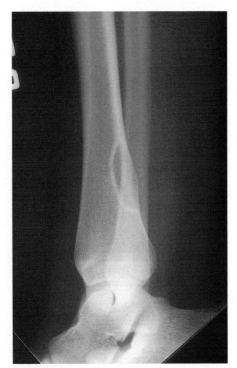

Fig. 3-50 Lateral ankle radiograph: Well-defined lytic lesion with sclerotic border along posterior metadiaphysis of distal tibia. Nonossifying fibroma.

- May see fragment in dependent part of cyst: fallen fragment sign
- Called "simple cysts" of bone, often appear multilocular

b. Fibroma, myxofibroma
- Benign, fibrous lesion
- Same location and appearance as bone cyst

c. Nonossifying fibroma **[Fig. 3-50; see also Fig. 1-76]**
- Benign, cortically based lesion
- Lytic with surrounding sclerosis in metadiaphysis
- Fibrous stroma, scattered xanthoma and giant cells
- Fills in and may appear diffusely sclerotic in older teens

d. Fibrosarcoma
- Malignant; metadiaphysis-diaphysis; very rare in children

e. Fibrous dysplasia **[Fig. 3-51]**
- Proliferation and maturation of fibroblasts ("woven bone")
- Classically described as "ground glass," but has widely variable appearance
- Expansile, scalloping of inner cortex
- Femoral neck involvement causes "Shepherd's crook" deformity
- Can cause pseudoarthroses
- Skull: expanded sclerotic outer table, little involvement inner table, may obliterate sinuses, cranial nerve foramina
- Most common cause of expansile focal rib lesion
- Malignant degeneration rare

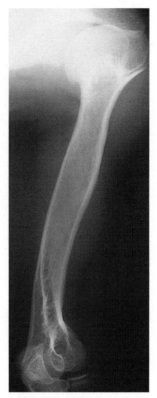

Fig. 3-51 AP humerus radiograph: Abnormal modeling of humeral shaft and neck, "ground glass" appearance in medullary cavity, thin cortex. Fibrous dysplasia.

    f. Polyostotic fibrous dysplasia, McCune-Albright syndrome
- See dysplasia section
5. Round cell tumors of bone
    a. Ewing's sarcoma **[Figs. 1–41 and 2–112]**
- Second most common primary malignancy of bone
- Patients are frequently systemically ill
- Pain and swelling are common
- Most common 5 to 15 years of age
- 90% involve diaphysis of bone, 10% involve metaphysis
- Most frequently femur, pelvis, tibia, humerus
- Two-thirds involve lower extremity and pelvis
- Typical radiographic appearance: permeative appearance of bone with laminated periosteal new bone formation

       60% lytic

       25% lytic with sclerotic reactive new bone

       15% sclerotic

       Codman triangle caused by interruption of laminated periosteal new bone is suggestive but not specific for Ewing's
    b. Neuroblastoma/leukemia **[Figs. 3-52 and 3-53; see also Fig. 8-11]**
- Leukemia: skeletal involvement in children in 50 to 70%

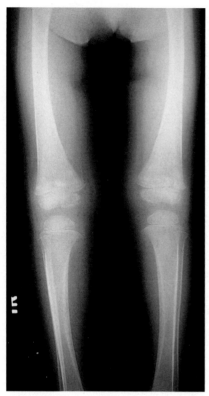
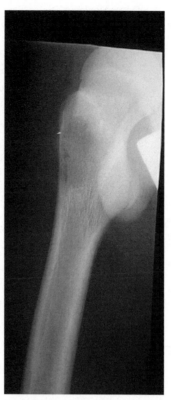

Fig. 3-52 AP lower extremity radiograph: Poorly-defined metaphyseal lucencies best seen in proximal tibial metaphyses. Leukemia.

Fig. 3-53 AP hip radiograph: Ill-defined poorly marginated lytic lesion in proximal femur. No tumor new bone formation. Leukemia.

- Lucent metaphyseal bands (transverse), osteolysis, osteosclerosis (unusual), subperiosteal new bone formation
- Also periosteal new bone formation, "moth-eaten pattern"
- Neuroblastoma findings identical to leukemia

c. Lymphoma
- Mixed lytic-sclerotic

d. Langerhans cell histiocytosis of bone (LCH) **[Fig. 3-54; see also Fig. 8-19]**

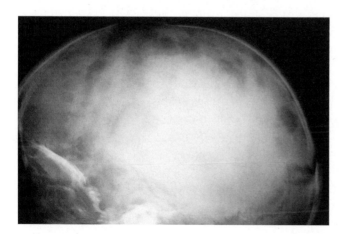

Fig. 3-54 Lateral skull radiograph: Numerous lytic lesions in calvaria producing geographic pattern. LCH.

- Previously called histiocytosis X
- Old classification
  - Letterer Siwe disease
    - Infants with disseminated disease
    - Wasting, lymphadenopathy, anemia
    - Bone lesions rare
  - Hand-Schüller-Christian disease
    - Young children
    - Multiple bony lesions, especially skull, frequently mastoids
    - Diabetes insipidus
  - Eosinophilic granuloma
    - Focal bony lesion
- Current classification
  - Restricted LCH
    - Skin rash alone
    - Bone lesions not involving more than two bones or two lesions in one bone
    - May have rash or localized lymphadenopathy, diabetes insipidus
  - Extensive LCH
    - 2a: visceral involvement without organ dysfunction
    - 2b: visceral involvement with organ dysfunction
- Bone lesions of LCH
  - Round/oval or geographic lesions of skull, beveled edges due to greater involvement of outer than inner table
  - Lytic lesions of metaphysis and diaphysis of long bones ± sclerosis
  - Periosteal new bone common, may see sequestra
  - Skull > long bones > ribs > pelvis > spine responsible for 90%
  - Mandible 2%, but "floating teeth" suggest LCH

6. Vascular lesions of bone
   a. Angiomas
      - Hemangioma, hemangiopericytoma, hemangiosarcoma
      - Usually multiple focal lytic defects
      - Angiomatous tumors can cross joint spaces to involve contiguous bones
   b. Aneurysmal bone cyst **[Fig. 3-55]**
      - Two-thirds associated with preexisting lesion, such as simple bone cyst, fibroxanthoma, chondroblastoma, giant cell tumor
      - One-third of cases have no underlying bone lesion
      - Lytic, bubbly-appearing, expansile, benign
      - MRI shows hematocrit levels in cysts
   c. Metastatic tumors to bone in children
      - Rhabdomyosarcoma
      - Retinoblastoma
      - Primitive neuroectodermal tumor (PNET)
      - Osteosarcoma

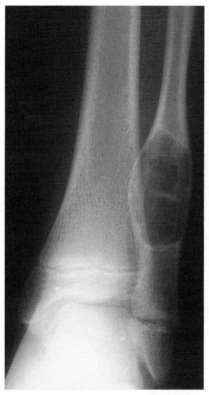

Fig. 3-55 AP ankle radiograph: Expansile, bubbly, lytic lesion of distal fibula. Margin is well-defined. Aneurysmal bone cyst.

- Ewing sarcoma
- Wilms' tumor (<5%; unfavorable histology)
- Present with metaphyseal rarefaction, rarely focal lytic lesions
- Diffuse periosteal new bone can be seen

XII. TRAUMA

A. Physeal fractures

1. The surrounding tendons and ligaments are more than twice as strong as the physis
2. Physeal fractures are more common than sprains in children
3. Physeal fractures can result in growth deformity after fractures heal **[Fig. 3-56]**
4. Salter-Harris (SH) classification **[Fig. 3-57]**
   - Increasing grade correlates with increasing risk of deformity
   - Risk of deformity also varies by joint. Risk of deformity in SH II distal femur >> distal radius
   a. SH I:
      - Fracture through the physis only **[Fig. 3-58]**
      - If nondisplaced, focal soft-tissue swelling suggests diagnosis
      - May be completely radiographically occult
      - Deformity is rare
   b. SH II:
      - Fracture through physis then obliquely through the metaphysis;

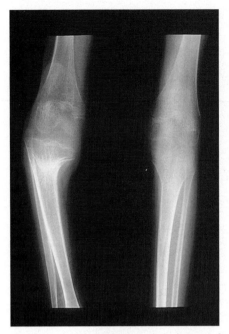

Fig. 3-56 AP knee radiograph: Tethering of growth plate centrally in proximal tibial physis due to previous fracture. Note effect on growth of tibia as well as generalized osteopenia. Physeal growth disturbance.

the physeal fracture extends through most of the physis **[Figs. 3-59 and 3-60]**

- Deformity is more common than with SH I, but still unusual

c. SH III:
- Fracture through a portion of the physis, then longitudinally through the epiphysis **[Fig. 3-61]**
- The physeal fracture is limited to the physis bordering the epiphyseal fracture fragment
- The fragment must be reduced into near anatomic position, otherwise deformity or degenerative change may occur
- Distal tibia is most common site

d. SH IV:
- Fracture extends through epiphysis, physis, and metaphysis **[Figs. 3-62 and 3-63]**

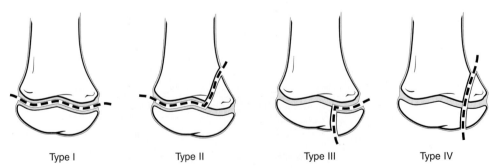

Type I   Type II   Type III   Type IV

Fig. 3-57   Schematic drawing indicating Salter-Harris fractures, Types I-IV.

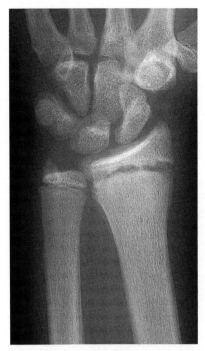

Fig. 3-58 AP wrist radiograph: Irregular widening of growth plate in distal radius. Compare with normal growth plate width in ulna. Salter I fracture.

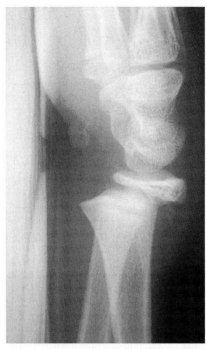

Fig. 3-59 Lateral wrist radiograph: Fracture through growth plate of distal radius with displacement. Note small ossified metaphyseal component attached to epiphysis. Salter II fracture.

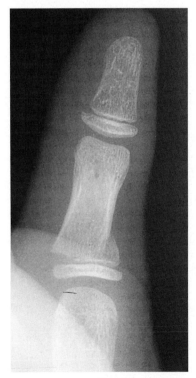

Fig. 3-60 AP thumb radiograph: Angulated Salter II fracture of proximal phalanx of thumb.

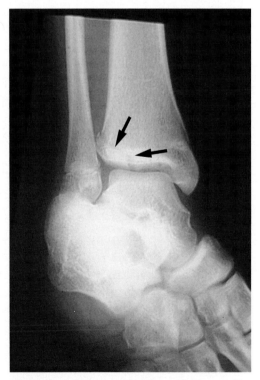

Fig. 3-61 Oblique ankle radiograph: Fracture line through growth plate and epiphysis (arrows). Salter III fracture.

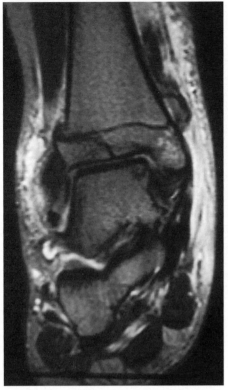

Fig. 3-62 Coronal T2-weighted MRI of ankle: Fracture through metaphysis, growth plate, and epiphysis in sagittal plane. Note high signal hemorrhage or edema in surrounding soft tissues and medial malleolus. Salter IV fracture.

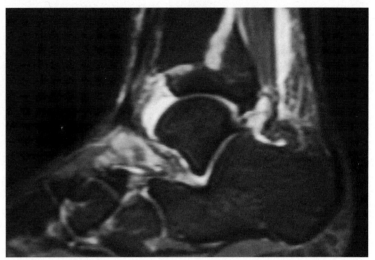

Fig. 3-63 Sagittal STIR MRI of ankle: Same patient as in Figure 3-62. Fracture through anterior growth plate and coronal fracture through metaphysis of distal tibia. Note high signal hemorrhage or edema in ankle joint anterior to talus ("tear drop sign"). Salter IV fracture, triplane fracture.

- Lateral condyle of the humerus is most common site
- Open reduction usually required to avoid deformity

e. SH V:
- Fracture of physis that destroys growth potential
- Occult at time of injury
- Identified only by growth failure following injury
- Extremely rare
- Additional classes are less frequently used

f. SH VI:
- Damage to the perichondrial ring surrounding the physis
- Ogden (1990) described subgroups of the Salter-Harris classification and added additional classes:

g. SH VII:
- Fracture of the epiphysis that does not involve the physis

h. SH VIII:
- Metaphyseal fracture interrupting vascular supply to the physis

i. SH IX:
- Severe diaphyseal injury destroying a large amount of periosteum

5. Slipped capital femoral epiphysis (SCFE) **[Fig. 3-64]**
   a. Salter I fracture through the proximal femoral physis

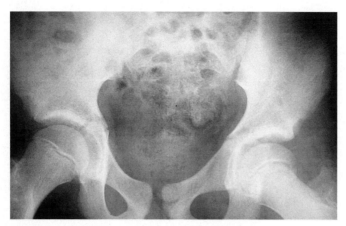

Fig. 3-64 AP pelvis radiograph: Offset between cortex of left femoral head and femoral neck. Lateral slipped capital femoral epiphysis.

  b. Femoral head slips backward more than medially, making frog-leg view more sensitive than AP

  c. Normal AP does not exclude SCFE

  d. A line drawn along the superior cortex of the femoral neck (Klein's line) should intersect a portion of the femoral head. In medial SCFE the line extends above the femoral head

  e. 10% bilateral at diagnosis

  f. 60% develop bilateral disease at some time

  g. Classically obese prepubertal boys, rarely younger than age 10 years

 6. Stubbed toe fracture **[Fig. 3-65]**

  a. Salter II fracture of distal phalanx of finger or toe with associated nailbed injury

  b. The periosteum of the physis is contiguous with the nailbed, so skin bacteria may be injected into the fracture site

  c. Should be treated as an open fracture with antistaphylococcal antibiotics

B. **Fractures of children's flexible bones**

 1. Stress on flexible bones causes a predictable spectrum of bone damage from slight flexion without fracture through complete transection

 2. Bending causes compression force on the concave side, tension force on the convex side

 3. Mild force causes deformation, which returns to original position; no bony injury occurs in this case

 4. The following fractures occur with increasing force:

  a. Plastic bowing fracture **[Fig. 3-66]**

   • Microfractures occur along the convex side

   • Bone distorts, curving without a cortical break

   • Usually heals without callus or sclerosis

  b. Buckle fracture **[Fig. 3-67]**

   • Focal cortical angulation on the compression side without visible cortical break

   • These fractures are less likely to develop deformity as the fracture heals than greenstick fractures

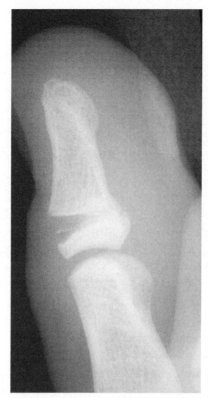

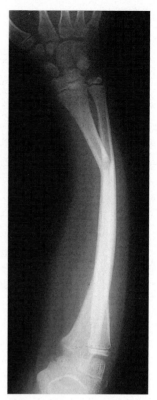

Fig. 3-65 Lateral radiograph of great toe: Salter II fracture of distal phalanx. This is called the "stubbed toe fracture," referring to the mechanism of injury. If associated with subungual hematoma, this fracture has a high incidence of osteomyelitis and should be treated as an "open fracture equivalent."

Fig. 3-66 Lateral forearm radiograph: Angulated fracture of radius, bowing of entire forearm including soft tissues. Trace cortex of ulna. Note bowing of ulnar cortical margin. Plastic bowing fracture of ulna.

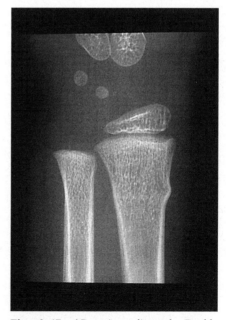

Fig. 3-67 AP wrist radiograph: Buckle fracture of distal radius.

     c. Greenstick fracture
- Fracture of the cortex on the extension side, without fracture of the opposite cortex

     d. Complete fracture
- Due to strong periosteum, complete fractures are less likely to displace in children than in adults

5. A very common pediatric fracture is the distal radial buckle fracture; always look closely at the dorsal distal radial cortex on lateral view as the fracture is easily missed due to superimposition of the radius and ulna.

6. Fractures frequently are combinations of these types, particularly combined buckle and greenstick fracture.

C. Toddler fracture

1. Mechanism of injury is twisting with foot fixed in position
2. Oblique or spiral fracture through lower one-third of the tibia
3. Occult on AP/lateral in one-third
4. Focal tenderness over anterior lower tibia is invariably present

D. Ring bone fractures

1. At any site where the bones form a ring, or where two bones are attached together at both ends, it is more common to see two fractures or a fracture and a dislocation than a single fracture. Always look for the second fracture.

     a. Pelvis

     b. Mandible

     c. Radius and ulna
- Monteggia fracture/dislocation—ulnar fracture with radial head dislocation [Fig. 3-68]
- Galeazzi fracture/dislocation—radial fracture with distal ulnar dislocation

     d. Tibia and fibula

E. Nonaccidental trauma (child abuse, battered child syndrome, trauma X)

1. One-third of children with child abuse will have fractures

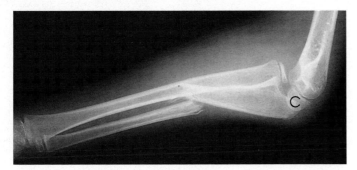

Fig. 3-68 Lateral forearm radiograph: Obvious angulated ulnar fracture. Note radial head is anterior to capitellum (C), indicating radial head dislocation. Monteggia fracture-dislocation.

2. ABSENCE OF FRACTURES DOES NOT IMPLY ABSENCE OF ABUSE
3. Fractures are far more common during the first year of life
4. The most common child abuse fracture is the diaphyseal fracture, indistinguishable from an innocent fracture
5. Highly specific fractures are less common, but must be recognized
   a. Metaphyseal fractures **[Fig. 3-69]**
      - Corner fractures
      - Bucket handle fractures
   b. Posterior rib fractures **[Fig. 8-3]**
   c. The 3 Ss:
      - Sternum
      - Scapula
      - Spinous processes
6. Frequently, fractures are inconsistent with the history, or with good care
   a. Neglected fractures
      - Abnormal alignment
      - Exuberant callus
   b. Multiple fractures of different ages **[Fig. 3-70]**

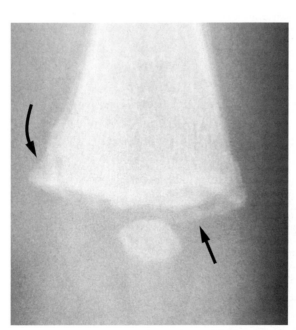

Fig. 3-69 Coned-down radiograph: Classic buckethandle (arrow) and corner fracture (curved arrow) due to jerking of extremity. Child abuse.

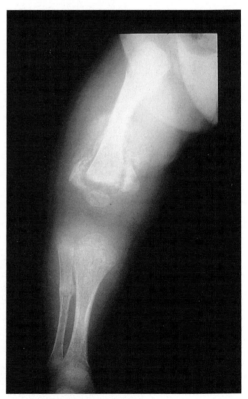

Fig. 3-70 AP lower extremity radiograph: Multiple fractures in different stages of evolution. Note fluffy callus along distal right femur, high density surrounding hemorrhage or calcification in soft tissues, and more completely healed fracture of mid-fibula. Child abuse.

7. Fractures due to sufficient force rarely seen in typical household injuries
   a. Complex skull fractures **[Fig. 1-30]**
   b. Vertebral body fractures and subluxations **[Fig. 8-2]**
   c. Complete physeal separation
8. History is critical. An otherwise innocent fracture may be strongly suggestive of child abuse if an appropriate history of trauma is absent

F. **Osteochondroses**
1. Osteonecrosis
   a. Also called ischemic or avascular necrosis (AVN)
   b. Decreased blood supply causes osteocyte death
   c. Site of obstruction anywhere between extraosseous vessel and medullary sinusoids
   d. All radiologic changes relate to bone repair; osteocyte death alone causes no radiographic changes
   e. Different classifications exist, but four stages can be identified in all osteonecroses
      - Initial phase
        Pathology
        – Osteocyte death
        Radiology
        – No radiographic abnormality
      - Early phase
        Pathology
        – Revascularization of bone
        – Fissures in necrotic bone
        – Cartilage (supplied by synovium) continues to grow
        Radiology
        – Increased bone density
        – Bone growth stops, resulting in decreased size of ossified bone relative to unaffected bones
        – "Crescent sign," other fractures
        – Cartilage growth results in increased apparent joint space
      - Intermediate phase
        Pathology
        – Necrotic bone resorption and new bone formation
        – Resorption predominates initially; new bone formation predominates later
        Radiology
        – Mixed lucency and sclerosis
        – Lucency predominates initially, increased density predominates later
        – Reconstitution of more normal bone shape late in intermediate phase
      - Late phase
        Pathology
        – Mature Haversian systems develop

Radiology
    – Amorphous bone remodels into mature cancellous bone
  f. MRI appearance of osteonecrosis
    • Early changes
      Marrow edema (nonspecific finding)
      Decreased marrow enhancement following gadolinium administration (more specific finding)
    • Later changes
      "Double line sign" on T2-weighted images of hip
        – Low signal peripheral rim with underlying line of high signal
        – Specific for osteonecrosis
        – Likely corresponds to early-intermediate pathologic phases
  g. Bone scintigraphy in osteonecrosis
    • Pinhole images necessary for greatest accuracy
    • Early
      Well-defined area of decreased isotope uptake
    • Late
      Isotope uptake becomes normal or increased as bone revascularizes
  h. Differential diagnosis of osteonecrosis of femoral head
    • Corticosteroids
    • Sickle cell disease (SCD)
      Three to five times more frequent in Hemoglobin SC than Hemoglobin SS type
      AVN also occurs in other bones
        – AVN of humerus can be seen as incidental finding on chest radiograph in patients with SCD
        – Bone infarct(s) may be initial presentation in infant with SCD [Fig. 8-16]
    • Following treatment of hip dislocation or SCFE
    • Trauma
    • Osteomyelitis
    • Gaucher's disease
2. Legg-Perthes disease [Figs. 3-71 and 3-72]
  a. Idiopathic AVN of the femoral head
  b. 3 to 12 years of age, most commonly 6 to 8 years of age
  c. M:F = 5:1
  d. Frequent delayed skeletal maturation
  e. 10% bilateral
  f. Rare in blacks
  g. MRI and bone scintigraphy both > 95% sensitive and specific in symptomatic children
  h. Radiographs
    • Flattening and sclerosis most common findings
    • Subchondral fracture stage rarely appreciated
    • As disease progresses, a medial metaphyseal lucency develops; femoral neck becomes widened and shortened

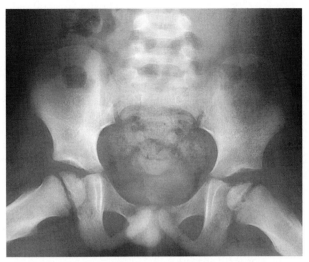

Fig. 3-71 AP pelvis radiograph: Left femoral head is smaller and somewhat more sclerotic than the right femoral head. Legg-Perthes disease.

i. Bone scintigraphy
  • Early in process, there is decreased uptake diffusely in femoral head or localized to anterolateral femoral head
  • Size of defect correlates with later radiographic abnormality
  • Two patterns in ensuing process
     Focal increased activity in lateral column (indicates better prognosis)
     Band of increased activity across base of epiphysis (worse prognosis)
j. MRI
  • Marrow edema pattern
     Decreased signal on T1-weighted images, without signal change on T2-weighted images

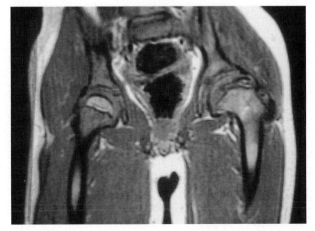

Fig. 3-72 Coronal T1-weighted hip MRI: Normal right hip. Deformed, widened left femoral neck and acetabulum. Note hypointense (sclerotic), flattened left femoral head. Legg-Perthes, late.

Early, but nonspecific, finding; may be transient, with no sequelae
- Decreased femoral head enhancement
  Must compare marrow signal on T1-weighted fat-suppressed images before and after gadolinium administration
  Decreased enhancement reflects decreased blood flow
  Early and specific finding
- Double line sign
  Later, but highly sensitive and specific, finding
3. Freiberg disease
   a. Posttraumatic osteonecrosis of second (3/4) or third (1/4) metatarsal heads
   b. Late childhood to early adolescence
   c. F:M = 3:1
4. Kohler disease
   a. Osteonecrosis of tarsal navicular
   b. Early school age
   c. F:M = 4:1
   d. Easily confused with normal variant (irregular ossification of navicular)
   e. Diagnosis supported by typical progression of osteonecrotic changes
   f. Nuclear medicine bone scintigraphy can confirm diagnosis
5. Osteochondritis dissecans [Figs. 3-73 and 3-74]
   a. Subchondral lucency at joint surface on plain radiograph

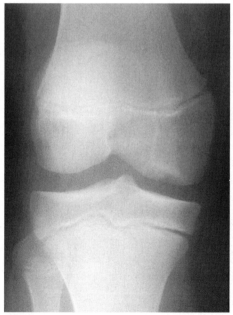

Fig. 3-73   AP knee radiograph: Crescentic defect in medial femoral condyle. Osteochondritis dissecans.

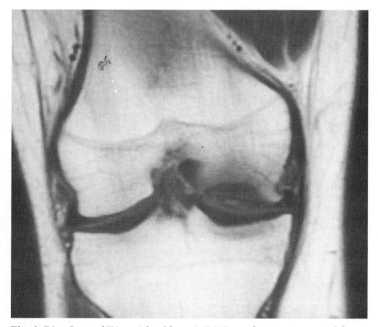

Fig. 3-74   Coronal T1-weighted knee MRI: Bony fragment separated from femoral condyle. Osteochondritis dissecans.

b. MRI better demonstrates extent, free fragment

c. Contrast in joint space improves detection of free fragment with CT or MRI

d. Common locations

- Knee, anteromedial articular surface of medial condyle
- Talar dome
- Metatarsal head

6. Blount disease **[Fig. 3-75]**

a. Also called tibia vara

b. Depression and fragmentation of the medial tibial metaphysis causes genu varum

c. Metaphyseal-diaphyseal angle (between lateral diaphyseal cortex and a line drawn perpendicular to a line between the medial and lateral margins of the metaphysis) >11 degrees suggests progression

- Infantile

    Develops between 2 to 5 years of age

    More common than adolescent form

    Must be distinguished from physiologic bowing

- Adolescent

    10 to 15 years of age

    More severe than infantile form

- Physiologic bowing

    Normal variant

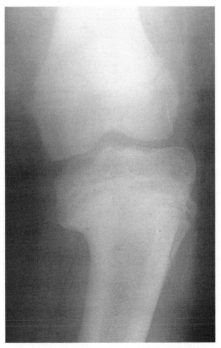

Fig. 3-75 AP knee radiograph: Angulation of medial tibia and varus knee deformity. Blount's tibia vara.

Bowed legs without metaphyseal abnormality

Resolves without treatment over time

7. Skeletal abnormalities associated with neuromuscular diseases

a. Paralytic arthropathy

- Recurrent trauma in disused bones can result in changes essentially identical to hemophilic arthropathy
- Can simulate osteogenesis imperfecta (OI) or child abuse
- Disuse causes demineralization and gracile long bones
- Fractures occur due to delicate bones and difficulty handling patients
- Fractures can be very difficult to identify due to demineralization
- Examples:

Meningomyelocele

Cerebral palsy

b. Congenital insensitivity to pain

- Fractures
- Charcot joints

c. Premature infants

- Fractures due to physiotherapy

Chest percussion can result in rib fractures or new bone formation

- Metaphyseal rarefaction

Nearly universal in ill premature infants due to nutritional deficiency

- Fractures may present with minimal symptoms

XIII. **METABOLIC/ENDOCRINE**

A. **Rickets [Fig. 3-76]**

1. Radiographic appearance

a. Flared, cupped, and frayed metaphyses

b. Broad physis

c. Changes appear first in most rapid growth areas

d. Evaluation in young children easiest in wrist

2. Causes

a. Renal tubular disease most common cause

b. Drugs

c. Hepatic disease, especially biliary disease

d. Associated with prematurity

e. Vitamin D deficiency rare cause

B. **Hypothyroidism**

1. Congenital hypothyroidism = cretinism

2. Striking delayed bone maturation, especially proximal humerus and at knee

3. Proximal femoral epiphysis may not ossify until child >2 years old

4. Epiphyseal dysgenesis: irregular or fragmented epiphyses

5. Mental retardation or developmental delay

C. **Hypoparathryoidism**

1. In children probably frequently due to circulating antibodies

2. F > M

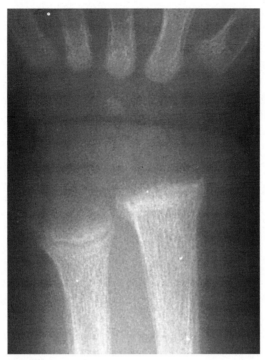

Fig. 3-76 AP wrist radiograph: Osteopenia, widening, flaring, and cupping of distal radius and ulna. Rickets.

3. Results in hypocalcemia
4. Osteosclerosis
5. Calvarial thickening
6. Premature physeal closure
7. Soft tissue and basal ganglia calcification

D. **Pseudohypoparathyroidism**
 1. End-organ resistance to parathormone
 2. In addition to findings of hypoparathyroidism see:
   a. Short stature
   b. Cone epiphyses
   c. Brachydactyly

E. **Pseudo-pseudohypoparathyroidism**
 1. Normocalcemic pseudohypoparathyroidism

F. **Hypophosphatasia**
 1. May have the same appearance as rickets, but normal calcium and phosphorus
 2. Infantile lethal type
   a. Poorly mineralized skull
   b. Thin, poorly mineralized ribs
   c. "Absent" vertebral bodies
 3. Childhood type
   a. Bowed bones
   b. Deep central defects extending into the metaphyses from the physes distinguish from rickets

G. **Scurvy**
1. Deficiency in vitamin C
2. Not seen in infants <6 months of age
3. Infants fed boiled milk most at risk as boiling destroys vitamin C
4. Dense provisional zones of calcification form spurs at the margins of the physes
5. "Scurvy line" is a lucency beneath the dense line at the metaphysis, usually seen at only one margin
6. Large subperiosteal hemorrhages may occur

FURTHER READING

Ablin DS, Greenspan A, Reinhart M, Grix A: Differentiation of child abuse from osteogenesis imperfecta. AJR 1990;154:1035–1046.

Berquist TH. Magnetic Resonance imaging of primary skeletal neoplasms. Radiol Clin North Am 1993:31:411–424.

Bufkin WJ. The avulsive cortical irregularity. Am J Roentgenol, Radium Therapy & Nucl Med. 1971;112:487–492.

Caffey J. Multiple fractures in the long bones in infants suffering from subdural hematoma. AJR 1946;56:163–173.

Egeler RM, D'Angio GJ. Langerhans' cell histiocytosis. J Pediatr 1995;127:1–11.

Gerscovich EO. A radiologist's guide to the imaging in the diagnosis and treatment of developmental dysplasia of the hip. Skeletal Radiol 1997;26:447–456.

Graf R. Guide to Sonography of the Infant Hip. New York: Thieme Medical Publishers; 1987.

Greenspan A. Benign bone-forming lesions: osteoma, osteoid osteoma, and osteoblastoma. Clinical, imaging, pathologic, and differential considerations. Skeletal Radiol 1993;22:485–500.

Greulich WW, Pyle SI. Radiographic Atlas of Skeletal Development of the Hand and Wrist, 2nd ed. Stanford, CA: Stanford University Press; 1959.

Helms CA. Skeletal "don't touch" lesions. Applied Radiol 1992; 21:16–21.

Jaramillo D, Treves ST, Kasser JR, et al. Osteomyelitis and septic arthritis in children: Appropriate use of imaging to guide treatment. AJR 1995;165:399–403.

John DS, Wherry K, Swischuk LE, Phillips WA. Improving detection of pediatric elbow fractures by understanding their mechanics. RadioGraphics 1996;16:1443–1460.

Johnson ND, Wood BP, Jackson KV. Complex infantile and congenital hip dislocation: Assessment with MR imaging. Radiology 1988;168:151–156.

Keats TE. Atlas of Normal Roentgen Variants that may Stimulate Disease, 5th ed. St. Louis: Mosby; 1992.

Kleinman PK. Diagnostic Imaging of Child Abuse. Baltimore, MD: Williams and Wilkins, 1987.

Laor T, Chung T, Hoffer FA, Jaramillo D. Musculoskeletal magnetic resonance imaging: How we do it. Pediatr Radiol 1996;26:695–700.

Laor T, Jaramillo D, Hoffer FA, Kasser JR. MR imaging in congenital lower limb deformities. Pediatric Radiol 1996;26:381–387.

Majd M, Frankel RS. Radionuclide imaging in skeletal inflammatory and ischemic disease in children. AJR 1976; 126:832–841.

Merten DF, Radkowski MA, Leonidas JC. The abused child: a radiological reappraisal. Radiology 1983;146:377–381.

Nelson JD. Acute osteomyelitis in children. Infect Dis Clin North Am 1990;4:513–522.

Oestreich AE. How to Measure Angles from Foot Radiographs. New York: Springer-Verlag, 1990.

Ogden JA. Skeletal Injury in the Child, 2nd ed, Philadelphia: WB Saunders, 1990.

Ozonoff MB. Pediatric Orthopedic Radiology, 2nd ed. Philadelphia: WB Saunders, 1992.

Pinckney LE, Currarino G, Kennedy LA. The stubbed great toe: a cause of occult compound fracture and infection. Radiology 1981;138:375–377.

Poznanski AK, Gartman S. A bibliography covering the use of metacarpophalangeal pattern profile analysis in bone dysplasias, congenital malformation syndromes, and other disorders. Pediatr Radiol 1997;27:358–365.

Resnick D, Kyriakos M, Greenway GD. Tumors and tumor-like lesions of bone: Imaging and pathology of specific tumors. In: Resnick D., ed. Diagnosis of Bone and Joint Disorders, 3rd ed. Philadelphia: WB Saunders, 1995:3662–3697.

Ricci C, Cova M, Kang YS, et al. Normal age-related patterns of cellular and fatty marrow distribution in the axial skeleton: MR imaging study. Radiology 1990;177;83–88.

Rogers LF. The radiography of ephiphyseal injuries. Radiology 1994;191:297–308.

Salter RB, Harris R. Injuries involving the epiphyseal plate. J Bone Joint Surg 1963;5:587–602.

Sundar M, Carty H. Avulsion fractures of the pelvis in children: a report of 32 fractures and their outcome. Skeletal Radiol 1994;23:85–90.

Taccone A, Oddone M, Dell'Acqua A, Occhi M, Ciccone MA. MRI "road map" of normal age-related bone marrow. II. thorax, pelvis and extremities. Pediatr Radiol 1995;25:596–606.

Taybi H, Lachman R. Radiology of Syndromes, Metabolic Disorders and Skeletal Dysplasias, 3rd ed. Chicago: Year Book Medical, 1990.

Wilkinson RH. Epiphyseal injuries. Applied Radiology 1989;18:13–18.

CHAPTER FOUR   CARDIOVASCULAR SYSTEM

I. **ORDERED EVALUATION OF THE CHEST RADIOGRAPH
   FOR CARDIAC DISEASE**
   A. **Heart**
      1. Size
      2. Position
      3. Configuration
   B. **Pulmonary vascularity [Figs. 4-1 through 4-3]**
      1. Increased or decreased
      2. Well- or ill-defined

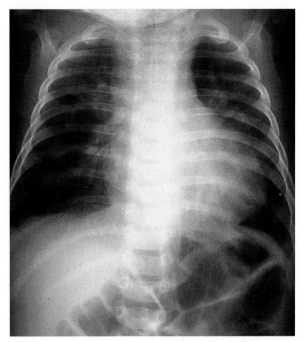

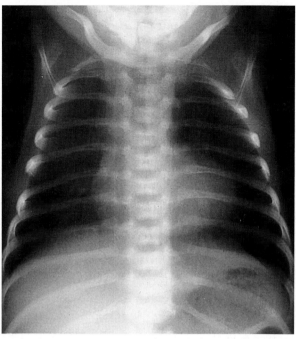

Fig. 4-1 Posteroanterior (PA) chest radiograph: Mild cardiac enlargement, symmetric and increased pulmonary arterial blood flow. Note that pulmonary vessel margins are sharp, indicating absence of pulmonary venous congestion. VSD.

Fig. 4-2 PA chest radiograph: Horizontal cardiac axis and symmetric but decreased pulmonary arterial blood flow, indicating outflow obstruction to pulmonary artery. Note increased density overlying left vertebral pedicles, indicating left descending aorta. Tetralogy of Fallot.

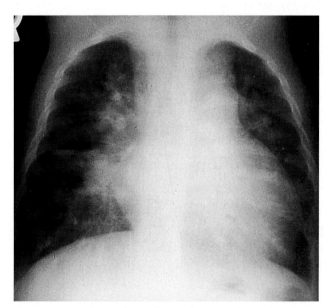

Fig. 4-3 PA chest radiograph: Moderate cardiac enlargement, definitely increased and symmetric pulmonary arterial blood flow. Pulmonary vessels are unsharp. Fluid in minor fissure. Left-to-right shunt (VSD) with pulmonary venous congestion.

    3. Collateral vessels

    4. Symmetrical/asymmetrical

    5. Main pulmonary artery (MPA) increased/decreased

  C. **Aortic arch**

    1. Position

    2. Size

  D. **Pulmonary edema**

    1. Septal lines

    2. Peribronchial thickening

    3. Pleural effusion

  E. **Ribs**

    1. 11 or 13

    2. Notching

  F. **Additional observations**

    1. Bifid manubrial ossification center (80% of trisomy 21, 20% of normal children)

    2. Spinal anomalies

    3. Scoliosis increased in congenital heart disease (CHD)

    4. Malformations in VATER (vertebral defects, anal atresia, tracheoesophageal fistula with esophageal atresia, and radial and renal anomalies) association

    5. Liver size

    6. Abdominal situs

    7. Postsurgical changes

II. **NORMAL CHEST RADIOGRAPH OF THE INFANT AND CHILD**

  A. **Cardiac size [Figs. 1-1, 1-2, 1-4, and 1-5]**

    1. Lateral film is more useful than frontal film

    2. Cardiothoracic ratio may exceed 50% in normal children

    3. In young children diagnose cardiomegaly only if the posterior cardiac margin approaches the spine

    4. Thymus frequently obscures the entire cardiac margin in infants; again lateral view correlation helpful

  B. **Cardiac configuration**

    1. Cardiac axis and shape are variable. The thymus fills in the retrocardiac space in young children, obscuring the right ventricle. Many normal infants have cardiac configurations not unlike those seen with CHD.

    2. The right margin of the left atrium is visible in one-third of normal children.

  C. **Pulmonary vascularity**

    1. Pulmonary vascularity in children is both more prominent and less well-defined than in adults

    2. Pulmonary arteries (PAs) should be the same size as accompanying bronchi

    3. The right descending PA should be $\leq$ the width of the trachea above the aortic arch.

    4. Pulmonary vessels should not be seen in the peripheral third of the lung

   5. If necessary, a series of normal chest radiographs (CXRs) can be maintained to "calibrate" your eyes when needed

D. **Aorta**

   1. Aortic knob often difficult to see in the first 3 months of life
   2. The trachea deviates away from the aortic knob, so should be located to the right of midline in normal children
   3. The ascending aorta is never prominent in normal children
   4. The descending aorta can frequently be identified by finding increased density overlying the pedicles or paraspinous area on the side of the descending aorta

III. **EVALUATING PULMONARY VASCULARITY**

A. **Description of pulmonary vascularity [Figs. 4-1 through 4-3]**

   1. Increased, decreased, or normal
   2. Well-defined or ill-defined
   3. Symmetric or asymmetric **[Fig. 1-6]**
   4. Pulmonary vascular branching pattern or collateral vessels

B. **This determination is the most difficult part of assessing the CXR**

C. **Interval changes best evaluated by comparison of the same area on sequential CXR**

D. **The experienced reader's impression is more accurate than any rule, but here are some suggestions:**

   1. Peripheral PAs should be the same size as their accompanying bronchus; larger arteries suggest increased blood flow
   2. Normally, lung markings should not be seen in peripheral one-third of the lung; visible peripheral vessels suggest increased blood flow.
   3. A descending right PA larger than the trachea above the aortic arch indicates increased pulmonary blood flow. This requires a marked increase in pulmonary blood flow, so blood flow may be increased without enlargement of the descending PA to this degree.
   4. Hyperlucent lungs with normal lung volume and decreased lung markings often have decreased blood flow

E. **Well-defined large vessels suggest increased flow**

F. **Ill-defined large vessels suggest edema secondary to venous hypertension**

   1. The margins of well-defined vessels can be traced with a sharp pencil
   2. Ill-defined central vessels often have a frondlike or masslike appearance
   3. The margins of individual vessels are indistinct and cannot be separated from adjacent vessels
   4. The hila on lateral view often show this difference better than vessels seen on the frontal view

G. **Assess symmetry by comparing the vessels in the same area of each lung**

H. **In the normal branching pattern, the largest vessels are in the hila; branch vessels taper toward the periphery**

I. **Collateral vessels often form a reticular pattern with little difference in vessel size in the central third and middle third of the lung**

J. **Pulmonary edema [Figs. 5-46 and 5-47]**
1. Kerley lines are less common in children than adults
    a. When present, they may be best seen behind the sternum on lateral view
2. Edema is frequently diffuse rather than central
3. A hazy appearance of the lungs diffusely with normal or increased lung volumes (sixth anterior rib crosses diaphragm) is often the only indication of interstitial pulmonary edema

IV. **CONGENITAL HEART DISEASE: INCIDENCE**
A. **Incidence: 1% of live births**
B. **The top 10 in incidence:**
1. Ventricular septal defect (VSD): 20 to 25%
2. Tetralogy of Fallot: 10 to 15%
3. Patent ductus arteriosus (PDA): 10 to 15%
4. Atrial septal defect (ASD): <10%
5. Pulmonic stenosis (PS): >5%
6. Coarctation of aorta: >5%
7. Transposition of great vessels (TGV): 5%
8. Endocardial cushion defect (ECD): <5%
9. Aortic stenosis (AS): <5%
10. Total anomalous pulmonary venous connection (TAPVC): 1 to 2%

C. **Bicuspid aortic valve (2% of population) not included**

V. **PHYSIOLOGY HELPFUL IN UNDERSTANDING CONGENITAL HEART DISEASE**
A. **Increased volume, not increased pressure, causes chamber enlargement**
B. **Shunt lesions are described by the ratio of pulmonary to systemic blood flow ($\dot{Q}P : \dot{Q}S$), which is usually stated as a "two to one shunt," for example**

    A $\dot{Q}P : \dot{Q}S$ ratio of 2 to 2.5 : 1 is necessary to detect an increase in pulmonary blood flow

    One-third of systemic blood must cross from the systemic to the pulmonary system to produce a 2 : 1 shunt

C. **The radiographic appearance of almost all CHD is variable, depending on the amount of abnormal blood flow**

D. **Prenatal/perinatal physiology**
1. Prenatally, 90% of blood flow bypasses the lungs through the foramen ovale
2. The right and left ventricular pressures are similar; the ventricular walls are similar in thickness at birth

3. Pulmonary vascular resistance equals or exceeds systemic resistance at birth

4. Pulmonary vascular resistance decreases rapidly in the first few days of life and continues to decrease for 4 to 6 weeks before reaching an adult ratio of pulmonary to systemic pressure.

5. The ductus arteriosus closes functionally in the first day of life, but can reopen for several weeks. Permanent ductus closure progresses from the aorta toward the PA and is complete by 6 to 8 weeks.

VI. **CLINICAL INFORMATION**

   A. **Clinical information as to whether a patient is cyanotic or acyanotic must be obtained before attempting to diagnose a specific lesion in CHD**

   B. **Neither a heart murmur nor an abnormal CXR is found in all patients with CHD. Transposition usually presents without a murmur, and the radiograph is frequently normal.**

VII. **ACYANOTIC CONGENITAL HEART DISEASE**

   A. **Acyanotic with increased blood flow – left to right shunts**

     1. ASD

       a. Right sided enlargement rotates heart, straightens left cardiac margin; superior vena cava (SVC) overlies the spine and is not seen on frontal film in two-thirds

       b. No left chamber enlargement

       c. Location

- Secundum, at foramen ovale: 60%
- Primum, below foramen ovale: 35%
    A component of endocardial cushion defect
- Sinus venosus, posterior to foramen ovale: 5%
    Frequently associated with partial anomalous venous connection

     2. VSD [Figs. 4-1 and 4-3]

       a. Right sided enlargement balanced by left sided enlargement

       b. Enlarged left atrium (LA)

       c. Location

- Membranous: 75 to 80%
- Muscular: 10 to 15%
- Supracristal or conal: 5 to 10%
- Atrioventricular (AV) canal defect has a posterior VSD

     3. PDA [Figs. 4-4 and 4-5]

       a. Enlarged aorta

       b. Enlarged LA and left ventricle (LV)

     4. ECD [Figs. 4-6 and 4-7]

       a. During development, the endocardial cushions separate the four cardiac chambers

       b. Defects range from an ostium primum ASD only to complete AV canal

       c. Variable appearance, right atrial (RA) enlargement may be strik-

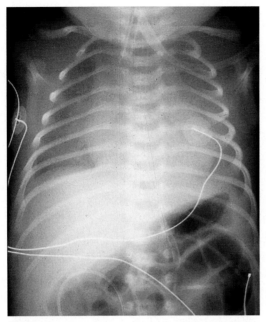

Fig. 4-4 PA chest radiograph: Two days after Survanta therapy for hyaline membrane disease (HMD). Cardiac enlargement, pulmonary edema. Surfactant decreases atelectasis, decreases pulmonary vascular resistance, and allows a patent ductus arteriosus (PDA) to shunt left-to-right. PDA.

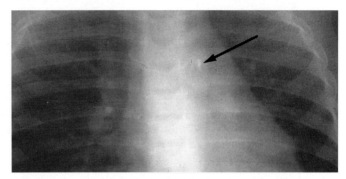

Fig. 4-5 PA chest radiograph: Calcification (arrow) in closed ductus arteriosus. Pulmonary vascularity is normal.

ing due to continuity between all four chambers with maximal flow between the highest and lowest pressure chambers (LV to RA)

   d. Patient with AV canal has the largest heart of this group.

   e. The right heart has a globular contour while the left heart is normal in appearance

   f. Most common cardiac anomaly in trisomy 21

B. **Acyanotic with normal flow—outflow obstruction lesions**

- Newborn with high grade obstruction, especially left-sided, may present with congestive heart failure (CHF)

1. Aortic stenosis
   a. Valvular
      - Most common (two-thirds of AS)
      - Usually normal CXR; may see dilated ascending aorta
   b. Supravalvular
      - Williams syndrome in one-third
   c. Subvalvular
      - Membranous
      - Usually thin membrane 1 cm below aortic valve
   d. Muscular
      - Idiopathic hypertrophic subaortic stenosis

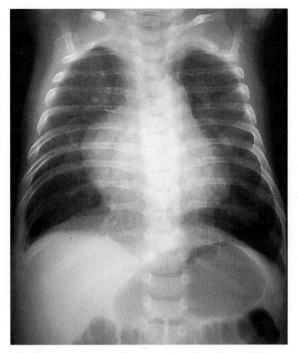

Fig. 4-6 PA chest radiograph: Bilateral pulmonary hyperinflation, increased pulmonary vascularity, and bulbous enlargement of right cardiac border, indicating right atrial enlargement. This pattern is typical for atrioventricular canal (AVC). Right atrial enlargement and decreased pulmonary vascularity suggest pulmonic atresia with intact ventricular septum, Ebstein's anomaly, or persistent fetal circulation (PFC) with tricuspid regurgitation.

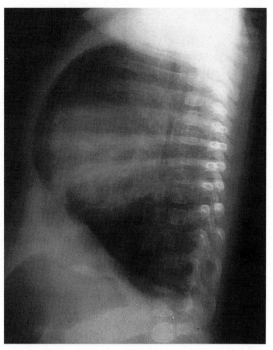

Fig. 4-7 Lateral chest radiograph: Marked pulmonary hyperinflation. Hyperinflation suggests air trapping due to airways disease (bronchiolitis, reactive airways disease, cystic fibrosis, bronchopulmonary dysplasia). Pulmonary hyperinflation can also be seen with large left-to-right shunts. AVC.

2. Pulmonic stenosis
   a. 90% due to fused leaflets
   b. 10% due to generalized dysplasia
   c. Generally asymptomatic
   d. May see poststenotic dilatation of MPA and left pulmonary artery (LPA)
3. Absent pulmonic valve
   a. Small annulus causes severe pulmonic stenosis
   b. Striking poststenotic dilatation causes obvious mediastinal contour abnormality
4. Aortic coarctation **[Figs. 4-8 through 4-10]**
   a. Children may present at any age with a murmur and upper extremity hypertension
   b. Closure of PDA narrows aortic lumen and can result in severe lower body ischemia at several months of age; presents with acute onset of sepsis-like picture
   c. Associated cardiac disease frequent
      • PDA: two-thirds

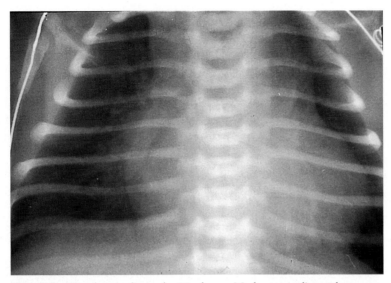

Fig. 4-8 PA chest radiograph: Newborn. Moderate cardiac enlargement, normal pulmonary vascularity. This pattern is seen with myocardial dysfunction, infant of diabetic mother, hypervolemia, left heart obstruction. Infantile aortic coarctation.

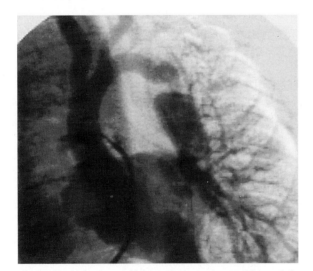

Fig. 4-9 Left ventriculogram: Same patient as Figure 4-8. Infantile aortic coarctation.

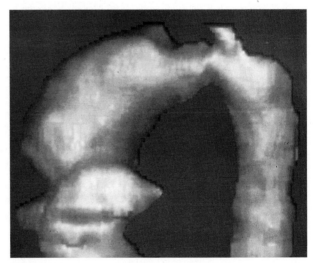

Fig. 4-10 Three-dimensional (3D) MRI: focal preductal coarctation.

- VSD: one-third
- Bicuspid aortic valve: 50%

d. "Three" sign
- Upper convexity—dilated subclavian artery
- Narrow point at coarctation
- Lower convexity—poststenotic dilatation

e. Rib notching usually seen by 6 to 8 years of age
- Inferior rib margin often irregular; rib notching should be diagnosed only if the margin is sclerotic

5. Pseudocoarctation
   a. Very high aortic arch, often accompanied by "three" sign
   b. Caused by kinked but nonobstructing aorta

C. **Nonobstructive lesions**
1. Endocardial fibroelastosis
   a. Simulates cardiomyopathy
   b. Thickened and stiff endocardium causes ventricular dysfunction with a dilated and poorly functioning LV
   c. LV almost always involved
   d. LA involved in 50%
   e. Right ventricle (RV) involved in <25%
   f. Associated CHD in 75%
   g. CHF usually develops in the first months of life

VIII. **CYANOTIC CONGENITAL HEART DISEASE**
- There is increasing recognition that the division of cyanotic heart disease by blood flow is limited by the fact that many lesions have a variable appearance.
- The divisions in this section represent the traditional descriptions of these lesions.
- The gamuts at the end of this chapter identify those lesions with a variable appearance.

A. **Cyanotic CHD with increased blood flow**
1. Admixture lesions
   a. Transposition
      - Transposition is highly variable in its appearance and is therefore difficult to classify
      - Pure transposition isolates the pulmonic and systemic circulations without admixture, but is incompatible with life
      - Pulmonary blood flow varies depending on the degree of admixture, the relative pressures of the right and left heart, and the presence of additional lesions
      - d-Transposition **[Fig. 4-11]**
         Aorta connected to RV, PA to LV
         Aorta located anterior to PA
         Normal heart size
         Blood flow may be normal or increased
         Appearance described as "an egg on a string"
         - Aorta directly in front of MPA narrows mediastinum
         - Normal cardiac axis, so "egg" angles downward to left

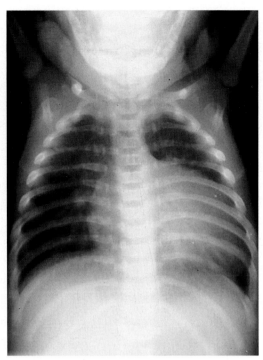

Fig. 4-11 PA chest radiograph: Moderate cardiac enlargement, normal-to-increased pulmonary vascularity. Note very narrow mediastinum. d-Transposition of great vessels.

Right arch in 75% of transposition with PS, otherwise rare (<5% overall)
- l-Transposition **[Fig. 4-12]**
  Ventricles and great vessels are both transposed
  Normal path of blood flow
  Almost all have associated CHD
  If isolated, l-TGV usually asymptomatic, may be autopsy finding in elderly
  Abnormal convex left heart border due to abnormal position of ascending aorta; often the only finding in isolated l-TGV
b. Truncus arteriosus **[Fig. 4-13]**
- A single vessel originates from both ventricles
- 35% have right arch
- Truncal valve may have up to six leaves
- Types:
  1: MPA takes off from side of trunk
  2: Separate PAs from back of trunk
  3: One PA from each side of trunk
  4: "PAs" from descending aorta (pseudotruncus); this is actually pulmonary atresia with bronchial collateral vessels

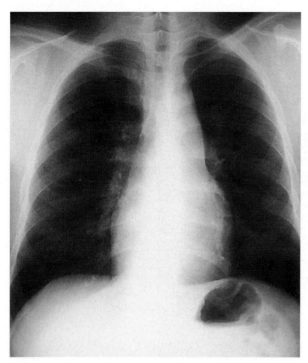

Fig. 4-12 PA chest radiograph: Unusual convex contour of left upper mediastinum. Pulmonary vascularity is normal. Congenitally corrected transposition of the great vessels (l-transposition).

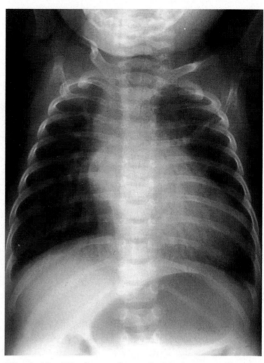

Fig. 4-13 PA chest radiograph: Moderate cardiac enlargement, increased pulmonary arterial blood flow, and right aortic arch. Truncus arteriosus.

c. Total anomalous pulmonary venous connection (TAPVC) **[Fig. 4-14]**
  - Pulmonary blood flow returns to RA rather than LA
  - Three types
    1: Supracardiac: 50%, drains into innominate vein through a vertical vein
    2: Cardiac: one-third, drains into coronary sinus
    3: Infracardiac: veins drain into inferior vena cava (IVC) or hepatic veins
  - Combinations may be called type 4
  - Infracardiac are always obstructed; others may be either obstructed or nonobstructed
  - Without obstruction, see only increased right-sided blood flow
  - Obstruction causes pulmonary venous hypertension
  - Pulmonary venous congestion with normal heart size strongly suggests Type III TAPVC
    Differential diagnosis (DDx) includes congenital pneumonia, pulmonary lymphangiectasia, pulmonary vein stenosis or atresia, cor triatriatum

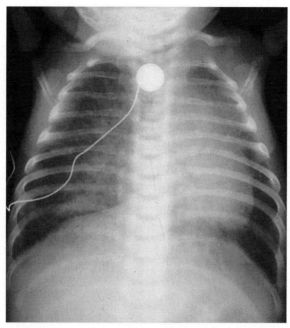

Fig. 4-14 PA chest radiograph: Normal cardiac size, pulmonary hyperinflation, and pulmonary venous congestion. Infradiaphragmatic TAPVC Type III.

- "Snowman heart" describes the appearance of Type 1 TAPVC in older children

    The dilated vertical vein that gives this appearance takes months to years to develop and with early correction is rarely seen today

d. Double outlet right ventricle (DORV)
  - Aorta and PA originate from RV
  - Mixing generally results in increased pulmonary blood flow
  - Appearance depends on presence of PS or AS
  - VSD always present
  - Single ventricle with common AV valve is less common
  - Double outlet left ventricle extremely rare
  - Taussig-Bing

    DORV with side-by-side great vessels

B. **Cyanotic CHD with decreased blood flow**
  1. Right-sided obstructive lesions
    a. Tetralogy of Fallot **[Figs. 4-15 through 4-18]**
      - Most common cyanotic CHD
      - Right arch in 25%
      - Normal heart size
      - Four components

        RV outflow obstruction

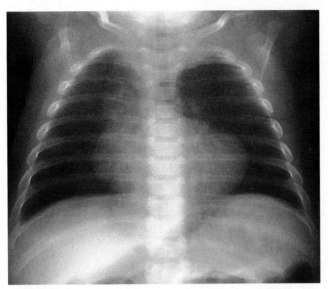

Fig. 4-15 PA chest radiograph: Horizontal cardiac axis, right aortic arch, normal-to-mildly decreased pulmonary arterial blood flow. Pulmonic atresia with VSD (tetralogy of Fallot).

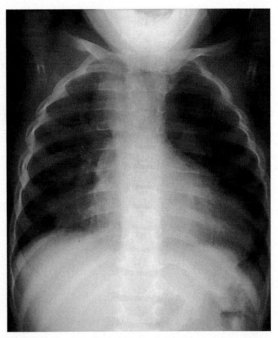

Fig. 4-16 PA chest radiograph: Mild cardiac enlargement, right aortic arch, and asymmetric pulmonary blood flow, right greater than left. Tetralogy of Fallot with asymmetric blood flow.

<ul>
<li>   − 75% infundibular</li>
<li>   − 25% valvular</li>
</ul>

       Right ventricular hypertrophy (RVH)

       VSD

       Overriding aorta

- Boot-shaped heart or "coeur en sabot"

       Concave PA segment due to decreased MPA flow

       Right sided enlargement elevates cardiac apex

- Degree of cyanosis depends on severity of RV outflow obstruction
- Acyanotic "pink tets" occur when there is little right to left shunt
- "Tet spells"

       Seen only in untreated cases

       Acute cyanosis and distress caused by change in the balance of pulmonary and systemic pressures

       Treated with morphine and oxygen

b. Tricuspid atresia

- No flow from RA to RV
- RV develops only if VSD present
- Types

       1: Normal great vessels

       2: With d-transposition

       3: With l-transposition

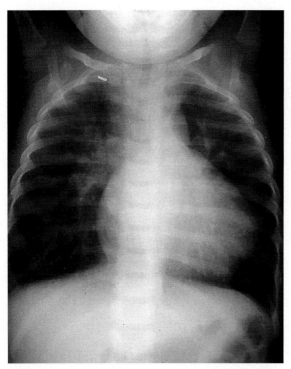

Fig. 4-17 PA chest radiograph: Normal cardiac size, asymmetric pulmonary blood flow, right greater than left. Note surgical clip in right upper mediastinum. Tetralogy of Fallot, post right B-T shunt (subclavian artery-pulmonary artery shunt). Note alteration in cardiac contour compared to previous non-shunted Tetralogy images.

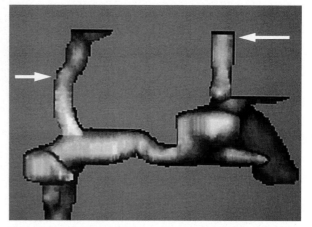

Fig. 4-18 3D MRI: Right and left pulmonary arteries connected to bilateral Blalock-Taussig shunts (arrows). Tetralogy of Fallot, B-T shunts.

    c. Pulmonary atresia
       • With intact ventricular septum
          Decreased pulmonary vascularity (all flow is from PDA)
          Right ventricular size depends on tricuspid regurgitation
          – 80% minimal regurgitation
          – Normal heart size
          – Tiny RV
          20% have tricuspid regurgitation and enlarged RV and RA
          – Increased heart size
       • With VSD
          Severe form of tetralogy of Fallot
    d. Ebstein anomaly **[Fig. 4-19]**
       • Tricuspid valve leaflets enlarged, malformed, and displaced into RV
       • Discoordinated contraction
       • Both obstruction and regurgitation
       • Marked cardiac enlargement, especially RA
IX. **GREAT VESSEL ANOMALIES**
    A. **Left arch with aberrant right subclavian**
      1. Most common arch anomaly

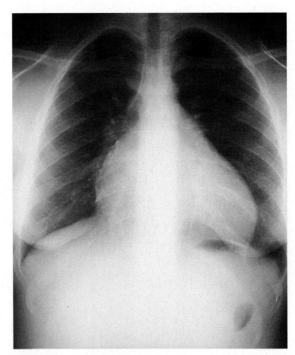

Fig. 4-19 PA chest radiograph: Mild cardiac enlargement with predominant enlargement of right atrium. Pulmonary vascularity mildly decreased. Ebstein's anomaly.

    2. 0.5% of population

    3. Usually asymptomatic

    4. Posterior impression on mid-esophagus

B. **Innominate artery compression syndrome [Fig. 4-20]**

    1. Innominate artery originates left of midline, passes in front of trachea

    2. Anterior tracheal impression 2 cm above carina

    3. May be symptomatic in infants, otherwise an incidental finding

    4. Rarely requires treatment

C. **Right arch without aberrant vessels**

    1. Mirror image of left arch

    2. CHD in >95%, usually cyanotic

D. **Rings and slings**

    1. True ring completely encircles trachea and esophagus and is usually symptomatic (80%)

    2. True ring may be completed by ligamentous remnant of ductus and can appear incomplete on imaging

    3. Presence of ring best established with suspicious anatomy and findings of tracheal and esophageal narrowing

    4. A normal esophagram virtually excludes a vascular ring

    5. Abnormal esophagram best followed by MRI for complete evaluation

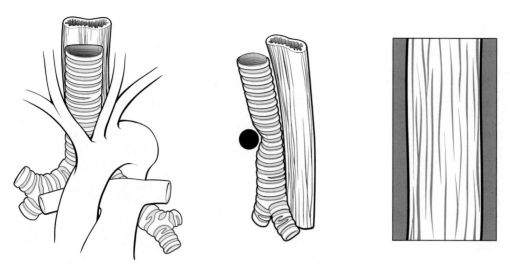

Fig. 4-20 Innominate artery compression. Diagram shows normal aortic branching. On lateral image the innominate artery is closely apposed to the anterior tracheal wall. On fluoroscopy, tracheomalacia may be identified. There is no mass effect on the esophagus.

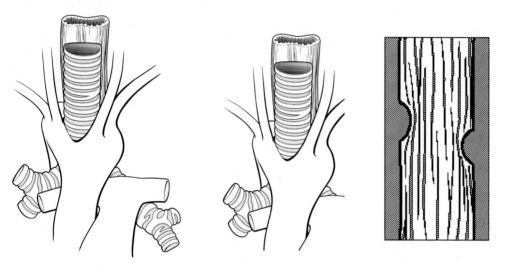

Fig. 4-21 Double aortic arch (DAA). The ascending aorta bifurcates into right and left arches that surround the trachea and esophagus. The two arches recombine to form a descending aorta. In this example of DAA, the descending aorta is on the right; more commonly in DAA, the descending aorta is on the right. On a lateral view, there are anterior and posterior indentations on the trachea and esophagus, respectively. An anteroposterior (AP) esophagram shows two indentations on the esophagus. The more superior is caused by the right arch, the more inferior by the left arch.

E. **Double arch [Figs. 4-21 through 4-24]**
   1. Left arch passes anterior to trachea, right arch posterior
   2. Right usually larger and higher than left
   3. Both limbs may be patent, or left limb atretic with a fibrous remnant
F. **Right arch with aberrant left subclavian [Figs. 4-25 through 4-28]**
   1. Rarely associated with CHD
   2. Ring completed by ligamentum arteriosum
   3. Posterior impression on mid-esophagus

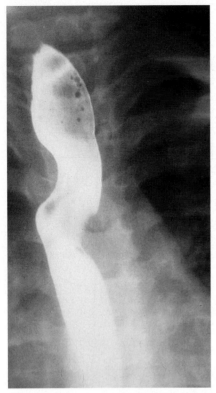

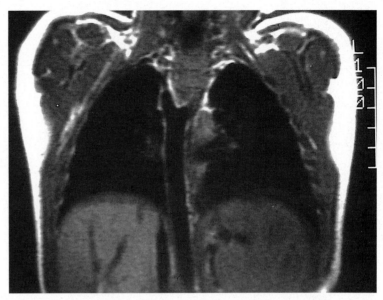

Fig. 4-22 AP esophagram: Indentations on the esophagus. The more superior indentation is on right, more inferior indentation on left. Vascular ring, DAA.

Fig. 4-23 Coronal T1-weighted MRI: DAA with descending aorta on right.

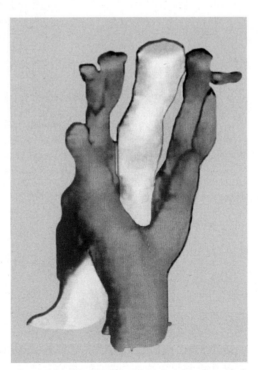

Fig. 4-24 3D CT (frontal image): Trachea (dark area), aorta (light area). Complete DAA encircling trachea. **(See Color Plate 1.)**

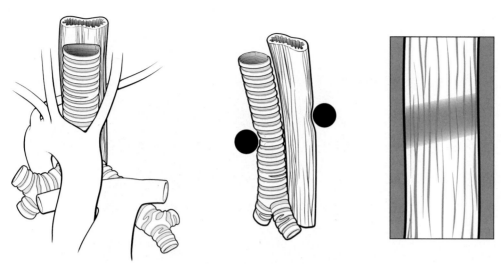

Fig. 4-25 Right aortic arch with aberrant left subclavian artery (SCA). Note the branching pattern of vessels from the right aortic arch (left common carotid is first). The left SCA extends from the posterior arch on the right behind the esophagus, and produces an oblique indentation seen on AP esophagram. On lateral view fluoroscopy, the anterior aorta may produce an indentation on the anterior wall of the trachea or tracheomalacia (without vascular indentation) may be identified. The posterior esophageal indentation is produced by the origin of the left SCA (called the diverticulum of Kommerell). Vascular ring.

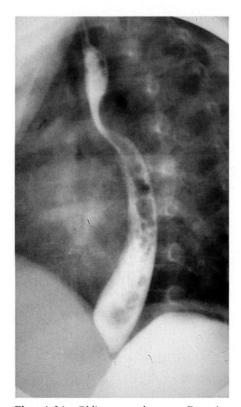

Fig. 4-26 Oblique esophagram: Posterior indentation on esophageal barium column. Note narrowing of adjacent trachea. Retro-esophageal SCA. Tracheomalacia.

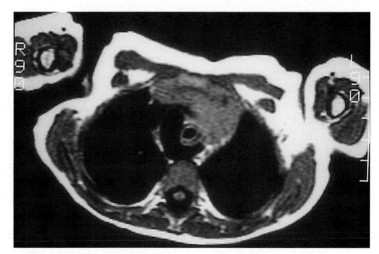

Fig. 4-27 Axial T1-weighted MRI: Same patient as Figure 4-26. Vascular ring, right aortic arch, aberrant left subclavian artery.

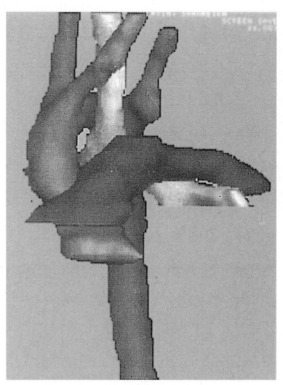

Fig. 4-28 3D MRI (oblique image): Trachea (white), pulmonary artery (black), aorta (gray). Note the left subclavian artery arising posterior to the trachea in this patient with right aortic arch. Ligamentum arteriosum (not seen) completes the vascular ring. **(See Color Plate 2.)**

    G. **PA sling [Figs. 4-29 through 4-32]**
        1. Aberrant origin of the LPA from the right pulmonary artery (RPA)
        2. LPA between trachea and esophagus as it passes from right to left
          a. In newborn, right mainstem bronchus may be narrowed by aberrant LPA
          b. This can cause an initially opaque lung followed by hyperexpansion
          c. This appearance can be confused with congenital lobar emphysema
  X. **CARDIAC AND VISCERAL MALPOSITION**
    A. **Cardiac position**
        1. Dextrocardia: location of the heart to the right of midline
        2. Dextroversion: heart on right due to abnormal cardiac development
        3. Dextroposition: normal heart displaced to right
    B. **Abdomen**
        1. Situs describes the abdominal viscera
          a. Situs solitus: normal
          b. Situs inversus: mirror image

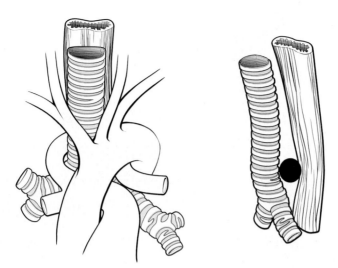

Fig. 4-29 Pulmonary artery sling. The main pulmonary artery (PA) does not branch immediately into right and left branches. Instead, the main PA gives rise to the right PA. The left PA arises from the right PA. The left PA courses from right to left, around the trachea, between the trachea and esophagus. Lateral fluoroscopy identifies an *anterior* indentation on the esophagus. Depending on anatomic variations, the PA sling can obstruct the right main bronchus, trachea, or even the left main bronchus.

C. **Heterotaxy: bilateral right or left sidedness**
D. **Evaluation by plain film:**
    1. Cardiac apex
        a. Left—levocardia
        b. Right—dextrocardia
    2. Stomach and liver
        a. Normal location: situs solitus
        b. Reversed: liver left, stomach right: situs inversus
        c. Transverse liver or midline stomach—indeterminate situs

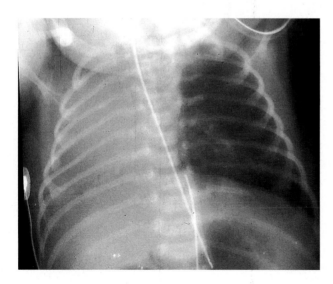

Fig. 4-30 AP chest radiograph: Atelectasis of the right lung with displacement of heart and mediastinum to right. Pulmonary artery sling. The aberrant left pulmonary artery hooks the trachea or bronchus, causing obstruction and collapse.

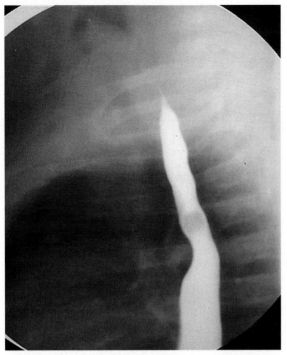

Fig. 4-31 Lateral esophagram: Anterior indentation on esophagus with soft tissue mass interposed between tracheal air column and esophagus. Pulmonary artery sling.

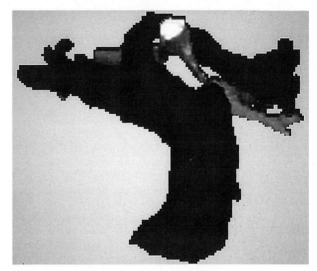

Fig. 4-32 3D MRI: Aberrant left pulmonary artery arising from right pulmonary artery. Note the narrowed bronchus. Pulmonary artery sling.

E. **Left atrium is concordant with the stomach, so thoracoabdominal discordance frequently accompanied by complex CHD**
1. Situs solitus totalis—normal: 1% CHD
2. Situs inversus and dextrocardia (situs inversus totalis)—complete mirror image: 2% CHD
   a. Abdominal situs (stomach bubble), cardiac apex concordant
   b. CHD usually common anomalies, such as VSD, tetralogy of Fallot, etc.
3. Dextrocardia and situs solitus (right-sided apex, left-sided stomach): 80% CHD
4. Levocardia and situs inversus (left-sided apex, right-sided stomach): 100% CHD
   a. Abdominal situs (stomach bubble), cardiac apex discordant
   b. CHD usually uncommon anomalies, combinations of lesions, and cyanotic in type, such as single ventricle with transposition, double outlet ventricle, etc.
F. **Situs indeterminus or visceral heterotaxy**
1. Asplenia **[Figs. 4-33 and 4-34]**
   a. Bilateral right sidedness
   b. Asplenia
   c. Transverse (symmetrical) liver
   d. Bilateral right lung morphology
   e. Cyanotic CHD
      • Anomalous systemic venous return

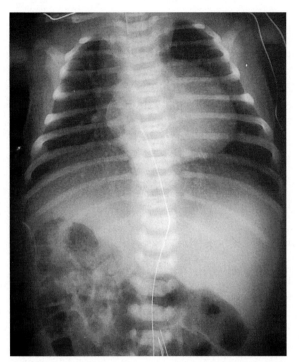

Fig. 4-33 AP chest radiograph: Liver spans midline of abdomen. Globular heart with mildly decreased pulmonary vascularity. Asplenia.

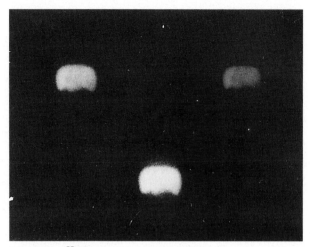

Fig. 4-34 99mTechnetium sulfur-colloid liver spleen scan: Midline liver, absence of uptake in spleen. Asplenia.

- Total anomalous pulmonary venous connection
- Transposition of great vessels
- Single ventricle
- 90% have significant obstruction to pulmonary blood flow

     f. Identified clinically by evaluating peripheral blood smear for Howell-Jolly and Heinz bodies, pitted erythrocytes

2. Polysplenia **[Figs. 4-35 and 4-36]**
     a. Bilateral left-sidedness

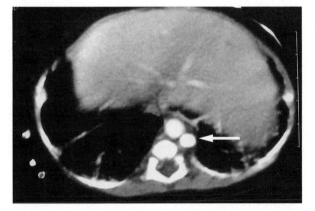

Fig. 4-35 Abdomen CT: Left-sided IVC (arrow), lack of communication between hepatic veins and IVC, midline liver. Polysplenia.

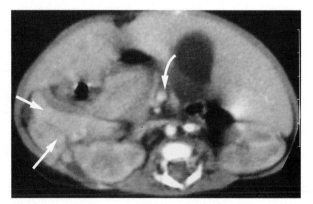

Fig. 4-36 Abdomen CT: Multiple right-sided splenic lobules (arrows), right renal vein enters left-sided IVC. Superior mesenteric vein (curved arrow) anterior to superior mesenteric artery, suggesting malrotation. Polysplenia.

   b. Polysplenia

   c. Biliary anomalies

   d. Bilateral left lung morphology

   e. Interrupted IVC

   f. Congenital heart disease, usually acyanotic

    • ASD, VSD, AV canal, partial anomalous pulmonary venous connection

  3. Asplenia associated with abnormal immune system and frequent infections, more complex CHD and worse overall prognosis

  4. Imaging evaluation:

   a. Ultrasound (US) for morphology of liver and spleen

   b. Liver/spleen scan to confirm absence of spleen

XI. **OPERATIVE PROCEDURES FOR CONGENITAL HEART DISEASE**

 A. **Blalock-Taussig (B-T) Shunt**

  1. Originally end-to-side anastomosis of subclavian artery to PA. Loss of subclavian flow to the arm caused a small arm in some patients. Rib notching was seen in some cases.

  2. Today, the modified B-T is used with a graft placed between the subclavian artery and PA.

 B. **Jatene arterial switch**

  1. Definitive d-transposition repair

  2. PA and aorta are returned to normal position

  3. The coronary arteries must be transplanted, so aberrant coronary artery anatomy can exclude this procedure

  4. Must be performed in early infancy, otherwise the left ventricle "deconditions" and will not support systemic pressures

 C. **Senning procedure**

  1. d-Transposition repair using an atrial baffle to redirect flow from pulmonary veins to tricuspid valve and from systemic veins to mitral valve.

  2. Baffle formed from infolded atrial wall.

 D. **Mustard procedure**

  1. Similar to Senning, but uses pericardium or synthetic graft material as baffle

 E. **Glenn shunt**

  1. SVC to RPA anastomosis

  2. Originally used in tricuspid atresia, now becoming more popular to increase PA size prior to definitive correction of right outflow obstruction

  3. Originally the PA was divided, removing connection with the MPA

  4. Bidirectional Glenn retains the continuity of the PA system

 F. **Fontan procedure**

  1. Right atrium to PA anastomosis

  2. Direct anastomosis, or valved or nonvalved conduit

3. With this procedure the LV is the only pump for both systemic and pulmonic circuits.
4. Elevated central venous pressure is common and patients frequently develop chronic pleural effusions.

G. **Rastelli procedure**
   1. Corrective procedure in d-transposition and VSD
   2. LV blood flows through VSD to aorta

H. **Norwood procedure**
   1. Three-step procedure to correct hypoplastic left heart
      a. Step 1: at birth
         - Atrial septectomy
         - Aorta enlarged with graft
         - MPA divided, aorta sutured to base of MPA
         - Systemic blood flow: RV to base of MPA to anastomosed aorta
         - Systemic shunt to distal MPA to provide pulmonary blood flow
         - PDA ligated
      b. Step 2: at age 3 to 9 months
         - Bidirectional Glenn placed
         - Systemic to pulmonary shunt closed
      c. Step 3: by 2 years of age
         - Glenn converted to Fontan

XII. **POSTOPERATIVE THORACOTOMY DEFORMITY**
   A. **Right thoracotomy**
      1. Blalock–Taussig shunt
      2. Esophageal atresia repair (associated with CHD in VATER association)
   B. **Left thoracotomy**
      1. B–T shunt
      2. PDA closure
      3. Coarctation repair
      4. PA band
   C. **Median sternotomy**
      1. All other repairs including Glenn shunt

XIII. **NEONATAL HEART DISEASE**
   A. **Neonatal physiology**
      1. 90% of fetal blood flows through the foramen ovale; only 10% goes through the lungs
      2. All newborns can shunt RA to LA and between PA and aorta
      3. At birth, PA pressure = aortic pressure
      4. PA pressure decreases over 6 to 8 weeks after birth
      5. Fetal left-sided cardiac output is half of right-sided output. The relatively underused LV markedly increases work at birth in the normal infant. Any stress, including outflow obstruction, high-flow states, or metabolic stress frequently results in left-sided failure. The RV better tolerates stress.

B. **Persistent fetal circulation (primary pulmonary hypertension)**
  1. Persistence of the high pulmonary pressures of the fetus, blood shunts right to left through PDA, bypassing the lungs
  2. Cyanosis, pulmonary oligemia

C. **Hypoplastic left heart syndrome**
  1. Underdeveloped left-sided structures
  2. Extent of hypoplasia is variable
  3. Aorta always severely hypoplastic
  4. Systemic blood flow is from PA via PDA
  5. Up to 50% are detected after 3 days of age, so patient may have been discharged from hospital and return in shock
  6. Infant classically described as gray rather than truly cyanotic
  7. Heart size variable, pulmonary edema is extreme in late cases

D. **Poor myocardial function in newborn [Fig. 4-37]**
  1. Frequent cause of cardiomegaly and CHF
  2. DDx of poor myocardial function in newborn
     a. Hypoxia

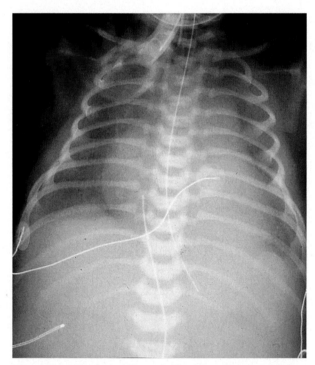

Fig. 4-37 AP chest radiograph: Two-day-old infant. Moderate-marked cardiac enlargement, pulmonary edema. DDx includes myocardial dysfunction (due to asphyxia, hypoglycemia, hypocalcemia, infant of diabetic mother with glycogen infiltration of heart or asymmetric septal hypertrophy, arrhythmia, carnitine deficiency), left ventricular obstruction, polycythemia, fluid overload. Perinatal asphyxia with myocardial dysfunction.

  b. Hypoglycemia

  c. Hypocalcemia

  d. Infant of diabetic mother

  e. Anemia

  f. Dysrhythmia

   • Congenital heart block (maternal lupus)

  g. Mitochondrial dysfunction

   • Carnitine deficiency

 E. **Peripheral arteriovenous malformation (AVM)**

  1. Mild to moderate CHF

  2. Bruit should be audible clinically

  3. With vein of Galen malformation, see wide superior mediastinum

  4. With hepatic hemangioendothelioma, expect large liver

XIV. **ACQUIRED HEART DISEASE**

 A. **Kawasaki disease**

  1. Coronary artery aneurysms and thrombosis

  2. Aneurysms usually resolve spontaneously

  3. Myocardial infarction occurs rarely

  4. Myocarditis may occur

 B. **Cardiomyopathy**

  1. Viral

   • Coxsackie virus

   • Mumps

   • Ebstein–Barr virus

  2. Rheumatic heart disease

  3. Connective tissue disease

  4. Rheumatoid arthritis

  5. Familial/hereditary

  6. Muscular dystrophies

  7. Friedereich's ataxia

  8. Pompe's disease

 C. **Cor pulmonale**

  1. Cystic fibrosis

  2. Bronchopulmonary dysplasia

 D. **Eisenmenger's physiology [Figs. 4–38 and 4–39]**

  1. Increased pulmonary blood flow and pressure cause irreversible pulmonary hypertension with reversal of shunting and right to left shunt

  2. Rarely seen today with early detection and treatment of CHD

 E. **Rheumatic heart disease**

  1. Immune reaction to group A beta-hemolytic *streptococcus* infection

  2. Myocardial disease seen acutely

  3. Valvular disease seen with chronic rheumatic fever

  4. Mitral stenosis, regurgitation, or both

  5. Aortic involvement similar, less common than mitral valve

 F. **Arrhythmogenic right ventricular dysplasia**

  1. Teens and young adults

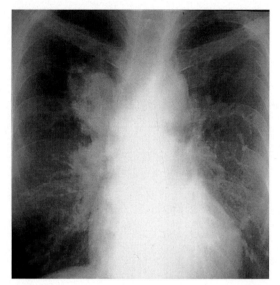

Fig. 4-38 PA chest radiograph: Young adult. Marked enlargement of central pulmonary arteries with abrupt arterial tapering in midlung fields. History of unoperated tetralogy of Fallot with systemic-to-pulmonary collaterals. Note rib notching. Pulmonary artery hypertension.

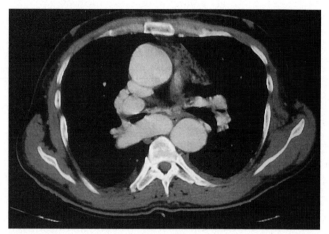

Fig. 4-39 Chest CT: Same patient as Figure 4-38. Marked enlargement of ascending and descending aorta. Main pulmonary artery is absent. Note extensive aorto-pulmonary collateral vessels. Severe tetralogy of Fallot (pulmonary atresia with VSD) with extensive aorto-pulmonary collaterals.

      2. Syncope, arrhythmias

      3. Fatty replacement of RV myocardium

      4. Magnetic resonance imaging (MRI) diagnosis

XV. **CARDIAC TUMORS**

  A. **80% cardiac, 20% pericardial**

    1. Cardiac

      a. Rhabdomyoma

        • Tuberous sclerosis in 50%

      b. Fibroma

        • Left ventricular myocardium

      c. Rhabdomyosarcoma

      d. Metastatic

    2. Pericardial

      a. Usually of mesenchymal origin or teratomas

      b. Metastatic

      c. Frequently cause effusions

XVI. **PERICARDIUM**

  A. **Absent left pericardium [Fig. 4-40]**

    1. Congenital defect in the pericardium

    2. Left atrial appendage herniates through defect

    3. Abnormal prominence of left cardiac contour

    4. Fluoroscopy shows striking cardiac motion in this area

    5. Today more often diagnosed with MRI

    6. Usually asymptomatic, rarely herniation through defect and resulting strangulation can be life-threatening

B. **Pericardial effusion [Figs. 4-41 through 4-43]**
   1. Globular enlargement of cardio-pericardial silhouette
      a. Resembles "water bottle"
      b. DDx: cardiomyopathy
   2. US best modality to confirm diagnosis
C. **Pericardial cyst**
   1. May cause focal contour abnormality
   2. Usually not associated with pericardial effusion
D. **Pericardial tumors**
   1. 20% of cardiac tumors
      a. Teratoma
      b. Fibroma
      c. Lipoma
   2. Frequently produce pericardial effusion
E. **Pericarditis**
   1. Inflammation of pericardium
      a. Always associated with pericardial effusion
      b. Friction rub heard on auscultation
   2. Viral most common etiology
      a. Coxsackie virus
   3. Bacterial rare in children
F. **Post-pericardiectomy syndrome**
   1. Pericardial effusion following cardiac surgery
   2. Responds to nonsteroidal antiinflammatory drugs

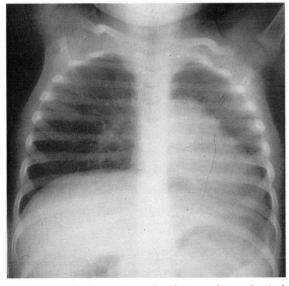

Fig. 4-40 PA chest radiograph: Classic cardio-mediastinal contour of partial absence of left pericardium.

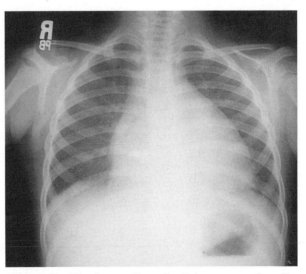

Fig. 4-41 PA chest radiograph: Enlargement of cardio-pericardial silhouette. Pulmonary vascularity is normal. Pericardial effusion.

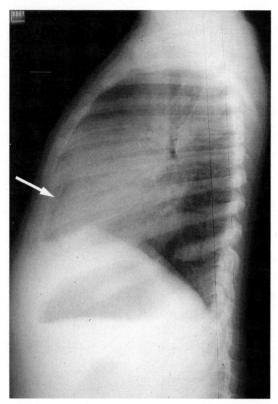

Fig. 4-42 Lateral chest radiograph: Same patient as Figure 4-41. Epicardial fat (arrow) with fluid or soft tissue density anterior, indicating pericardial effusion. This pattern is unusual in children with pericardial effusion and is more likely to be seen in adults with pericardial effusion.

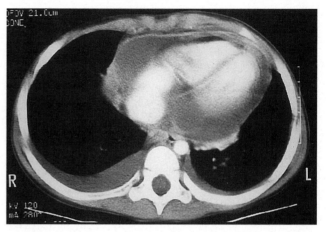

Fig. 4-43 Chest CT: Same patient as Figure 4-41. Large pericardial effusion and bilateral pleural effusions.

XVII. **GAMUTS**
- These gamuts are not exhaustive
- They include the types of CHD most commonly found in each group
- Within each group they are listed in order of decreasing frequency (most common first)

A. **Acyanotic CHD with increased flow**
  1. VSD
  2. ASD
  3. PDA
  4. ECD

B. **Acyanotic CHD with normal flow**
  1. PS
  2. AS
  3. Coarctation of the aorta

C. **Cyanotic CHD with decreased flow**
  1. Normal heart size
     a. Tetralogy of Fallot

        b. Pulmonary atresia with VSD

        c. Complex CHD with pulmonic obstruction

    2. Large heart

        a. Ebstein anomaly

        b. Pulmonary atresia with intact ventricular septum and tricuspid regurgitation

D. **Cyanotic CHD with increased flow**

    1. Truncus arteriosus

    2. Total anomalous pulmonary venous return without obstruction

E. **Cyanotic CHD with variable pulmonary blood flow**

    1. d-Transposition

    2. Tricuspid atresia

    3. DORV

F. **CHD associated with a right-sided aortic arch (RAA)**

    1. Tetralogy of Fallot accounts for 65% of CHD with RAA

    2. Truncus arteriosus accounts for 15% of CHD with RAA

    3. Tricuspid atresia accounts for 10% of CHD with RAA

    4. d-Transposition accounts for 5% of CHD with RAA

    5. Other CHD accounts for 5% of CHD with RAA

    6. In complex CHD, a right arch is often associated with PS

G. **Pulmonary venous congestion in the newborn**

    1. First week

        a. Hypoplastic left heart

        b. Severe aortic stenosis

        c. Fluid overload

        d. Myocardial insult

          • Hypoglycemia

          • Hypocalcemia

          • Asphyxia

        e. Obstructed TAPVC

        f. Arrhythmia

        g. Peripheral AV shunting

          • Vein of Galen malformation

          • Hepatic hemangioendothelioma

    2. Second to sixth week

        a. Left ventricular outflow obstruction

          • Severe coarctation

          • Interrupted aortic arch

          • Severe aortic stenosis

         b. Endocardial fibroelastosis

        c. Anomalous origin of left coronary artery

        d. Cor triatriatum

XVIII. **CAUSES OF CONGESTIVE HEART FAILURE AT DIFFERENT AGES**

    A. **Premature infant**

        1. Fluid overload

        2. PDA

        3. Bronchopulmonary dysplasia (cor pulmonale)

B. **Term newborn**
  1. Asphyxia
  2. Infant of diabetic mother
      a. Asymmetric septal hypertrophy
      b. Glycogen infiltration
      c. Hypoglycemia
      d. Hypocalcemia
  3. Critical left-sided obstruction
      a. Coarctation or aortic stenosis
      b. Hypoplastic left heart
  4. Transposition of great vessels
  5. Single ventricle physiology
  6. AVM
      a. Vein of Galen malformation
      b. Hepatic hemangioendothelioma
C. **Child several months of age**
  1. VSD
  2. AVM
D. **Older child**
  1. Renal disease
  2. Viral myocarditis
  3. Kawasaki disease

Further Reading

Amparo EG, Higgins CB, Shafton EP. Demonstration of coarctation of the aorta by magnetic resonance imaging. AJR 1984;143:1192–1194.

Amplatz K, Moller JH. Radiology of Congenital Heart Disease. St. Louis, MO: Mosby-Yearbook, 1993.

Bank ER. Magnetic resonance of congenital cardiovascular disease: An update. Radiol Clin North Am 1993; 31:553–572.

Berdon E, Baker DH. Vascular anomalies and the infant lung: rings, slings, and other things. Semin Roentgenol 1972;7:39–64.

Coussement AM, Gooding CA. Objective radiographic assessment of pulmonary vascularity in children. Radiology 1973;109:649.

Donnelly LF, Hurst DR, Strife JL, Shapiro R. Plain film assessment of the neonate with D-transposition of the great vessels. Pediatr Radiol 1995;25:195–197.

Fellows KE, Weinberg PM, Baffa JM, Hoffman EA. Evaluation of congenital heart disease with MR imaging: current and coming attractions. AJR 1992;159:925–931.

Jatene AD, Fontes VF, Souza LC, et al. Anatomic correction of transposition of the great arteries. J Thorac Cardiovasc Surg 1982;83:20–26.

Kuhn MA, Latson LA, Cheatham JP, et al. Management of pediatric patients with isolated valvar aortic stenosis by balloon aortic valvulopasty. Cathet Cardiovasc Diagn 1996;39:55–61.

Morrow WR, Vick GW III, Nihill MR, et al. Balloon dilation of unoperated coarctation of the aorta: short- and intermediate-term results. J Am Coll Cardiol 1988;11: 133–138.

Rosario-Medina W, Strife JL, Dunbar JS. Normal left atrium: Appearance in children on frontal chest radiographs. Radiology 1986;161:345–346.

Sano S, Brawn WJ, Mee RB. Total anomalous pulmonary venous drainage. J Thorac Cardiovasc Surg 1989;97:886–892.

Swischuk LE. Plain Film Interpretation of Congenital Heart Disease, 3rd ed. Baltimore, MD: Williams and Wilkins, 1985.

Swischuk LE, Stansberry SD. Pulmonary vascularity in pediatric heart disease. J Thorac Imaging 1989;4:1–6.

Winer-Muram HT, Tonkin IL. The spectrum of heterotaxia syndromes. Radiol Clin North Am 1989;27:1147–1170.

CHAPTER FIVE   CHEST AND RESPIRATORY SYSTEM

I. **THE NEWBORN CHEST**

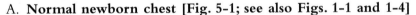

    A. **Normal newborn chest [Fig. 5-1; see also Figs. 1-1 and 1-4]**
        1. Shape
           a. Broader than adult, with near parallel lateral margins
           b. Bell-shaped chest suggests neuromuscular disease or paralysis
        2. Heart size
           a. Normal cardiothoracic ratio up to 60%
           b. Obtain lateral view if confirmation of cardiomegaly needed
           c. If the posterior cardiac margin is not close to the anterior margin of the vertebral bodies, the heart is not enlarged
        3. Thymus
           a. Wavy edge due to anterior rib end impressions
           b. No mass effect
           c. Variable size
             • May extend to diaphragm
             • Even extreme asymmetry in thymic lobes is normal
             • Stress atrophy with marked decrease in size of thymus can occur within 12 hours of onset of stress
        4. Vascularity
           a. Centrally less well-defined than adult
           b. Appears more prominent than in older children/adults

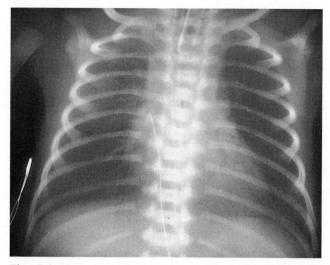

Fig. 5-1 Anteroposterior (AP) chest radiograph: Endotracheal tube, feeding tube present. Umbilical venous catheter (UVC) in right atrium. Lungs well-inflated. Vascular markings well-seen. Cardiothymic silhouette normal. Notice slightly increased density along left pedicles of vertebrae, indicating left descending aorta. Normal newborn chest radiograph.

5. Chest wall
   a. Ribs
      • Thin, horizontal ribs with prominent rib ends
   b. Soft tissues
      • Usually less than 5 mm thick over the ribs in full term
      • Thickened soft tissue
         Anasarca
         Infant of diabetic mother
         Soft tissue edema, pulmonary edema, no bowel gas: consider
            Pavulon paralysis of sick premature (Pavulon causes third-
            spacing of fluid)

B. **Neonatal lung disease**
   1. Four patterns of neonatal lung disease
      • Neonatal lung disease differs markedly from that occurring at any other age. The following descriptions facilitate a useful differential of the radiographic appearances typical of neonatal lung disease.
      a. Fine granular opacities, evenly distributed **[Figs. 5-2, 5-3, and 5–11]**
         • Hyaline membrane disease
         • Group B streptococcal pneumonia
            Consider if >34 weeks, pleural fluid present, uneven distribution
      b. Linear opacities radiating from hila
         • Retained fetal lung fluid
            Resolves within 3 days

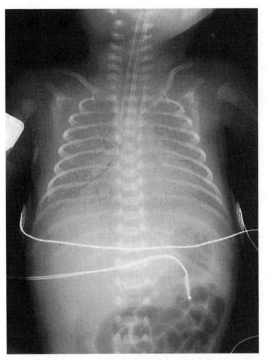

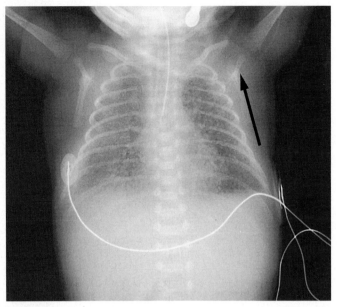

Fig. 5-2 AP chest radiograph: Premature infant. Diffuse granularity of lungs with bilateral air bronchograms, cardiac contour difficult to appreciate due to parenchymal haze. Fine granular opacities. HMD.

Fig. 5-3 AP chest radiograph: Numerous circular or rod-like lucencies in perihilar areas bilaterally. Air bronchograms in right upper lobe. Rounded lucencies denote PIE (PIE darker than and fail to branch like air bronchograms). Note peripherally inserted central catheter (picc) line overlying left axilla (arrow). Fine granular opacities in right lung with air bronchograms. HMD.

    c. Coarse linear and reticular opacities, evenly distributed **[Fig. 5-4]**
- Meconium aspiration
  Term or postterm infants
  Often complicated by air leak
- Neonatal pneumonia
- Severe retained fetal lung fluid
- Bronchopulmonary dysplasia (BPD) (classic form)
  Only infants > 3 weeks of age
- Wilson–Mikity disease

    d. Confluent opacities, unevenly distributed
- Neonatal pneumonia
- Pulmonary hemorrhage

C. **Specific pathologies of neonatal lung disease**
1. Hyaline membrane disease (HMD) or respiratory distress syndrome (RDS)
   a. Surfactant deficiency due to immature type II alveolar cells
   b. Evenly distributed ground glass appearance due to alveolar collapse
   c. Low lung volumes are classically described, but this finding may be altered by ventilator settings
   d. Rare after 36 weeks gestation
   e. Pleural effusions should not be seen with HMD
   - HMD appearance with effusions suggests group B streptococcal pneumonia

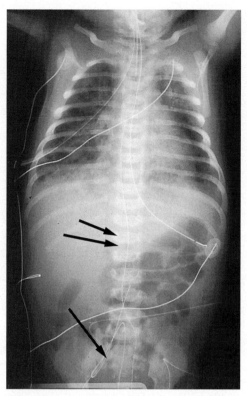

Fig. 5-4 AP chest radiograph: Term newborn. Hyperinflated lungs, nodular interstitial opacities bilaterally. Note umbilical artery catheter (UAC) (arrow) coursing downward into pelvis then upward into aorta (umbilical artery is branch of internal iliac artery), and umbilical venous catheter (double arrow) coursing cephalad. Coarse linear-reticular opacities. Meconium aspiration.

   f. Surfactant treatment of HMD
- Exogenous surfactant administered intratracheally
- Usually markedly improves radiographic and clinical HMD
- Surfactant may be readministered if little response
- Poor response frequently associated with worse clinical course
- Radiographs obtained immediately after surfactant administration may show streaky linear densities radiating from hila as fluid is absorbed into lymphatics
- Effect of surfactant may be patchy or non-uniform if surfactant is not distributed evenly throughout tracheobronchial tree

2. Transient tachypnea of newborn
   a. Better called "retained fetal lung fluid"
   b. Caused by inadequate clearance of lung fluid prior to first breath
- Precipitous delivery
- Cesarean section

   c. Fluid moves into lymphatics and pleural space
   d. Linear densities radiating from hila, thick fissures, small effusions

3. Neonatal pneumonia
   a. In the differential of most abnormal neonatal lung appearances; Gram negative organisms more common than at any other age
   b. Group B streptococcal pneumonia can simulate RDS
4. Congenital diaphragmatic hernia **[Figs. 5-5 and 5-6]**
   a. Prognosis depends primarily on degree of pulmonary hypoplasia
   b. Presents as opaque hemithorax or bowel loops in the chest
   c. Scaphoid abdomen seen clinically
   d. Can present at or after birth
      - Bochdalek—posterior and lateral (Bochdalek = behind)
        Most frequent and most severe
      - Morgagni—anterior and medial (Morgagni = medial)
        Rarely presents clinically at birth
      - Immediate presentation
        left (L) ≫ right (R)
        Congenital diaphragmatic defect
      - Delayed presentation
        R > L
        Associated with group B streptococcal pneumonia
5. BPD **[Figs. 5-7 through 5-9]**
   a. Abnormal chest radiograph (CXR) and oxygen requirement after 28 days of life or 36 weeks gestational age
   b. First described by Northway et al. (1967) as having four stages:
      - 1 = RDS, first week
      - 2 = White out, 4 to 10 days

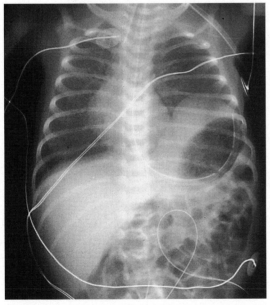

Fig. 5-5 AP chest radiograph: Newborn with abnormal left hemidiaphragm, unusual course of feeding tube. Congenital diaphragmatic hernia.

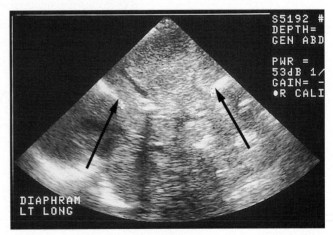

Fig. 5-6 Parasagittal ultrasound through left hemidiaphragm: Same patient as Figure 5-5. Discontinuity of echogenic diaphragm (between arrows). Left lobe of liver protrudes within diaphragmatic defect. Congenital diaphragmatic hernia.

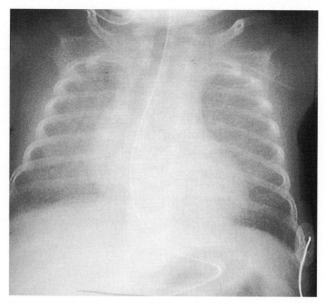

Fig. 5-7 AP chest radiograph: 1-month-old former premie. Diffuse fine interstitial pattern. Note picc line overlying left axilla. BPD, diffuse. Differential diagnosis (DDx): "leaky lungs" or pulmonary edema.

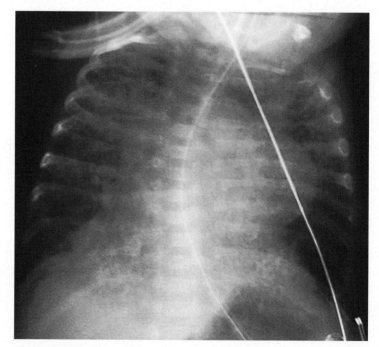

Fig. 5-8 AP chest radiograph: 2-month-old former premie, following chronic ventilator therapy. Marked hyperinflation, flattened diaphragm, coarse interstitial opacities, air trapping. BPD, disorganized pattern.

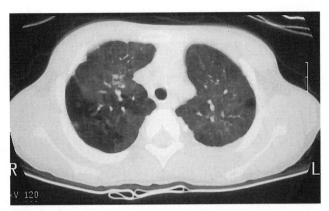

Fig. 5-9   HRCT: 4-year-old with BPD. Juxta pleural scarring, focal air trapping, mosaic parenchymal pattern. Hyperlucent areas represent air trapping in small airways.

- 3 = Bubbly-appearing lungs due to inflammation with areas of atelectasis and emphysema, 10 to 20 days
- 4 = Bubbly-appearing lungs with development of fibrosis, > one month

  c. Due to marked changes in neonatal care since 1967, this regular progression is now rarely seen
  - Formerly, radiographic BPD pattern seen after 30 days of life
  - Currently, with improved treatment, tinier newborns with immature lungs are rescued. Pulmonary immaturity + oxygen and/or barotrauma results in earlier appearance of BPD (approximately 10 days of age)
  d. Swischuk (1996) has suggested that premature lung disease should be classified into three categories:
  - Surfactant deficiency disease (RDS)
  - Leaky lung syndrome (pulmonary edema pattern)
  - BPD (bubbly-appearing lungs) seen at any age
  e. Clinical course is more important than radiographic appearance, as there is often poor correlation between clinical status and the severity of CXR changes
  f. BPD changes often long-standing (years)
  - Best shown by high resolution computed tomography (HRCT)
6. Wilson-Mikity syndrome
  a. Wilson and Mikity (1959) reported five infants with a CXR appearance suggesting BPD. There was no history of ventilator support, and CXRs in some showed a BPD appearance at a very young age
  b. Appearance of coarse opacities similar or identical to BPD can appear within the first week of life
  c. Currently this remains an idiopathic entity
  d. 75% recover, 25% die
7. Meconium aspiration syndrome **[Fig. 5-4]**
  a. Rare in preterm infants; suggests Listeria infection in this group

    b. Term or postterm neonates aspirate meconium–containing amniotic fluid

    c. Bile acids and particulate material cause small airway inflammation and obstruction

    d. Hypoxia worsens rapidly during the first hours of life

    e. May develop severe pulmonary hypertension

8. Persistent fetal circulation

    a. High pulmonary vascular resistance causes right to left shunt across ductus

    b. Severe hypoxia

    c. CXR frequently normal

    d. May see prominent right cardiac contour due to tricuspid regurgitation

    e. May see pulmonary oligemia

9. Extracorporeal membrane oxygenation (ECMO) **[Fig. 5-10]**

    a. Pulmonary bypass

    b. Requires systemic heparinization

       • Head ultrasound (US) required to exclude hemorrhage that could extend after heparinization

    c. Venovenous

       • Right atrium (RA) → membrane oxygenator → venous system

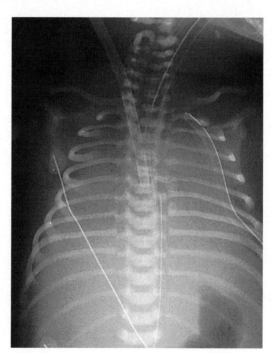

Fig. 5-10 AP chest radiograph: Newborn with completely opaque lungs. Note large bore catheter along right side of neck. Venovenous ECMO. Arteriovenous ECMO requires two catheters, one in internal jugular vein and one in carotid artery.

d. Arteriovenous
- RA → oxygenator → carotid artery
- Arteriovenous provides cardiac as well as pulmonary bypass

e. Carotid artery was sacrificed in earlier methods, but now can be preserved

10. Chylothorax

a. Most common cause of large pleural effusion in newborn

b. Does not develop until child ingests lipids and forms chyle

D. **Air leak in neonates**

1. Pneumothorax **[Figs. 5-11 through 5-13; see also Figs. 1-17 and 1-18]**

a. Pleural line often difficult to see

b. Often located at anterior lung bases

c. May appear as lucency along cardiac margin resembling an abnormally wide Mach line

d. Suspect in hyperlucent lung

2. Pneumomediastinum **[Fig. 5-14; see also Figs. 1-15 and 1-16]**

a. "Sail sign" of elevated thymus

b. Extension of air into neck rare in infants

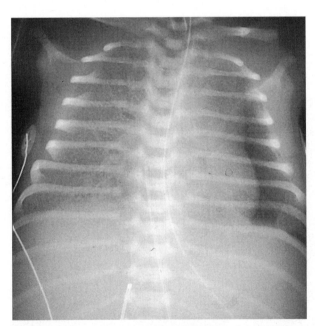

Fig. 5-11 AP chest radiograph: Newborn with HMD. Note lucency adjacent to left heart border. Lung markings seen through area of lucency. Anterior pneumothorax. Remember, film is taken supine. Image is a two-dimensional representation of a three-dimensional object. Pneumothorax is anterior. Air in lung parenchyma is posterior. Small wedge of hazy lung in left costophrenic angle.

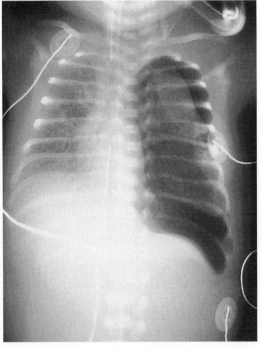

Fig. 5-12 AP chest radiograph: Newborn with HMD. Obvious lucency in left hemithorax, depression of left hemidiaphragm, widening of rib interspaces, and displacement of mediastinum to right. Note failure of left lung to completely deflate (poorly compliant or stiff lung). Small cardiac size indicates decreased venous return to atria, decreased cardiac output. This is a medical emergency. Tension pneumothorax.

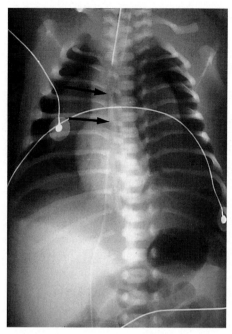

Fig. 5-13 AP chest radiograph: Newborn with HMD. Bilateral lucency, depression of both hemidiaphragms, widening of rib interspaces, and small cardiac size. Vertical line (arrows) indicates anterior junction line outlined by air in bilateral tension pneumothoraces.

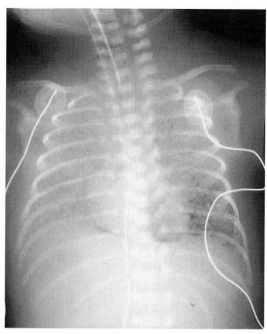

Fig. 5-14 AP chest radiograph: Newborn with HMD. Numerous rounded lucencies in left lung (PIE), curvilinear lucency around base of heart (Pneumomediastinum).

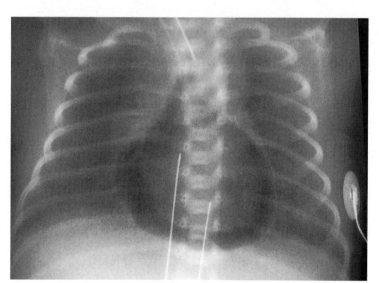

Fig. 5-15 AP chest radiograph: Newborn with HMD. Air completely encircles heart. Note cephalad extent around great vessels. Pneumopericardium.

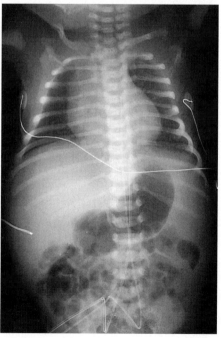

Fig. 5-16 AP chest radiograph: Newborn with two UACs. Note course of UAC, which enters pelvis then extends cephalad into aorta. Umbilical artery to internal iliac artery to common iliac artery to aorta. UAC.

  c. Difficult to distinguish from anterior pneumothorax

  d. Rarely symptomatic

 3. Pneumopericardium **[Fig. 5-15]**

 4. Pulmonary interstitial emphysema (PIE) **[Figs. 1-13, 5–3 and 5–14]**

  a. Barotrauma causes alveolar tears with air tracking into perivascular spaces and lymphatics

  b. Small, sharply defined, round and rod-shaped lucencies

  c. Darker than air bronchograms

  d. Does not taper like air bronchograms

  e. PIE can coalesce into cystic air collections

  f. Frequently complicated by pneumomediastinum or pneumothorax

E. **Umbilical arterial and venous catheters**

 1. Arterial **[Fig. 5-16]**

  a. Course: Umbilical artery to hypogastric (internal iliac) to aorta

  b. Correct position of tip

   • High position: T6 to T9

   • Low position: L3 to L4

  c. Identified by caudad course from umbilicus with sharp bend near superior margin of sacroiliac joint

 2. Venous **[Figs. 5-17 and 5-18]**

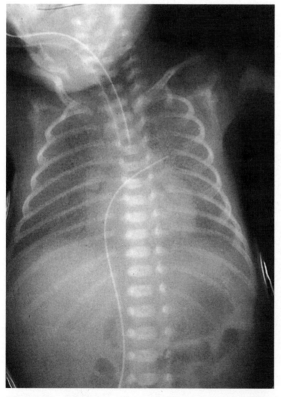

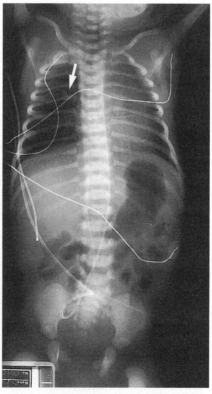

Fig. 5-17 AP chest radiograph: Newborn with HMD. Note course of UVC, which crosses midline into left atrium via foramen ovale, extends beyond border of heart to enter left upper pulmonary vein. UVC.

Fig. 5-18 AP chest radiograph: Newborn with HMD. Note course of UVC, which crosses midline into left atrium via foramen ovale, loops within left atrium, and extends into right upper pulmonary vein (arrow). UVC.

a. Course: Umbilical vein to ascending left portal vein to ductus venosus to inferior vena cava (IVC) to right atrium
b. Correct position of tip: above diaphragm in right atrium
c. Craniad direction from umbilicus
d. Beware of loops in catheter outside the patient that can confuse the intravascular course of the catheter
e. Common malpositions
- Tip overlying right upper quadrant (RUQ) directed right—right portal vein
- Abrupt caudad reversed direction below diaphragm—middle hepatic vein
- Advancement beyond RA most often crosses foramen ovale into left atrium, and tip frequently enters pulmonary vein

II. **NORMAL CHEST IN THE OLDER CHILD [Fig. 5-19; see also Figs. 1-2 and 1-5]**

A. **Sternum**
1. Five ossification centers by age 6 months
2. Bifid manubrial ossification center in 80% Down's syndrome, 20% normal children
3. Sternal fusion in 50% children with cyanotic congenital heart disease

B. **Thymus**
1. Thymus changes little in size during childhood
2. Proportionately largest in infancy
3. Enlarges until puberty, but decreases in relative size
4. Extreme variability limits value of "normal dimensions"
5. Asymmetry is common

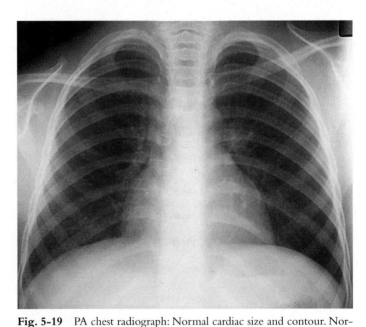

Fig. 5-19 PA chest radiograph: Normal cardiac size and contour. Normal pulmonary vascularity. Trachea deviated slightly to left, indicating right aortic arch. Otherwise normal chest radiograph in a 4-year-old child.

6. Commonly extends behind superior vena cava (SVC) into middle mediastinum
7. Visible on CXR in 5 to 10% of 5-year-olds
8. Usually visible on CT/magnetic resonance imaging (MRI) through pediatric age
9. Size of thymus on MRI
   a. Thickness of lobes remains constant at approximately 2 cm at all ages
   b. Left lobe length increases from 3 cm in infants to 4.5 cm in teens
   c. Right lobe length increases from 2.5 cm in infants to 3.0 cm in teens

III. **CONGENITAL MALFORMATIONS**
- No single theory accepted to explain malformations
- Insult can affect vascular, bronchial, or parenchymal components of the lung singly or in combination
- Additional spectrum of malformations including tracheoesophageal fistula arises from incomplete separation of primitive gut and respiratory tract
- Timing of insult may be important factor in determining type of malformation

A. **Pulmonary agenesis or aplasia [Fig. 5-20]**
   1. Total absence of lung
   2. Frequency: R = L
   3. In agenesis, contralateral lung is large and has twice the number of alveoli of a normal lung
   4. Agenesis—no bronchus
   5. Aplasia—atretic bronchus present

B. **Pulmonary hypoplasia**
   1. Unilateral or bilateral small lung
   2. In unilateral hypoplasia, small or absent pulmonary artery
   3. On lateral view extrapleural areolar tissue causes a soft-tissue stripe anterior and/or posterior to the small lung

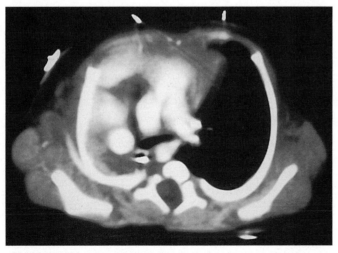

Fig. 5-20 Chest CT: Right pulmonary agenesis. Note abrupt termination of tracheobronchial tree and absence of right pulmonary artery.

4. Bilateral can be difficult to detect
   a. Look for low lung volumes without vascular crowding or atelectasis
5. Suspect bilateral hypoplasia in neonate with any of the following:
   a. Small chest
   b. Spontaneous pneumothorax, especially bilateral
   c. Oligohydramnios or renal dysfunction
   d. Any intrathoracic mass
6. Hypoplasia may be due to:
   a. Decreased number of airway branchings
   b. Decreased alveolar size
   c. Both
7. Hypoplasia can be congenital or acquired
   a. Acquired causes:
      - Postinfectious (Swyer-James syndrome)
      - Radiation
      - Scoliosis

C. **Tracheal atresia**
   1. Entire trachea usually absent
   2. Bronchi or distal trachea connected to esophagus

D. **Bronchial atresia**
   1. Often segmental interruption; therefore, may see mucous-filled bronchi distal to the atresia
   2. In newborn may present as fluid-filled lung that later clears by collateral ventilation
   3. May be seen in association with bronchopulmonary foregut malformations
   4. Left upper lobe (LUL) most common location; RUL next most common

E. **Tracheal stenosis**
   1. 50% focal or segmental
   2. 30% diffuse tracheal narrowing
   3. 25% cone-like, with normal wide upper trachea and narrow lower trachea
   4. Usually presents in infancy
   5. Associations include tracheal bronchus, pulmonary hypoplasia, VATER (Vertebral defects, Anal atresia, Tracheoesophageal fistula with Esophageal atresia, and Radial and/or Renal anomalies) or VACTERL (VATER + Cardiac + Limb anomalies) association

F. **Bronchopulmonary foregut malformations**
   1. Sequestration
      a. Lung without airway connection to rest of lung; systemic arterial supply
      b. Aeration by collateral ventilation (pores of Kohn)
      c. Medial lung base L > R
      d. Intralobar
         - No pleural separation from lung
      e. Extralobar
         - Pleura separates from rest of lung, cannot aerate or become infected

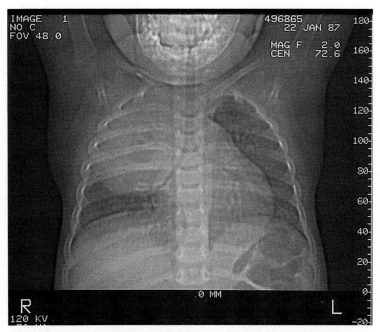

Fig. 5-21 AP scoutview for CT: Mass in right upper lobe. Note depression of right bronchus, air within mass. Infected parenchymal bronchogenic cyst.

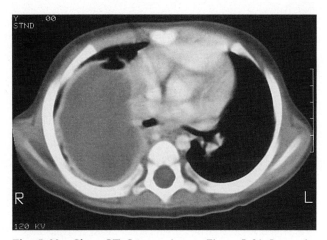

Fig. 5-22 Chest CT: Same patient as Figure 5-21. Large air-containing mass in right hemithorax with thick, enhancing rim. Infected parenchymal bronchogenic cyst.

2. Bronchogenic cyst **[Figs. 5-21 through 5-23]**
   a. Equal incidence mediastinum and lung
   b. CT/MRI: smoothly marginated, thin walled, homogeneous
   c. CT attenuation may be high
3. Cystic adenomatoid malformation **[Fig. 5-24]**
   a. Abnormal organization of lung tissue elements
   b. Three types
      • I = Few or solitary large cyst(s)

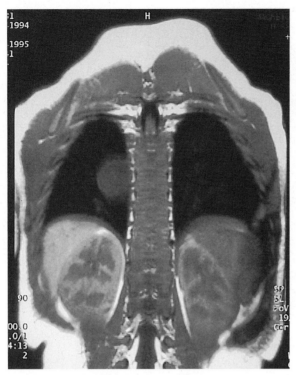

Fig. 5-23 Coronal T1-weighted MRI: Rounded mass adjacent to spine. Mediastinal bronchogenic cyst

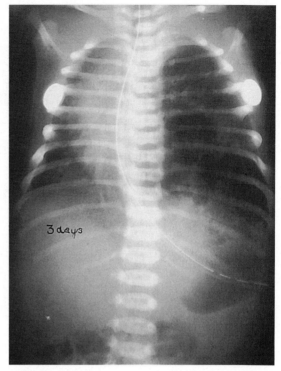

Fig. 5-24 AP chest radiograph: 3-day-old with respiratory distress. Multiple cysts in left lower lobe, displacement of mediastinum to right, intact left hemidiaphragm. Cystic adenomatoid malformation

- II = Multiple small cysts
- III = Solid
  c. Unilateral, can affect entire lung
  d. Equally distributed throughout different lobes
  e. High association with extrathoracic malformations in type II
4. Congenital lobar emphysema **[Fig. 5-25]**
   a. Initially opaque due to slow clearance of fetal lung fluid; clears over first days of life then hyperinflates
   b. LUL most common site, then right middle lobe (RML), then right upper lobe (RUL)
   c. Lower lobes account for only 10%
   d. Majority present in neonatal period
5. Venolobar syndrome **[Fig. 5-26]**
   a. Also called scimitar or hypogenetic lung syndrome
   b. Right lung usually affected
   c. Abnormal pulmonary drainage into IVC or hepatic vein
   d. Draining pulmonary vein forms the scimitar
   e. Always associated with hypoplastic lung
   f. Atrial septal defect (ASD) in 25%
G. **Tracheal bronchus**
   1. RUL apical segmental bronchus originates from trachea rather than right UL bronchus

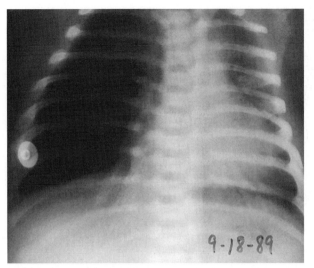

Fig. 5-25 AP chest radiograph: Newborn. Well-defined lucency in right hemithorax. Displacement of mediastinum to left, widened right rib interspaces, intact right hemidiaphragm. Congenital lobar emphysema, right middle lobe

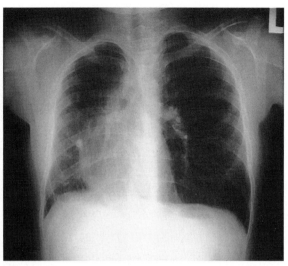

Fig. 5-26 PA chest radiograph: Displacement of heart to right. The right hemithorax is hypoplastic. Note unusual vessel resembling a Turkish scimitar in right lower thorax. Venolobar (scimitar) syndrome

    2. Also called a pig bronchus since RUL bronchus normally arises from trachea in the pig.

    3. Can be associated with tracheal stenosis

    4. Usually replaces RUL apical segmental bronchus with no other apical segmental bronchus present

    5. Rarely may be a duplicated bronchus with a normally located RUL apical segmental bronchus present as well

  H. **Lymphangiectasia**

    1. Very rare anomaly of the lymphatic system with abnormal lymphatic drainage

    2. Lungs show a coarse reticular pattern of increased density

      a. Resembles type III total anomalous pulmonary venous connection

IV. **INFLAMMATION**

  A. **Infection**

    1. Airway inflammation more often clinically significant in children than adults due to:

      a. Small size of airways

      b. More mucous glands

      c. Increased bronchial reactivity

    2. Differentiation of viral and bacterial pneumonia:

      a. Radiographic appearance is not highly specific

      b. Pleural effusions are rare in viral pneumonia

      c. Clinical information is essential for useful differential

  B. **Bacterial pneumonia**

    1. Consolidative pneumonia **[Fig. 5-27; see also Fig. 1-8]**

      a. Segmental or lobar opacity without volume loss

      b. *Streptococcus pneumoniae* (pneumococcus)

        • Accounts for more than 90% of pediatric bacterial pneumonia

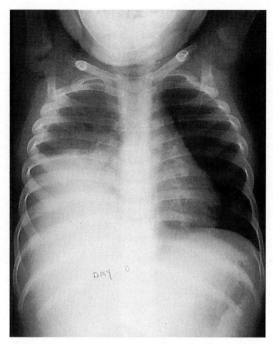

Fig. 5-27 PA chest radiograph: Consolidation of right middle and right lower lobes. Lobar pneumonia.

- Effusion frequent
- High fever and high white count

c. *Staphylococcus aureus*
  - 70% patients less than one year of age
  - High mortality unless treated early
  - Infection rapidly progresses to abscess with secondary empyema **[Fig. 5-28]** early and pneumatoceles later as disease progresses

d. *Haemophilus influenzae*
  - Increasingly rare due to *Haemophilus influenzae* Type B (HIB) vaccine
  - Gradual onset
  - Often clinically unimpressive

e. *Klebsiella pneumoniae*
  - Sporadic or epidemic in neonates
  - Rare in older immune-competent children
  - "Bulging fissure sign" suggests diagnosis

2. Round pneumonia **[Figs. 5-29 and 5-30]**
   a. Well-defined, masslike appearance
   b. Usually pneumococcus
   c. Almost always lower lobes
   d. Rare after 8 years of age; in older children round densities suggest unusual organisms, especially fungi
   e. Child with clinical pneumonia and an isolated parenchymal mass should be treated for pneumonia, with CXR repeated in 2 weeks

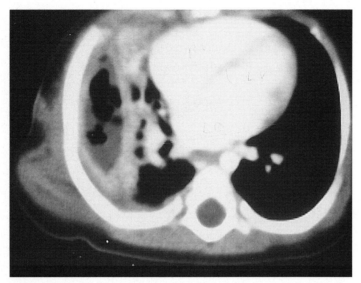

Fig. 5-28 Chest CT: Thickening and enhancement of visceral and parietal pleura adjacent to pneumonia. Bubbles of gas within infected pleural space. Empyema.

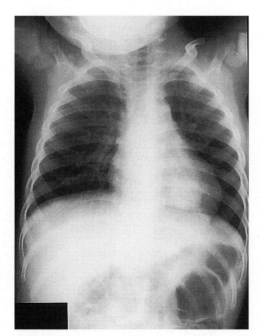

Fig. 5-29 PA chest radiograph: Round opacity behind heart. Round pneumonia.

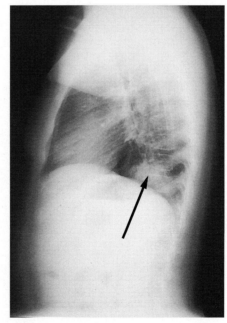

Fig. 5-30 Lateral chest radiograph: Round opacity (arrow) overlying vertebral column superior to hemidiaphragms. As your eye tracks down along vertebral column, notice parenchyma becomes whiter (this is abnormal) instead of darker. Lower lobe pneumonia.

3. Bronchopneumonia
   a. Scattered subsegmental infiltrates, frequently perivascular distribution
   b. *Bordetella pertussis*
      - Whooping cough
      - Incompletely immunized or very young infants
      - "Shaggy heart" caused by central patchy infiltrates and bronchial wall thickening
   c. *Chlamydia trachomatis* [**Fig. 5-31**]
      - Transvaginal inoculation at birth
      - Infants, 6 to 12 weeks of age
      - Afebrile, barking cough, eosinophilia
      - Frequently associated with conjunctivitis
      - Appearance suggests viral pneumonia
   d. *Mycoplasma pneumoniae* [**Fig. 5-32**]
      - Most common cause of pneumonia in children
      - Rarely younger than school age
      - Interstitial infiltrates to dense consolidation
      - Often multifocal
      - Effusions in 20%, almost never large
      - Hilar adenopathy not uncommon
4. Lung abscess
   a. Thick irregular walls ± air/fluid level or mobile debris
   b. Pneumatoceles have thin walls, may have air/fluid levels
   c. May heal completely or leave residual pneumatocele

C. **Viral pneumonia**
   1. Appearance
      a. Hyperinflation, peribronchial thickening, scattered bilateral subsegmental infiltrates

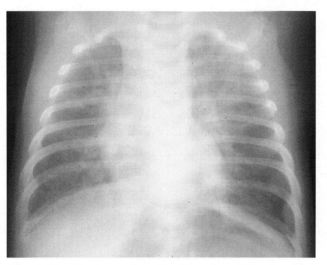

Fig. 5-31 AP chest radiograph: Bilateral perihilar interstitial opacity with nearly diffuse interstitial thickening. Linear opacities; interstitial pneumonia, Chlamydia.

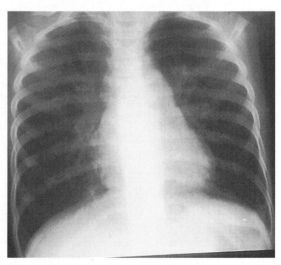

Fig. 5-32 PA chest radiograph: Bilateral perihilar interstitial opacities radiating from hila. For this pattern, consider chlamydia in infants 4 weeks to 4 months of age, respiratory syncytial virus in all infants, mycoplasma in older children. Bronchopneumonia—mycoplasma.

2. Respiratory syncytial virus (RSV)
   a. Most common cause of lower respiratory infection in children under 2 years of age
   b. Rarely fatal
   c. Resolution of symptoms often requires weeks
   d. Radiologic appearance may not correlate with clinical severity
3. Adenovirus
   a. Most frequent viral pneumonia with adenopathy
   b. Sequelae include bronchiolitis obliterans, Swyer-James syndrome, bronchiectasis
4. Varicella
   a. Rare, often seen with systemic involvement
   b. Diffuse reticulonodular infiltrates
   c. May heal with multiple small calcifications
5. Measles
   a. Acute
      • Rare except in immunocompromised children
      • Diffuse reticulonodular infiltrates
      • Adenopathy
   b. Atypical
      • Patients given killed vaccine then exposed to measles or given live vaccine
      • Rarely seen in pediatrics as killed vaccine not used since 1970
      • Extensive infiltrates, frequent adenopathy, effusion

D. **Tuberculosis (TB) [Figs. 5-33 and 5-34]**
   1. Adult TB is reactivation disease
   2. Pediatric TB is primary disease
      a. Primary complex
         • Hilar adenopathy
         • Nonspecific, usually peripheral, infiltrate
      b. Pleural fluid: high protein, low glucose, few organisms
      c. Rarely large effusions present with chest pain as primary symptom
      d. Most young children are asymptomatic
      e. Probably no difference in clinical course between TB with and without pulmonary involvement
      f. Endobronchial involvement often simulates chronic foreign body
      g. Progressive primary pulmonary TB
         • Primary complex enlarges, cavitates, and ruptures into bronchus
         • Presents as pneumonia, does not respond to usual antibacterial treatment

E. *Pneumocystis carinii* **infection [Fig. 5-35]**
   1. Protozoan
   2. Hypoxia out of proportion to symptoms
   3. Immunodeficient patients
   4. Subtle interstitial infiltrates
   5. CT may show peripheral small cysts

F. **Fungal infection**
   1. Usually suspected in:
      a. Immunocompromised patients

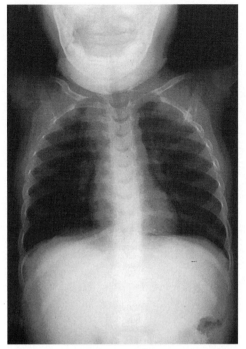

Fig. 5-33 PA chest radiograph: Right paratracheal mass deviating trachea to left and narrowing proximal right bronchus. Hyperlucency of right lung due to partial right bronchial obstruction. Primary TB.

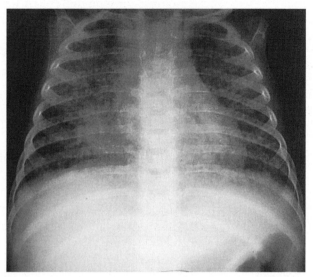

Fig. 5-34 PA chest radiograph: Multiple diffuse nodular and interstitial opacities, right middle lobe airspace opacity. Miliary TB.

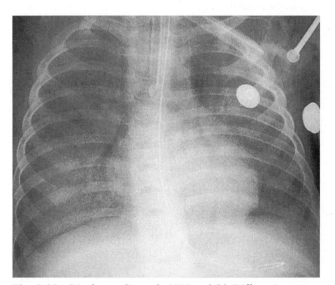

Fig. 5-35 PA chest radiograph: HIV+ child. Diffuse airspace or alveolar opacity with bilateral air bronchograms. *Pneumocystis carinii* pneumonia. DDx includes various causes of noncardiogenic pulmonary edema.

     b. Hilar adenopathy

     c. Pneumonia unresponsive to conventional therapy

2. Appearance of fungal pneumonia is rarely specific or even strongly suggestive of fungal infection

3. Actinomycosis

     a. Pleural and nodal involvement

     b. Frequent chest wall involvement

4. Blastomycosis

     a. Massive lymph node enlargement

     b. Parenchymal involvement usually minimal

     c. May see miliary pattern from hematogenous spread

5. Cryptococcus

     a. Large areas of dense consolidation without cavitation

6. Candida albicans

     a. Nonspecific pulmonary infiltrates

7. Aspergillosis **[Fig. 5-36]**

     a. Frequently affects preexisting cavities

     b. May involve chest wall

     c. Rare except in immunosuppressed children

     d. Allergic bronchopulmonary aspergillosis

        • Mucous plugs secondary to endobronchial inflammation

        • Steroid therapy decreases progression

        • Diagnosis

            Known asthma or cystic fibrosis (CF)

            Elevated eosinophils and IgE

            Aspergillus skin reactivity and precipitating antibodies

            Bronchiectasis

8. Histoplasmosis

     a. Endemic midwest and southeast

     b. Commonly seen as multiple calcifications

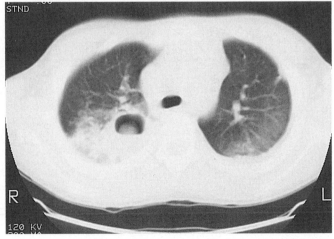

Fig. 5-36 Chest CT: Patient with leukemia. Airspace opacity in right lung. Note soft tissue mass surrounded by crescent of air within cavitary lesion. Aspergillosis.

       c. Primary infection rarely symptomatic

       d. Multiple nonspecific infiltrates, adenopathy

   9. Coccidioidomycosis

       a. Endemic southwest and California

       b. Rarely symptomatic

       c. Radiographic appearance often simulates TB

       d. If symptomatic, may see large area consolidation with adenopathy

G. **Acquired immunodeficiency syndrome (AIDS) (see Chapter 8)**

   1. Infection

       a. *Pneumocystis carinii* occurs in 1/3 to 1/2

       b. Viral infection

       c. TB, including atypical

       d. Any bacterial pathogen

   2. Lymphocytic interstitial pneumonitis **[Fig. 5-37; see also Fig. 8-21]**

       a. Small nodular densities and hilar adenopathy classic

       b. Patchy infiltrates frequently superimposed on interstitial opacities

       c. Specific diagnosis by lung biopsy

   3. Lymphoma

       a. Rapidly progressive nodular lung disease

H. **Organisms causing pneumonia at different ages**

   1. Premature infants

       a. Group B *streptococcus*

       b. *E. coli*

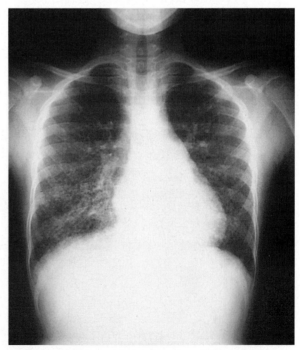

Fig. 5-37 PA chest radiograph: HIV+ child. Bilateral interstitial opacities. Notice numerous rounded interstitial opacities resembling "bagels" or "doughnuts." Lymphocytic interstitial pneumonitis.

    c. *Listeria* species

    d. Cytomegalovirus (CMV)

  2. Infants

    a. RSV

    b. *Chlamydia*

    c. *Streptococcus pneumoniae*

    d. *Haemophilus influenzae* type B (now much decreased due to widespread vaccination)

  3. School age

    a. Mycoplasma

    b. Influenza A

    c. *Streptococcus pneumoniae*

I. **Reactive airways disease (RAD) [Fig. 5-38]**

  1. Asthma diagnosed when RAD recurs; cannot diagnose asthma in the first year

  2. RSV and Aspergillus have been suggested as precipitating infections

  3. Radiographic appearance

    a. Peribronchial thickening

    b. Hyperinflation

    c. Small parenchymal opacities are far more likely due to atelectasis rather than pneumonia

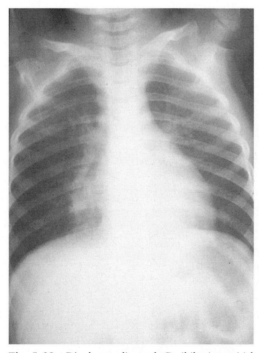

Fig. 5-38 PA chest radiograph: Perihilar interstitial thickening, indicating airways disease (asthma, bronchitis, CF, BPD, chronic aspiration) with superimposed airspace opacity in right middle, right lower, left lower lobes. Airways disease with superimposed multifocal atelectasis.

4. Apparent severity on radiographs does not correlate with clinical severity
5. CXR useful to detect unsuspected abnormalities
    a. Pneumomediastinum
    b. Pneumothorax
    c. Lobar consolidation, especially with effusion suggesting pneumonia
    d. Asymmetric appearance suggesting foreign body

J. **Bronchiectasis**
1. In otherwise normal children, probably most frequently occurs as a sequela of viral disease
2. Immunodeficiency
3. Chronic infection
4. Secondary to foreign body

K. **CF (see Chapter 8) [Figs. 5-39 and 5-40]**
1. Autosomal recessive inheritance
2. 1:3000 in Caucasian population, less common in other races
3. Abnormality of CF transmembrane regulator (CFTR) causes abnormal transmembrane transport of Na^+ and Cl^-
4. Gene located on chromosome 7
5. More than 600 different defects have been identified
6. Diagnosed by sweat test: $Cl^->60$ positive >40 equivocal
7. Average life expectancy, 30 years
8. Clinical course
    a. Lungs initially normal
    b. Abnormal chloride secretion results in viscid airway mucus
    c. Infection, inflammatory response, and airway obstruction cause progressive small and large airways disease

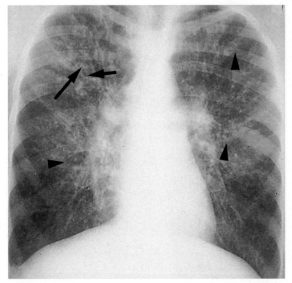

Fig. 5-39 PA chest radiograph: Pulmonary hyperinflation, extensive interstitial opacities, bronchial dilatation and thickening along long axis (arrows) and short axis (arrowheads), prominent hila, small heart. CF.

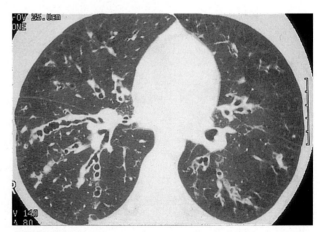

Fig. 5-40 HRCT: CF, bronchiectasis. Dilated and beaded bronchi, bronchial wall thickening, and peripheral bronchial mucous plugging.

      d. Bronchial wall thickening progresses to bronchiectasis

      e. Chronic obstruction causes hyperinflation

      f. Hilar enlargement due to adenopathy and later pulmonary hypertension with dilated central pulmonary arteries

      g. Increasing cardiac size indicates cor pulmonale and poor survival without transplantation

      h. Pneumomediastinum and pneumothorax occur

      i. Lobar pneumonia very rare in established cases

      j. CXRs do not reflect clinical changes in acute exacerbations

L. **Immotile cilia**

    1. Situs inversus in 50%

    2. Expect sinus disease as well as pulmonary disease

    3. Deafness and infertility also occur

    4. Kartagener's syndrome

      a. Situs inversus

      b. Sinus disease

      c. Bronchiectasis

M. **Swyer-James syndrome**

    1. Unilateral hyperlucent lung

    2. Postinfectious bronchiolitis obliterans prior to complete development of alveoli (age 8 years), especially following adenovirus infection

    3. Lung volume decreased or equal to normal lung

    4. Decreased perfusion and expiratory air trapping

V. **NEOPLASMS**

A. **Malignant**

    1. Pulmonary blastoma

      a. Rare, rapidly progressive primary pulmonary malignancy

      b. Heterogeneous enhancing focal mass

    2. Mesenchymal sarcoma

      a. Associated with congenital lung lesions

    3. Lymphoma/leukemia

      a. Isolated pulmonary involvement extremely rare

      b. Mediastinal lymphatic obstruction more common than lymphatic involvement of lung

    4. Metastases **[Fig. 5-41]**

      a. Osteogenic sarcoma

      b. Wilms' tumor

      c. Ewing sarcoma

      d. Rhabdomyosarcoma

B. **Benign**

    1. Postinflammatory pseudotumor

      a. Also called xanthogranuloma, fibrous histiocytoma, and plasma cell granuloma

      b. Unknown cause, but likely reaction to inflammation

      c. Arises in pulmonary parenchyma, may invade pleura or mediastinum

      d. Two-thirds respiratory symptoms, one-third asymptomatic

      e. Calcifications in 20%

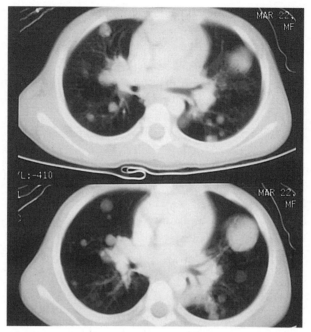

Fig. 5-41 Chest CT: Patient with rhabdomyosarcoma. Numerous pulmonary nodules of various sizes. Pulmonary metastases.

2. Bronchial adenoma
   a. May be classified as low grade malignancy
   b. 90% carcinoid type; carcinoid syndrome rare in children
   c. 10% salivary gland type, most adenoid cystic
3. Pulmonary hamartoma
   a. Abnormal arrangement of normally occurring pulmonary tissues
   b. Usually <2 cm, smooth, lobular margins
4. Laryngeal papilloma **[Fig. 5-42]**
   a. Spread to lungs rare
   b. Nodular, frequently cavitary, parenchymal lesions

VI. **TRAUMA**
   A. **Pulmonary laceration is likely responsible for most of the findings seen with blunt chest trauma**
   B. **Pulmonary contusion:**
      1. Small lacerations with bleeding into alveoli, or crush injury with edema
      2. Presents as patchy infiltrate that clears in days
   C. **Pulmonary hemorrhage:**
      1. Larger lacerations with more focal blood than seen with contusion
      2. Presents as dense, focal opacity
      3. Requires weeks for clearing
   D. **Pneumatocele**
      1. Secondary to lacerations with elastic recoil of lung creating an air-containing space within the parenchyma
      2. Can be seen acutely, but more common during recovery
      3. Usually slowly decreases in size over months to years

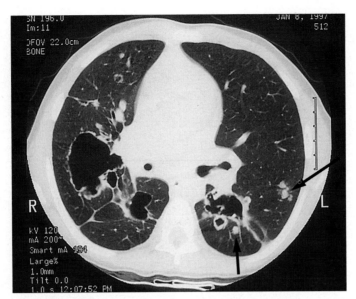

Fig. 5-42   HRCT: Pulmonary cysts of various sizes, nodules (arrows), and cavitary lesions. Note narrowing of left main bronchus. Tracheo-bronchial papillomatosis.

E. **Types of air leak**
  1. Pneumothorax
  2. Pneumomediastinum **[Fig. 1-14]**
     a. Asthma
     b. Foreign body
     c. "Continuous diaphragm" sign
  3. Pulmonary interstitial emphysema
  4. Bronchopleural fistula
  5. Fracture of tracheobronchial tree

F. **Airway foreign body [Figs. 5-43 through 5-45]**
  1. Most common between one and two years of age
  2. Right and left sided involvement nearly equal
  3. 90% distal to the trachea
  4. Foreign bodies usually nonradiopaque
  5. Two-thirds present with hyperlucency
  6. Aspirated foreign bodies frequently form a "check valve" with air entry during inspiration when negative intrathoracic pressure enlarges bronchus, but obstruction during expiration with resultant hyperinflation distal to the foreign body
  7. Chronic foreign bodies can present as atelectasis, recurrent pneumonia, or bronchiectasis
  8. Imaging evaluation
     a. Air trapping best evaluated with inspiratory/expiratory or decubitus radiographs
     b. Plain radiographic findings:
        • One-third focal hyperlucency
        • 25% atelectasis

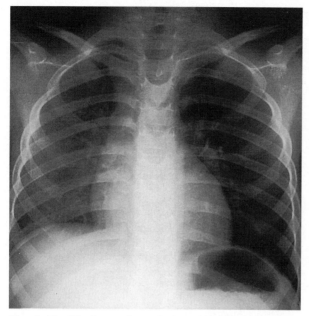

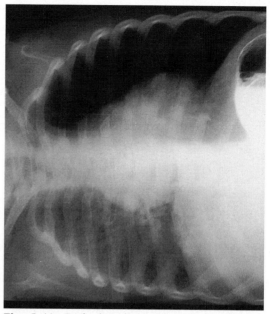

Fig. 5-43 PA chest radiograph: Asymmetric pulmonary lucency. Hazy right lung, which is in exhalation, lucent left lung, which is over-inflated. Left bronchial obstruction due to foreign body aspiration.

Fig. 5-44 Right lateral decubitus chest radiograph (right side down) obtained through chest anterior to posterior: Same patient as Figure 5-43. The dependent right lung is hazy, in expiratory phase. The nondependent left lung is well-inflated. This appearance is normal for a decubitus chest radiograph. Foreign body aspiration-decubitus radiograph.

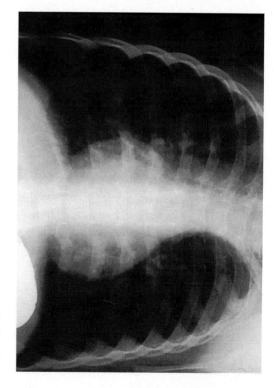

Fig. 5-45 Left lateral decubitus chest radiograph (left side down) obtained through chest anterior to posterior: Same patient as Figure 5–43. The dependent left lung is over-inflated. The nondependent right lung is also well-inflated. This appearance is abnormal for a decubitus chest radiograph, indicating air trapping in dependent left lung due to left bronchial obstruction. Foreign body aspiration-decubitus radiograph.

c. Interruption of normal air column in foreign bodies in larger airway causes "missing segment sign"; this is difficult to appreciate in most cases

d. Fluoroscopy useful in equivocal cases
  - Abnormal mediastinal motion indicating subtle air trapping or bilateral obstruction
  - Mobile foreign bodies; especially tracheal

e. CT provides the most sensitive detection of obstruction, but is not usually required to make diagnosis

G. Aspiration pneumonia
1. Acute
   a. Diffuse (Mendelson syndrome)
     - Liquid distributed widely into alveoli
     - Pulmonary edema pattern, but more focal confluence and slow clearing over 1 to 2 weeks
   b. Focal
     - Material aspirated into one or more lobe(s)
     - RUL and lower lobes most common sites
2. Chronic
   a. Often presents as airways disease
   b. May see alveolar or interstitial opacities
   c. Evaluate for tracheoesophageal fistula, gastroesophageal reflux, and abnormal swallowing

H. Hydrocarbon aspiration
1. Gasoline, kerosene, household cleaners, and polishes
2. Aspiration following emesis after swallowing hydrocarbon
3. Illness rare if CXR normal 6 hours after ingestion
4. Patchy airspace disease, often basilar and symmetrical
5. Pneumatoceles may develop as sequelae

I. Near drowning
1. Pulmonary edema appearance
2. Usually present on first CXR, but may be delayed >24 hours

J. Posttraumatic bronchial stenosis
1. Often due to frequent suctioning during intubation; RUL most common
2. DDx
   a. Postinfectious, especially TB
   b. Chronic foreign body

K. Posttraumatic diaphragmatic hernia
1. L ≫ R
2. Suspect in posttraumatic opacified lung with mass effect and loculated air collections
3. Fluid in affected hemithorax suggests vascular compromise of herniated bowel
4. Delayed presentations occur, especially with small defects and bowel strangulation

L. Complications of tubes and lines
1. Endotracheal tube
   a. Position tip halfway between thoracic inlet and carina

b. Flexing the neck moves the endotrachial tube tip caudad, extending the neck moves the tip cephalad

c. Low lung volumes and air-distended upper gastrointestinal tract suggest esophageal intubation

2. Enteric tubes

a. Tracheal or pulmonary malposition

b. Perforation

- Hypopharyngeal perforation

  Small infants

  Frequently dissects into mediastinum, may simulate normal esophageal location

  May enter pleural space

- Small bowel perforation

  Most common at duodenal bulb or junction of descending and transverse duodenum

  Catheters stiffen with age, increasing risk

  Stiffening wires increase risk, especially if not removed immediately after placement

M. **Drug reactions**

1. Bronchospasm

   a. Aspirin

   b. Penicillin, other antibiotics

2. Noncardiogenic pulmonary edema

   a. Heroin

   b. Contrast media

   c. Salicylate overdose

3. Interstitial fibrosis

   a. Bleomycin

   b. Methotrexate

VII. **MISCELLANEOUS**

A. Idiopathic pulmonary hemosiderosis

1. Recurrent bleeding into alveoli

2. Frequently presents without clinical pulmonary hemorrhage

3. Acute appearance resembles pulmonary edema

4. Chronic appearance: reticular interstitial disease

5. Diagnosis confirmed with MRI demonstrating hemosiderin or bronchoscopy showing hemosiderin-laden macrophages

B. **Collagen vascular disease**

1. Juvenile rheumatoid arthritis

   a. Effusions, pericarditis

2. Lupus erythematosus

   a. Effusions

C. **Spontaneous pneumothorax**

1. Teenagers

2. Symptomatic treatment unless recurrent

D. **Pulmonary edema**

1. Cardiogenic **[Fig. 5-46; see also Fig. 4-4]**

   a. Enlarged heart may be less evident than in adults

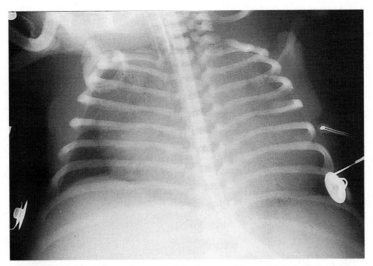

Fig. 5-46 AP chest radiograph: Newborn with marked cardiac enlargement, indistinct pulmonary vascularity. Cardiogenic pulmonary edema. DDx includes myocardial dysfunction (myocarditis or cardiomyopathy), left heart obstruction (hypoplastic left heart, infantile aortic coarctation), polycythemia, cerebral or hepatic arteriovenous fistula, fluid overload.

      b. In infants the lungs often demonstrate diffuse, rather than central opacity

  2. Noncardiogenic **[Fig. 5-47]**

    a. Near drowning

    b. Smoke inhalation

    c. High altitude

    d. Head trauma

    e. Increased intracranial pressure

    f. Organophosphate poisoning

    g. Pulmonary re-expansion following pneumothorax treatment

    h. Upper airway obstruction and acute relief of upper airway obstruction

E. Histiocytosis [Fig. 8-18]

  1. Pulmonary involvement is rare in children (usually age 20 to 40 years)

    a. Associated with smoking history

    b. May present with spontaneous pneumothorax

  2. Interstitial disease

    a. Centrilobular nodules on high resolution computed tomography (HRCT)

    b. Cysts of variable size and shape

  3. Indicates extensive involvement (Grade 2)

    a. 2a if no symptoms of organ dysfunction

    b. 2b with organ dysfunction

VIII. **THE MEDIASTINUM**

  A. **Anatomy**

    1. Classic divisions:

      a. Superior: above line between sternal angle and T4-5 disk space

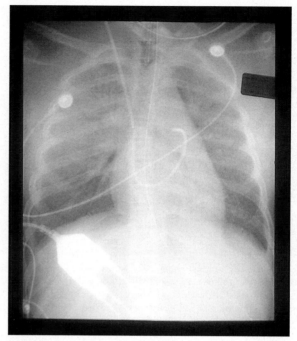

Fig. 5-47 AP chest radiograph: Normal cardiac size, diffuse air space opacity, air bronchograms in all lobes, right pleural effusion. Noncardiogenic pulmonary edema. DDx includes narcotic overdose, neurogenic pulmonary edema, toxic inhalation, salicylate or organophosphate intoxication, high altitude, near-drowning, overwhelming pneumonia or aspiration.

    b. The remaining compartments are below this line
- Anterior: in front of the heart
- Middle: containing the heart
- Posterior: behind the heart

  2. Kirks and Korobkin (1981) have modified this system to make it more useful for children **[Figs. 5-48 and 5-49]**

    a. Posterior: behind a line drawn along the anterior cortex of the vertebral bodies

    b. Anterior: in front of a line drawn from the top of the sternum to the diaphragm parallel to the above line

    c. Middle: between the two lines described above

B. Mediastinal lesions by location

  1. The thymus frequently extends into all three divisions

  2. Pathology that occurs in all divisions:

    a. Lymphoma/leukemia

    b. Adenopathy

    c. Mediastinitis

    d. Hematoma

  3. Pathology occurring in specific divisions:

    a. Anterior **[Figs. 5-50 through 5-55; see also Fig. 8-9]**
- Teratoma

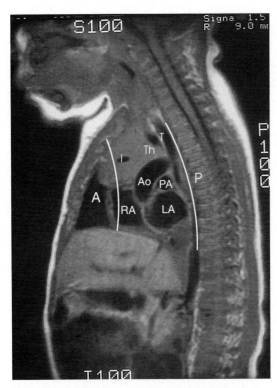

Fig. 5-48 Sagittal T1-weighted MRI: Note thymus (Th), innominate vein (I), innominate artery anterior to trachea (T), right atrium (RA), left atrium (LA), aorta (Ao), pulmonary artery (PA). Curved lines separate anterior (A), middle, and posterior (P) mediastinum. Thymus in this patient extends into the middle mediastinum. Mediastinal anatomy.

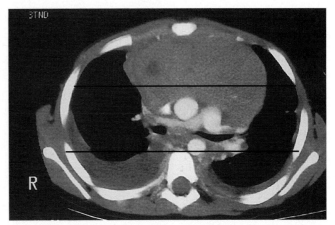

Fig. 5-49 Chest CT: Heterogeneous mass in anterior mediastinum, bilateral pleural effusions. Lines separate anterior, middle, and posterior mediastinum. Mediastinal anatomy. Anterior mediastinal mass. Lymphoma.

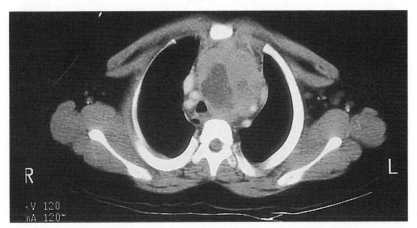

Fig. 5-50 Chest CT: Heterogeneous mass in anterior and middle mediastinum. Note tracheal deviation, left axillary adenopathy. Mediastinal germ cell tumor.

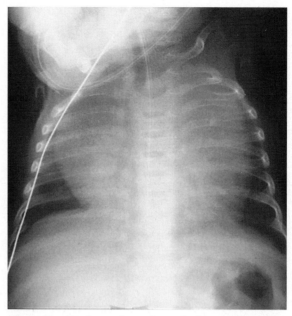

Fig. 5-51 AP chest radiograph: Markedly enlarged cardio-thymic silhouette. Anterior mediastinal mass. Thymic hyper-plasia.

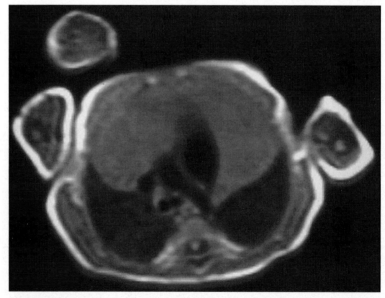

Fig. 5-52 Axial T2-weighted MRI: Same patient as Figure 5-51. Homogeneous anterior and middle mediastinal mass comprised of thymus. Anterior mediastinal mass. Thymic hyperplasia.

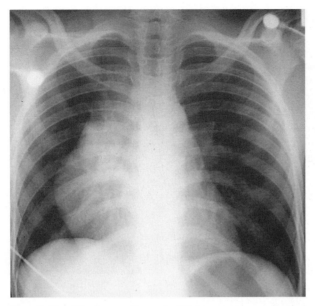

Fig. 5-53 PA chest radiograph. Right anterior mediastinal mass abutting heart and obliterating right cardiac border. Anterior mediastinal Hodgkin's disease.

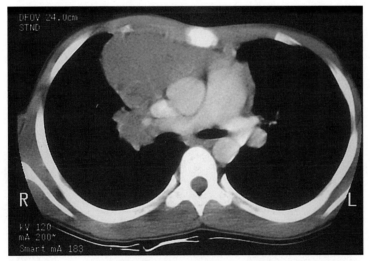

Fig. 5-54 Chest CT: Same patient as Figure 5-53. Right anterior mediastinal mass with right hilar component. Anterior mediastinal Hodgkin's disease.

- Thyroid
- Thymoma
  b. Middle **[Fig. 5-56]**
  - Bronchopulmonary foregut malformations
  - Hiatal hernia, other gastric or esophageal abnormality
  - Cardiac/pericardiac tumors and cysts
  - Great vessel aneurysms/anomalies
  c. Posterior **[Figs. 5-57 and 5-58; see also Figs. 2-126 and 8-5]**

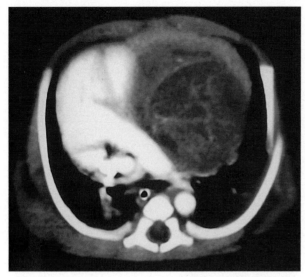

Fig. 5-55 Chest CT: Left anterior and middle mediastinal mass with heterogeneity, hypervascularity, and stippled calcification. Mediastinal teratoma.

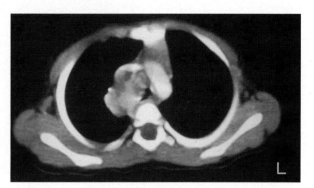

Fig. 5-56 Chest CT: Heterogeneously enhancing right paratracheal mass indenting trachea. Deviation and flattening of superior vena cava. Middle mediastinal mass. Primary TB.

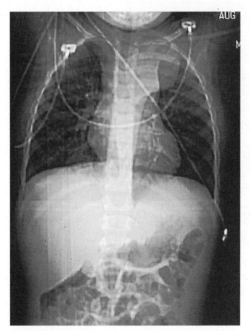

Fig. 5-57 Scoutview from chest CT: Left superior mediastinal mass. Note extension of mass above level of clavicle, indicating posterior location. Posterior mediastinal mass. Ganglioneuroblastoma.

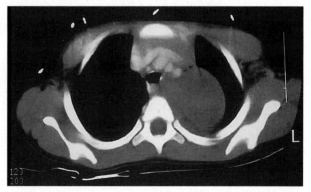

Fig. 5-58 Chest CT: Same patient as Figure 5-57. Middle and posterior mediastinal mass abutting posterior pleura. Posterior mediastinal mass. Ganglioneuroblastoma.

- Neurogenic tumors
- Neurenteric cysts
- Lateral meningoceles
- Spinal tumors/osteomyelitis/discitis
- Descending aortic or azygous anomaly or aneurysm
- Extramedullary hematopoiesis

4. Ductus calcification **[Fig. 4-5]**
  a. A calcification several mm in size that sometimes forms in the closed ductus arteriosus
  b. Rarely visible on plain film, more commonly seen on CT
  c. No associated mass
  d. Should not be confused with pathologic calcification

IX. **THE CHEST WALL IN THE OLDER CHILD**
  A. **Chest wall masses**
  - Incidentally palpated chest wall mass frequently due to congenital rib abnormalities
  - Palpable asymptomatic anterior chest wall masses usually do not require evaluation beyond CXR
  1. Askin tumor **[Fig. 5-59]**
    a. Aggressive tumor of the chest wall
    b. Now classified as a primitive neuroectodermal tumor
    c. Destructive and invasive, calcification rare

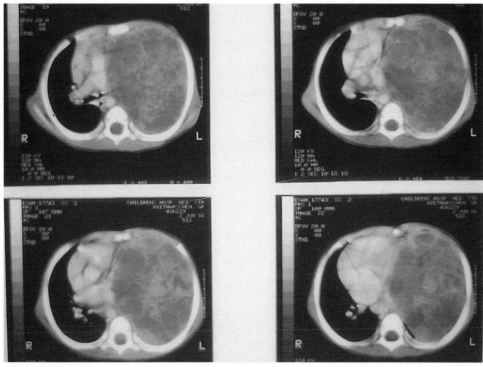

Fig. 5-59 Multiple images from chest CT: Large heterogeneous mass fills left hemithorax, displaces heart and mediastinum to right. Askin tumor.

2. Pectus excavatum
    a. Depressed sternum
    b. On frontal CXR often displaces heart slightly to the left, with the right cardiac margin ill-defined, simulating RML pneumonia
    c. Usually asymptomatic
    d. Rarely may be associated with respiratory difficulty, and surgical correction performed
    e. Usually isolated, may be seen in Marfan's syndrome and rickets
3. Pectus carinatum
    a. Pigeon breast
    b. Prominence of sternum and costal cartilage

Further Reading

Ablow RC. Radiologic diagnosis of the newborn chest. Curr Probl Pediatr 1971; 1:1–55.

Ablow RC, Gross I, Effmann EL, et al. The radiographic features of early onset group B streptococcal neonatal sepsis. Radiology 1977;124:771–777.

Burton EM, Brick WG, Hall JD, et al. Tracheobronchial foreign body aspiration in children. South Med J 1996;89:195–198.

Clements BS, Warner JO. Pulmonary sequestration and related congenital bronchopulmonary-vascular malformations: nomenclature and classification based on anatomical and embryological considerations. Thorax 1987;42:401–408.

Cremin BJ. Tuberculosis: the resurgence of our most lethal infectious disease-a review. Pediatr Radiol 1995;25:620–626.

Donnelly LF, Taylor CNR, Emery KH, Brody AS. Asymptomatic, palpable, anterior chest wall lesions in children: is cross-sectional imaging necessary? Radiology 1997;202:829–831.

Edwards DK, Hilton SVW, Merritt TA, et al. Respiratory distress syndrome treated with human surfactant: radiographic findings. Radiology 1985;157:329–334.

Gooding CA, Gregory GA. Roentgenographic analysis of meconium aspiration of the newborn. Radiology 1971;100:131–140.

Griscom NT. Pneumonia in children and some of its variants. Radiology 1988; 167:297–302.

Guckel C, Benz-Bohm G, Widemann B. Mycoplasmal pneumonias in childhood. Roentgen features, differential diagnosis and review of literature. Pediatr Radiol 1989;19:499–503.

Kirks DR, Korobkin M. Computed tomography of the chest in infants and children: techniques and mediastinal evaluation. Radiol Clin North Am 1981;19:409–419.

Kuhn JP. Pediatric thorax. In: Naidich DP, Zerhouni EA, Siegelman SS. eds. Computed Tomography and Magnetic Resonance of the Thorax, 2nd ed. New York: Raven Press; 1991:503–555.

Manson D, Reid B, Dalal H, Roifman CM. Clinical utility of high-resolution pulmonary computed tomography in children with antibody deficiency disorders. Pediatr Radiol 1997;27:794–798.

McSweeney WJ. Radiologic evaluation of the newborn with respiratory distress. Semin Roentgenol 1972;7:65–83.

Northway WH Jr, Rosan RC. Radiographic features of pulmonary oxygen toxicity in the newborn: bronchopulmonary dysplasia. Radiology 1968;91:49–58.

Pickhardt PJ, Siegel MJ, Gutierrez FR. Vascular rings in symptomatic children: frequency of chest radiographic findings. Radiology 1997;203:423–426.

Stickney RH, Bjelland JC, Capp MP, et al. Chlamydia trachomatis: a cause of an infantile pneumonia syndrome. AJR 1978;131:914–915.

Swischuk LE, John SD. Immature lung problems: can our nomenclature be more specific? AJR 1996;166:917–918.

Swischuk LE. Transient respiratory distress of the newborn (TRDN). A temporary disturbance of a normal phenomenon. AJR 1970;108:557–563.

Wood BP, Anderson VM, Mauk JE, Merritt TA. Pulmonary lymphatic air: locating "pulmonary interstitial emphysema" of the premature infant. AJR 1982;138: 809–814.

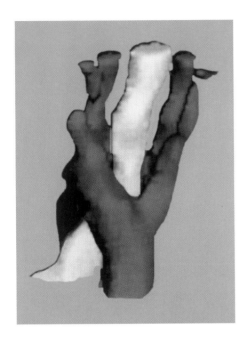

Color Plate 1. 3D CT (frontal image): Trachea (red), aorta (white). Complete DAA encircling trachea. *(See Chapter 4, Figure 4-24.)*

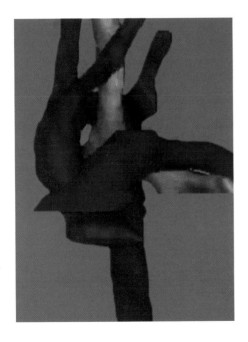

Color Plate 2. 3D MRI (oblique image): Trachea (pink), pulmonary artery (purple), aorta (red). Note the left subclavian artery arising posterior to the trachea in this patient with right aortic arch. Ligamentum arteriosum (not seen) completes the vascular ring. *(See Chapter 4, Figure 4-28.)*

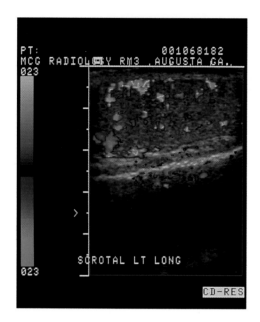

Color Plate 3. Longitudinal US of the left testis with color-flow Doppler: Note ovoid testis with homogeneous echogenic texture and bright speckles indicating vascularity. Normal testis-color flow Doppler. *(See Chapter 7, Figure 7-51.)*

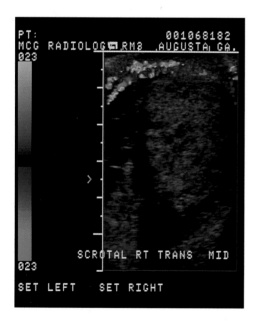

Color Plate 4. Transverse US of right testis with color-flow Doppler: Same patient as Color Plate 3. Testis with heterogeneous echogenicity and absence of central vascular speckles. Blood flow is around testis. Testicular torsion-color flow Doppler. *(See Chapter 7, Figure 7-52.)*

CHAPTER SIX   GASTROINTESTINAL SYSTEM

I. **ESOPHAGUS**
   A. **Anomalies**
      1. Esophageal atresia (EA) **[Figs. 6-1 and 6-2]**
         a. Most common anomaly of esophagus and trachea
         b. Failure of endodermal recanalization into trachea and esophagus during 4th-5th weeks gestation
         c. Types:
            • EA and distal tracheo-esophageal (TE) fistula (85%)
               Gas present in distal gastrointestinal (GI) tract
            • EA without TE fistula (5 to 10%)
               Gasless abdomen
            • H-type TE fistula without atresia (1 to 5%)
               Usually presents with aspiration or cyanosis on feeding
            • EA and proximal and distal TE fistula (1 to 2%)
               Gas present in distal GI tract
               Proximal TE fistula may be suspected at surgery
               – After intubation, air will bubble into proximal esophageal pouch if small amount of saline placed in upper pouch as child is ventilated
            • EA and proximal TE fistula (1 to 2%)
               Gasless abdomen
               Proximal fistula may be suspected at time of surgery (see above)

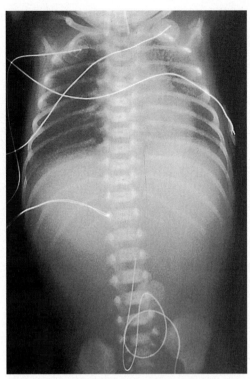

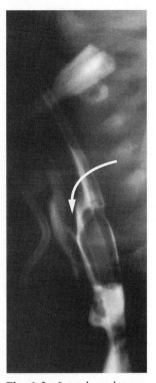

Fig. 6-1 Chest and abdomen radiograph in 4-day-old infant: Endotracheal tube in place and catheter in upper esophageal pouch. No gas in abdomen. EA without distal TE fistula.

Fig. 6-2 Lateral esophagram postesophageal atresia repair: Central catheter in superior vena cava (SVC), catheter in esophagus above anastomosis. Contrast injected above anastomosis crosses fistula (curved arrow) into trachea. Note: proximal TE fistula in upper esophagus looks like an "N" rather than an "H".

    d. Anastomotic stricture develops in 35 to 50%

    e. Tracheomalacia, hypoperistalsis, gastroesophageal reflux (GER) common in EA

    f. Esophagography to study EA after repair:

- Use feeding tube with end hole to place contrast directly into area of interest (just above anastomosis)

        Feeding tube with side hole only will back-fill proximal esophagus, possibly causing aspiration at level of vocal cords

        Do not study infant with recent EA repair by bottle feeding

        Infants with EA often have swallowing dysfunction, will aspirate and confound study

- Study performed with patient in right lateral position
- Inject small amount (0.5 cc) of barium

        Larger amount may backfill, especially if obstruction present, and cause aspiration at level of vocal cords

    g. Recurrent fistula in 8 to 10%; may be delayed by years

2. VATER association
   a. Vertebral, Anal atresia, Tracheoesophageal (TE) fistula, Renal anomalies
   b. For additional cardiac anomaly, VACTER
   c. For additional limb anomaly, VACTERL
3. Esophageal duplication cyst
   a. A type of bronchopulmonary foregut malformation (BPFM)
      • BPFM also includes bronchogenic cyst, neurenteric cyst
   b. May mimic vascular ring on barium swallow [can distinguish by computed tomography (CT) or magnetic resonance imaging (MRI)]
4. Esophageal impressions on esophagogram **[Figs. 4-22, 4-26, and 4-31]**
   • Posterior impression + left aortic arch = aberrant right subclavian artery (normal variant—0.5%)
   • Posterior + right aortic arch = vascular ring (right arch, left subclavian artery + left ligamentum arteriosum, or double aortic arch)
   • Anterior esophageal impression + posterior tracheal impression = pulmonary sling
      Left pulmonary artery (PA) arises from right PA, hooks trachea or bronchus **[Fig. 4-30]**
      May present in newborn with hyperinflated or fluid-filled lung
      − Do not confuse with congenital lobar emphysema

B. **Inflammation, dysfunction**
   1. Esophagitis **[Fig. 6-3; see also Fig. 8-22]**
      a. Usually secondary to gastroesophageal (GE) reflux
      b. Also due to caustic ingestion, infectious [candida, herpes, cytomegalovirus (CMV)], epidermolysis bullosum
   2. Gastroesophageal Reflux (GER)
      a. Very common in infancy due to immature lower esophageal segment
      b. Usually resolves by 18 months
      c. Associated with esophagitis, iron deficiency anemia, failure to thrive (FTT), abdominal pain in older children (epigastric)
      d. Trigger for asthma, bronchospasm, stridor

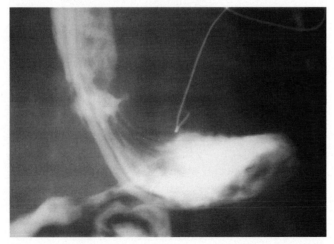

Fig. 6-3 Catheter in stomach. Note patulous GE junction with esophageal ulceration. Reflux esophagitis.

3. Hiatal hernia (HH) **[Fig. 6-4]**
   a. Most common in middle age and in infants
   b. In infants, HH associated with pyloric stenosis, malrotation, duodenal web
   c. When present in children, HH virtually always accompanied by GER
4. Barrett esophagus
   a. Classically, stricture or ulceration of mid-esophagus
   b. Higher incidence with scleroderma, myotomy for achalasia, previous gastric surgery, indwelling esophageal feeding tube
   c. Columnar epithelium

C. **Trauma**
   1. Foreign body
      a. Most common site of obstruction is at thoracic inlet
      b. Coin in esophagus
         • On anteroposterior (AP) chest film, flat side of coin visualized
           Lateral film of airway must be obtained to:
           (1) Identify multiple coins or other foreign body that resembles a coin
              – Camera battery will have a flange
           (2) Evaluate tracheal air column
              – Patient may present with "croup"
              – Inflammation from metallic foreign body in esophagus will

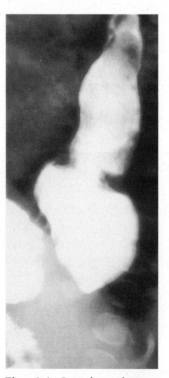

Fig. 6-4 Lateral esophagram: Large sliding HH and markedly distended lower esophagus.

thicken soft tissue between esophagus and trachea, and cause tracheal narrowing

Do not attempt Foley balloon removal of coin in esophagus if air column is narrowed

    – Controlled removal under endoscopic visualization

  2. Perforation

    a. Usually due to instrumentation; retching

      • May produce pseudo-diverticula

      • Cause of pneumomediastinum

D. **Obstruction**

  1. Achalasia **[Fig. 6-5]**

    a. Failure of relaxation of lower esophagus; <5% of patients are children

    b. Manometry may distinguish from spasm

    c. Esophagram shows distal obstruction with "rat-tail appearance"

  2. Stricture

    a. Following esophageal atresia repair at anastomosis

    b. Caustic ingestion **[Fig. 6-6]**

    c. Associated with esophagitis, GER

    d. Epidermolysis bullosum dystrophica (rare)

E. **Swallowing dysfunction**

  1. Sucking

    a. Coordinated mandibular and tongue movement

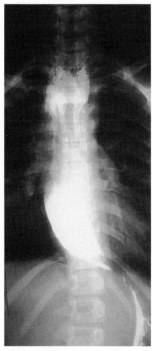

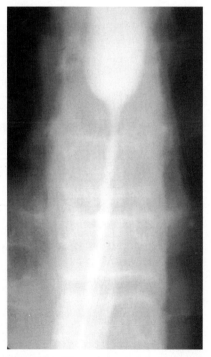

Fig. 6-5 AP esophagram: Markedly distended esophagus through cardiac shadow. Note narrowed distal segment resembling a "rat tail." Achalasia.

Fig. 6-6 AP esophagram: Long segment esophageal stricture. Caustic esophageal stricture.

2. Swallowing [Fig. 1-52]
   a. Pharyngeal movement
   b. Note palatal and epiglottal closure
   c. In patients at risk for aspiration (mental retardation, ex-premies, neuromotor dysfunction), study swallowing when evaluating for GER
   d. Swallowing dysfunction may be seen in otherwise normal infants
      • Clinical symptoms: choking with feeding, "bronchitis" or "asthma" in infant <6 months of age, hoarseness, wheezing, stridor
      • Evaluate swallowing in lateral projection by barium esophagram
         Cord penetration, tracheal aspiration may be fleeting
      • Modified barium swallow with speech pathologist
         Videotape study
         Infant placed in chair or appropriate seat to simulate home feeding
         Various consistencies fed to child
            − Thin liquid, thick liquid, puree or pudding, solids (crackers or cookies)
3. Dysmotility
   a. Typical in patients with esophageal atresia
   b. Abnormal peristalsis also reported in chronic granulomatous disease (CGD)

II. **STOMACH**
   A. **Anomalies**
      1. Duplication cyst
         a. Noncommunicating cyst lined by intestinal, pancreatic, or gastric epithelium
         b. Most common location is greater curve
         c. Rarely communicates
         d. Presents as obstructing mass
      2. Volvulus
         a. Mesentero-axial rotation
            • Perpendicular to long axis of stomach
            • Associated with diaphragmatic hernia or eventration; may cause high-grade gastric inlet obstruction, gastric necrosis
               Necrosis may manifest as gastric or small bowel pneumatosis, with/without perforation
         b. Organo-axial rotation
            • Parallel with long axis
            • Associated with hiatal hernia
            • Obstruction may be intermittent
   B. **Inflammation**
      1. Granulomatous
         a. Tuberculosis, syphilis, herpes simplex, sarcoid
         b. Unusual in children
         c. Crohn's and CGD of childhood may produce antral narrowing
      2. Toxic
         a. Acid, alkali, iron salts (ferrous), salicylates
      3. Menetrier's disease (MD) and eosinophilic gastroenteritis (EG)
         a. These disorders are indistinguishable radiographically when changes are limited to the stomach

    b. Hypertrophic folds in fundus, body of stomach

    c. Childhood MD may cause protein-losing enteropathy, but does not carry increased risk of cancer

    d. Differential diagnosis (DDx): hypertrophic gastritis, lymphoma

C. **Trauma**

    1. Gastric rupture

       a. Most common cause of pneumoperitoneum in term infants **[Figs. 1–23 and 1–24]**

       b. Associated with perinatal asphyxia/ischemia, occasionally with proximal small bowel obstruction (SBO)

       c. Upright/decubitus plain film shows free air without air–fluid level in stomach

    2. Bezoars

       a. Lactobezoar (milk curd) in infants, trichobezoar (swallowed hair) in older children

    3. Gastric atony **[Fig. 6-7]**

       a. Hypotonia and functional gastric outlet obstruction in postoperative patient, or as consequence of trauma, electrolyte disturbance, neurologic disorder, or acute starvation

       b. May occur as part of child abuse/neglect

       c. Also seen in patients with bulimia, anorexia nervosa

D. **Tumors**

    1. Teratoma is most common gastric tumor

       a. Found most commonly in males less than one year of age

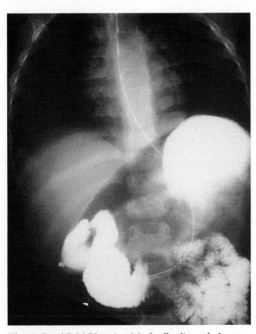

Fig. 6-7 AP UGI series: Markedly distended stomach. Duodenum is also distended at the level of the spine. This child had been starved recently. Gastric atony, hypoperistalsis.

2. Heterotopic pancreas most often in duodenum and distal stomach
    a. Resembles ulcer on upper GI series (UGI)

E. **Ulcers [Fig. 6-8]**
    1. Gastric ulcers less common than duodenal ulcers in children
    2. In infants, secondary to stress induced by sepsis, burns, trauma, surgery, congestive heart failure, or hypoxia

F. **Gastric Outlet Obstruction**
    1. Functional
        a. Gastric atony
    2. Pylorospasm
        a. Rate of gastric emptying in infants and children is variable
        b. The pyloric channel may be narrowed, but mass effect on antrum and duodenum is not seen with pylorospasm, as in hypertrophic pyloric stenosis (HPS), nor is pyloric channel narrowing persistent
    3. HPS
        a. Incidence = 1.26 : 1000 in whites and 0.48 : 1000 in blacks
        b. Male:female = 4 : 1
        c. Developmental disorder noted at 2 - 12 weeks of age
        d. Manifested by non-bilious vomiting
        e. Typical is hypokalemic, hypochloremic alkalosis
        f. Appearance on UGI simulated by chronic prostaglandin therapy
        g. Radiographic findings include marked gastric dilatation disproportionate to small bowel gas **[Fig. 6-9]**

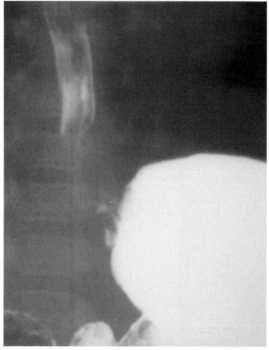

Fig. 6-8 AP UGI series: Sharply demarcated gastric fundus "collar button" and distal esophageal ulcers.

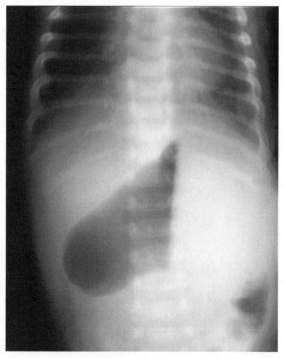

Fig. 6-9 Left lateral decubitus abdomen radiograph: Distended stomach with paucity of distal bowel gas. Hypertrophic pyloric stenosis.

h. UGI **[Fig. 6-10]**
  - Most important is mass effect on antrum and duodenum, producing pyloric tit or beak
  - Single or double track in elongated pylorus is evidence of hypertrophied muscle compressing mucosa
  - Use of nasogastric tube is recommended to:
    Empty stomach of retained food and secretions
    Control barium-air instillation (do not overfill; too much barium will obscure pylorus)
    Air bolus added to barium may facilitate visualizing "string" sign
    Empty stomach of excess barium when study is completed

i. Ultrasound (US) **[Fig. 6-11; see also Fig. 1-67]**
  - Most reliable sign is hypertrophy of hypoechoic muscle > 3.0 mm
  - Next most reliable sign is elongation of pylorus (true pyloric length > 1.7 cm)
  - Major pitfall is failure to image pylorus adequately, either due to operator inexperience or to curvature of pylorus preventing proximal and distal portions seen within plane of focus

j. Imaging DDx includes:
  - EG
  - Chronic prostaglandin administration (to maintain ductus arteriosus patency in cyanotic heart disease)

III. SMALL INTESTINE

A. Congenital

1. Duplication cyst **[Fig. 6-12]**
   a. On mesenteric border of GI tract
     - Colon duplication cyst may be on anti-mesenteric border
   b. Most common location is ileal (35% of alimentary tract duplications)
     - Esophageal (19%), colonic or appendiceal (18%), gastroduodenal (15%), jejunal (9%)

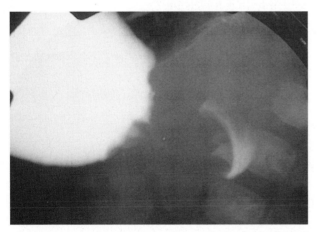

Fig. 6-10 UGI series: Elongated, narrowed pyloric channel with "string sign." Note mass effect upon duodenal bulb. Hypertrophic pyloric stenosis.

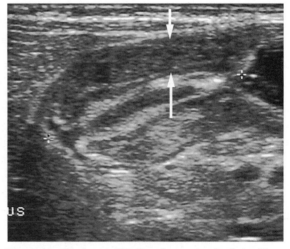

Fig. 6-11 Transverse US along long axis of pylorus: Electronic cursors indicate pyloric length. Wall thickness determined between arrows. Hypertrophic pyloric stenosis.

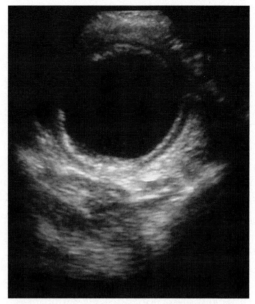

Fig. 6-12 Transverse abdomen US: Cystic mass. Note hyperechoic rim indicating mucosa and hypoechoic cyst wall identical to sonographic appearance of gastrointestinal viscus. SB duplication cyst.

    c. Usually presents with GI obstruction or palpable mass

    d. Usually does not communicate with lumen

    e. Gastric duplication cyst on greater curvature

- Cyst may actually be separate from stomach
- Can simulate pancreatic pseudocyst

  2. Meckel's diverticulum

    a. On antimesenteric border of GI tract

    b. Presents with painless bleeding

- Diverticulum with gastric mucosa causes ulceration on opposite wall of bowel, which produces bleeding
- Bleeding is not from diverticulum itself

    c. Diagnosis by nuclear Meckel scan

- Pertechnetate uptake can be virtually anywhere in abdomen if bowel is mobile
- If bowel is fixed, uptake usually in right lower quadrant

    d. Rule of 2's

- 2% of population
- 2 feet from ileocecal valve
- 20% contain gastric mucosa
- 2 hard 2 find

B. **Inflammation**

  1. Proximal small bowel

    a. Pancreatitis, *Giardia lamblia,* Ascariasis, *Strongyloides*

  2. Terminal ileum

    a. Crohn's disease, tuberculous, *Yersinia enterocolitica,* Behcet's, trichuriasis

3. Graft versus host (GVH)
   a. Infiltration of engrafted lymphocytes into host tissue
   b. Occurs 10 to 50 days posttransplant
   c. Clinically, patient has morbilliform rash, mouth ulcers, abdominal pain, diarrhea, liver dysfunction, malabsorption
   d. UGI/small bowel (SB) series:
      • Abrupt transition at jejuno-ileal junction to widely separated edematous ileal loops devoid of mucosal markings
      • Very rapid mouth-anus transit

C. **Tumors**
   1. Peutz-Jeghers syndrome
      a. Sessile or pedunculated hamartomas, without malignant potential
   2. Gardner's syndrome
      a. Adenomatous polyps in SB may occur without other signs of Gardner's
      b. Osteomas, abdominal desmoid
      c. Autosomal dominant
   3. Osler-Weber-Rendu syndrome
      a. Telangiectasias anywhere in SB
      b. Pulmonary arteriovenous malformations
      c. Central nervous system (CNS), conjunctival telangiectasias
   4. Sturge Weber syndrome
      a. Cavernous hemangiomata
   5. Others:
      a. Cronkhite-Canada, neurofibromatosis, Turner's syndrome, tuberous sclerosis, Klippel-Weber-Trenaunay
   6. Lymphoma **[Figs. 6-13 and 6-14; see also Fig. 8-10]**
      a. Most common SB malignancy in children
      b. Most often non-Hodgkin's lymphoma (NHL)

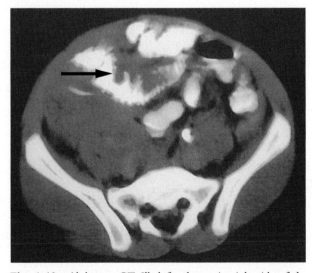

Fig. 6-13 Abdomen CT: Ill-defined mass in right side of abdomen. Note infiltration of SB wall (arrow) and of psoas muscle. SB lymphoma.

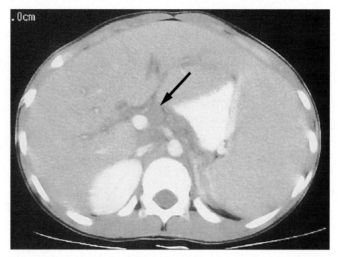

Fig. 6-14 Abdomen CT: Splenomegaly, adenopathy in gastrohepatic ligament (arrow). SB lymphoma.

    c. Peak age, 5 to 8 years of age; M : F = 9 : 1
    d. Most often arises in terminal ileum or cecum, presenting occasionally as lead point in intussusception, but may diffusely involve mesentery and/or retroperitoneum
    e. Burkitt type tends to be anterior, involving mesentery, and relatively spares perivascular areas
    f. Non-Burkitt NHL may present in any location
    g. Clinical presentation
      • Insidious weight loss, fatigue, vomiting secondary to obstruction, abdominal pain or mass
      • Fever and night sweats uncommon
      • Rarely, as malabsorption
    h. Radiographic appearances
      • Diffuse polypoid mucosal folds
      • Bowel wall thickening
      • Featureless bowel with aneurysmal dilatation
      • Polypoid mass
      • Mesenteric mass
  7. Other malignancies
    a. Carcinoid
      • Appendix most common location
    b. Others
      • Leiomyosarcoma, rhabdomyosarcoma, etc.

D. **Trauma**
  1. Locations susceptible to shearing forces are fixed locations such as duodenum, duodenojejunal junction (DJJ), and terminal ileum
  2. Rupture may occur as lap-belt injury in motor vehicle accident, iatrogenic event, child abuse
  3. Intramural hematoma, often seen in proximal SB, may be secondary to Henoch-Schonlein purpura, hemophilia, hemolytic uremic syndrome, or abuse

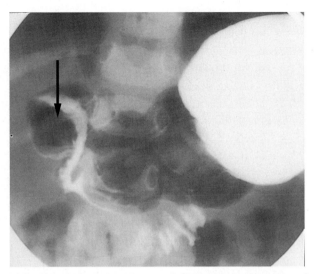

Fig. 6-15   UGI series: History of physical abuse. Deviation of descending duodenum due to intramural mass (arrow) on antimesenteric border, thickening of mucosal folds in third-fourth part of duodenum. Duodenal hematoma.

4. Child abuse
   a. Visceral injuries associated with 50% mortality
   b. Duodenal hematoma, usually in lateral wall, may appear as mural nodule **[Figs. 6-15 and 6-16]**
      • UGI shows mucosal thickening or "stacked coin" appearance
      • US shows complex mass adjacent to pancreas
E. **SB patterns**
   1. Dilated, folds not thickened (SOS)
      a. Celiac disease (Sprue)
      b. Tropical sprue

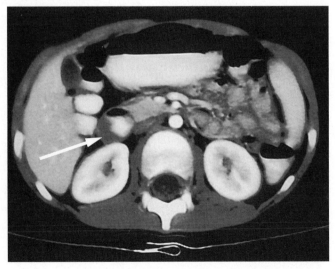

Fig. 6-16   Abdomen CT: Lapbelt injury in auto accident. Hypodense lesion (arrow) in lateral wall of duodenum. Duodenal hematoma.

    c. Obstruction (SBO) or ileus **[Fig. 6-17]**

    d. Scleroderma

    e. SB diverticulosis

      • All are usually associated with increased secretions

2. Slightly dilated, thick folds, no nodules

    a. SB edema secondary to decreased serum albumen (cirrhosis, congestive heart failure, nephrotic syndrome, GI protein loss)

      • Rarely in Whipple's, amyloidosis, lymphangiectasia

3. Minimal dilatation, thick folds, increased secretions

    a. Lymphangiectasia

    b. Menetrier's or Zollinger-Ellison (also involves stomach)

    c. Occasionally, Whipple's disease or lymphoma

4. Thick, irregular folds (WAGEL)

    a. Whipple's (most marked proximally)

    b. Amyloidosis

    c. Giardiasis (proximal)

    d. Eosinophilic enteritis

    e. Lymphoma

5. Thick folds, granular (small nodules) (LLMM)

    a. Lymphoid hyperplasia (benign or secondary to decreased immunoglobulins)

    b. Lymphoma (nodules are usually larger than hyperplasia)

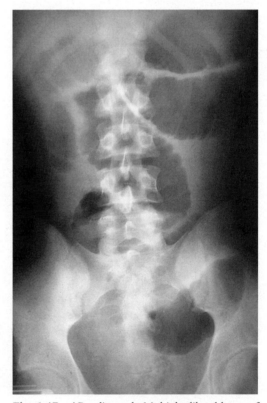

Fig. 6-17 AP radiograph: Multiple dilated loops of small bowel, paucity of gas in colon. SBO.

     c. Mastocytosis

     d. Macroglobulinemia with steatorrhea

  6. Segmental SB disease

     a. Regional enteritis (Crohn's)

     b. Intramural hemorrhage or infarction

     c. Metastatic disease

     d. Lymphoma

     e. Edema secondary to adjacent inflammation

     f. Radiation enteritis

  7. Diffusely abnormal SB with gastric involvement (ZELMA)

     a. Zollinger-Ellison syndrome

     b. Eosinophilic gastroenteritis

     c. Lymphoma (nodules)

     d. Menetrier's disease

     e. Amyloidosis

Diffuse Involvement

	Dilated	**Not Dilated**
Thick Folds	↓Protein	ZELMA
No Thick Folds	SOS	NORMAL

Irregularly Thickened Folds = WAGEL
Large or Small Nodules = LLMM
+ Gastric Involvement = ZELMA
Segmental Involvement
    Blood
    Neoplasm
    Radiation
    Regional enteritis

F. **Cystic Fibrosis (CF)**

  1. Newborn

     a. Autosomal recessive disorder occurring in 1 : 3000 live births

     b. Meconium ileus (MI) **[Figs. 6–18 through 6–20; see also Fig. 1–62]**

        • Mode of presentation for 10 to 20% of patients with CF

        • Microcolon and meconium plugs in terminal SB

        • Radiographic findings

          SBO with lack of air-fluid levels suggests MI

        • 50% uncomplicated (treated by radiologist), 50% complicated (treated surgically)

        • Uncomplicated MI

          Patency from dilated SB to rectum, treated medically

PITFALL

- You cannot differentiate dilated SB from dilated large bowel by cnventional radiographs.

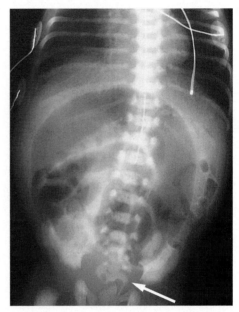

Fig. 6-18 AP radiograph: Dilated bowel loops in central abdomen. Although largest of these loops resembles transverse colon, it is SB. Small bowel and large bowel difficult to discriminate in newborn. Note small caliber of contrast-filled rectum (arrow). Microcolon-meconium ileus.

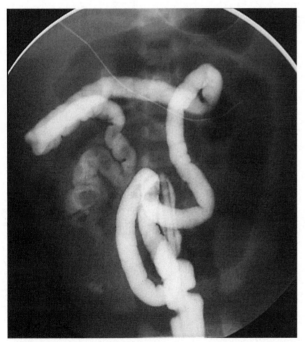

Fig. 6-19 Water soluble contrast enema: Narrowed caliber and redundant colon. Note disproportionately dilated SB. Distal SB atresia, total colon Hirschsprung's disease in DDx of microcolon. Microcolon-meconium ileus.

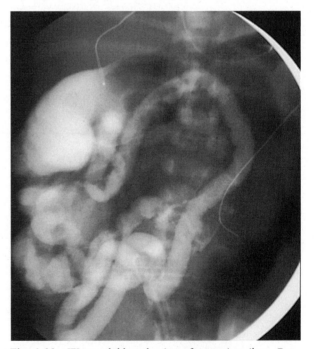

Fig. 6-20 Water soluble reduction of meconium ileus. Contrast in microcolon enters dilated SB loop in right upper quadrant.

15% Hypaque enema for diagnosis

Then 25% Hypaque ± 1% mucomyst enema for treatment

Use heated fluid to 37°C to reduce heat loss from cold enema fluid

May require daily enemas with fluoroscopic guidance to resolve

Treatment requires close clinical cooperation to manage fluids, heat loss in radiology suite, etc.

- Complicated MI

  Volvulus, SB ischemia, perforation, meconium peritonitis (MP) common

  Calcification in MP may occur as early as 12 hours after in-utero perforation

  MI with pseudocyst may present in newborn as abdominal mass — Associated with SB atresia and/or volvulus and in-utero perforation

2. Older child **[Fig. 8-13]**

   a. Meconium ileus equivalent
      - Now termed distal intestinal obstructive syndrome (DIOS)
      - Inspissated fecal mass in cecum and ascending colon
      - Presents as abdominal mass or abdominal pain suggesting appendicitis

   b. Intussusception
      - 1% of patients with CF
      - Most are ileo-colic, although ileo-ileal and colo-colic types reported
      - Usually in children >4 years of age; may be subacute or chronic

   c. Other SB patterns of CF
      - Malabsorption
      - Pneumatosis, with or without rectal prolapse
      - Mucosal changes **[Fig. 8-12]**

        Thickened folds and hypertrophied bowel wall, most commonly seen in duodenum, also noted in SB and colon

G. **Obstruction**

1. Most common causes of GI obstruction
   a. Hypertrophic pyloric stenosis
   b. Intussusception
   c. Intestinal atresia
   d. Incarcerated hernia
   e. Imperforate anus
   f. Hirschsprung's disease

2. Congenital
   a. Duodenal obstruction
      - Atresia (50%) **[Fig. 6-21]**

        25% preampullary

        Annular pancreas in 21% of atresias

        Down's syndrome in 25% of patients with atresia
      - Diaphragm or web (40%)
      - Stenosis (10%)

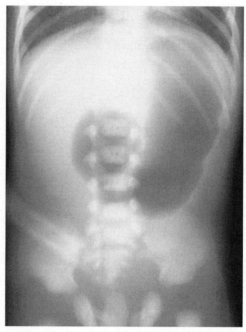

Fig. 6-21 AP radiograph: "Double bubble" sign of duodenal atresia. Note flared iliac wings and flattened acetabular roof in pelvis, indicating Down's syndrome.

- Preduodenal portal vein
    Rare anomaly whose associations (intrinsic duodenal anomaly or malrotation with Ladd's bands) responsible for duodenal obstruction
- Annular pancreas
    Secondary anomaly associated with intrinsic duodenal obstruction or malrotation
- Radiographic findings
    "Double bubble" sign by prenatal US or postnatal plain film, polyhydramnios, absence or paucity of SB gas
- Clinical findings
    Infant presents in first few days of life with bilious vomiting
    Emergency UGI necessary to rule out malrotation and midgut volvulus, which may have an identical appearance to duodenal atresia by plain film.
  b. Malrotation (MR), midgut volvulus (MV) **[Figs. 6-22 through 6-25; see also Figs. 1-53 and 1-55]**
    - Typical presentation of MR/MV is acute bilious vomiting few days to several weeks of life
        One-third of patients with MR and vomiting have nonbilious vomiting
    - Can occur in person of *any* age, including adults
    - Radiographic patterns
    (1) Normal

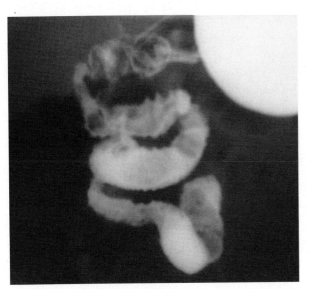

Fig. 6-22 UGI series: "Corkscrew" appearance of duodenum without obvious obstruction. Malrotation.

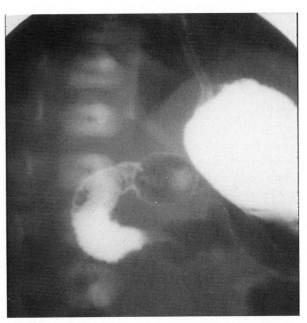

Fig. 6-23 UGI series: Obstruction in third portion of duodenum. Note "beaked" appearance at site of obstruction. Malrotation with midgut volvulus.

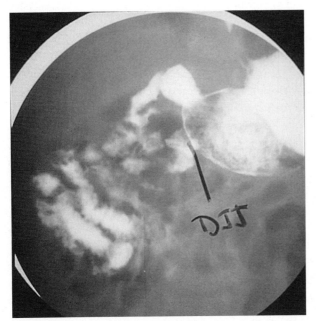

Fig. 6-24 UGI series: Position of DJJ inferior to duodenal bulb, overlies right pedicle of vertebral column; jejunum is to right of spine. Malrotation.

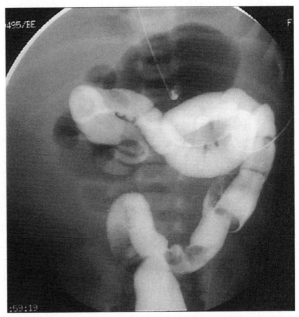

Fig. 6-25 Contrast enema: Medial position of cecum. Note position of appendix. The air-filled stomach and proximal SB overlie the cecum, indicating shortened mesentery. Malrotation.

PITFALL IN INTERPRETING MR BY BE

- The cecum that is positioned "high" relative to the iliac wing found in normal children (up to 8 years of age)

- The cecum in patients with MR is not only high but the tip is directed superiorly or transversely

PITFALL IN INTERPRETING MR BY UGI

- Overfilling the stomach (usually by allowing the infant to drink from a bottle) may prevent visualizing the position of the ligament of Treitz (DJJ).

- UGI using a nasogastric tube provides the radiologist with control of the study. Once a small amount of barium (10 cc) reaches the second portion of the duodenum, place the infant in the supine position and follow the barium bolus to the DJJ.

- The normal position of the DJJ is to the left of the spine at the level of the duodenal bulb or proximal second portion of duodenum.

(2) Duodenal obstruction
(3) Apparent low SB obstruction, with air-fluid levels
  - Indicates bowel ischemia due to venous congestion
  - MR/MV with bowel ischemia is a cause of pneumatosis
(4) Gasless abdomen
  UGI is preferred to barium enema (BE) if MR/MV is considered
  - Sutton's (of bank robbing fame) law: "Go where the money is"
  BE diagnostic of MR in 2/4 newborns and 3/6 older patients in one study
  Diagnosis by UGI in 15/16 newborns and 7/7 older patients in one study
  - Classic appearance of downward spiralling "corkscrew" of duodenum and proximal jejunum
- Chronic MR/MV may be cause of malabsorption, hypoproteinemia, and recurrent or "cyclic" vomiting.
- Intestinal dilatation may cause inferior displacement of DJJ or superior displacement of the stomach, mimicking MR
- Transverse stomach and superiorly-directed duodenal bulb can also mimic abnormal DJJ relationship; DJJ should remain left of midline

c. Jejuno-ileal atresia
- Incidence = 1 : 1000 live births, occurring as consequence of in utero vascular accident
- Associated with MR/MV, CF with MI, omphalocele, or gastroschisis
- 25% are in preterm newborns
- Clinical presentation
  First day of life with bilious vomiting and/or abdominal distention
- Radiographs
  SBO with air-fluid levels characteristic
  Calcified MP in 12%
  - Distal SB atresia associated with microcolon
  - Proximal SB atresia usually is not
    Presence of succus entericus in distal SB prevents unused colon appearance of microcolon

d. Intussusception (INT) **[Figs. 6-26 through 6-28; see also Figs. 1-60 and 1-61]**
- Idiopathic INT occurs in infants with peak age of 9 months to 2 years
- Greater than 90% ileo-colic
- Lead points (2.5 to 5% of cases) most commonly found in infants < 6 months and children > 3 years.
  Meckel's diverticulum and SB tumors are most common lead points
- Proximal SB INT:
  Diagnosis by UGI/SB series
  - Narrowed barium channel, mass at distal end of channel, and/or "coiled spring" around channel
  Lead point usually found
  - Peutz-Jegher or adenomatous polyp cause jejuno-jejunal INT

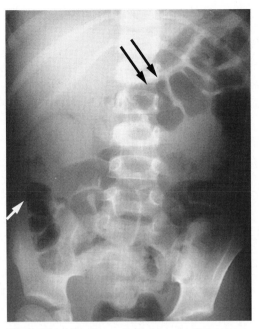

Fig. 6-26 AP radiograph: Elongated soft tissue mass in right upper quadrant bounded by air-filled SB (arrow) and air-filled transverse colon (two arrows). Air is present within mass in intussusceptum. Transverse colon is intussuscipiens (*recipient*). Intussusception.

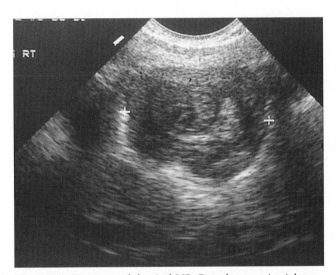

Fig. 6-27 Transverse abdominal US: Complex mass in right upper quadrant. Mass has whorl-like character with alternating layers of echogenic and echolucent material. Note crescentic central echoes representing mesenteric fat. Intussusception.

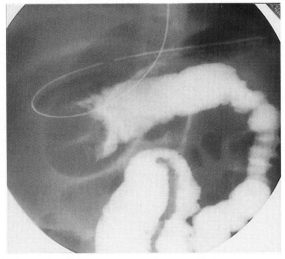

Fig. 6-28 Contrast enema: Abrupt termination of contrast column with contrast in interstices of intussusceptum and widening of contrast column where intussusceptum meets intussuscipiens. Intussusception.

– Henoch-Schonlein-induced intramural hematoma in 50% of ileoileal INT
- Clinical findings:
  Abdominal pain (97%), vomiting (78%), bloody stool (42%)
- Plain film findings of INT
  Soft tissue mass (60%)
  – Mass seen only on horizontal cross-table lateral radiograph in 12/24 cases in which mass was visualized
  SB obstruction
- Sonographic findings of INT
  "Pseudokidney sign" perpendicular to long axis
  – Looks like target with multiple concentric rings of variable echoes
  Tubular lesion with mutiple layers of variable echoes along long axis
- Reduction of INT (see Quick Start chapter)

e. Superior Mesoenteric Artery (SMB) pseudo-obstruction
- Recurrent abdominal pain and distention resembling SBO, but due to dysmotility
- Biopsy shows myopathy or segmental muscular thinning.
- Associated with gastroschisis, megacystis-microcolon, and "prune belly" in female infant

f. Superior Mesenteric Artery (SMA) syndrome
- Functional or mechanical obstruction as third portion of duodenum or proximal SB crosses spine
  Seen in patients with acute weight loss
  – Recent surgery
  – Bulimia, anorexia nervosa, starvation

IV. **COLON**
   A. **Anomalies**
      1. Imperforate anus (IA) **[Figs. 6-29 and 6-30]**
         a. Relation to pubococcygeus (levator sling) indicates whether "high" or "low"
- Associated genitourinary (GU) anomalies are seen in 25% of "low" and 40% of "high" IA
- Sacral anomalies also more common in "high" than in "low" lesions
- IA may be present as part of VATER association or Currarino triad (IA, presacral meningocele, sacral dysgenesis)

         b. Radiologic evaluation
- Includes renal and spinal US in newborn
  10 to 30% of IA have spinal cord abnormality
  – Wedge-shaped conus medullaris
  – Tethered cord (below L3 in newborn)
- Distance from rectum to perineum can be measured by placing transducer directly on perineum and identifying meconium-filled rectum

   B. **Inflammation**
      1. Necrotizing enterocolitis (NEC) **[Figs. 6-31 and 6-32]**
         a. Underlying etiology is perinatal hypoxia/ischemia

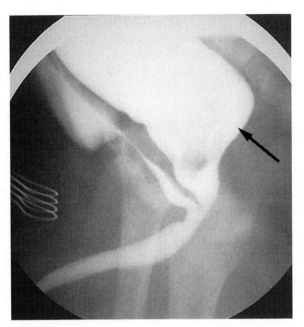

Fig. 6-29 Antegrade mucous fistulogram: Contrast in rectum (arrow). Note communication with urethra and backfilling into urinary bladder. Imperforate anus with rectourethral fistula.

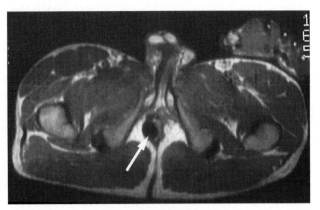

Fig. 6-30 Axial T2-weighted MRI: History of previous rectal pullthrough surgery for imperforate anus. Note air-filled rectum (arrow) surrounded by muscle on left and absence of levator tissue on right. Patient was incontinent due to insufficent levator tissue.

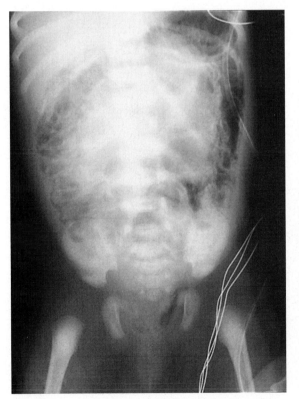

Fig. 6-31 AP abdomen radiograph: Extensive pneumatosis intestinalis. Note air coursing along bowel wall in right colon and stippled along left colon. Curvilinear pneumatosis in left upper quadrant. NEC.

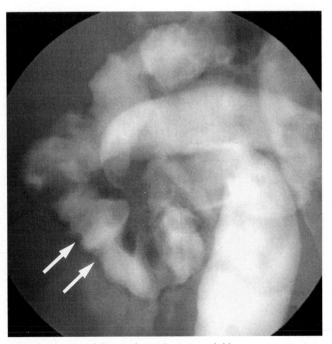

Fig. 6-32 Carefully performed water soluble contrast enema: Contrast is in lumen of colon, but air is in wall. Note minithumbprinting along lateral wall of right colon (arrows). NEC.

b. Most common sites are ileum and ascending colon

c. Early changes of mucosal edema and hemorrhage manifest by bowel wall thickening and irregular dilatation of gut

d. Submucosal pneumatosis due to gas produced by bacteria

e. Clinical signs
- Abdominal distention, bloody stools, gastric retention, temperature instability, lethargy, unexplained acidosis, thrombocytopenia
- Age of onset: 1 to 60 days of life

f. Early radiographic signs
- Disorganized bowel gas pattern, particularly with dilated centrally placed loops, thickened bowel wall displacing loops
- Pneumatosis and perforation, with or without portal venous gas, are late signs
- Perforation usually occurs within 30 hours of diagnosis
   Obtain supine and left lateral decubitus radiographs q6–8 hours from time of diagnosis until bowel gas pattern improves
- Stricture formation in 6 to 33% of survivors
   One to 20 months (mean 1.3 months) after acute NEC; 80% of strictures are colonic, 30% left-sided, 15% multiple

2. Granulomatous ileocolitis (Crohn's disease) **[Fig. 6-33]**
   a. Presents with growth failure, fever of unknown origin, bloody diarrhea, abdominal pain
   b. Ileocolic area most commonly affected
   c. Asymmetric or discontinuous lesions of deep or aphthous ulcers

3. Ulcerative colitis (UC)

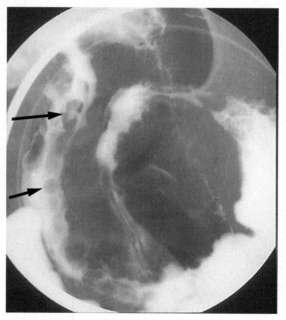

Fig. 6-33 Coned-down view SB followthrough: Geographic separation of bowel loops in distal ileum ("omega sign"). Note aphthous ulcerations (arrows). Granulomatous colitis.

a. Usually presents with acute bloody diarrhea
- Associated with growth failure
- Arthritis in 20%; may precede UC

b. Superficial ulcers, mucosal granularity or edema, or symmetric or continuous lesions

c. Early changes of granulomatous and ulcerative colitis are more accurately diagnosed by double contrast BE
- Advanced disease of both detected equally well by single and double contrast BE

4. Pseudomembranous colitis
a. Associated with *Clostridium difficile*

5. Milk-induced colitis
a. Eosinophilia on colon biopsy
b. Contrast enema normal or nonspecific inflammation

6. Typhlitis (Neutropenic colitis) **[Fig. 6-34]**
a. Associated with leukemia, neutropenia, *Pseudomonas spp.*
b. CT shows focal bowel wall thickening in colon, intramural gas, infiltration of mesenteric fat, and/or abscess
- Not confined to cecum; can involve multiple sites in colon

7. Appendicitis in children **[Figs. 6-35 through 6-37; see also Figs. 1-68 and 1-69]**
a. Factors that contribute to lack of timely diagnosis and associated appendiceal perforation
- Lack of specific signs/symptoms that indicate appendicitis
- Young age of the patient
- Duration of symptoms prior to correct diagnosis
- History negative for appendicitis in other family members
b. Increased risk of appendiceal perforation and abscess formation directly related to delay in diagnosis

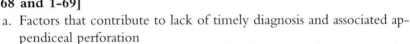

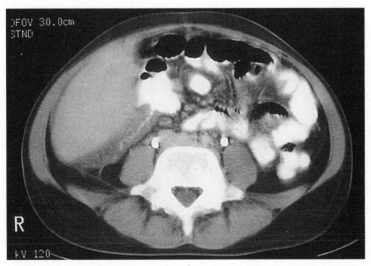

Fig. 6-34 Abdomen CT: Patient with leukemia. Well-demarcated zone of bowel wall thickening in right colon. Note thin intraluminal contrast column. Sigmoid (not shown) was also involved. Typhlitis (neutropenic colitis).

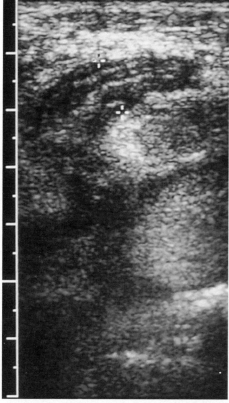

Fig. 6-35 Transverse right lower quadrant US: Abnormally distended appendix, measuring 9.9 mm from wall to wall. Usually sharply defined echogenic peritoneum is ill-defined, indicating localized peritonitis. Appendicitis.

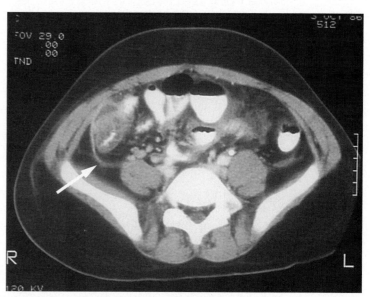

Fig. 6-36 Abdomen CT: Localized inflammation in right lower quadrant, thickened peritoneum (arrow). Appendicitis.

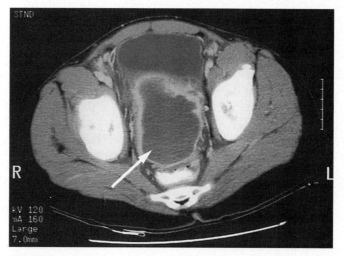

Fig. 6-37 Abdomen CT: Fluid-filled bladder anterior, contrast-filled rectum posterior, abscess (arrow) with enhancing, irregularly thickened wall in cul de sac. Appendicitis, abscess.

- The rate of perforation increases from 8% in patients symptomatic for less than 20 hours to 87% in patients symptomatic for >80 hours

c. Likelihood of perforation inversely related to age
  - Incidence of rupture in patients with appendicitis 93% in patients ≤ 2 years of age, 71% in children 3 to 5 years of age, 40% in those 6 to 10 years of age, and 33% in > 10 years

d. Appendicitis may be presenting complaint in CF

e. Radiographs
  - Appendicoliths detected by film radiography one-third of the time they are present
  - Appendiceal calculi are seen in 10 to 14% of cases of appendicitis and are associated with perforation in 50%

f. Contrast enema
  - Hallmark is nonfilling of appendix
    BE fails to fill appendix in 8 to 20% of normal patients
  - With perforation, abscess typically produces mass effect on cecum or rectosigmoid (cul de sac abscess)
  - Residual barium from contrast enema may degrade or preclude subsequent CT scan

g. US
  - Specificity, sensitivity, and accuracy in diagnosis of acute appendicitis in children 81 to 95%, 80 to 86%, and 82 to 90%, respectively
  - Criterion for diagnosis of uncomplicated acute appendicitis
    Noncompressible appendix ≥7 mm in wall-to-wall diameter
  - Appendiceal perforation
    Loculated pericecal fluid collection, prominent pericecal fat over 10 mm, and circumferential loss of submucosal layer of the appendix
    Loculated pericecal fluid collection is 100% specific for perforation
  - US is of greatest value in diagnosing those patients who have equivocal clinical signs and symptoms of acute appendicitis

h. CT
  - Diagnosis of acute appendicitis is based on:
    Visualization of the abnormal appendix as a small tubular structure with contrast-enhancing, slightly thickened wall and periappendiceal inflammatory change, or by depicting inflammatory changes, a phlegmon, or a pericecal or retrocolic abscess accompanied by calcified appendicolith
    Specificity, sensitivity, and accuracy of CT in the diagnosis of acute appendicitis is 83%, 98%, and 93%, respectively

8. Posttransplant pneumatosis
  a. Associated with steroid use
  b. Onset 10 to 63 days posttransplant
  c. Lasts 2 to 16 days
  d. Resolves without stricture, following conservative management

C. **Motility disorders**

1. Hirschsprung's disease (HD) **[Figs. 6-38 through 6-40; see also Figs. 1-58 and 1-59]**

a. Arrest of the cranio-caudal migration of ganglion cells in submucosa

b. Distribution
   - Short segment recto-sigmoid 80%
   - Long segment proximal to recto-sigmoid 10 to 15%
   - Total colon aganglionosis 5 to 10%

c. Indicators of HD
   - Combination of recto-sigmoid transition zone, retention of barium, and mixing of barium with stool
   - Irregular contractions in aganglionic segment
   - Abnormal postevacuation clearance (24 to 48 hours)
   - Spontaneous complete evacuation in HD has been reported

d. Clinical
   - In infancy, presents with bilious vomiting, possible SBO
   - Clinical DDx includes midgut volvulus, meconium plug syndrome, small left colon, distal bowel atresia

e. Radiographs
   - May appear as SBO
   - Diminished gas in rectum and/or colon on prone cross-table lateral

f. BE
   - Colon narrowed distally compared to more proximal colon

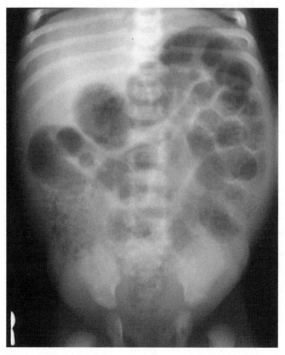

Fig. 6-38 AP abdomen radiograph: Multiple dilated bowel loops including air mixed with fecal material in colon and SB dilatation. Hirschsprung's disease.

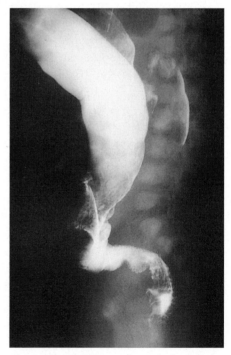

Fig. 6-39 BE: Abnormal recto-sigmoid relationship. Rectum is considerably smaller than sigmoid. Note funnel-shaped transition zone; spiculation in rectum due to unrestrained contractions. Hirschsprung's Disease.

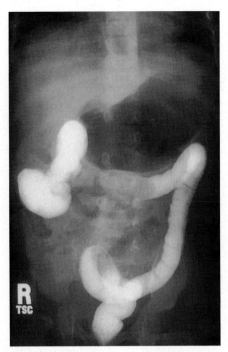

Fig. 6-40 Contrast enema: Caliber is equal thoughout entire colon. Flexures somewhat shortened. Total colonic Hirschsprung's Disease.

- Abnormal recto-sigmoid ratio, irregular contour with spiculations
- Delayed emptying proximal to distal
- Enterocolitis
- Pneumatosis
  g. Total colonic aganglionosis
    - Shortened colon
    - Simple, uncoiled flexures
    - Near normal, uniform caliber throughout colon
    - Excessive SB reflux
    - One-third of contrast enemas normal in total colon HD
    - Disproportionate distention of SB
2. Pseudo-HD
  a. Clinical and radiographic appearance of HD, with dysplastic and/or disorganized ganglion cells on rectal biopsy
3. Meconium plug syndrome **[Fig. 6-41]**
  a. Clinical
    - Failure to pass meconium in 24 hours in term and 48 hours in preterm newborn
  b. Associated with maternal toxemia and/or magnesium therapy
  c. Cannot be differentiated from total colonic aganglionosis
4. Neonatal small left colon syndrome **[Fig. 6-42]**
  a. Abrupt transition at splenic flexure; consider long-segment HD
  b. Occurs in infant of diabetic mother
    - Functional disorder
    - Resolves spontaneously in 2 to 3 weeks

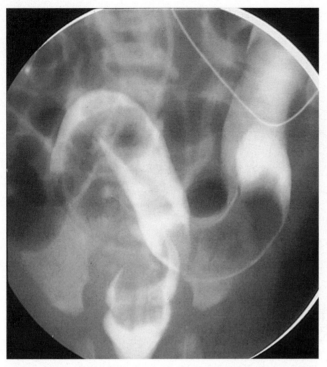

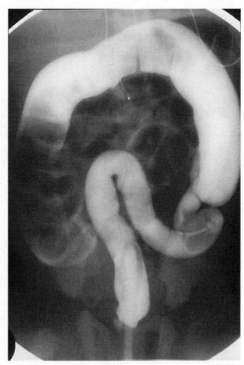

Fig. 6-41 Contrast enema: Long cylindrical filling defect, caliber of rectum and sigmoid approximately equal. Study does not exclude HD; rectal biopsy recommended. Meconium plug.

Fig. 6-42 Contrast enema: Transition between dilated proximal colon and smaller descending colon at splenic flexure. Long segment HD cannot be excluded. Neonatal small left colon.

5. Microcolon
   a. Distal SB atresia
   b. Total colonic aganglionosis
   c. MI
   d. Microcolon of prematurity (nonbilious vomiting)
      • Low birthweight infants (920 to 1320 g) with abdominal distention and failure to pass meconium
      • Bilious vomiting absent (bilious vomiting present in distal SB atresia, MI, and total colon HD)
      • Association with maternal toxemia and/or magnesium therapy
      • Following conservative therapy, bowel function returns to normal within 2 weeks of initial studies
      • CF and HD should be excluded
      • Rectal biopsy shows immature ganglion cells

D. **Tumors**
   1. Juvenile polyps **[Fig. 6-43]**
      a. Most are located in sigmoid and rectum
      b. Present with acute rectal bleeding
      c. 25% are multiple
      d. No risk of malignant transformation
   2. Polyposis syndromes
      a. Familial polyposis and Gardner's syndrome are autosomal dominant disorders associated with malignant risk

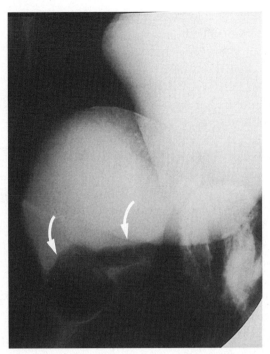

Fig. 6-43 Dilute BE: Mushroom-shaped filling defect (curved arrows) in rectum. Juvenile polyp.

    b. Juvenile polyposis characterized by numerous polyps of juvenile type predominantly in colon
- No malignant transformation, but there is increased risk of bowel cancer in families of affected patients

3. Others
    a. Cronkhite–Canada syndrome
- Alopecia, nail changes, skin pigmentation

    b. Turcot syndrome
- Polyposis, CNS tumors

    c. Intestinal ganglioneuromatosis
- Polypoid mucosa, thyroid carcinoma, pheochromocytoma

4. Colon carcinoma in children
    a. Most common primary cancer of GI tract in children
    b. Most common location is rectum and sigmoid
    c. Most are colloid mucin-producing adenocarcinoma
    d. High-grade biologic activity
    e. May develop after uretero-sigmoidostomy
    f. In children, usually *no association with polyposis syndromes*
- Polyposis-induced colon carcinoma usually occurs in young adults

V. LIVER
A. Congenital
1. Situs abnormalities
    a. Midline liver in asplenia/polysplenia syndromes
2. Alagille syndrome
    a. Most common syndrome of intrahepatic cholestasis

      b. Paucity of bile ducts, pulmonary stenosis, butterfly vertebrae, short ulna, short distal phalanges, retarded bone age

  3. α1-Antitrypsin deficiency

      a. Autosomal recessive

      b. 10 to 20% of neonatal jaundice

      c. Diminished or hypoplastic bile ducts in 28%

  4. Metabolic disorders

      a. Galactosemia: neonatal hypoglycemia

      b. Tyrosinemia: increased incidence of hepatocellular carcinoma

  5. CF

      a. Inspissated bile syndrome indistinguishable from biliary atresia (BA) by nuclear scan or ultrasound

      b. 2.2% incidence of symptomatic liver disease in patients with CF

B. Inflammation

  1. Hepatitis

      a. Neonatal **(Table 6–1),** A, B, C, etc.

      b. Mononucleosis: consider if spleen enlarged, adenotonsillitis

  2. Abscess: pyogenic **[Fig. 6-44]**

      a. Associated with sepsis, omphalitis, CGD of childhood, immunosuppression

      b. *S. aureus* most common

      c. Single, multiple, various sizes

  3. Abscess: granulomatous

      a. CGD of childhood

         • Granulomas often calcify; X-linked recessive; nitroblue tetrazolium (NBT) test positive

         • Leukocytes can engulf microorganisms, but cannot kill them

         • Organisms include *S. aureus, Serratia marcescans,* Candida

      b. Fungal (Candida) **[Fig. 6-45]**

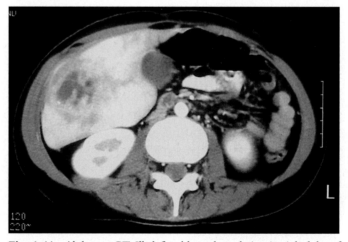

Fig. 6-44 Abdomen CT: Ill-defined hypodense lesion in right lobe of liver. Note thickening of liver capsule and inflammatory effect in soft tissues of abdominal wall. Bacterial hepatic abscess.

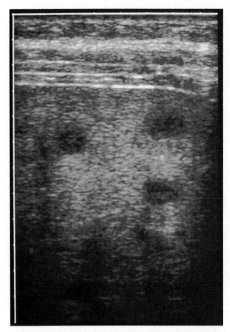

Fig. 6-45 High-resolution liver US: Several small well-defined hypoechoic lesions with "spokewheel" appearance. Candida liver abscess.

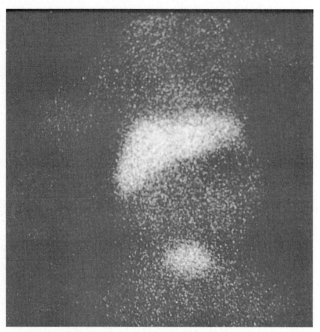

Fig. 6-46 ⁹⁹ᵐTechnetium hepatobiliary scan: Tracer uptake in liver and urinary excretion into bladder. No tracer excretion from biliary system into SB. Biliary atresia.

Table 6-1. Neonatal Hepatitis vs. BA [see also Fig. 6-46]

HEPATITIS	BA
Males, premature newborns	Females
TORCH infections	Polysplenia
Skeletal abnormalities	Choledochal cyst

Jaundice after first week of life in both; conjugated hyperbilirubinemia.

Both considered within spectrum of neonatal obstructive cholangiopathy.

Patient with initial diagnosis of neonatal hepatitis may progressively obstruct biliary system and develop BA.

Close follow-up critical

Normal gall bladder ≥ 15 mm does not exclude BA.

In BA, Kasai 17% successful after 3 months; 40 day rule: successful Kasai procedure more likely if diagnosis and surgery of BA made by 40 days of age.

Must exclude CF in patients thought to have BA.

Phenobarbital prep 5 mg/kg/d × 5 d improves sensitivity of hepatobiliary scan.

- "Spoke-wheel" by US, multiple, same size (microabscesses), immunosuppression, on antibiotics
  c. Cat-scratch disease, tuberculosis, histoplasmosis
4. Hyperalimentation-induced cholestasis
   a. Cholestasis in 20 to 30% of premies on total parenteral nutrition (TPN)
   b. Incidence is 50 to 60% if body weight is <1000 g
   c. Onset 7 to 10 days after TPN onset
   d. Clinical, lab abnormalities resolve in 1 to 4 weeks
      - Biopsy abnormal for months

C. **Trauma**
1. Management determined by clinical signs, symptoms; in children, usually conservative
2. Lacerations simple, complex, right or left lobe **[Fig. 6-47]**
3. Associated injuries: kidney, spleen, lung ipsilateral to liver injury
   a. Left lobe injury associated with pancreas, duodenal injuries
4. Biloma: bile duct disruption, pain, jaundice, fever; hepatobiliary scan positive for bile collection

D. **Benign tumors**
1. Hemangioma
   a. Association with cutaneous hemangiomas
   b. Most common benign liver tumor
   c. Usually <4 cm diameter; large lesions may have central fibrous scar
   d. Hyperechoic on US
   e. CT
      - Hypodense on noncontrast CT and fills in with intravenous (IV) contrast
      - Progressive filling from periphery to center
      - 85% will fill in completely

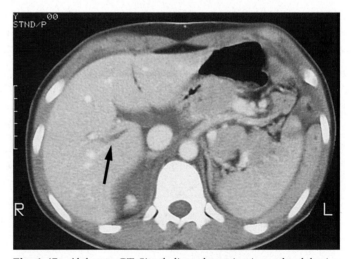

Fig. 6-47 Abdomen CT: Simple linear laceration in caudate lobe (arrow) and anterior spleen. Also hemorrhage in porta hepatis and right adrenal fossa. Liver laceration.

f. MRI
- Hypointense on T1-weighted image (T1WI); markedly hyperintense on T2WI
- Progressive enhancement with gadolinium from periphery to center within 15 minutes

2. Hemangioendothelioma **[Fig. 6-48]**
   a. >85% in children <6 months
   b. Twice as common in females
   c. Newborn presents with heart failure, bruit
   d. Diffuse or localized
   e. US
   - Hypo- or hyperechoic
   f. CT
   - Hypervascular
   - Change in aortic caliber at level of liver as flow is siphoned into high-flow lesion
   - Patchy or homogeneous enhancement, "lacelike"
   g. MRI
   - Heterogeneous, multinodular on T1WI and T2WI
   - If fibrotic, decreased signal on T2WI

3. Focal nodular hyperplasia (FNH)
   a. Hyperplasia of liver cells, with bile ducts; contains Kupffer cells
   b. Second most common benign tumor of liver
   c. Usually solitary, <5 cm diameter
   d. Central fibrous scar
   e. Association with glycogen storage disease, type I
   f. US
   - Homogeneous; hypo-, iso-, hyperechoic

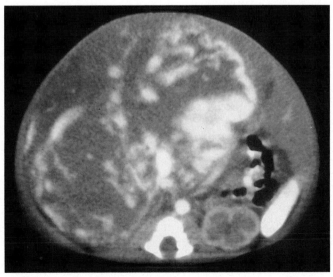

Fig. 6-48 Abdomen CT: Hypervascular lesion with neovascularity virtually replacing enlarged liver. Hemangioendothelioma

    g. CT
- Slightly hypodense, enhances to iso- or hyperdensity

    h. MRI
- Variable signal on T1WI and T2WI
  Central scar hyperintense on T2WI
  Marked enhancement

    i. Nuclear medicine
- Sulfur colloid uptake in 40 to 70% of FNH
  No uptake in adenoma
  Uptake can occur in hepatoblastoma

4. Adenoma
   a. Normal liver cells, no bile ducts
   b. Oral contraceptives, anabolic steroids
   c. Tendency to hemorrhage
   d. Surrounded by capsule
   e. Association with glycogen storage disease, types I or VI
   f. Normal level of α-fetoprotein
   g. US
      - Homogeneous or heterogeneous; hypo-, iso-, hyperechoic
   h. CT
      - 50% have calcification
      - Hypodense, variable enhancement
   i. MRI
      - Heterogeneous on T1WI and T2WI due to presence of fat, hemorrhage, necrosis
      - Usually poor uptake with gadolinium
      - May not be distinguished from hepatocellular carcinoma

5. Mesenchymal hamartoma
   a. Large, multiloculated cystic lesion
      - Cystic or solid (if mesenchymal components predominate)
   b. 10% exophytic
   c. CT or MRI
      - Large (>10 cm) cystic and solid tumor
      - Loculated with septations

E. **Malignant tumors**
   1. Hepatoblastoma (HBL) **[Fig. 6-49]**
      a. Most common symptomatic malignant liver tumor <5 years of age
      b. Epithelial type
         - Fetal or embryonal hepatocytes
         - Necrotic, hemorrhagic
      c. Mesenchymal type
         - Primitive, osteoid
      d. + α-fetoprotein in 60 to 90%
      e. Chunky calcification in 80% (AFIP data)
      f. Can present with paraneoplastic syndrome or precocious puberty
   2. Hepatocellular carcinoma (HCC)
      a. Increased incidence in cirrhosis, tyrosinemia, anabolic steroids, previous hepatitis

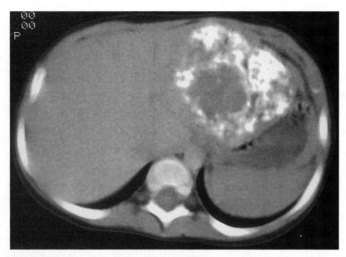

Fig. 6-49 Non-contrast abdomen CT: Enlarged left lobe of liver, which contains heterogeneous mass with chunky calcification. Hepatoblastoma.

    b. Older children than HBL
    c. Elevated α-fetoprotein
    d. Focal, multifocal, diffuse, satellite lesions
    e. CT
        • Patchy or homogeneous enhancement
    f. MRI
        • Variable appearance on T1WI
        • Mild hyperintensity on T2WI, with areas of increased signal representing necrosis
        • Enhancement with gadolinium
        • Vascular invasion
  3. Fibrolamellar hepatocarcinoma
    a. Young adults
    b. Better prognosis than HCC
    c. Normal α-fetoprotein
    d. Large, solitary mass; satellite lesions occasionally
    e. Hemorrhage, necrosis uncommon
    f. Central fibrous scar
    g. MRI
        • Hypointense central scar on T1WI and T2WI
            Central scar of FNH hyperintense on T2WI
        • Remainder of tumor usually hypointense on T1WI and mildly hyperintense on T2WI
  4. Metastatic
    a. Wilms' tumor
    b. Neuroblastoma
        • Stage IVS
    c. Rhabdomyosarcoma, osteosarcoma
    d. Leukemia/lymphoma **[Fig. 6-50]**
F. **Acute portal vein thrombosis [Figs. 6-51 and 6-52]**
  1. Associated with GI inflammation (appendicitis, pancreatitis)

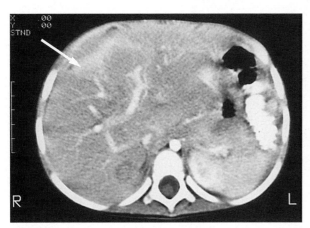

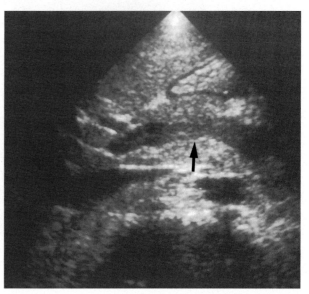

Fig. 6-50 Abdomen CT: Hypodense lesion involving nearly entire liver. Note small area of relatively normal-appearing parenchyma (arrow). Hepatic lymphoma.

Fig. 6-51 Transverse US: Echogenic thrombus (arrow) in splenic vein, which extended into portal vein. Acute splenic and portal vein thrombosis.

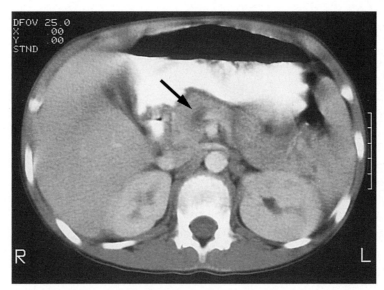

Fig. 6-52 Abdomen CT: Filling defect in superior mesenteric vein (arrow). Note subtle enhancement around thrombus, as well as cut-off of contrast in splenic vein. Acute superior mesenteric vein thrombosis.

2. Associated with clotting abnormalities
   a. Protein C or S deficiency, antithrombin III deficiency
3. Insidious signs, symptoms
   a. Abdominal pain, distention, ascites, splenomegaly
4. Radiology
   a. Thrombus can be identified by US, CT
   b. If flow preserved around clot, MRI may be misleading
5. Treatment medical, directed at restoring portal vein patency

G. **Chronic portal vein thrombosis [Fig. 6-53]**
1. Secondary to umbilical vein catheterization or omphalitis in newborn
2. Idiopathic
3. Signs and symptoms
   a. GI hemorrhage, hematemesis, esophageal varices, hemorrhoids, hypersplenism, ascites
4. Radiology
   a. Thrombus usually not identified
   b. "Normal" portal vein replaced by fibrous cord or cavernomatous transformation (collateral flow)
   c. US, CT, or MRI can show portal vein abnormalities
   d. Treatment surgical, portal-systemic shunting

VI. **GALL BLADDER AND BILIARY SYSTEM**
A. **Congenital**
1. Choledochal cyst **[Figs. 6-54 through 6-56]**
   a. Four times more common in females
   b. 30% <1 year of age, 80% <10 years of age
   c. Abdominal pain in 70%, jaundice in 50%
   d. NB: congenital
   e. Older children: possibly due to pancreatic juice reflux into common bile duct (CBD)

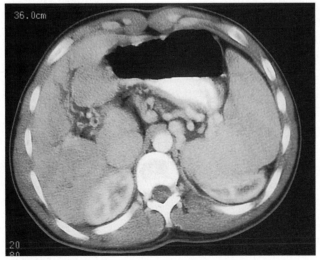

Fig. 6-53 Abdomen CT: Splenomegaly, nodular liver with left lobe atrophy. Note collateral vessels posterior to stomach and replacement of portal vein by small portal collaterals. Chronic portal vein thrombosis; cavernomatous transformation of portal vein.

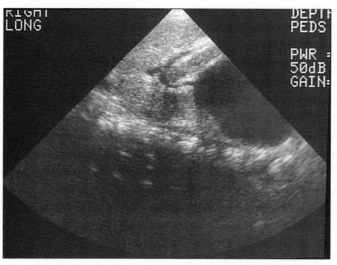

Fig. 6-54 Parasagittal US: Dilated biliary ducts leading into cystic lesion. Choledochal cyst.

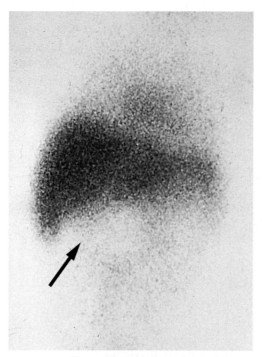

Fig. 6-55 ^{99m}Technetium hepatobiliary scan: 10 minutes after injection, tracer in cardiac blood pool, in liver, and hypoattenuated mass (arrow) inferior to liver. Choledochal cyst.

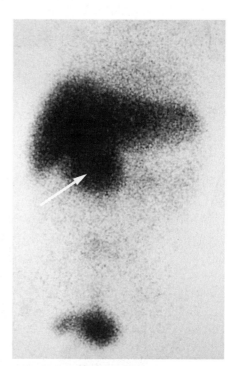

Fig. 6-56 ^{99m}Technetium hepatobiliary scan: 24 hours after injection, tracer accumulates in previously hypoattenuated mass (arrow) inferior to liver. Choledochal cyst.

f. Cyst + dilated intrahepatic ducts
- Type I: Fusiform dilatation of CBD
- Type II: Eccentric diverticulum of CBD
- Type III: Choledochocele at CBD-duodenal junction
- Type IV: Caroli's; intrahepatic BD dilatation
  - Association with autosomal recessive polycystic kidney disease (ARPKD) (congenital hepatic fibrosis)

B. **Inflammation**
1. Hydrops
   a. Associated with sepsis, leptospirosis, Kawasaki's
2. Cholecystitis
   a. Associated with sickle cell disease, hemolytic anemia
3. Cholangitis
   a. Ascending
      - Gall stones, CBD stricture, post-Kasai or liver transplant
   b. Sclerosing
      - Associated with inflammatory bowel disease
      - Diagnosis by endoscopic retrograde cholangiopancreatography (ERCP) or cholangiography
4. Gall stones **[Fig. 6-57; see also Fig. 2-66]**
   a. Associated with hemolytic disease, especially sickle cell disease

VII. **PANCREAS**
A. **Congenital**
1. Pancreas divisum
   a. Most common pancreatic anomaly
   b. Wirsung (main pancreatic duct) and Santorini (accessory) unfused
   c. Wirsung drains inferior head and uncinate process
   d. Santorini drains superior head, body, tail

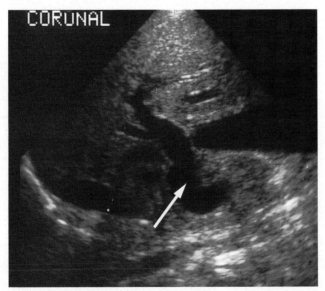

Fig. 6-57 Transverse US at level of pancreatic head: Dilated hepatic ducts and common bile duct (arrow) terminate abruptly. Obstruction due to common bile duct stone.

2. Annular pancreas
   a. Second most common pancreatic anomaly
   b. Faulty fusion of ventral and dorsal portions of pancreas
   c. Encircles second part of duodenum
   d. Up to 75% associated anomalies
      • EA/TE fistula, Down's syndrome, intrinsic duodenal anomaly, malrotation
3. CF
   • Hyperechogenic, fatty replacement
4. Schwachman-Diamond syndrome
   a. Metaphyseal dysplasia in 25%
   b. Cyclic neutropenia
   c. Pancreatic insufficiency, fatty replacement **[Fig. 6-58]**

B. **Inflammation**
   1. Pancreatitis in childhood
      a. Multisystem disease (35%)
         • Viruses
         • Sepsis
      b. Trauma (15%)
      c. Idiopathic (25%)
      d. Metabolic (10%)
         • CF
         • Hyperlipidemia
      e. Anomaly (10%)
      f. Drugs (3%)
         • Steroids
         • Asparaginase
      g. Focal or diffuse enlargement
      h. Pancreatic duct >2 mm
      i. Pseudocyst(s) **[Fig. 6-59]**

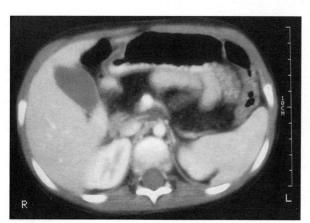

Fig. 6-58 Abdomen CT: Markedly hypodense pancreas anterior to splenic vein; DDx includes CF, Pearson syndrome. Pancreatic lipomatosis (Schwachman syndrome).

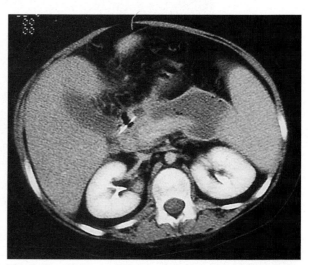

Fig. 6-59 Abdomen CT: Irregularly shaped hypodense lesion with thickened, enhancing rim in tail of pancreas. Pancreatic pseudocyst.

C. **Tumors**
   1. Rare
   2. Clinical indicators of underlying pancreatic neoplasm
      a. Hypoglycemia, profuse diarrhea, abdominal mass, Cushing syndrome, peptic ulceration

VIII. **SPLEEN**
   A. **Congenital**
      1. Situs: asplenia, polysplenia
      2. Accessory spleen
   B. **Splenomegaly in childhood**
      1. Spleen tip palpable in 30% of normal newborns
      2. Spleen tip palpable in 15% of normal infants < 6 months
      3. Spleen edge > 1 cm below left costal margin in those > 6 months old is abnormal
      4. Hemolytic diseases
         a. Spherocytosis
         b. Thalassemia
         c. Sickle cell anemia
            • Splenic sequestration
      5. Toxic causes of splenomegaly
         a. Hemochromatosis
      6. Cardiovascular causes of splenomegaly
         a. Hyperkinetic hypertension
            • Arteriovenous malformation, hemangioendothelioma
         b. Hepatic venous hypertension
         c. Congestive heart failure
         d. Pericardial tamponade
         e. Hepatic vein thrombosis (Budd-Chiari)
         f. Portal vein thrombosis
         g. Portal hypertension
         h. Cirrhosis
            • BA
            • CF
            • α1-Antitrypsin deficiency
      7. Metabolic and syndromic causes of splenomegaly
         a. Storage diseases
            • Gaucher's
            • Niemann-Pick
            • Mucopolysaccharidoses
            • Wilson's disease
            • Tyrosinosis
   C. **Small or absent spleen**
      1. Postsurgical
      2. Sickle cell anemia
         a. Occasionally calcified (Zuckergüss, or "sugar-coated")
      3. Hypovolemic shock
   D. **Inflammation**
      1. Abscess
         a. Similar to hepatic lesions

2. Granulomatous
   a. Histoplasmosis, tuberculosis, cat-scratch, CGD
3. Others
   a. Toxoplasmosis, other infections, rubella, cytomegalovirus infection, and herpes simplex (TORCH) infections, infectious mononucleosis, subacute bacterial endocarditis (SBE), malaria, acquired immunodeficiency syndrome (AIDS), juvenile rheumatoid arthritis (JRA), systemic lupus erythematosus (SLE)

E. **Trauma**
1. Management determined by clinical signs, symptoms; in children, usually conservative
2. Lacerations simple, complex, fractures, maceration **[Figs. 6-60 and 6-61; see also Figs. 1-73 and 1-74]**
3. Associated injuries: left kidney, left lung
4. Sensitivity: CT > US
5. Hypovolemic shock **[Fig. 6-62]**
   a. Small, hyperdense spleen due to splanchnic vasoconstriction
   b. Also marked contrast enhancement of bowel wall, kidneys, pancreas, dilated fluid-filled bowel, small caliber aorta, and inferior vena cava (IVC)
      • If these findings are present, fluid resuscitation is urgent. As soon as possible, return the child to clinical management from the CT scan suite!!

F. **Tumors**
1. Cyst
   a. Posttraumatic > congenital
   b. Hydatid is most common worldwide
   c. Cystic hygroma

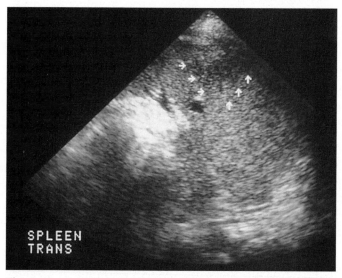

Fig. 6-60 Transverse spleen US: Poorly defined hypoechoic wedge-shaped area (outlined by electronic cursors) in lateral spleen. Spleen laceration.

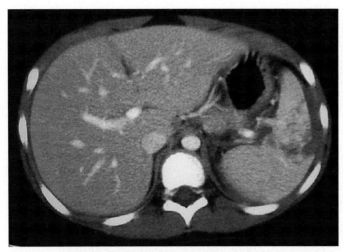

Fig. 6-61   Abdomen CT: Same patient as Figure 6-60. Clearly defined fracture in midportion of spleen, anterior spleen contusion, and subcapsular hematoma. Spleen laceration.

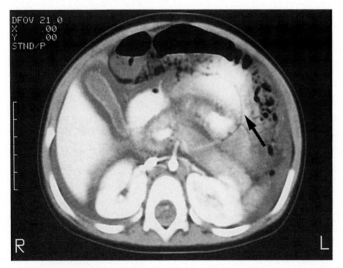

Fig. 6-62   Abdomen CT: Child abuse. Pneumatosis in transverse colon, air in mesenteric vessels (arrow), tiny spleen (splanchnic vasoconstriction), small aorta and inferior vena cava. Bowel hypoperfusion; hypovolemic shock.

   2. Malignant
      a. Lymphoma **[Fig. 8-10]**
IX. **PERITONEUM AND RETROPERITONEUM**
  A. **Peritoneum [Figs. 6-63 and 6-64; see also Figs. 1-26 and 7-4]**
    1. Most dependent portion of peritoneal cavity is the cul de sac
      a. Between bladder and rectum in male, uterus and rectum in female
      b. First place for free fluid, pus, cells in peritoneum to localize
        • Ruptured appendiceal abscess often found in cul de sac
    2. Fluid from cul de sac ascends along right paracolic gutter to Morison's pouch (hepatorenal fossa)

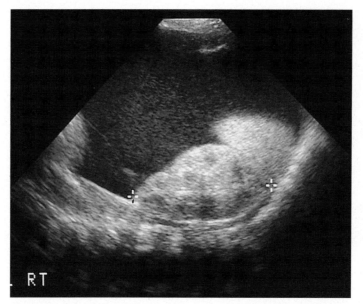

Fig. 6-63 Parasagittal abdomen US: Large amount of ascites anterior to right kidney (outlined by electronic cursors). Note multiple echoes in ascites. Echogenic ascites = hemoperitoneum, malignant ascites, chylous ascites, or peritonitis.

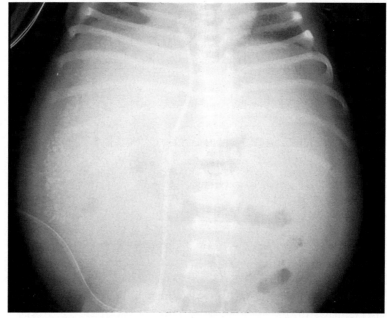

Fig. 6-64 Abdomen radiograph: Marked abdominal protuberance, widely separated bowel loops, stippled calcifications in right flank. Also note falciform ligament, outlined by intraperitoneal air, indicating bowel perforation and postpartum pneumoperitoneum. MP.

3. Ascites on US: anechoic if transudate, intermediate-level echoes if chylous, hemorrhagic, inflammatory, or malignant

4. Normal peritoneum thin, nonenhancing on CT, sharply echogenic on high resolution US
   a. Lumpy, thickened, enhancing peritoneum is abnormal
   b. Consider peritonitis, neoplastic implants
   c. Correlate with clinical findings

5. Peritoneal reflections (omentum, ligaments, mesenteries)
   a. Also called subperitoneal space
      - Includes gastrocolic ligament, hepatoduodenal ligament, transverse mesocolon, SB mesentery
   b. Contain nerves, blood vessels, lymphatics
   c. Connector between peritoneum and retroperitoneum
   d. Provide pathway for spread of disease
      - Pancreatitis
      - Lymphoma
      - Sarcoma, carcinoma

6. Cysts
   a. Lymphangioma (cystic hygroma) **[Figs. 6-65 and 6-66]**
      - Abdominal distention, palpable mass
      - Multiseptated, noncalcified
   b. Enteric duplication cyst
      - Painful, palpable mass
      - Unilocular, noncalcified
        Anechoic, unless infected or hemorrhagic
   c. Meconium pseudocyst
      - Associated with in-utero perforation and/or bowel atresia/volvulus
      - Usually unilocular, contains echoes, debris

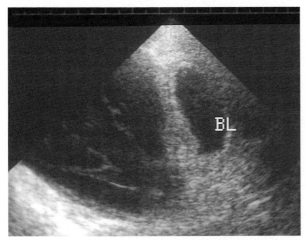

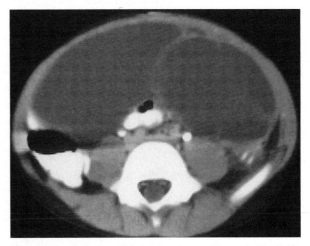

Fig. 6-65 Transverse abdomen US: Multiseptated hypoechoic abdominal mass superior to urinary bladder. Mesenteric cystic hygroma.

Fig. 6-66 Abdomen CT: Same patient as Figure 6-65. Multiseptated cystic abdominal mass. Mesenteric cystic hygroma.

B. **Retroperitoneum**
1. Anterior pararenal space
   a. Between posterior parietal peritoneum and anterior renal fascia
   b. Contains pancreas, retroperitoneal portions of GI tract (part of duodenum, ascending, descending colon)
   c. Fluid in this space is vertically oriented
      - Retroperitoneal bowel displaced anteriorly
2. Perirenal space
   a. Within Gerota's fascia (anterior and posterior renal fascia)
   b. Contains kidney, adrenal, proximal renal collecting system
   c. Fluid in this space is vertically oriented, extends down into pelvis
3. Posterior pararenal space
   a. Between posterior renal fascia and transversalis fascia
   b. Contains no organs
   c. Fluid in this space obliterates properitoneal fat stripe
      - Retroperitoneal bowel displaced antero-medially
4. Multiple space involvement not uncommon in children
   a. Omentum may not extend into right lower quadrant in children <4 years of age
      - Appendicitis and appendiceal rupture poorly localized in young children
         Accounts for nonspecific symptoms, signs, delayed diagnosis, high incidence of perforation, abscess formation
   b. Hemoretroperitoneum and hemoperitoneum in blunt abdominal trauma

FURTHER READING

Bower RJ, Sieber WK, Kiesewetter WB. Alimentary tract duplications in children. Ann Surg 1978;669–674.

Burton EM, Babcock DS, Heubi JE, Gelfand MJ. Neonatal jaundice: clinical and ultrasonographic findings. South Med J 1990;83:294–302.

Houston CS, Wittenborg MH. Roentgen evaluation of anomalies of rotation and fixation of the bowel in children. Radiology 1965;84:1–17.

Kirks DR, Coleman RE, Filston HC, et al. An imaging approach to persistent neonatal jaundice. AJR 1984;142:461–465.

Meyers MA. Dynamic Radiology of the Abdomen. Normal and Pathologic Anatomy, 2nd ed. New York: Springer-Verlag 1982.

Meyers MA, Oliphant M, Berne AS, Feldberg MAM. The peritoneal ligaments and mesenteries: pathways of intraabdominal spread of disease. Radiology 1987; 163:593–604.

Oliphant M, Berne AS. Computed tomography of the subperitoneal space: demonstration of direct spread of intraabdominal disease. J Comput Assist Tomogr 1982;6:1127–1137.

Powers C, Ros PR, Stoupis C, et al. Primary liver neoplasms: MR imaging with pathologic correlation. RadioGraphics 1994;14:459–482.

Puylaert JBCM. Acute appendicitis: US evaluation using graded compression. Radiology 1986;158:355–360.

Rappaport WD, Peterson M, Stanton C. Factors responsible for the high peforation rate seen in early childhood appendicitis. The Amer Surgeon 1989;55:602–605.

Ros PR, Olmsted WW, Moser, Jr. RP, Dachman AH, Hjermstad BH, Sobin LH. Mesenteric and omental cysts: histologic classification with imaging correlation. Radiology 1987; 164:327–332.

Siegel MJ. Acute appendicitis in childhood: the role of US. Radiology 1992; 185:341–342.

Sivit CJ, Newman KD, Boenning DA, et al. Appendicitis: usefulness of US in diagnosis in a pediatric population. Radiology 1992;185:549–552.

Snyder WH, Chaffin L. Embryology and pathology of the intestinal tract: presentation of 40 cases of malrotation. Ann Surg 1954;140:368–379.

Stringer DA. Pediatric Gastrointestinal Imaging. Toronto: B. C. Decker, Inc.; 1989.

Taylor GA, Fallat ME, Eichelberger MR. Hypovolemic shock in children. Radiology 1987;164:479–481

I. **KIDNEY**
  A. **Congenital**
    1. Horseshoe kidney **[Fig. 7-1]**
       a. Kidneys fuse in midline prior to embryologic ascent from pelvis; ascent limited by position of inferior mesenteric artery
       b. Association: Turner's syndrome (45,XO)
       c. Increased incidence of Wilms' tumor and primary renal carcinoid tumor
       d. Intravenous urography (IVU)
          • Medial position of calyces, ureters arise more anterior than normal, visible isthmus
       e. Sonography
          • Abnormal axis of kidneys with medial position of lower poles; soft tissue isthmus crosses midline
          • May be difficult to identify kidney crossing in front of spine
              Angle probe inferiorly, push gently to displace air-filled gut, or image from posterior
    2. Crossed ectopy
       a. Ureter crosses from ectopic kidney to enter bladder on contralateral side

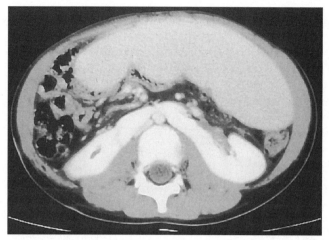

Fig. 7-1 Abdomen CT: Renal tissue crosses midline anterior to aorta. Note anterior location of left renal pelvis. Incidentally noted splenomegaly and portal collateral blood vessels in patient with portal vein thrombosis. Horseshoe kidney.

  b. Ectopic kidney is caudal; fused in 85 to 90% of cases
  c. Fusion of metanephric blastema occurs after metanephric ducts join renal tissue
  d. Ureters arise from mesonephric ducts, which then form metanephric ducts
  e. IVU
  - Fused renal mass and proximal collecting systems on same side
  - Ureter of ectopic kidney crosses midline to enter bladder from contralateral side of kidney
3. Pelvic kidney
  a. Failure of embryologic ascent of unfused kidney
  b. Increased incidence of vesicoureteral reflux
4. Single kidney
  a. First, exclude pelvic kidney or fused kidney
  b. Unilateral renal agenesis, 1:500 births
  c. Occasionally, multicystic dysplastic kidney may regress completely, simulating congenital solitary kidney
  d. Solitary kidney and Müllerian anomalies related
5. Duplication **[Figs. 7-2 and 7-3]**
  a. Embryology
  - Ureteral bud arises from dorsal surface of lower end of Wolffian duct by 30th–35th day of gestation
  - If two ureteral buds arise from one Wolffian duct, ureteral duplication occurs
  - Lower ureteral bud progresses upward and outward and becomes absorbed into vesicourethral canal
  - Upper ureteral bud migrates medially and downward
  - In 85% of cases of ureteral duplication, the ureter draining the upper pole opens below and medial to that draining the lower pole (Weigert-Meyer rule).

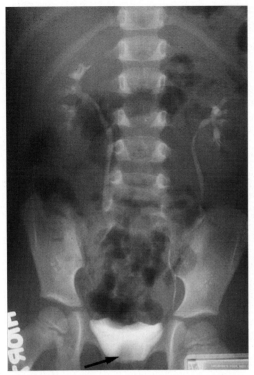

Fig. 7-2 Intravenous pyelogram (IVP): Lateral position of ureter draining left lower pole. Downward displacement of lower pole moiety of left kidney ("drooping lily"). Filling defect in base of urinary bladder (arrow). Renal duplication with ectopic ureterocele

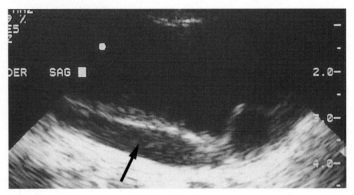

Fig. 7-3 Left parasagittal US: Dilated ureter (arrow). Rounded structure within bladder is ectopic ureterocele

- Upper pole ureteral orifice can open in urinary bladder base, posterior urethra in males, or distal to the external sphincter in females.
- Obstruction of the ectopic ureter results from persistence of an embryonic membrane or failure of expansion of the ectopic ureteral orifice.
- Occasionally, the ectopic ureteral orifice is widely patent and incompetent.
- Ectopic ureterocele 6.5 times more common in girls than in boys
- When present in boys, the anomaly is often complex:
  Bilateral ureteroceles, eversion of ureterocele, or elongation of posterior urethra that resembles posterior urethral valves

b. IVU
- "Drooping lily sign" due to inferior displacement of lower moiety by upper moiety, which often does not opacify due to poor excretory function
- Lateral displacement of renal pelvis by interposed dilated upper moiety ureter

c. Sonography
- Renal sinus echoes separated by renal parenchyma in mid-portion of kidney; kidney usually elongated

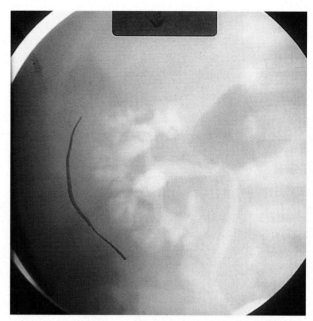

Fig. 7-4 Coned-down view from VCUG: Normal right renal pelvis with excessive number of calyces of geometric appearance. Normal infundibula and renal contour. Congenital megacalyces

- "Pseudocyst" produced by calyceal dilatation of obstructed upper moiety
- Ectopic ureterocele seen as "cystic" structure protruding into bladder at ureteral orifice

6. Congenital megacalyces **[Fig. 7-4]**
   a. Polygonal enlargement of calyces, hypoplasia or flattening of medullary pyramids, renal pelvis normal
   b. Unilateral or bilateral
   c. Short, broad infundibula
   d. Kidneys may be large; fetal lobulation present
   e. No obstruction or reflux

B. **Inflammation**

1. Urinary tract infection (UTI)
2. Vesicoureteral reflux (VUR)
3. UTI and VUR: Current concepts **[Figs. 7-5 through 7-12]**
4. VUR
   a. Grade I: Ureter only
   b. Grade II: Ureter, pelvis, calyces without dilatation
   c. Grade III: II + dilatation and slight blunting
   d. Grade IV: More pronounced pyelocalyceal dilatation, ureteral tortuosity, marked calyceal fornix blunting
   e. Grade V: Marked dilatation and ureteral tortuosity
   f. VUR is due to immaturity or maldevelopment at the ureterovesical junction (UVJ)

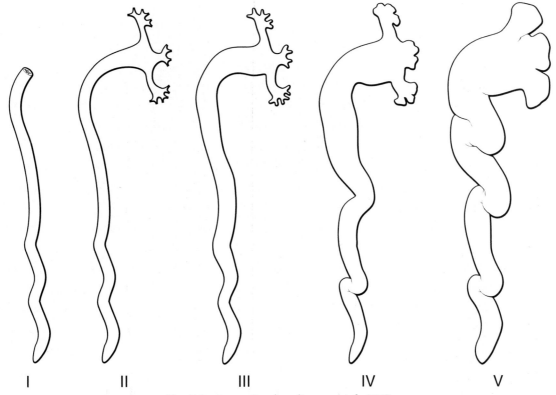

| I | II | III | IV | V |

Fig. 7-5 International grading system for VUR.

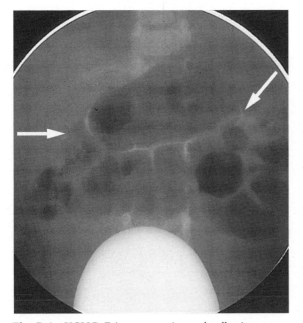

Fig. 7-6 VCUG: Faint contrast in renal collecting system bilaterally (arrows). No dilatation of collecting structures. Bilateral grade II VUR.

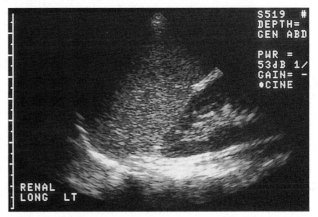

Fig. 7-7 Longitudinal US left kidney: Normal hypoechoic parenchyma, echogenic renal sinus. Normal renal US in patient with grade III VUR.

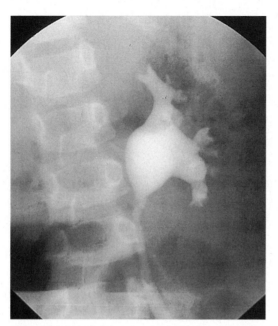

Fig. 7-8 VCUG 10 minutes after Figure 7-7: Contrast in dilated renal collecting system with slight blunting of calyces. Grade III VUR.

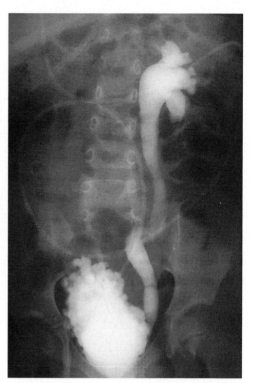

Fig. 7-9 VCUG: Patient with neurogenic bladder. Markedly trabeculated bladder. Dilatation and tortuosity of ureter, dilatation and blunting of calyces. Grade IV VUR.

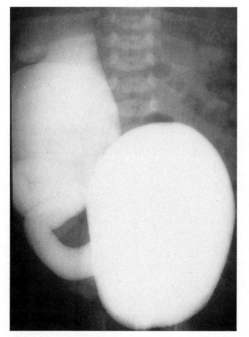

Fig. 7-10 VCUG: Markedly dilated, tortuous right ureter and dilated renal pelvis, ballooned calyces. Grade V VUR.

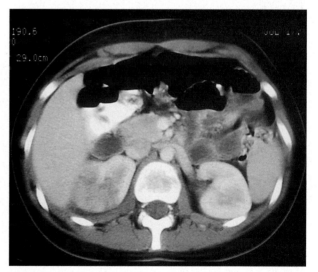

Fig. 7-11 Abdomen CT: Wedge-shaped hypodense lesion in right kidney. Note fine vascular striations within lesion. Acute pyelonephritis.

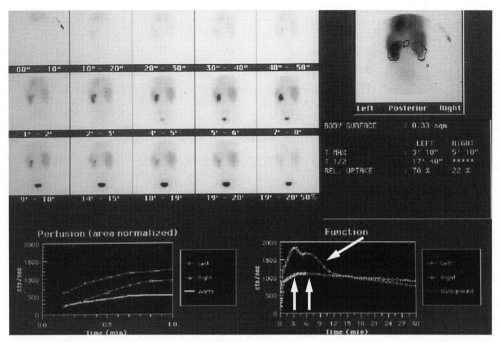

Fig. 7-12 Nuclear renal scan: Grade IV VUR on right. Normal uptake and excretion on left (arrow). Nearly flat time-activity curve on right indicating poor uptake and excretion on right (double arrow). Reflux nephropathy.

- Lower grades of reflux tend to subside by 2 years of age
- VUR can occur in children of all ages, including teenagers

g. Reflux nephropathy is a significant cause of chronic renal disease, hypertension

h. Reflux + UTI = scarring; pyelonephritis without VUR may = scarring

i. Not all pyelonephritis is due to reflux; reflux found in 30 to 35% of patients with pyelonephritis

j. Acute pyelonephritis in absence of demonstrable VUR is common

k. Infection does not cause reflux; voiding cystourethrogram (VCUG) can be performed when child is asymptomatic and urine is sterile

l. Study the first documented UTI in children

m. Highest intravesical pressure during voiding; static or non-voiding cystography limited in evaluating VUR.

n. US is very insensitive to identify VUR in children of all ages
   - VCUG is the gold standard [**Figs. 7-7 and 7-8**]

o. Renal parenchymal scarring can occur independent of presence or degree of reflux at time of presentation of first documented episode of pyelonephritis
   - Acute pyelonephritis and scarring are best identified by renal cortical scintigraphy with ^{99m}Tc-DMSA or glucoheptonate [**Figs. 1-81 and 1-82**]
   - Scarring is poorly evaluated by US

5. UTI in febrile infants
   a. Overall prevalence = 5.3%

   b. <2 months of age with presumed sepsis = 4.6%
   c. >2 months of age; no source of fever; UTI suspected = 5.9%
   d. >2 months of age; no source of fever; UTI not suspected = 5.1%
   e. Incidence of UTI
      • White female infants with temp >39 ≫ males and black infants
6. Antenatal hydronephrosis
   a. Prenatal grading of fetal pyelocaliectasis:
      • Grade I: Renal pelvis ≤1 cm, normal calyces
      • Grade II: Renal pelvis 1–1.5 cm, normal calyces
      • Grade III: Renal pelvis >1.5 cm, calyces slightly dilated
      • Grade IV: Renal pelvis >1.5 cm, calyces moderately dilated
      • Grade V: Renal pelvis >1.5 cm, calyces severely dilated + atrophic cortex
   b. Vesicoureteral reflux is a common cause of fetal renal pyelectasis
      • Prenatal hydronephrosis + normal postnatal kidney = VUR in 25%
   c. Neonates with antenatally detected hydronephrosis should be routinely screened for reflux with VCUG
      • Postnatal ultrasound is no substitute for properly performed VCUG; sonography does not correlate with reflux
      • VCUG should be performed several days after delivery
         If reflux is found postnatally, prophylaxis should be started and continued until reflux subsides
      • US should be obtained at 1 to 2 weeks of age if prenatal sonogram shows hydronephrosis
         US on day 1 to 2 of life may underestimate degree of hydronephrosis
         – Newborn infants are relatively dehydrated and glomerular filtration rate is low. Hydronephrosis, especially UPJ obstruction, may be masked by low urine output.

C. **Renal Trauma [Figs. 7–13 through 7–16]**
1. Indications for abdominal/renal computed tomography (CT) evaluation
   a. Hemodynamically stable with suspected significant abdominal injury
   b. Multisystem trauma (especially head trauma) with difficult or impossible abdominal physical examination
   c. Hypotension responsive to fluids without obvious blood loss
   d. Symptomatic hematuria
2. Grading scheme for renal trauma
   a. Grade I: Small parenchymal injury; no subcapsular or perirenal fluid
   b. Grade II: Incomplete renal laceration; subcapsular or small amount of perirenal fluid
   c. Grade III: Extensive laceration or fracture; large perirenal collection
   d. Grade IV: Multiple renal fragments (shattered)
   e. Grade V: Vascular injury

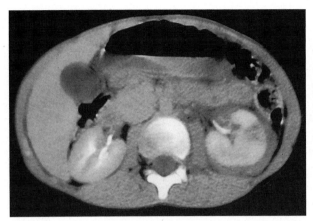

Fig. 7-13 Abdomen CT: Abdominal trauma. Wedge-shaped hypodense lesion in left kidney. Left perirenal fluid collection. Renal contusion.

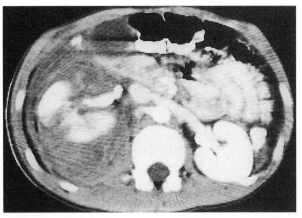

Fig. 7-14 Abdomen CT: Trauma. Right renal fracture, perirenal fluid collection. Renal fracture-early CT.

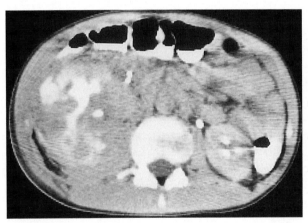

Fig. 7-15 Abdomen CT: Same patient as Figure 7-14, 10 minutes later. Note extravasation of contrast into perirenal space. In setting of renal trauma and perirenal fluid, delayed imaging 5 to 10 minutes after contrast administration necessary to identify extravasation. Renal fracture-delayed CT.

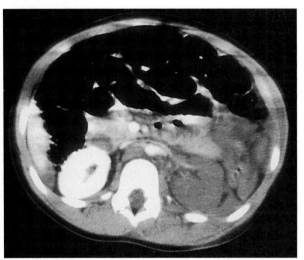

Fig. 7-16 Abdomen CT: Abrupt termination of left renal artery, diffuse hypodensity of left kidney. Vascular striations within left kidney and left renal vein from flow in capsular vessels. Renal pedicle injury.

    3. Renal pedicle injury
        a. In patients with renal injury, 3.6% have renal pedicle injury
        b. Gross hematuria in 40%
        c. Microscopic hematuria in 20%
        d. Hematuria absent in 40%
        e. Restoration of normal or near normal renal function in pedicle injury unusual
        f. Hypertension in 50% of survivors of pedicle injury
  D. **Renal vascular abnormalities**
    1. Renal artery stenosis (RAS)
        a. Fibromuscular hyperplasia = most common cause

    b. Neurofibromatosis

    c. Williams' syndrome (idiopathic hypercalcemia of infancy)

    d. Middle aortic syndrome

    e. Takayasu's arteritis

    f. Posttransplant

    g. Clinical
- Listen for abdominal bruit with stethoscope

    h. US
- Difficult and time-consuming study
- Increase volume of Doppler US to localize abdominal bruit, if present
- Dampening of peak systolic velocity seen with Doppler US ("pulsus tardus")
  - Provoked by captopril administration
  - Curving inflection and delay in upstroke before peak systole

    i. Nuclear imaging
- Delay in tracer uptake on involved side
- Worsening of renal function following captopril administration

        In RAS, renal perfusion and function maintained by renin-angiotensin autoregulation

        Captopril (angiotensin-converting enzyme inhibitor) prevents formation of angiotensin II

        Lack of angiotensin II decreases transcapillary pressure gradient, reduces renal function in RAS

- DTPA + captopril imaging in RAS

        Captopril given 1 hour prior to study

        Decreased extraction and delayed appearance of isotope in collecting system

- MAG_3 + captopril imaging in RAS

        Captopril given 1 hour prior to study

        Prolonged retention of isotope in renal parenchyma

2. Renal artery thrombosis

    a. Secondary to blunt trauma to renal pedicle

    b. Secondary to left-sided cardiac thromboemboli

    c. Secondary to right-sided cardiac thromboemboli + patent ductus arteriosus and/or intracardiac right-to-left shunt

    d. Secondary to umbilical artery catheterization

3. Renal vein thrombosis

    a. Usually begins in arcuate and interlobular veins and extends to renal vein, inferior vena cava (IVC)

    b. Nephrotic syndrome

    c. Protein C or S, or antithrombin III deficiency

    d. Dehydration, especially hypernatremic

    e. Polycythemia

    f. Burns

    g. Left adrenal hemorrhage
- Left adrenal vein is branch of left renal vein
- Thrombosis of left renal vein due to left adrenal vein thrombosis

- IVC thrombosis due to extension of adrenal vein thrombus
h. Posttransplant
i. US
    - Kidney enlarged acutely, hyperechogenic; loss of corticomedullary differentiation, echogenic interlobular streaking
    - Depending on severity, some kidneys may recover; others become atrophic and echogenic, or involute

E. **Medical Renal Disease**
1. Normal renal sonographic appearance unique to pediatrics: **[Figs. 1-63 through 1-65]**
2. Premature newborns: cortex hyperechogenic, prominent renal pyramids, no sinus fat
3. Term newborns: cortex slightly hyperechogenic or isoechoic relative to liver or spleen, prominent renal pyramids, no sinus fat
4. Between 1 and 6 months of age: cortex isoechoic, prominent renal pyramids, no sinus fat
5. Between 6 and 12 months of age: cortex becomes hypoechoic, prominent renal pyramids, no sinus fat
6. 2 to 5 years of age: cortex hypoechoic, prominent renal pyramids, little sinus fat
7. More than 10 years of age: Pyramids become less prominent, sinus fat increases
8. Medical renal disease defined by generally hyperechogenic renal cortex relative to liver or spleen **[Figs. 7-17 and 7-18]**
    a. Acute tubular necrosis (ATN)
    b. Nephrosis
    c. Renal vascular disease

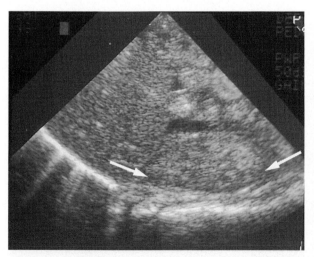

Fig. 7-17 Longitudinal US of right kidney: Echogenic kidney (between arrows) without cortico-medullary differentiation. Medical renal disease-chronic renal disease.

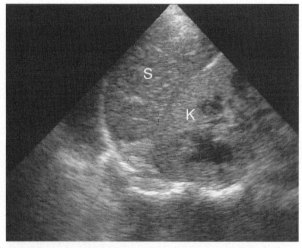

Fig. 7-18 Longitudinal US of left kidney: Echogenic kidney compared to spleen. Cortico-medullary differentiation preserved. DDx includes glomerulonephritis, pyelonephritis, renal infiltration, or storage disease. Medical renal disease-acute tubular necrosis.

d. Renal vein thrombosis

e. Transplant rejection/chemotherapy

f. Sickle cell disease

g. Storage diseases
   - Glycogen storage disease
   - Mucopolysaccharide disease
   - Diabetes mellitus

h. Inflammatory disease
   - Pyelonephritis
   - Glomerulonephritis
   - Henoch-Schonlein purpura
   - Hemolytic uremic syndrome
   - Human immunodeficiency virus (HIV)-associated nephropathy
   - Kawasaki's disease

i. End stage renal disease

j. Reflux nephropathy

F. **Nephrocalcinosis, nephrolithiasis [Figs. 7-19 and 7-20]**

1. Diuretic therapy

   a. Especially in former prematures with bronchopulmonary dysplasia

2. Renal tubular acidosis

3. Idiopathic hypercalciuria

4. Oxalosis

5. Bartter's syndrome

6. Hypophosphatasia

7. Glycogenosis type I

8. Hypervitaminosis D

9. Hyperparathyroidism

10. Medullary sponge kidney

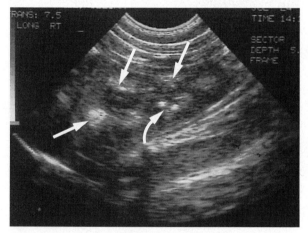

Fig. 7-19 Longitudinal US of right kidney: Echogenic medullary pyramids (arrows) as well as parenchymal calculi (curved arrow). Nephrocalcinosis.

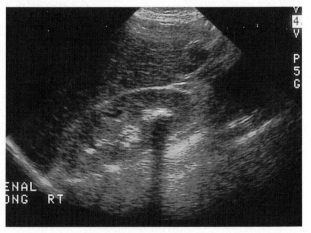

Fig. 7-20 Longitudinal US of right kidney: Echogenic foci with posterior acoustic shadowing within lower pole collecting system. Renal calculi.

11. US
    a. Normal medullary pyramids hypoechoic
    b. In nephrocalcinosis, pyramids hyperechoic
        • Calcification conforms to distribution of medullary pyramids

G. **Renal cystic disease [Table 7–1, p. 397]**
    • Potter Type I: Infantile; autosomal recessive polycystic kidney disease (ARPKD)
    • Potter Type II: Multicystic dysplastic kidney (MDK)
    • Potter Type III: Adult; autosomal dominant polycystic kidney disease (ADPKD)
    • Potter Type IV: Cystic renal dysplasia (associated with distal obstruction, such as posterior urethral valves (PUV)

    1. Autosomal recessive polycystic kidney disease (ARPKD) **[Fig. 7-21]**
        a. In utero onset of renal dysfunction due to ARPKD
        b. Oligohydramnios, pulmonary hypoplasia, and clubfeet (Potter's syndrome)
            • Death from respiratory insufficiency is the usual outcome of Potter's syndrome
        c. Newborn period
            • Usual presentation is bilateral nephromegaly
            • Less severely affected neonates with pulmonary hypoplasia and ARPKD may survive for variable periods
                Incidence of spontaneous pneumothorax is high in these patients
        d. ARPKD diagnosed later in the first year of life
            • These children have less renal enlargement and more hepatic fibrosis than those diagnosed as newborns
        e. ARPKD diagnosed after the first year of life
            • Milder renal involvement

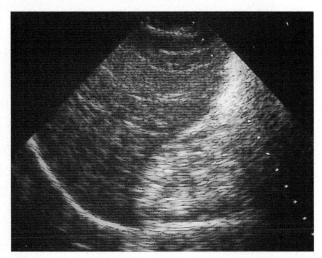

Fig. 7-21 Longitudinal US of right kidney: Markedly echogenic kidney compared to liver, without cortico-medullary differentiation. ARPKD.

- Hepatomegaly with or without portal hypertension
- This group formerly was classified as congenital hepatic fibrosis
- Cysts enlarge with age, becoming identifiable by US
 f. Liver involvement is present in all patients with ARPKD
- Manifested microscopically by bile duct hyperplasia and portal fibrosis
- Inversely related to severity of renal disease
- Cystic dilatation of intrahepatic bile ducts (Caroli's disease) has also been described with ARPKD
 g. IVU
- Streaky appearance due to stasis of contrast media in dilated collecting tubules
 h. CT following intravenous contrast
- Similar appearance of radial streaking
 i. US
- Bilaterally enlarged hyperechogenic kidneys
    Due to innumerable interfaces in parenchyma from microcysts in collecting tubules
- Occasionally macrocysts can be identified by US
    In older infant or child
2. Autosomal dominant polycystic kidney disease (ADPKD) **[Fig. 7-22]**
 a. Most common genetic renal disease
- Affects 300,000 to 400,000 Americans
- Responsible for 10% of end stage renal disease in adults
 b. Most patients first develop symptoms during 3rd–4th decades
- Can be symptomatic in the neonatal period
- Peak age of clinical detection of ADPKD in childhood is the neonatal period

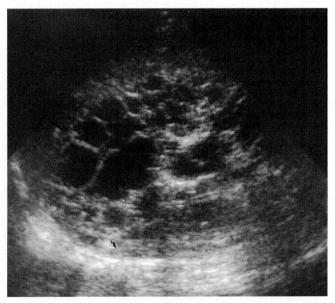

Fig. 7-22 Longitudinal US of kidney: Numerous cysts of various size scattered throughout kidney. ADPKD.

c. Gene responsible for ADPKD on short arm of chromosome 16
d. Kidneys markedly enlarged, normal renal contour distorted by large fluid filled cysts of varying size
e. Renal cysts develop in all nephron segments and enlarge in asymmetric fashion
   - Most commonly, cysts arise from Bowman's capsule, the angle of the loop of Henle, or from the proximal convoluted tubule
f. Hepatic cysts in up to 30%
g. Extra-renal cysts are also found in other organs (ovaries, pancreas, thyroid) in 3% of affected patients
h. Berry aneurysms in circle of Willis in 10%
   - Family history of deaths from cerebrovascular accident not uncommon
i. Most children present with abdominal or flank masses
j. IVU
   - Calyceal distortion
   - Collecting system appears stretched or displaced by multiple cysts, which impart a "Swiss cheese" appearance to nephrogram
k. US
   - Enlarged renal size, normal echogenicity, and cysts of varying size
   - Calcification in wall of cysts occasionally seen
l. ADPKD has been reported in the infant and fetus as early as 24 weeks gestation
   - In some instances, normal sonograms in second trimester, ADPKD in third trimester
   - Fetal US has demonstrated nephromegaly and diffuse hyperechogenicity, indistinguishable from ARPKD
   - Cortical cysts may not be visible
     As infant ages, number and size of parenchymal cysts increase
m. Note: Distinction between ARPKD and ADPKD may be difficult
   - In fetus or newborn, both may present as large, echogenic kidneys
   - In older infant or child, both may manifest numerous cysts resolvable by US
   - Diagnose by US of biological parents' kidneys and family history
     Parent may already know his/her diagnosis of ADPKD, or diagnosis of ADPKD in parent may ensue from diagnosis of ADPKD in child

3. Multicystic dysplastic kidney (MDK) [Fig. 7-23]
   a. Most common unilateral abdominal mass in neonatal period
   b. Due to failure of normal induction of the metanephric blastema by the ureteric bud
   c. Microscopically, renal parenchyma replaced by disorganized epithelial structures (primitive ducts) and cartilage
      - Primitive glomeruli, tubules, and ducts may be present and may have minimal function
      - There may be a few mature nephrons, accounting for faint uptake on renal scan

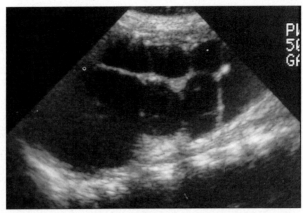

Fig. 7-23 Longitudinal US of kidney: Numerous cysts of various size without definable renal pelvis. No communication between cysts. Multicystic dysplastic kidney (MDK).

    d. Usually the ureter and renal pelvis are atretic, but occasionally the "hydronephrotic" type of multicystic dysplastic kidney is seen
- In this form, the ureter is atretic but renal pelvis and infundibula are present

    e. Up to one-third of patients with MDK have contralateral renal abnormalities, such as ureteropelvic junction (UPJ) stenosis, MDK, or renal ectopy

    f. MDK may involve entire kidney or portion of kidney in cases of segmental duplication

    g. US of the pelvoinfundibular type of MDK:
- Malformed kidney with multiple noncommunicating cysts
- Largest cysts are peripheral in location
- Noncystic portions of kidney hyperechogenic, due to renal parenchymal dysplasia

    h. In hydronephrotic type of MDK:
- Largest cyst is central in location and resembles dilated renal pelvis

    i. Nuclear renal scintigraphy with ^{99m}Tc-DTPA
- Absence of renal perfusion on early dynamic images
- Usually lack of renal function on later static images
- Rarely, faint renal parenchymal function is seen

II. **Genitourinary (GU) tumors**

  A. **Wilms' tumor [Figs. 7-24 through 7-26]**

    1. Most common primary renal tumor in childhood; peak age 2 to 3 years; 75% before age 5

    2. Arises in nephrogenic blastema

    3. Epithelial, stromal, blastemal (undifferentiated) components

    4. May contain primitive cartilage, osteoid, fat

    5. Histology

      a. Favorable: 88%
- Cure rate 90%

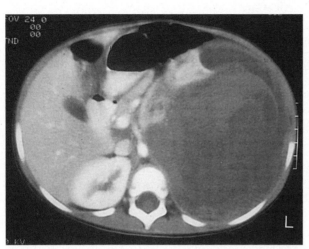

Fig. 7-24 Abdomen CT: Fairly homogeneous mass within left kidney. Enhancing normal renal parenchyma medial to lesion. Note displacement of aorta and superior mesenteric artery. Wilms' tumor.

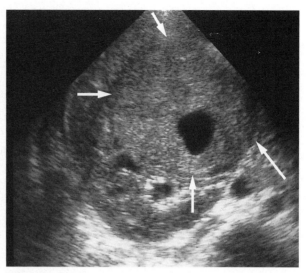

Fig. 7-25 Transverse US: Homogeneous renal mass with central necrosis or cyst formation. Note normal right kidney partially surrounding lesion ("claw" sign). Arrows around mass. Wilms' tumor.

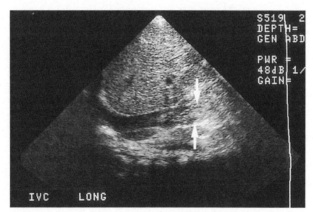

Fig. 7-26 Parasaggital US through IVC: Echogenic thrombus (arrows) within IVC in patient with Wilms' tumor.

b. Unfavorable:
- Anaplastic, 4%
  Cellular atypia
  More common in older children and African-Americans
- Clear cell sarcoma, 6%
  "Bone metastasizing renal tumor of childhood"
  Mortality, 50%
  Bone mets, 40%
  May be cystic
- Rhabdoid tumor, 2%
  Median age 13 months
  Mortality, 90%

Hypercalcemia

Early dissemination

6. Clinical

   a. Abdominal mass, fever, microscopic hematuria, hypertension (due to renal compression, vascular involvement or renin)

7. Associations

   a. Hemihypertrophy of any cause; Beckwith-Wiedemann syndrome

   b. Spontaneous aniridia: 33% incidence of Wilms' tumor

   c. Increased incidence in crossed renal ectopy and horseshoe kidney

8. Imaging

   a. Usually homogeneous tumor with areas of necrosis

   b. Calcification uncommon (5 to 10%)

   c. May be cystic

10. Staging

   a. I: Tumor limited to kidney, capsule intact

   b. II: Beyond kidney or into blood vessels; no adjacent organs or adenopathy; resectable

   c. III: Confined to abdomen, does not involve liver

   d. IV: Hematogenous mets: liver, lung, bone, brain; bone involvement a late phenomenon

   e. V: Bilateral renal involvement: 5 to 10%

B. **Nephroblastomatosis [Fig. 7-27]**

1. Persistent nodular blastema, or nephrogenic rests

2. Perilobar (subcapsular) or intralobar (virtually anywhere in kidney) nephrogenic rests

   a. Intralobar has higher incidence of multifocal or bilateral Wilms'

3. Nephrogenic rests present in 40% of unilateral Wilms', 100% of bilateral Wilms'

4. Premalignant

C. **Multilocular cystic nephroma**

1. Probably from undifferentiated blastema (similar to Wilms')

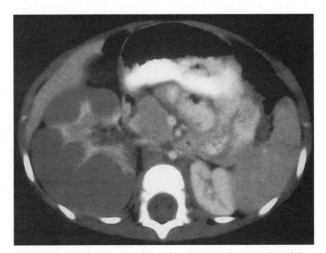

Fig. 7-27 Abdomen CT: Multiple right renal cortical nodules. Nephroblastomatosis.

2. Locules do not communicate
3. No calcification, hemorrhage, or necrosis
4. 98% benign
5. In children M > F; in adults, F > M
6. May herniate into pelvis (sausage configuration)

D. **Mesoblastic nephroma [Fig. 7-28]**
1. Most common solid renal mass in first 6 months of life
2. Interdigitates with nephrons, like scaffolding
3. Rarely calcifies
4. In first 3 months, usually does not recur unless incompletely resected
   a. Recent reports of distant metastases
   b. Current recommendation
      • Postoperative abdominal US monthly for first year

E. **Renal cell carcinoma [Fig. 7-29]**
1. Tumor of proximal convoluted tubules
2. In second decade, more common than Wilms'
3. Renal vein invasion; calcification in 25%
4. Associated with von Hippel–Lindau

F. **Neuroblastoma (NBL) [Figs. 7-30 through 7-34]**
1. Most common extracranial solid malignancy in children
2. Third most common malignancy after leukemia and brain tumor
3. Second most common abdominal malignancy, after Wilms'
4. Elevated catecholamines: vanillylmandelic acid (VMA), homovanillic acid (HVA)
5. Two-thirds arise in abdomen
6. Clinical
   a. Abdominal mass
   b. Unusual presentations
      • Myoclonus-ataxia-opsoclonus: "dancing eyes"
      • Intractable diarrhea due to vasoactive intestinal peptides (VIP)

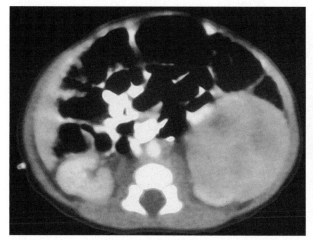

Fig. 7-28 Abdomen CT: Large homogeneous left renal mass in newborn. Note fine rim of enhancement around mass. Mesoblastic nephroma.

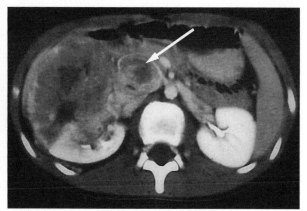

Fig. 7-29 Abdomen CT: Large, heterogeneous right renal mass. Tumor extends into and expands IVC (arrow). Renal cell carcinoma.

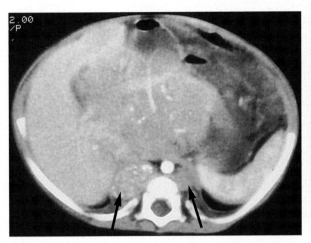

Fig. 7-30 Abdomen CT: Large mid-abdominal mass with stippled calcifications. Note encasement of celiac axis, calcified and non-calcified retrocrural adenopathy (arrows). Neuroblastoma.

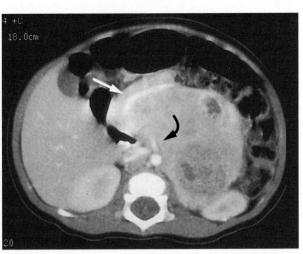

Fig. 7-31 Abdomen CT: Heterogeneous mass in mid and left abdomen with displacement of pancreas (arrow) and encasement of superior mesenteric artery (curved arrow). Left kidney is displaced. Neuroblastoma.

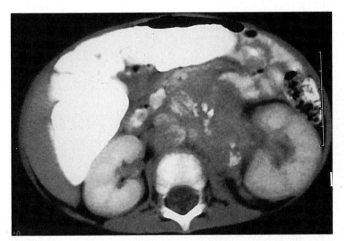

Fig. 7-32 Abdomen CT: Lobulated retroperitoneal mass. Lateral displacement of left kidney, chunky calcification, and anterior displacement of aorta and IVC. Neuroblastoma.

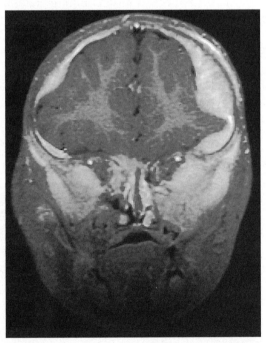

Fig. 7-33 Coronal gadolinium-enhanced T1-weighted MRI with fat saturation: Enhancing epidural lesions bilaterally, nearly completely surrounding the frontal lobes. Metastatic neuroblastoma.

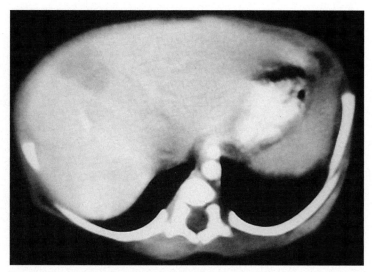

Fig. 7-34 Abdomen CT: Well-defined hypodense mass in right lobe of liver in newborn with abdominal NBL. Stage IV-S neuroblastoma.

7. Associated with fetal hydantoin and fetal alcohol syndromes
8. Better prognosis in thoracic NBL than in abdominal NBL
9. Imaging
   a. US: Echogenic with areas of calcification
   b. CT: Heterogeneous, calcification in 80%
   c. Magnetic resonance imaging (MRI): Best for intraspinal extension
10. Staging
    a. Stage I: Confined to organ or structure of origin
    b. Stage II: Does not cross midline; homolateral lymph nodes (LN) may be involved
    c. Stage III: Crosses midline
    d. Stage IV: Remote disease involving skeleton, organs, soft tissue, distant nodes
    e. Stage IVS: Less than 1 year of age, otherwise Stage I or II + liver, skin, bone marrow involvement (but not bone)
11. NBL vs. Wilms' tumor
    a. Relationship to vessels
       • NBL *ENCASES VESSELS*
       • WILMS' *DISPLACES VESSELS*
            Except when Wilms' nodes surround vessels
       • Wilms' also invades vessels, such as renal vein and IVC
    b. Metastatic patterns
       • NBL ⇒⇒ Bone, liver, LN, orbit, cranial sutures, skin **[Fig. 2-85]**
       • Wilms' ⇒⇒ Lung, liver, LN, vascular invasion, heart
       • But: NBL can go to lung late and Wilms' can go to bone late!
    c. "Claw" sign: Identifies organ as site of tumor origin
       • Note renal enhancement or calyces around intrarenal tumor

- But: NBL can invade kidney, usually on left side through renal hilum
    d. Calcification
        - Common in NBL, unusual in Wilms'
    e. Extrarenal Wilms'
        - Get serious, you won't make a correct preoperative specific diagnosis!
        - You will probably make radiologic diagnosis of (rhabdomyo)-sarcoma

G. **Pheochromocytoma**
    1. 5% bilateral, 10% familial
    2. Associated with neurofibromatosis, von Hippel-Lindau, multiple endocrine neoplasms (MEN II, or Sipple's; MEN III, mucosal neuromas)
        a. MEN II = Hyperparathyroidism, medullary carcinoma of thyroid, pheochromocytoma
    3. Hypoechoic on US
    4. Homogeneous on US, CT
    5. Calcification uncommon
    6. Uptake with ^{131}I-MIBG (metaiodobenzyl-guanidine)

H. **Adrenal hemorrhage [Figs. 7-35 through 7-37]**
    1. Associated with neonatal stress
    2. Initially complex mass that becomes "cystic" within 1 to 3 weeks
    3. Resolves in weeks-months; may become calcified
        a. Differential diagnosis (DDx) of adrenal calcification
            - Resolved adrenal hemorrhage
            - Wolman's syndrome
    4. Left-sided hemorrhage associated with adrenal vein, left renal vein, and IVC thrombosis
    5. Distinguish from congenital NBL by following evolution and resolution

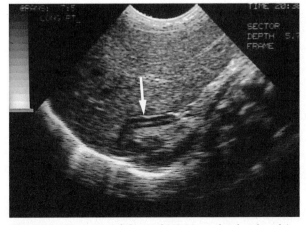

Fig. 7-35 Transverse abdominal US: Normal right adrenal (arrow). Note hypoechoic peripheral cortex, echogenic central medulla.

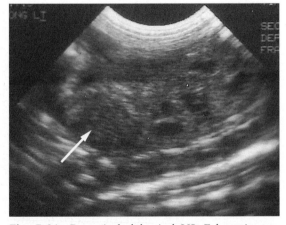

Fig. 7-36 Parasagittal abdominal US: Echogenic mass (arrow) in left suprarenal fossa in newborn. DDx includes congenital NBL. Adrenal hemorrhage-early.

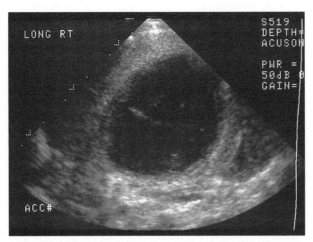

Fig. 7-37 Parasagittal abdominal US: 3-week-old infant. Hypoechoic mass in adrenal fossa. Previously, mass was echogenic. Adrenal hemorrhage-late.

   6. US
      a. Initially solid or complex mass, resembling NBL
      b. Repeat US in 10 to 14 days
      c. If NBL, no change
      d. If hemorrhage, mass will liquefy or become "cystic"
      e. May take months for adrenal hemorrhage to resolve
I. **Adrenal carcinoma**
   1. Virilization, Cushing's syndrome
   2. Associated with hemihypertrophy
   3. Venous invasion
   4. Calcification in 25%
   5. Lobulated
J. **Renal lymphoma [Fig. 7-38]**
   1. Generally portion of more extensive process

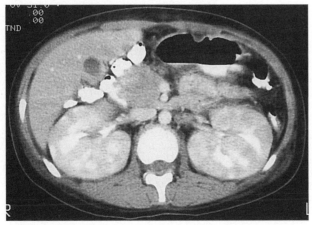

Fig. 7-38 Abdomen CT: Multiple hypodense lesions in parenchyma of both kidneys, which are enlarged. Note peripancreatic adenopathy. Renal lymphoma.

2. Non-Hodgkin's lymphoma (NHL)
3. Subcapsular
4. US
   a. Hypoechoic, or anechoic without through transmission
5. CT
   a. Hypodense

K. **Germ cell tumors**

1. Ovarian cyst
   a. In newborn **[Figs. 7-39 and 7-40]**
      - Abdomino-pelvic mass
      - Off-midline

2. Ovarian teratoma, dermoid **[Figs. 7-41 and 7-42]**
   a. Second to sacrococcygeal as site for teratoma
   b. Adolescent girls

3. Ovarian torsion
   a. Usually related to dermoid cyst, but can occur in normal ovary on a long pedicle
   b. Solid or heterogeneously echogenic mass of ovary of larger than expected size
   c. Associated with cul de sac fluid; confirm with color Doppler US

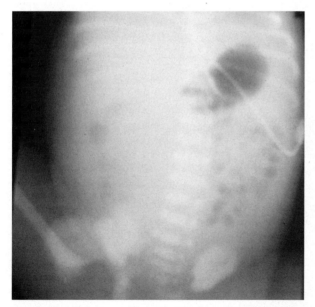

Fig. 7-39 Abdomen radiograph: Newborn. Displacement of loops of bowel by right paramedian abdominal mass. Neonatal ovarian cyst.

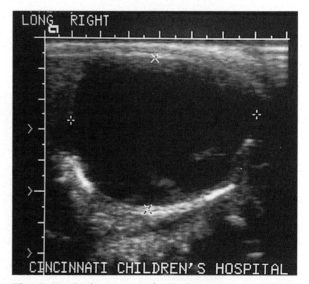

Fig. 7-40 Right parasagittal US: Same patient as Figure 7-39. Hypoechoic mass in right lower abdomen. Ovarian cyst.

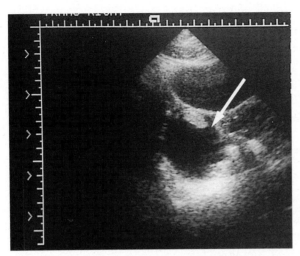

Fig. 7-41 Transverse pelvic US: Complex pelvic mass (arrow) composed of hypoechoic cyst posterior, echogenic fatty component anterior. Ovarian dermoid.

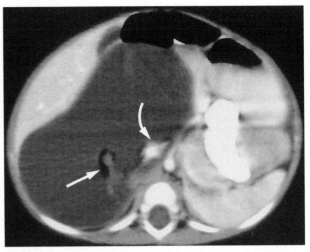

Fig. 7-42 Abdomen CT: Heterogeneous right abdominal mass. Hypodense fluid component, posterior hypodense fatty component (arrow), and chunky tooth-like calcification (curved arrow) in left side of mass. Ovarian teratoma.

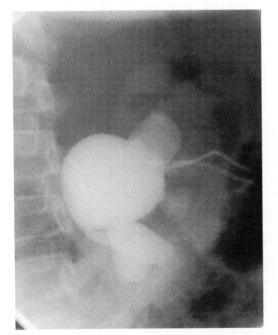

Fig. 7-43 Percutaneous pyelogram: Markedly dilated renal pelvis with virtually no emptying into ureter. Uteropelvic junction stenosis.

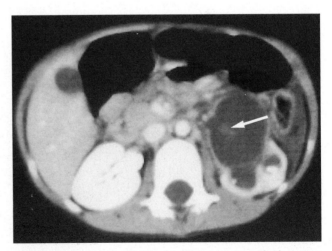

Fig. 7-44 Abdomen CT: History of minor trauma. Fluid–contrast level in calyx of left kidney and markedly dilated left renal pelvis. Note flash of contrast (arrow) into renal pelvis as well as nipple-like UPJ. Uteropelvic junction stenosis.

III. **URETER**
A. **Ureteropelvic junction (UPJ) stenosis [Figs. 7-43 and 7-44]**
1. Males > females; Left > right
2. More common in ectopic kidney
3. Probably due to in utero vascular insult, extrinsic crossing vessel, or fibrous band
4. Mass due to hydronephrosis, hypertension, or hematuria following minor trauma
5. Can co-exist with UVJ and/or vesicoureteral (VU) reflux
6. US
   a. Pyelocaliectasis with nonvisualized ureter
7. Lasix nuclear renogram
   b. Delayed excretion with persistence of activity in collecting system
B. **Ureterovesical junction (UVJ) stenosis [Fig. 7-45]**
1. "Primary megaureter or megaloureter"
2. Functional obstruction similar to Hirschsprung's
3. Aperistaltic distal ureteral segment
4. May be found in patients with VU reflux
5. Distal segment appears stenotic by imaging, in contrast to VUR
   a. Reflux
     • Dilated lowermost portion of ureter
   b. Congenital megaloureter (UVJ stenosis)
     • Narrowed lowermost portion of ureter
     • Dilated distal ureter > ± dilated upper ureter
C. **Prune belly syndrome**
1. Eagle Barrett, or Triad syndrome
2. Absent abdominal musculature
3. Cryptorchidism

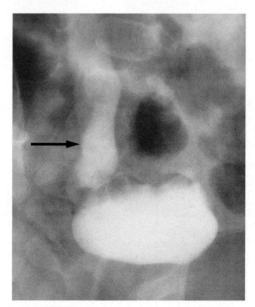

Fig. 7-45 Coned-down view from IVP: Dilated distal ureter (arrow) and narrowed UVJ. Primary megaureter. Uteropelvic junction stenosis.

4. Urethral obstruction or dysfunctional bladder emptying
5. Hydroureteronephrosis
6. Pulmonary hypoplasia, Potter's syndrome
7. Associated anomalies:
   a. Malrotation, intestinal atresia, imperforate anus, congenital heart disease

IV. BLADDER

A. Exstrophy, epispadias

1. Failure of closure of anterior wall of bladder
2. Incidence 1:30,000; M:F = 3:1
3. Associated with epispadias, pubic diastasis, anorectal malformation, spinal dysraphism, hydrometrocolpos
4. Normal pubic symphysis 5 to 9 mm in <2 yr; 4 to 8 mm 2 to 13 yr
   a. Pubic diastasis also seen with cleidocranial dysostosis, trauma
5. Urinary bladder open, small

B. Bladder wall thickening

1. Normal wall thickness <3 mm in distended state, <5 mm in collapse
2. Diffuse thickening
   a. Cystitis
      - Infectious, including viral
      - Postirradiation or chemotherapy (especially cytoxan)
3. Focal thickening
   a. Postsurgical (ureteral re-implantation)
   b. Small ureterocele
   c. Neoplasm
      - Neurofibroma
      - Rhabdomyosarcoma
         Sarcoma botryoides
         Intraluminal component lobulated
         This appearance simulated by hematoma, severe cystitis

C. Trauma

1. Extravasation **[Fig. 7-46]**
   a. Cystogram or delayed (5 to 10 minutes) CT after intravenous contrast

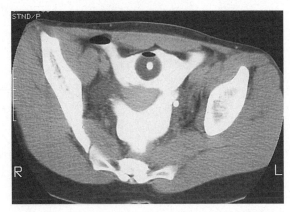

Fig. 7-46   Abdomen CT: Contrast in urinary bladder anterior and large contrast collection in cul de sac posterior. Note Foley catheter in bladder (CT cystogram can be performed if Foley is clamped). Bladder extravasation.

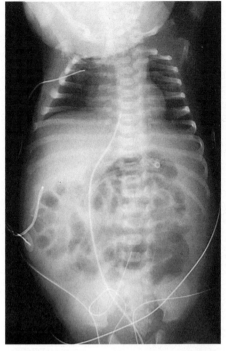

Fig. 7-47 Abdomen radiograph: Newborn. Centrally placed loops of bowel indicate ascites; abdominal protuberance, elevation of both hemidiaphragms. Urinary ascites. Posterior urethral valves.

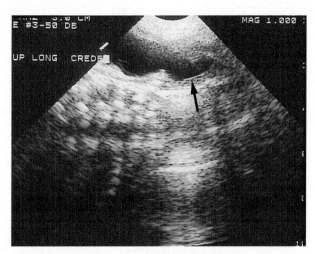

Fig. 7-48 Sagittal US of bladder: Dilatation of posterior urethra (arrow). Posterior urethral valves.

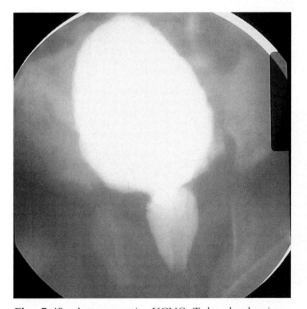

Fig. 7-49 Anteroposterior VCUG: Trabeculated urinary bladder, dilatation of posterior urethra. Note linear filling defects in urethra fanning out from central web-like opening. Posterior urethral valves.

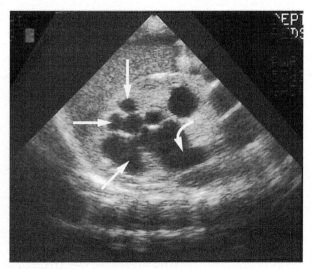

Fig. 7-50 Longitudinal US of kidney: PUV. Echogenic parenchyma, hydronephrosis. Note calyceal (arrows) and renal pelvis (curved arrow) dilatation. Renal dysplasia due to posterior urethral valves.

b. If Foley balloon in traumatized patient's bladder, keep catheter clamped to distend bladder

V. **URETHRA**

A. **PUV [Figs. 7-47 through 7-50]**

1. Folds of tissue below veru montanum that obstruct urethra
2. In utero hydronephrosis + dilated urinary bladder
3. Renal cystic dysplasia associated
4. Usually identified in newborns
5. Urinary ascites + pulmonary hypoplasia: think PUV
6. 35 to 50% have associated VUR
7. US
   a. Thick-walled trabeculated bladder
   b. Hydroureteronephrosis
   c. Hyperechogenic kidneys indicating dysplasia
   d. Renal cortical cysts
8. Voiding cystourethrogram (VCUG)
   a. Thick-walled trabeculated bladder
   b. VUR
   c. Distended posterior urethra with caliber change
   d. Thin linear filling defects converge at valve

VI. **ADRENAL**

- See GU tumors

VII. **TESTIS**

A. **Testicular torsion [Figs. 7-51 and 7-52]**

1. Acute pain; 6 hour window to preserve testis; urological emergency
2. Usually in boys 12 to 18 years of age; rarely in newborn
3. Associated with hydrocele
4. Doppler US or nuclear testicular scan for diagnosis
   a. Color flow Doppler shows no intratesticular flow; may show flow to scrotum around testis
   b. Normal nuclear scan or Doppler US does not exclude intermittent torsion

B. **Torsion of appendix testis**

1. Acute pain; not managed surgically
2. Usually in boys 10 to 13 years of age
3. Small hypervascular, hypoechoic structure at superior pole of testis
4. May be difficult to distinguish appendix testis from head of epidydimis

C. **Epidydimitis**

1. Associated with hydrocele
2. Doppler US shows hypervascular epidydimis, testis

D. **Neoplasm**

1. Germ cell tumors account for 60 to 70% testicular tumors
   a. Most common = embryonal carcinoma
   b. Yolk sac tumor, teratoma/teratocarcinoma, seminoma in descending order
2. Paratesticular tumors (rhabdomyosarcoma most common) = 10 to 15% of testicular tumors in children

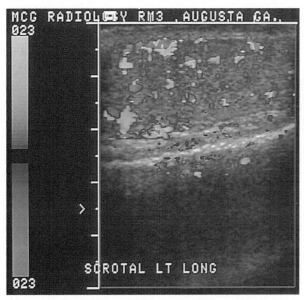

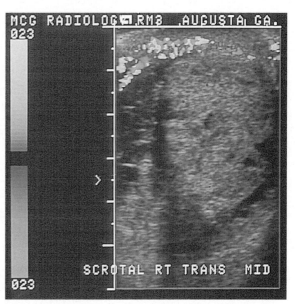

Fig. 7-51 Longitudinal US of left testis with color-flow Doppler: Note ovoid testis with homogeneous echogenic texture and bright speckles indicating vascularity. Normal testis-color flow Doppler. **(See Color Plate 3.)**

Fig. 7-52 Transverse US of right testis with color-flow Doppler: Same patient as Figure 7-51. Testis with heterogeneous echogenicity and absence of central vascular speckles. Blood flow is around testis. Testicular torsion-color flow Doppler. **(See Color Plate 4.)**

      3. Gonadal stromal tumors (Leydig or Sertoli cell tumors) = 5 to 10% of testicular tumors in children

      4. Lymphoma/leukemia = 5% of testicular tumors in children

   E. **Hernia, hydrocele**

      1. Patent processus vaginalis identified by US in longitudinal plane

   F. **Undescended testis**

      1. In US evaluation, place one finger at upper margin of inguinal canal and attempt to palpate testis, "milk" testis downward, or prevent retractile testis from disappearing

      2. Image along course of inguinal canal from distal to proximal while upper inguinal canal is compressed

VIII. **CLOACA**

   A. **Cloaca and variants**

      1. Cloaca from Latin = "Sewer"

      2. Common chamber for rectum, vagina, urethra

      3. Failure of urogenital and urorectal septa to form separate structures; one perineal opening

      4. Various types

        a. Associated with duplicate or septated bladder or vagina

      5. Initially, genitogram to define structures

      6. After colostomy, antegrade mucus fistulogram best to define anatomy

IX. **VAGINA**

   A. **Hydrometrocolpos [Fig. 7-53]**

      1. In newborn female, associated with vaginal atresia or stenosis

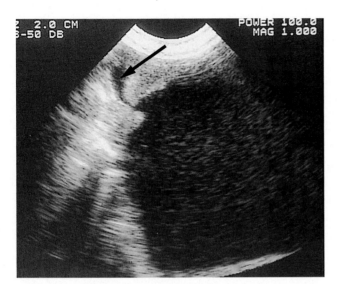

Fig. 7-53 Midline sagittal pelvic US: Newborn female. Echogenic material in markedly dilated vagina. Note fluid distending endometrial canal of uterus (arrow). Hydrometrocolpos.

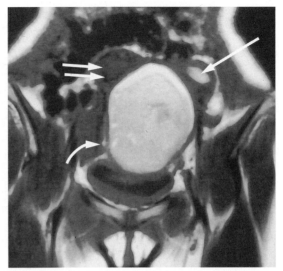

Fig. 7-54 Coronal proton density MRI: High signal in distended left vagina and left uterus (arrow). Note right uterine cavity (double arrow) and fluid in smaller right vagina (curved arrow). Uterus didelphys, septate vagina with left vaginal obstruction. Mayer-Rokitansky-Kuster-Hauser syndrome.

2. May be large enough to cause bladder outlet obstruction and hydro-ureteronephrosis
3. Large midline abdomino-pelvic mass
4. Sediment, debris in large chamber separate from and posterior to urinary bladder

B. **Müllerian anomalies [Fig. 7-54]**
  1. Mayer-Rokitansky-Kuster-Hauser
      a. Vaginal atresia + bicornuate or septate uterus
      b. Presents with hematometrocolpos as teenager or newborn or with lower abdominal/pelvic pain
      c. Unilateral renal anomaly in 50%
      d. Skeletal anomaly in 12%: vertebral, syndactyly

X. **AMBIGUOUS GENITALIA**
  A. **Normal male = 46 XY, gonad = testis; genitals = penis, scrotum, prostate, seminal vesicles, vas deferens, epidydimis**
  B. **Normal female = 46 XX, gonad = ovary; genitals = clitoris, labia minora and majora, vagina, uterus, Fallopian tubes**
  C. **Embryology**
    1. Genital ridge
        a. Becomes testis in male, ovary in female
    2. Wolffian duct
        a. Epidydimis, vas deferens, ejaculatory duct, seminal vesicle in male
        b. Vestigial Gartner's duct in female
    3. Müllerian duct
        a. Appendix testis, prostatic utricle, veru montanum in male
        b. Uterus, cervix, upper vagina, Fallopian tube in female

    4. Urogenital sinus

        a. Urethra, Cowper's glands, prostate in male

        b. Urethra, Bartholin's glands, lower vagina in female

    5. Genital tubercle

        a. Glans penis in male, clitoris in female

    6. Genital folds

        a. Penile urethra and shaft in male

        b. Labia minora in female

    7. Genital swelling

        a. Scrotum in male, labia majora in female

D. **Ambiguous genitalia**

- Three components of sex are incongruent (chromosomes, gonads, genitalia)
- Appearance of genitals indeterminate of sex designation

    1. In fetus, factors necessary for Wolffian duct structure development and normal male differentiation

        a. Testosterone must be secreted by fetal testis

        b. Testosterone must be converted to dihydrotestosterone

        c. Target organs must be sensitive to dihydrotestosterone

        d. In absence of androgen effect, female differentiation occurs

    2. True hermaphroditism

        a. Rare

        b. XX/XY mosaicism

        c. External genitalia variable

            - Labioscrotal fusion, hypospadias

            - Uterus usually present

        d. Gonadal tumors rare

    3. Female pseudohermaphroditism

        a. Normal ovaries and Müllerian structures (uterus present), XX, virilization of external genitalia

        b. Most common = congenital adrenal hyperplasia

            - 21-hydroxylase deficiency, most frequent enzyme defect

                − Salt-wasting in 30 to 65%

            - 11b-hydroxylase deficiency

                − Salt retention, hypertension

            - 3β-ol-dehydrogenase deficiency

                − Severe salt-wasting

                − Only enzyme defect to produce ambiguous genitalia in both boys and girls

                    Others produce ambiguous genitalia only in girls

        c. In utero exposure of female fetus to exogenous maternal progestogens

    4. Male pseudohermaphroditism

        a. On genitograms/cystograms, urethra is long and curved (male-type urethra)

        b. Without Müllerian structures

            - Testosterone synthesis defects

Table 7-1. Syndromes with Renal Cystic Disease

Acrocephalosyndactyly	Lissencephaly
Acro-renal-mandibular	Marden-Walker
Arthro-dento-osteodysplasia	Meckel-Gruber
Asphyxiating thoracic dysplasia, Jeune syndrome	Miranda
Cerebrohepatorenal syndrome of Zellweger	Noonan
Congenital nephrotic syndrome	Oral-facial-digital
Ehlers-Danlos	Peutz-Jeghers
Goldenhar	Roberts
Goldston	Short rib-polydactyly
Hadju-Cheney	Simopoulos
Ivemark	Trisomy 13, 18, 21
Kaufman-McKusick	Tuberous sclerosis [Fig. 8-4]
Laurence-Moon-Biedl	von Hippel-Lindau

- Androgen target organ failure
  - Complete testicular feminization
    - Looks like normal female, but no uterus
    - High incidence of gonadal malignancy
- Pituitary hormone deficiency
  - Microphallus, cryptorchidism
c. With Müllerian structures
- Gonadal dysgenesis
  - Uterus present in mixed gonadal dysgenesis
  - High incidence of gonadoblastoma or dysgerminoma

Further Reading

Blane CE, DiPietro MA, Zerin JM, et al. Renal sonography is not a reliable screening examination for vesicoureteral reflux. J Urol 1993;150:752–755.

Connor JP. DMSA scanning: a pediatric urologist's point of view. Pediatr Radiol 1995; 25:S50–S51.

Deal JE, Snell MF, Barratt TM, et al. Renovascular disease in childhood. J Pediatr 1992;121:378–384.

Dehner LP. Pediatric Surgical Pathology, 2nd ed. Baltimore: Williams & Wilkins. 1987.

DiPietro MA, Blane CE, Zerin JM. Vesicoureteral reflux in older children: concordance of US and voiding cystourethrographic findings. Radiology 1997;205:821–822.

Eklöf O, Löhr G, Ringertz H, et al. Ectopic ureterocele in the male infant. Acta Radiol: Diag 1978;19:145–153.

Grignon A, Filion R, Filiatraut D, et al. Urinary tract dilatation in utero: classification and clinical applications. Radiology 1986;160:645–647.

Halpern EJ, Needleman L, Nack TL, et al. Renal artery stenosis: should we study the main renal artery or segmental vessels? Radiology 1995;195:799–804.

Hoberman A, Chao HP, Keller DM, et al. Prevalence of urinary tract infections in febrile infants. J Pediatr 1993;123:17–23.

Karp MP, Jewett TC, Kuhn JP, et al. The impact of computed tomography scanning on the child with renal trauma. J Pediatr Surg 1986;21:617–623.

Kelalis PP, King LR, Belman AB, eds. Clinical Pediatric Urology, 3rd ed. Philadelphia: W. B. Saunders. 1992.

Lebowitz RL, Mandell J. Urinary tract infection in children: putting radiology in its place. Radiology 1987:165:1–9.

Majd M. In: Kelalis PP, King LR, Belman AB, eds. Clinical Pediatric Urology, 3rd ed. Philadelphia: W. B. Saunders. 1992:117–165.

O'Hara SM. Workup of febrile urinary tract infections. Pediatr Radiol 1996;26:497.

René PC, Oliva VL, Bui BT, et al. Renal artery stenosis: evaluation of Doppler US after inhibition of angiotensin-converting enzyme with captopril. Radiology 1995; 196:675–679.

Seigle R, Nash M. Is there a role for renal scintigraphy in the routine initial evaluation of a child with a urinary infection? Pediatr Radiol 1995;25:S52–S53.

Slovis TL. Is there a single most appropriate imaging workup of a child with an acute febrile urinary tract infection? Pediatr Radiol 1995;25:S46–S49.

Stables DP, Fouche RF, de Villiers van Niekirk JP, et al. Traumatic renal artery occlusion: 21 cases. J Urol 1976;115:229–233.

Taylor GA, Eichelberger MR, Potter BM. Hematuria. A marker of abdominal injury in children after blunt trauma. Ann Surg 1988;208:688–693.

Treves ST, Zurakowski D, Bauer SB, Mitchell KD, Nicholas DP. Functional bladder capacity measured during radionuclide cystography in children. Radiology 1996;198: 269–272.

Wright NB, Blanch G, Walkinshaw S, et al. Antenatal and neonatal renal vein thrombosis: new ultrasonic features with high frequency transducers. Pediatr Radiol 1996; 26:686–689.

CHAPTER EIGHT   MULTISYSTEM INVOLVEMENT IN PEDIATRIC IMAGING

I. **CHILD ABUSE**
   A. **Central nervous system (CNS)**
      1. Global hypoxic-ischemic encephalopathy
         a. Due to strangulation, drowning, asphyxiation
         b. Diffuse cerebral edema by computed tomography (CT) or magnetic resonance imaging (MRI) **[Fig. 8-1; see also Fig. 2-62]**
            • Loss of gray-white differentiation
            • Often preservation of cerebellum, brain stem
            • "Reversal sign" in which white matter is hyperdense relative to gray matter
      2. Acute and chronic subdural hematomas **[Fig. 2-61]**
         a. Especially anterior interhemispheric subdural hematoma
      3. Subarachnoid hemorrhage
      4. Focal infarcts
         a. Due to carotid dissection or direct vascular injury
      5. Skull fractures **[Fig. 1-30]**
         a. Often cross sutures or are stellate in pattern
      6. Spine
         a. Compression fractures **[Fig. 8-2]**
   B. **Chest**
      1. Rib fractures **[Fig. 8-3]**

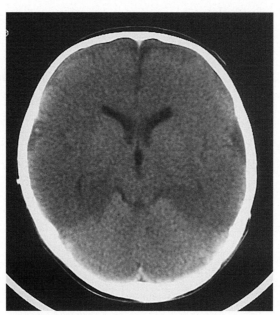

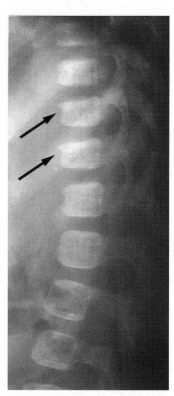

Fig. 8-1 Axial brain CT: Child abuse. Diffuse hypodensity in supratentorial compartment and lack of gray-white differentiation. Note discrepancy between density of cerebellum and cerebrum. Hypoxic-ischemic encephalopathy.

Fig. 8-2 Lateral thoracolumbar spine radiograph: Child abuse. Compression fractures (arrows) of T11 and T12.

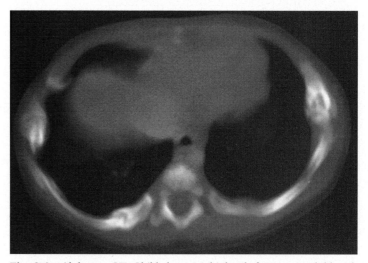

Fig. 8-3 Abdomen CT: Child abuse. Multiple rib fractures in child with liver laceration (not shown).

a. Difficult to visualize acutely; healing fracture identified by more bulbous appearance of involved rib than normal ribs

2. Acromion process fractures

C. **Gastrointestinal (GI)**

1. Solid organ injury
   a. Liver, spleen, pancreas
2. Duodenal hematoma **[Fig. 6-15]**
   a. Located on antimesenteric border
   b. Coiled-spring appearance on upper GI series (UGI) in acute phase; intramural mass, mucosal thickening seen as hematoma resolves
3. Bowel rupture
   a. On enhanced CT, peritoneal fluid, bowel wall enhancement and/or thickening, bowel dilatation
4. Mesenteric hematoma
5. Hypovolemic shock **[Fig. 6-62]**
   a. Due to internal injuries and hemorrhage
   b. CT
      • Small spleen (due to splanchnic vasoconstriction)
      • Small inferior vena cava (IVC) and aorta
      • Bright enhancement of pancreas, adrenals, bowel wall
6. Gastric atony **[Fig. 6-7]**
   a. Due to starvation

D. **Musculoskeletal**

1. "Corner" or "buckethandle" metaphyseal fractures **[Fig. 3-69]**
   a. Due to twisting or jerking of extremity
2. Fractures in different stages of healing **[Fig. 3-70]**
3. Diaphyseal fractures in young infants
   a. Radius, ulna, tibia, fibula, femur, humerus
   b. Fractures that cannot be explained by level of activity of child

II. **PHAKOMATOSES**

A. **Tuberous sclerosis (TS)**

1. Autosomal dominant, variable penetrance
2. Definitive diagnosis
   a. Cortical tubers or subependymal nodules **[Figs. 2-17 through 2-19]**
   b. Multiple renal angiomyolipomas
   c. Cardiac rhabdomyomas
   d. Adenoma sebaceum or subungual fibromas
   e. Subependymal giant cell tumors
3. Presumptive diagnosis (two of the following present):
   a. Hypopigmented macule ("ash-leaf spot")
   b. Shagreen patch
   c. Infantile spasms (hypsarrhythmia)
   d. Single retinal hamartoma
   e. Multiple renal cysts **[Fig. 8-4]**
      • Renal cystic disease of TS may be indistinguishable from that of autosomal dominant polycystic kidney disease (ADPKD)
   f. Cardiac rhabdomyoma
   g. First-degree relative with TS

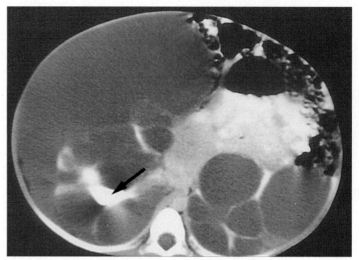

Fig. 8-4 Axial abdominal CT: Large, bilateral renal cysts virtually replace renal parenchyma. Note contrast excreted into right renal pelvis (arrow). Tuberous sclerosis. ADPKD can have identical appearance.

4. Skin lesions in 90%
5. Brain hamartomas in 90%
6. Retinal hamartomas in 50%
7. Renal hamartomas in 50 to 80%
8. Variability of symptoms from none to neurologically disabled
9. Other signs
   a. Lymphangiomyomatosis
   b. Osteosclerosis
   c. Bone involvement in TS in 10% of patients
   d. Cysts in small bones of hand or foot

B. **Neurofibromatosis: NF-1**
   1. Autosomal dominant, variable penetrance
   2. von Recklinghausen, peripheral neurofibromatosis
   3. 1 : 2000 to 3000 live births
   4. Long arm chromosome 17
   5. Two or more of following present:
      a. ≥ 6 cafe au lait spots, >5 mm before, >15 mm after puberty
      b. ≥ 2 neurofibromas **[Fig. 8-5]**
      c. ≥ 1 plexiform neurofibroma **[Fig. 8-6]**
      d. Axillary or inguinal freckling
      e. ≥ 2 iris hamartomas (Lisch nodules)
      f. ≥ 1 bone lesion (sphenoid dysplasia, pseudarthrosis, etc.)
      g. First-degree relative with NF-1
   6. Hamartomas
   7. Optic nerve glioma (15 to 40%) **[Fig. 2-20]**
      a. Low-grade pilocytic astrocytoma
   8. Parenchymal glioma (10%)
      a. Astrocytomas
   9. Malignant nerve sheath tumors (MNST)

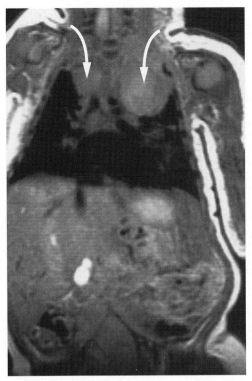

Fig. 8-5 Coronal T1-weighted brain MRI: Bilateral posterior mediastinal masses (curved arrows). NF-1.

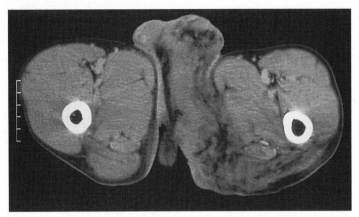

Fig. 8-6 Axial CT through perineum: Irregular, infiltrating mass in left posterior thigh, perineum, and scrotum. Plexiform neurofibroma.

      a. 50% occur in patients with NF-1

      b. Incidence of MNST in patients with NF-1 $\geq$ 5%

  10. Sphenoid dysplasia (pulsating exophthalmos) **[Figs. 2-21 and 2-22]**

  11. Lambdoid defect

  12. Dural ectasia of internal auditory canal (IAC), neural foramina

  13. Lateral meningocele

  14. Kyphoscoliosis

      a. Short-segment thoracic scoliosis (NF-1 or Marfan's)

  15. Pseudarthrosis of tibia

C. **Neurofibromatosis: NF-2**

  1. Autosomal dominant, variable penetrance

  2. Central neurofibromatosis

  3. Deletions on chromosome 22

  4. One of following present:

      a. Bilateral VIII nerve schwannomas **[Fig. 8-7]**

      b. First-degree relative with NF-2 + single VIII nerve mass or

      c. Any two of the following: schwannoma, neurofibroma, meningioma, glioma (ependymoma), juvenile posterior subcapsular lens opacity

D. **Sturge-Weber syndrome**

  1. Encephalotrigeminal angiomatosis

  2. Port-wine stain in cranial nerve V1 distribution + leptomeningeal angiomatosis

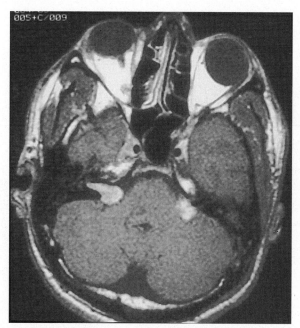

Fig. 8-7   Gadolinium contrast-enhanced axial T1-weighted brain MRI: Bilateral enhancing masses in IAC. Bilateral acoustic schwannoma, NF-2.

3. Facial or leptomeningeal angioma; unilateral (75%) or bilateral (25%)
    a. Usually occipital
4. Choroidal angioma: congenital glaucoma (buphthalmos)
5. Seizures in > 90%; retardation; hemiplegia
6. Hemiatrophy; Davidoff-Dyke-Masson
    a. Calvarial thickening ipsilateral to hemiatrophy
7. Abnormal venous drainage → progressive dystrophic gyral calcification
8. CT: Gyral calcification in dystrophic cortex **[Fig. 2-23]**
9. MRI: Atrophy; enhanced shows ischemic cortex
E. **von Hippel-Lindau (VHL) syndrome**
    1. Criteria for diagnosis
        a. More than one hemangioblastoma of CNS, or
        b. One CNS hemangioblastoma + visceral manifestation, or
        c. One manifestation of VHL + known family history
    2. CNS
        a. Cerebellar hemangioblastoma
            • 35 to 60% of patients with VHL
            • 80%: vascular nodule surrounded by fluid-filled cyst
            • 20% solid
            • Usually in cerebellar hemisphere
        b. Spinal hemangioblastoma
            • Lower cervical, lower thoracic spine most common locations
        c. Retinal hemangioblastoma
            • 50 to 67% of patients with VHL
            • Multiple in 50%; bilateral in 20 to 50%

3. GI
   a. Pancreatic cysts in 30%
      - May be extensive and replace pancreas
   b. Pancreatic malignancy
      - Includes pancreatic carcinoma, ampullary carcinoma, hemangio-blastoma, microcystic adenoma, nonfunctional islet cell tumor
4. Genitourinary (GU)
   a. Renal cell carcinoma
      - 30% of patients with VHL
      - Bilateral in 75%, multifocal in 87%
   b. Renal cysts
      - Most common single abdominal manifestation
      - 76% of patients with VHL
   c. Pheochromocytoma
      - 10% of patients with VHL; often bilateral

III. **LEUKEMIA/LYMPHOMA**
   A. **CNS**
      1. Calvarial or vertebral marrow infiltration **[Fig. 8-8]**
      2. Adenoidal mass
      3. Aggressive nasopharyngeal mass **[Fig. 2-105]**
         a. Similar imaging findings to rhabdomyosarcoma, carcinoma
      4. Aggressive orbital mass

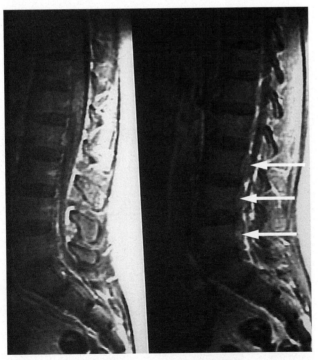

Fig. 8-8 Sagittal T1-weighted spine MRI: Patient with leukemia. Diffuse hypointensity of vertebral marrow indicating replacement of marrow. Note epidural soft tissue masses (arrows) posterior to several lumbar vertebral bodies. Bone marrow infiltration.

    B. **Chest**
        1. Anterior mediastinal mass **[Fig. 8-9; see also Figs. 5-49, 5-53, and 5-54]**
        2. Pleural thickening or effusion
        3. Sternal periosteal reaction
    C. **GI**
        1. Bowel wall thickening **[Fig. 6-13]**
        2. Mesenteric or retroperitoneal adenopathy **[Fig. 8-10; see also Fig. 6-14]**
        3. Hepatosplenomegaly
        4. Focal hypodense (CT) or hypoechoic (US) liver or spleen lesions **[Fig. 6-50]**
          a. Resemble "cysts"
    D. **GU**
        1. Focal hypodense or hypoechoic renal lesions **[Fig. 7-38]**
        2. Focal mass in ovary or testis
    E. **Musculoskeletal**
        1. Metaphyseal bands
        2. Osteopenia
        3. Focal lytic or sclerotic lesions **[Fig. 8-11; see also Figs. 3-52 and 3-53]**
        4. Periosteal reaction
IV. **CYSTIC FIBROSIS**
    A. **CNS**
        1. Chronic sinusitis

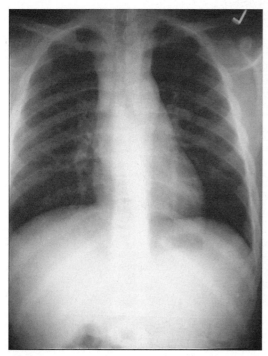

Fig. 8-9 Posteroanterior chest radiograph: Wide mediastinum, loss of normal paratracheal stripe. Mediastinal adenopathy, leukemia.

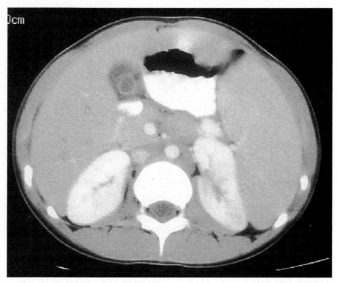

Fig. 8-10 Axial abdominal CT: Splenomegaly, retroperitoneal adenopathy, peritoneal implant indenting anterior wall of stomach. Also note fluid in gallbladder fossa. Lymphoma.

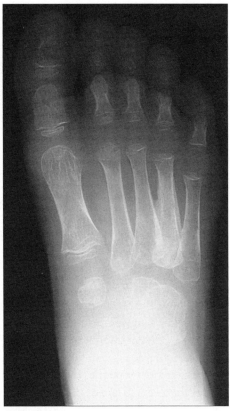

Fig. 8-11 Anteroposterior (AP) foot radiograph: Patient with leukemia. Periosteal reaction of fourth metatarsal.

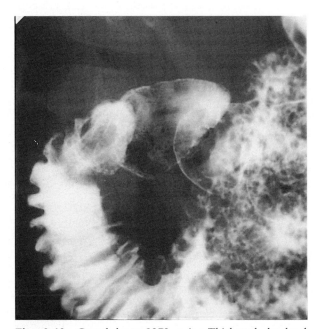

Fig. 8-12 Coned-down UGI series: Thickened duodenal folds. Cystic fibrosis.

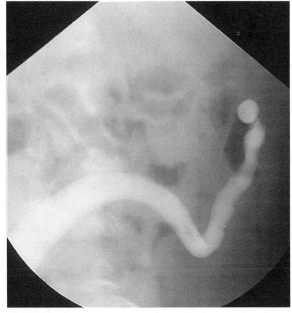

Fig. 8-13 Contrast enema: Patient with cystic fibrosis treated with high dose pancrease™. Diffuse narrowing and obliteration of contrast column in descending colon. Fibrosing colonopathy.

B. **Chest**
  1. Pneumonia
     a. *Staphylococcus aureus, Pseudomonas aeruginosa*
  2. Interstitial pattern **[Figs. 5-39 and 5-40]**
     a. Chronic bronchitis
     b. Bronchiectasis
        • Upper lobe predilection
        • Hemoptysis
            May require bronchial artery embolization
  3. Emphysema
C. **GI**
  1. Increased incidence of gastroesophageal reflux
  2. Thickened duodenal folds **[Fig. 8-12]**
  3. Meconium ileus **[Figs. 6-18 through 6-20]**
  4. Meconium ileus equivalent
  5. Congenital bowel atresia
  6. Meconium peritonitis
  7. Small bowel intussusception
  8. Appendiceal inspissation
     a. May present as appendicitis
  9. Rectal prolapse
  10. Fibrosing colonopathy **[Fig. 8-13]**
     a. Progressive fibrosis of colon associated with high dose Pancrease™
  11. Inspissated bile syndrome
     a. May simulate biliary atresia
  12. Chronic liver disease
     a. Cirrhosis
D. **GU**
  1. Infertility
E. **Cardiovascular (CV)**
  1. Pulmonary artery hypertension
  2. Cor pulmonale
F. **Musculoskeletal**
  1. Hypertrophic pulmonary osteoarthropathy

V. **SICKLE CELL DISEASE (SCD)**
A. **CNS**
  1. Stroke **[Figs. 2-65 and 2-66]**
     a. Most patients with SCD and stroke >5 years of age
     b. Large and small vessel disease, including moya-moya
        • Small vessel disease due to sludging
        • Large vessel disease due to endothelial proliferation, fibrosis in vessel wall
     c. Stroke Prevention Trial in Sickle Cell Anemia (STOP)
        • Maintenance of hemoglobin S below 30% reduced rate of cerebral infarction by 90% in children with elevated transcranial Doppler (TCD) velocity ($\geq$200 cm/sec)
        • TCD screening for children ages 2 to 16 years recommended every 6 months to identify those at high risk for first stroke

    2. Moya–moya

    3. Thickening of diploic space **[Fig. 8-14]**

B. **Chest**

    1. Acute chest syndrome

        a. Waste basket term that includes pneumonia (bacterial, viral, mycoplasma, etc.), and fat or bland emboli

    2. Myocardial ischemia

    3. Chronic anemia

    4. Sternal infarction

C. **GI**

    1. Hepatomegaly

    2. Gall stones or sludge

    3. Cholecystitis

    4. Biliary obstruction due to gall stones

    5. Small or inapparent spleen

    6. Functional asplenia on liver-spleen nuclear scan

    7. Splenic calcifications

    8. Splenomegaly

        a. Sequestration or splenic infarction

D. **GU**

    1. Bilateral nephromegaly

    2. Papillary necrosis

E. **Musculoskeletal**

    1. Osteomyelitis

        a. Most common etiology is *Staphylococcus aureus*

          • Metaphysis is most typical site

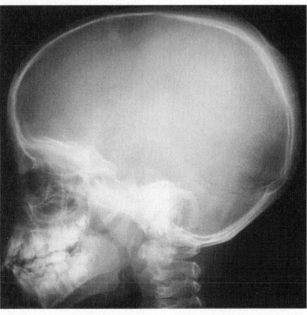

Fig. 8-14 Lateral skull radiograph: Thickened diploic space with "hair on end" appearance. Sickle cell disease. Differential diagnosis includes thalassemia.

b. Salmonella osteomyelitis more common in patients with SCD than in non-SCD patients
   - Infection of entire diaphysis suggests Salmonella **[Fig. 8-15]**

2. Infarction
   a. Long or flat bones
      - Depression of mid-portion of vertebral endplates produces "Lincoln log" appearance
   b. Metaphyseal, phalangeal infarcts
      - "Hand-foot syndrome" **[Fig. 8-16]**
         Occurs at ages 9 months to 3 years
         May be first manifestation of SCD
         Fever, swelling, redness
         Involved bone sclerotic, enlarged
         Associated periostitis
         Must still consider osteomyelitis
      - "Divot" in metaphysis from infarct
         This appearance also seen in child abuse

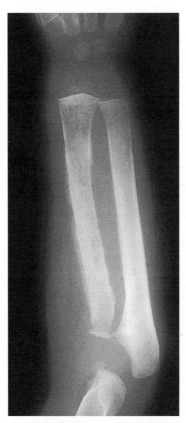

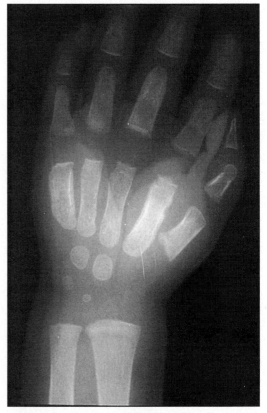

Fig. 8-15 Forearm radiograph: Patient with sickle cell anemia. Inhomogeneous lesion of radius, which is thickened, irregular in contour, and sclerotic. Note that periosteal reaction involves diaphysis and metaphysis. Salmonella osteomyelitis.

Fig. 8-16 AP hand radiograph: 9-month-old with sickle cell anemia. Thickened, sclerotic second and fifth metacarpals with periosteal reaction and overlying soft tissue swelling. Sickle cell dactylitis. Hand-foot syndrome.

c. Sternal infarcts **[Fig. 8-17]**
- Multiple ossification segments in child's sternum
- "Divot" in sternal ossification from infarct
  Appearance similar to vertebral endplate or metaphyseal infarct
- May be responsible for acute chest syndrome
  Usually visualized in conjunction with pulmonary lesions of acute chest syndrome

3. Methods to distinguish osteomyelitis from infarction
   a. Combined ^{99m}Tc and ^{67}Ga nuclear scans
      - Ga uptake $> ^{99m}$Tc uptake suggests osteomyelitis
      - Ga uptake $< ^{99m}$Tc uptake suggests infarction
      - Ga uptake $= ^{99m}$Tc uptake: indeterminate
   b. Serial radiographs, clinical evaluation, positive blood or lesion culture

4. Avascular necrosis (AVN)
   a. Femoral and humeral head most common sites

VI. LANGERHANS' CELL HISTIOCYTOSIS (LCH)
A. Restricted LCH
1. Biopsy-proven skin rash only, or monostotic or polyostotic lesions, ± diabetes insipidus, adjacent lymph node involvement or skin rash

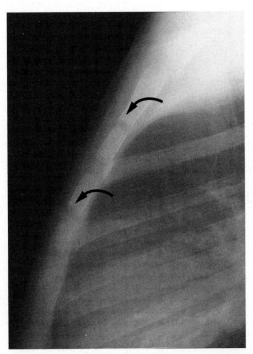

Fig. 8-17 Coned-down lateral sternum radiograph: "Divots," similar in appearance to infarcts in vertebral end plates or metacarpals in patients with SCD, in sternal manubrium and body (curved arrows). Sternal infarcts, Sickle cell disease.

B. **Extensive LCH**
1. Category 2a: Visceral organ involvement, ± bone lesions, diabetes insipidus, adjacent lymph node involvement and/or skin rash, without organ dysfunction of lung, liver, or bone marrow
2. Category 2b: Same as category 2a, but with organ dysfunction of lung, liver, or bone marrow
3. Highest mortality in youngest patients (80% in those 0 to 6 months of age)
4. Mortality = 90% if dysfunction involves 2 to 3 organ systems

C. **CNS**
1. Skull most common bone involved
2. Round or ovoid lytic lesions, well-defined, non-sclerotic margins
3. "Geographic skull" **[Fig. 3-54]**
4. "Bevelled edge"
5. Mandibular involvement produces "floating teeth"
6. Hypothalamic involvement
7. Thickening and enhancement of pituitary stalk
8. Absence of posterior pituitary bright spot
9. Erosion of temporal bone common, often bilateral
   a. Conductive hearing loss
   b. Otorrhea, VII nerve palsy

D. **Chest**
1. Reticular or reticulonodular opacities **[Fig. 8-18]**
2. Cysts or honeycombing
3. Upper lobes > lower lobes
4. Complete or partial regression common

E. **GI**
1. Hepatosplenomegaly
2. Periportal lymphadenopathy
3. Sclerosing cholangitis

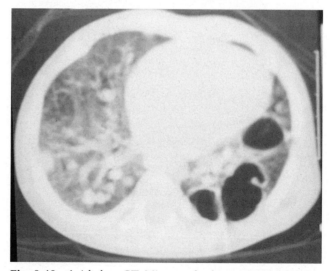

Fig. 8-18 Axial chest CT: Mixture of pulmonary nodules, interstitial opacities, and cysts. Langerhans' cell histiocytosis.

  F. **Musculoskeletal**

   1. Bone involvement most common manifestation **[Fig. 8-19]**

   2. Lytic, poorly or well-defined borders, with or without reactive sclerosis

   3. Laminated periosteal reaction

   4. "Bevelled edge"

   5. Diaphyseal location in long bone

   6. Uniform collapse of vertebral body (vertebra plana)

    a. LCH most common cause of vertebra plana in children

    b. Disc space preserved

VII. **ACQUIRED IMMUNODEFICIENCY SYNDROME (AIDS)**

  A. **80% of pediatric AIDS in USA is of perinatal transmission**

  B. **Rate of perinatal transmission approximately 30%**

  C. **Age at diagnosis for perinatal AIDS**

   1. 25% by age 6 months

   2. 50% by age 1 year

   3. 75% by age 2 years

   4. Incidence drops with increasing age; rare >9 years of age

  D. **Most common presentations are *Pneumocystis carinii* pneumonia (PCP), lymphocytic interstitial pneumonitis (LIP), wasting syndrome, encephalopathy**

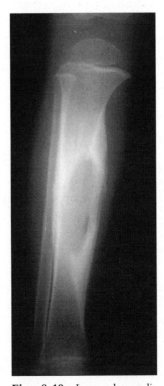

Fig. 8-19 Lower leg radiograph: Well-demarcated elliptical, lytic lesion in diaphysis with surrounding sclerosis and cortical thickening. Langerhans' cell histiocytosis, eosinophilic granuloma.

E. **Human immunodeficiency virus (HIV) infects CD4 molecule on surface of T4 helper-inducer lymphocyte**
  1. T4 cells normally induce variety of immune responses
  2. Destruction of T4 cells results in profound immunosuppression
F. **T lymphocyte level <400: patient at risk for opportunistic or pyogenic bacterial infection**
G. **Immunologic dysfunction**
  1. Reversed T4 : T8 ratio
  2. Hypergammaglobulinemia
H. **Provisional World Health Organization (WHO) clinical case definition for AIDS in children**
  1. Major signs
     a. Weight loss or failure to thrive
     b. Chronic diarrhea > 1 month
     c. Chronic fever > 1 month
  2. Minor signs
     a. Generalized lymphadenopathy
     b. Oral thrush
     c. Repeated common infections (otitis, pharyngitis)
     d. Generalized dermatitis
     e. Confirmed maternal HIV infection
  3. Pediatric AIDS suspected in child with ≥2 major signs associated with ≥2 minor signs in absence of known immunodeficiency
I. **Centers for Disease Control and Prevention (CDC) classification system for HIV infection in children**
  1. Class P-0. Indeterminate infection
     a. Infants <15 months born to infected mothers but without definitive evidence of HIV infection or AIDS
  2. Class P-1. Asymptomatic infection
     a. Subclass A. Normal immune function
     b. Subclass B. Abnormal immune function
        • Hypergammaglobulinemia, T4 lymphopenia, decreased T4 : T8 ratio, or absolute lymphopenia
     c. Subclass C. Immune function not tested
  3. Class P-2. Symptomatic infection
     a. Subclass A. Nonspecific findings (≥2 for ≥2 months)
        • Fever, failure to thrive, generalized lymphadenopathy, hepatomegaly, splenomegaly, enlarged parotid glands, persistent or recurrent diarrhea
     b. Subclass B. Progressive neurologic disease
        • Loss of developmental milestones or intellectual ability, impaired brain growth, or progressive symmetric motor deficits
     c. Subclass C. Lymphoid interstitial pneumonitis
     d. Subclass D. Secondary infectious diseases
        • Category D-1. Opportunistic infections
          Bacterial
          – Mycobacterial, nocardiosis

Fungal
- Candidiasis, coccidioidomycosis, histoplasmosis, crypto-coccosis

Parasitic
- *Pneumocystis carinii,* disseminated toxoplasmosis, chronic cryptosporidiosis or isosporiasis, extraintestinal strongyloidiasis

Viral
- Cytomegalovirus (CMV), chronic herpes, progressive multifocal leukoencephalopathy (PML)

- Category D-2. Unexplained, recurrent bacterial infections ≥2 within 2-year period
  Sepsis, meningitis, pneumonia, abscess of internal organ, bone/joint infection

- Category D-3. Other infectious diseases
  Persistent oral candidiasis, recurrent herpes stomatitis, disseminated herpes zoster

e. Subclass E. Secondary cancers
- Category E-1. Cancers with known AIDS association
  Kaposi's sarcoma
  B-cell, non-Hodgkin's lymphoma
  Primary lymphoma of brain
- Category E-2. Cancers with possible AIDS association

f. Subclass F. Other conditions possibly due to HIV infection
- Hepatitis
- Cardiomyopathy
- Nephropathy
- Hematologic disorders
- Dermatologic disorders

J. **CNS**
1. HIV encephalopathy
   a. CT
      - Atrophy, white matter hypodensity, basal ganglia and frontal white matter calcification
   b. MRI
      - Atrophy, T2 hyperintensity in white matter and/or basal ganglia
2. Growth retardation
3. Toxoplasmosis
   a. Usually multiple, small (<2 cm) hypo- or isodense lesions with variable enhancement
4. Non-Hodgkin's lymphoma **[Fig. 8-20]**
   a. Usually single lesion >3 cm
   b. Unresponsive to trial of anti-toxoplasmosis therapy
   c. CT
      - Hyperdense with or without surrounding edema
      - Can be hypo- or isodense with ring or periventricular enhancement, or diffuse infiltrating contrast-enhancing lesion

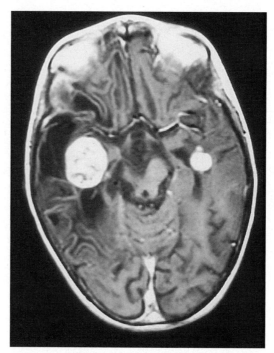

Fig. 8-20 Axial gadolinium-enhanced T1-weighted brain MRI: Patient with AIDS. Two round enhancing lesions in temporal lobes. Note infarction in right temporal lobe and atrophy in right cerebral peduncle. AIDS, non-Hodgkin's lymphoma.

    5. HIV vasculopathy
       a. Stroke
    6. PML
    7. Meningitis
    8. Recurrent otitis media
    9. Sinusitis
   10. CMV retinitis

K. **Chest**
    1. PCP **[Fig. 5–35]**
       a. Most common disease indicating AIDS
       b. Bilateral diffuse alveolar disease without hilar adenopathy
          • Initially perihilar, interstitial, rapidly becomes alveolar
          • Can be focal rather than diffuse
          • Cysts may be present
          • Pleural effusions uncommon
    2. Lymphocytic interstitial pneumonitis **[Fig. 8-21; see also Fig. 5-37]**
       a. Second most common disease indicating AIDS
       b. Reticulonodular pattern with or without hilar adenopathy
          • Persists for ≥2 months
          • Unresponsive to antimicrobial therapy
    3. CMV pneumonia
    4. Mycobacterium avium-intracellulare

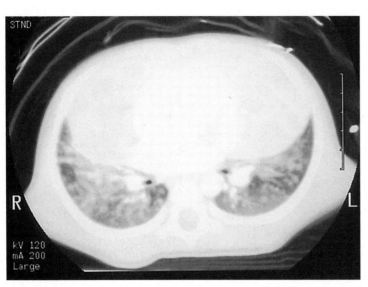

Fig. 8-21 Axial chest CT: Patient with AIDS. Small nodular, interstitial opacities. Mediastinum is wide, due to cystic HIV-related thymic mass. AIDS, Lymphocytic interstitial pneumonitis.

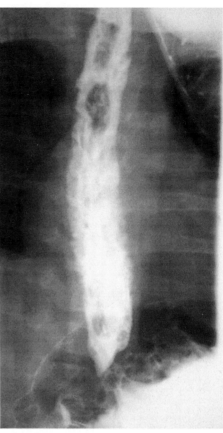

Fig. 8-22 Barium esophagram: Extensive, shaggy, coalescent esophageal erosions and ulcerations. AIDS, Candida esophagitis.

     5. Mycobacterium tuberculosis

     6. Repeated bacterial pneumonias

  L. **CV**

     1. HIV cardiomyopathy

     2. Septicemia

  M. **GI**

     1. Candida, herpes simplex esophagitis **[Fig. 8-22]**

     2. Intestinal cryptosporidiosis, isosporiasis

     3. Salmonella spp., Shigella spp., Clostridium difficile, Campylobacter

     4. Perirectal abscess

  N. **GU**

     1. HIV-associated nephropathy

       a. Proteinuria, nephrosis, nephritis

       b. Bilateral nephromegaly, medical renal disease by ultrasound

     2. Urinary tract infections

  O. **Musculoskeletal**

     1. Cellulitis, pyomyositis

FURTHER READING

Amundsen TR, Siegel MJ, Siegel BA. Osteomyelitis and infarction in sickle cell hemoglobinopathies: differentiation by combined technetium and gallium scintigraphy. Radiology 1984;153:807–812.

Anon. National Heart, Lung, and Blood Institute report. Stroke Prevention Trial in Sickle Cell Anemia (STOP). Sept. 18, 1997.

Egeler RM, D'Angio GJ. Langerhans' cell histiocytosis. J Pediatr 1995;127:1–11.

Moran CJ, Siegel MJ, DeBaun MR. Sickle cell disease: imaging of cerebrovascular complications. Radiology 1998;206:311–321.

Pizzo PA, Wilfert CM, eds. Pediatric AIDS. Baltimore, MD: Williams & Wilkins. 1991.

CHAPTER NINE CLINICAL PATHWAYS: GUIDELINES FOR APPROPRIATE IMAGING

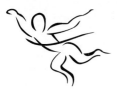

In this chapter, we present an ordered approach to imaging in the clinical diagnosis of several common pediatric problems. The algorithms represent practical recommendations for efficient and cost-effective imaging. These pathways are the result of our training and experience; we recognize that other approaches may be equally valid. While we have attempted to include most common diagnoses in our imaging pathways, it is impossible to designate all atypical presentations of common disorders and uncommon conditions that simulate more common diseases. We firmly believe, though, that the following will assist you to be more logical and expeditious when evaluating children with the clinical conditions we have described.

HYPOXIA-ISCHEMIA IN THE NEONATE

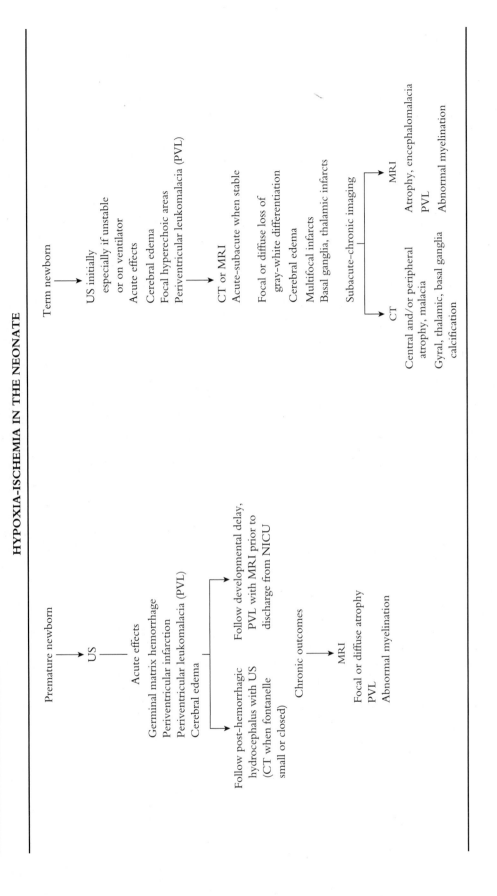

Premature newborn → US

Acute effects

Germinal matrix hemorrhage
Periventricular infarction
Periventricular leukomalacia (PVL)
Cerebral edema

Follow post-hemorrhagic
hydrocephalus with US
(CT when fontanelle
small or closed)

Follow developmental delay,
PVL with MRI prior to
discharge from NICU

Chronic outcomes → MRI

Focal or diffuse atrophy
PVL
Abnormal myelination

Term newborn →

US initially
especially if unstable
or on ventilator

Acute effects

Cerebral edema
Focal hyperechoic areas
Periventricular leukomalacia (PVL)

CT or MRI

Acute–subacute when stable

Focal or diffuse loss of
gray-white differentiation

Cerebral edema
Multifocal infarcts
Basal ganglia, thalamic infarcts

Subacute–chronic imaging

CT

Central and/or peripheral
atrophy, malacia
Gyral, thalamic, basal ganglia
calcification

MRI

Atrophy, encephalomalacia
PVL
Abnormal myelination

SEERURES

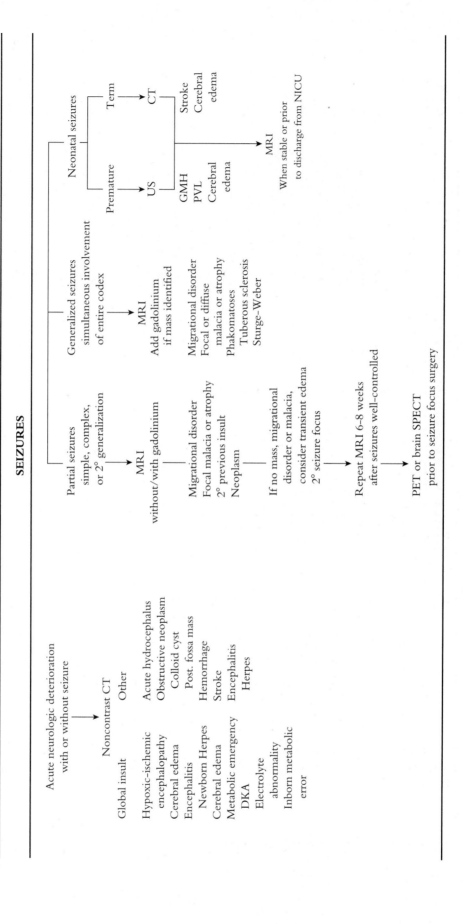

BACK PAIN

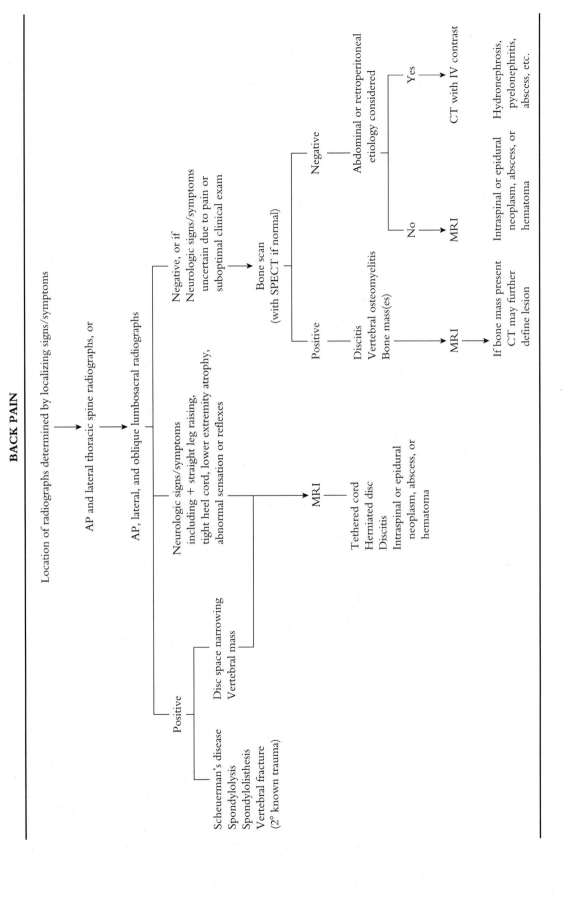

Location of radiographs determined by localizing signs/symptoms

AP and lateral thoracic spine radiographs, or

AP, lateral, and oblique lumbosacral radiographs

Positive
Scheuermann's disease
Spondylolysis
Spondylolisthesis
Vertebral fracture
(2° known trauma)

Disc space narrowing
Vertebral mass

Negative, or if
Neurologic signs/symptoms
including + straight leg raising,
tight heel cord, lower extremity atrophy,
abnormal sensation or reflexes

MRI

Tethered cord
Herniated disc
Discitis
Intraspinal or epidural
neoplasm, abscess, or
hematoma

Neurologic signs/symptoms
uncertain due to pain or
suboptimal clinical exam

Bone scan
(with SPECT if normal)

Positive
Discitis
Vertebral osteomyelitis
Bone mass(es)

MRI

If bone mass present
CT may further
define lesion

Negative
Abdominal or retroperitoneal
etiology considered

No → MRI
Intraspinal or epidural
neoplasm, abscess, or
hematoma

Yes → CT with IV contrast
Hydronephrosis,
pyelonephritis,
abscess, etc.

SCOLIOSIS

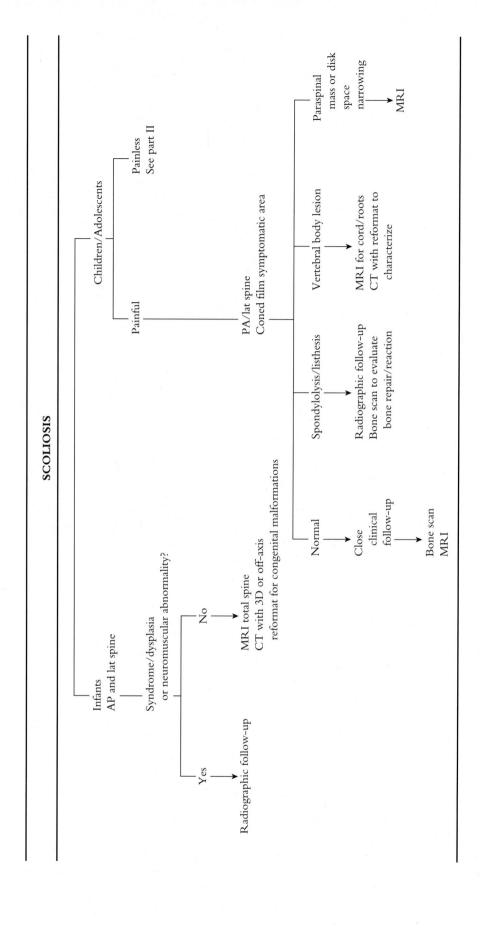

Infants
AP and lat spine

Syndrome/dysplasia
or neuromuscular abnormality?

Yes → Radiographic follow-up

No → MRI total spine
CT with 3D or off-axis
reformat for congenital malformations

Children/Adolescents

Painful

Painless
See part II

PA/lat spine
Coned film symptomatic area

Normal → Close
clinical
follow-up → Bone scan
MRI

Spondylolysis/listhesis → Radiographic follow-up
Bone scan to evaluate
bone repair/reaction

Vertebral body lesion → MRI for cord/roots
CT with reformat to
characterize

Paraspinal
mass or disk
space
narrowing → MRI

CHILDREN/ADOLESCENTS
PAINLESS SCOLIOSIS (PART II)

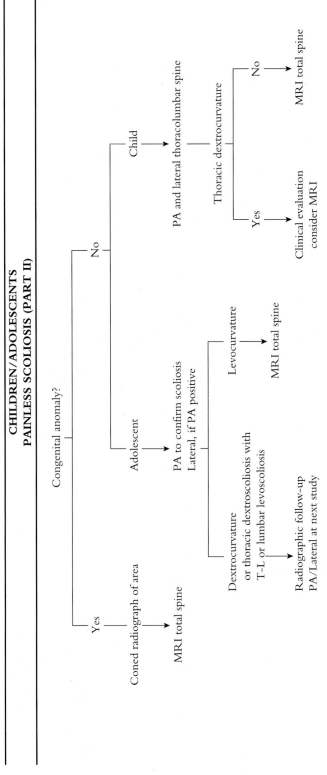

Clinically suspected scoliosis can be evaluated with frontal view only; lateral obtained immediately in all positive cases except adolescent idiopathic scoliosis. Any patient with neurological symptoms requires complete clinical evaluation and MRI if symptoms localized to spine. Long, arcuate curves suggest neuromuscular or CNS abnormality.

STRIDOR

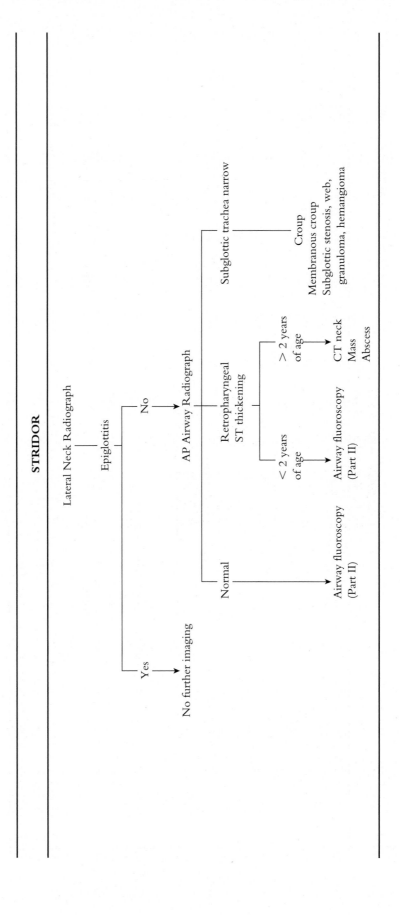

Lateral Neck Radiograph

Epiglottitis

Yes → No further imaging

No → AP Airway Radiograph

Normal → Airway fluoroscopy (Part II)

Retropharyngeal ST thickening
- < 2 years of age → Airway fluoroscopy (Part II)
- > 2 years of age → CT neck / Mass / Abscess

Subglottic trachea narrow
- Croup
- Membranous croup
- Subglottic stenosis, web, granuloma, hemangioma

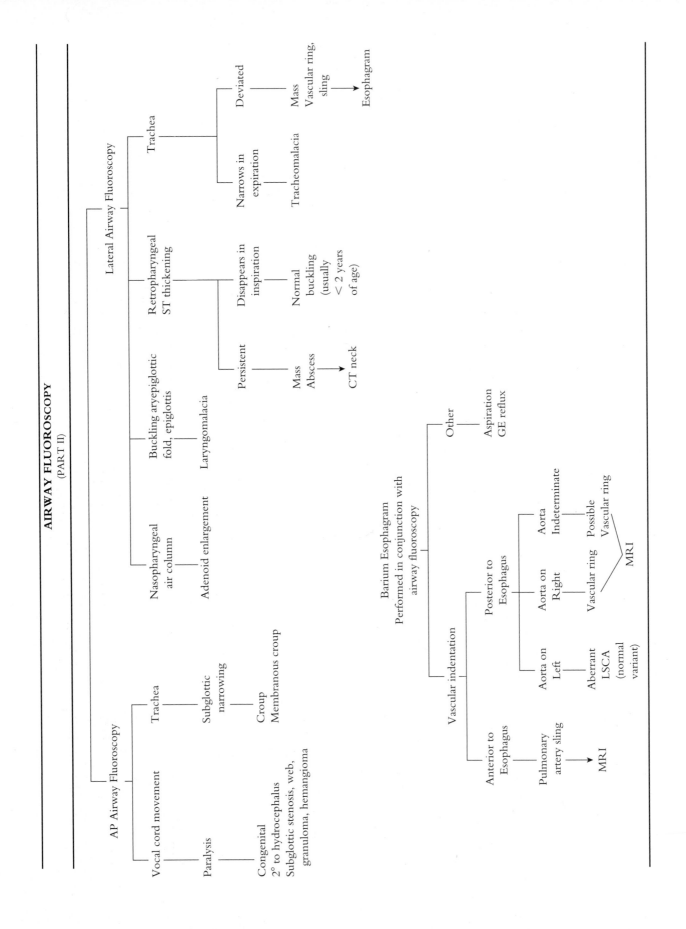

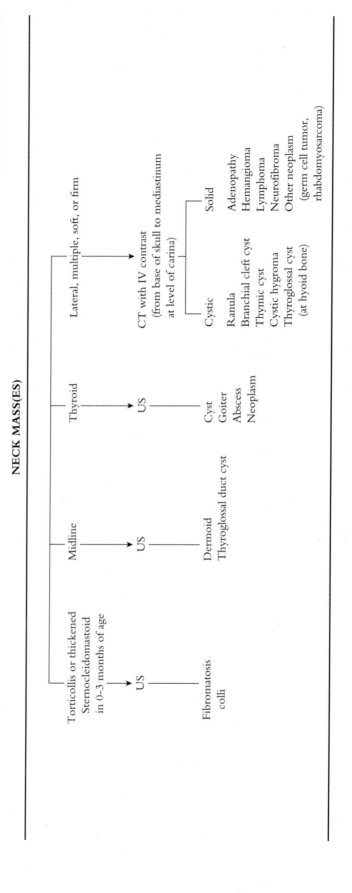

NECK MASS(ES)

Torticollis or thickened
Sternocleidomastoid
in 0–3 months of age

→ US — Fibromatosis
colli

Midline

→ US — Dermoid
Thyroglossal duct cyst

Thyroid

→ US — Cyst
Goiter
Abscess
Neoplasm

Lateral, multiple, soft, or firm

→ CT with IV contrast
(from base of skull to mediastinum
at level of carina)

Cystic
Ranula
Branchial cleft cyst
Thymic cyst
Cystic hygroma
Thyroglossal cyst
(at hyoid bone)

Solid
Adenopathy
Hemangioma
Lymphoma
Neurofibroma
Other neoplasm
(germ cell tumor,
rhabdomyosarcoma)

SINUSITIS

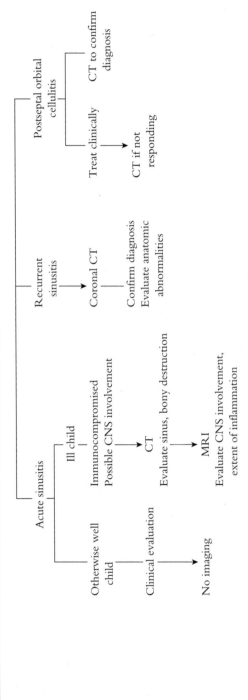

Acute sinusitis

Ill child
Immunocompromised
Possible CNS involvement
→ CT
Evaluate sinus, bony destruction
→ MRI
Evaluate CNS involvement,
extent of inflammation

Otherwise well child
Clinical evaluation
→ No imaging

Recurrent sinusitis
→ Coronal CT
Confirm diagnosis
Evaluate anatomic abnormalities

Postseptal orbital cellulitis

Treat clinically
→ CT if not responding

CT to confirm diagnosis

Soft tissue is found in the paranasal sinuses of more than 50% of children less than 1 year of age and remains common in young children. No imaging modality reliably diagnoses sinusitis in young children.

MINOR EXTREMITY TRAUMA

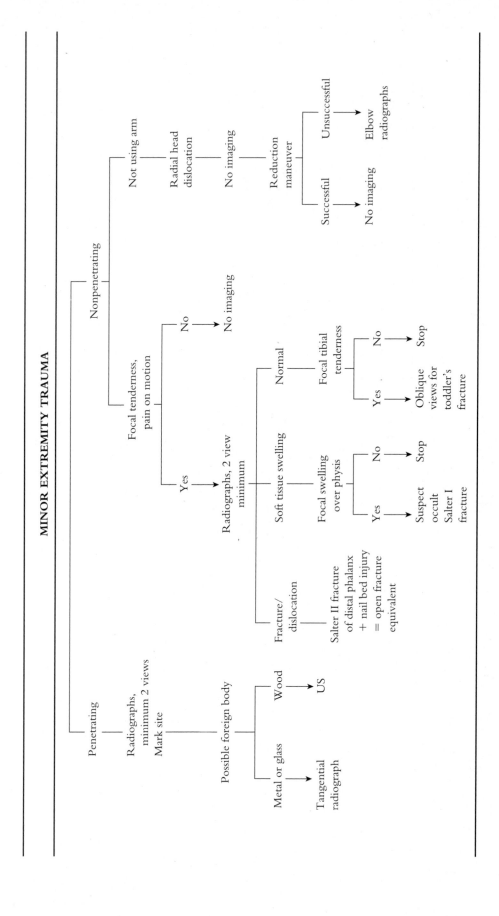

OSTEOMYELITIS

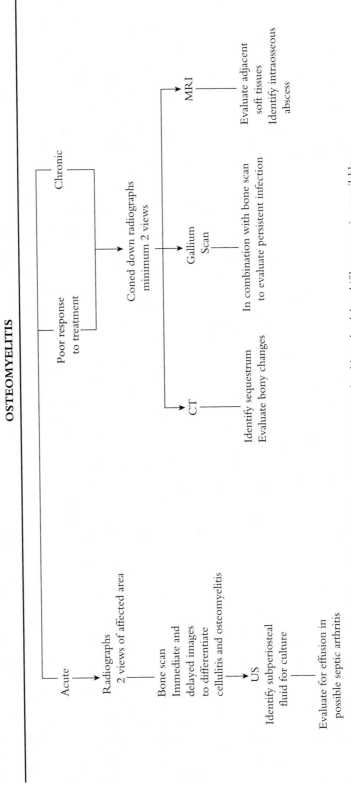

Acute

Radiographs
2 views of affected area

Bone scan
Immediate and
delayed images
to differentiate
cellulitis and osteomyelitis

US
Identify subperiosteal
fluid for culture

Evaluate for effusion in
possible septic arthritis

Chronic

Poor response
to treatment

Coned down radiographs
minimum 2 views

CT
Identify sequestrum
Evaluate bony changes

Gallium
Scan
In combination with bone scan
to evaluate persistent infection

MRI
Evaluate adjacent
soft tissues
Identify intraosseous
abscess

Bone scan remains diagnostic for > 3 days after beginning treatment. Treatment should not be delayed if bone scan is unavailable.
Bony changes may progress for weeks despite adequate treatment.

LIMP

Assessment of gait can limit diagnostic possibilities. Shoes should be examined for fit and abnormal wear and lower extremities observed for leg length discrepancy. Clinical evaluation should not be limited to the lower extremities. Discitis, appendicitis, and pyelonephritis can all present with limp.

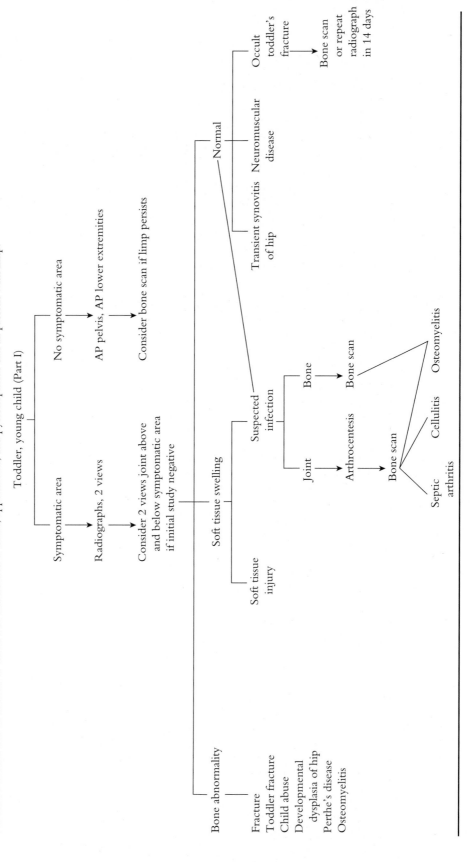

LIMP

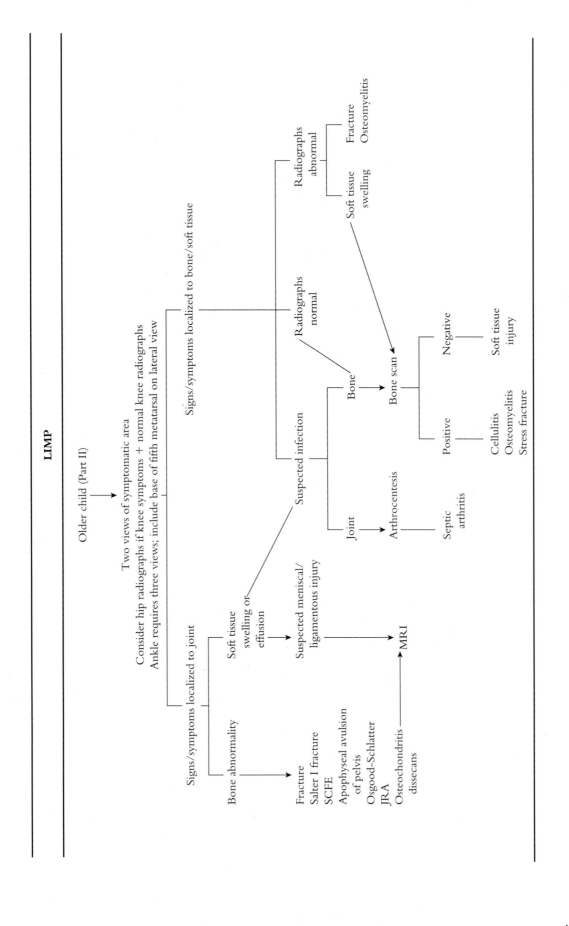

Older child (Part II)

Two views of symptomatic area
Consider hip radiographs if knee symptoms + normal knee radiographs
Ankle requires three views; include base of fifth metatarsal on lateral view

Signs/symptoms localized to joint

Signs/symptoms localized to bone/soft tissue

Bone abnormality

Fracture
Salter I fracture
SCFE
Apophyseal avulsion
of pelvis
Osgood-Schlatter
JRA
Osteochondritis
dissecans

Soft tissue
swelling or
effusion

Suspected meniscal/
ligamentous injury

MRI

Suspected infection

Joint

Arthrocentesis

Septic
arthritis

Bone

Bone scan

Positive

Cellulitis
Osteomyelitis
Stress fracture

Negative

Soft tissue
injury

Radiographs
normal

Radiographs
abnormal

Soft tissue
swelling

Fracture
Osteomyelitis

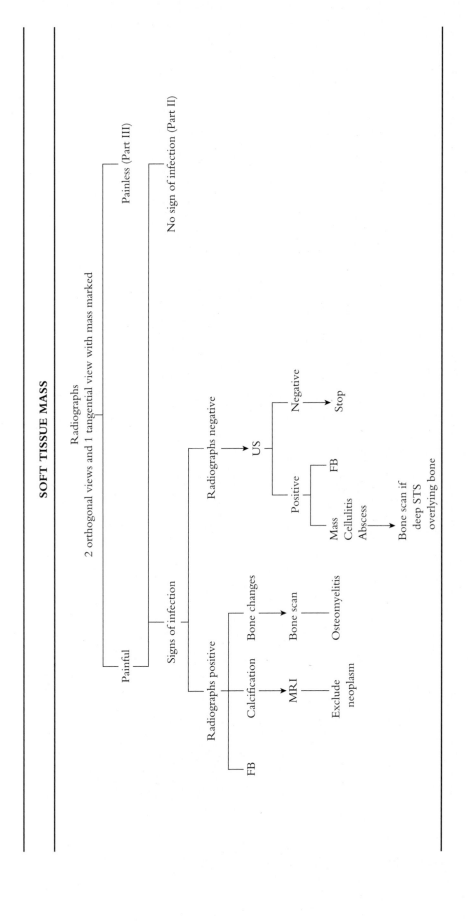

SOFT TISSUE MASS

Radiographs
2 orthogonal views and 1 tangential view with mass marked

Painful

Painless (Part III)

Signs of infection

No sign of infection (Part II)

Radiographs positive

Radiographs negative

FB

Calcification

Bone changes

MRI

Bone scan

Exclude neoplasm

Osteomyelitis

US

Negative → Stop

Positive

FB

Mass
Cellulitis
Abscess

Bone scan if deep STS overlying bone

SOFT TISSUE MASS

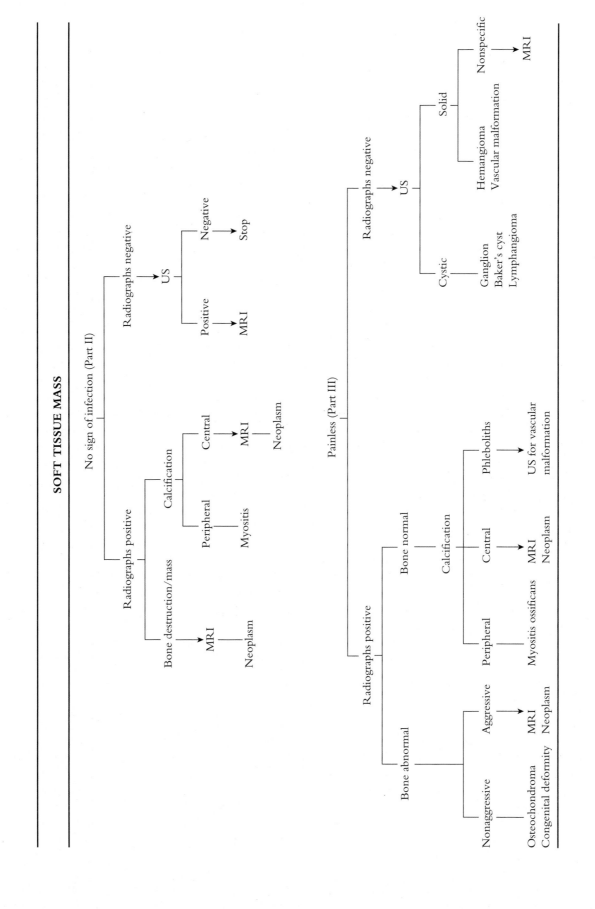

SUSPECTED HIP DYSPLASIA

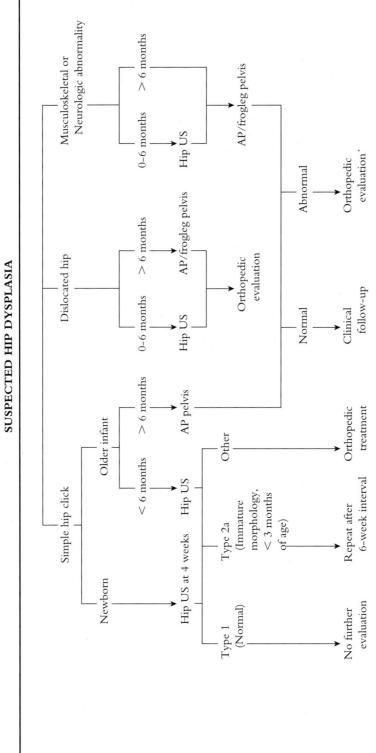

Delaying US in newborns until 4 weeks of age decreases number of repeat studies as type 2a morphology frequently matures to type 1 in this interval.

SUSPECTED CHILD ABUSE

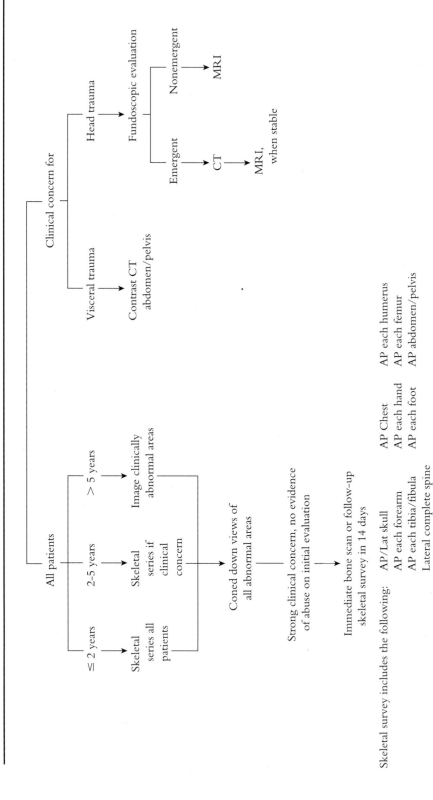

Clinical concern for

Visceral trauma → Contrast CT abdomen/pelvis

Head trauma → Fundoscopic evaluation

Emergent → CT → MRI, when stable

Nonemergent → MRI

All patients

≤ 2 years → Skeletal series all patients

2-5 years → Skeletal series if clinical concern

> 5 years → Image clinically abnormal areas

Coned down views of all abnormal areas

Strong clinical concern, no evidence of abuse on initial evaluation

Immediate bone scan or follow-up skeletal survey in 14 days

Skeletal survey includes the following:
AP/Lat skull
AP each forearm
AP each tibia/fibula
Lateral complete spine

AP Chest
AP each hand
AP each foot

AP each humerus
AP each femur
AP abdomen/pelvis

Imaging is one part of the team approach to child abuse evaluation.
If head CT obtained, skull series must also be obtained, since skull fractures are better detected on skull radiograph than on CT.
NORMAL IMAGING DOES NOT EQUAL ABSENCE OF ABUSE!

SHORT STATURE/BONE DYSPLASIA

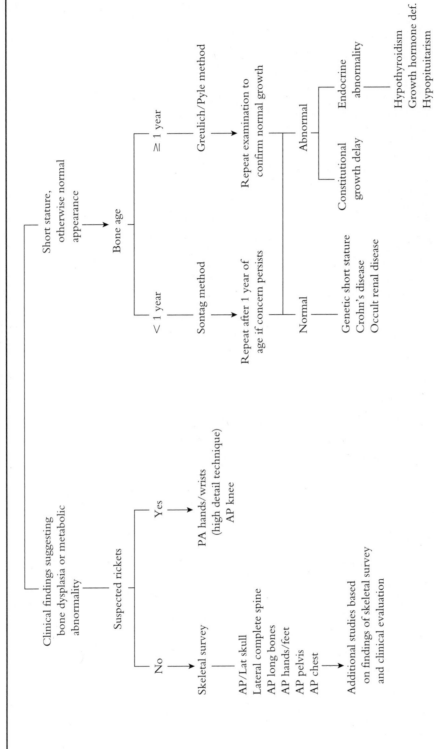

Clinical findings suggesting bone dysplasia or metabolic abnormality

Suspected rickets

No → Skeletal survey

AP/Lat skull
Lateral complete spine
AP long bones
AP hands/feet
AP pelvis
AP chest

Additional studies based on findings of skeletal survey and clinical evaluation

Yes → PA hands/wrists (high detail technique)
AP knee

Short stature, otherwise normal appearance → Bone age

< 1 year → Sontag method → Repeat after 1 year of age if concern persists

≥ 1 year → Greulich/Pyle method → Repeat examination to confirm normal growth

Normal
Genetic short stature
Crohn's disease
Occult renal disease

Abnormal

Constitutional growth delay

Endocrine abnormality
Hypothyroidism
Growth hormone def.
Hypopituitarism

Only a few examples of the many causes of short stature are given in this pathway. Over 300 skeletal dysplasias have been described. The reader is referred to the section on skeletal dysplasias for further information on some of the more common dysplasias and to Taybi's reference for a more complete description of dysplasias.

HYPERTENSION

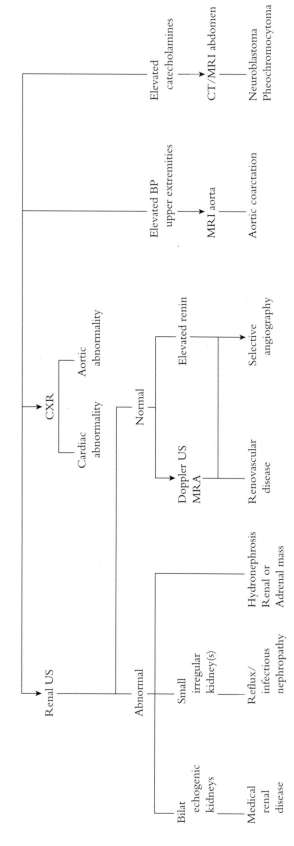

Essential hypertension is less common in children than in adults, but it remains the most common cause of systemic hypertension in children. Eighty percent of secondary hypertension in children is due to renal abnormality.

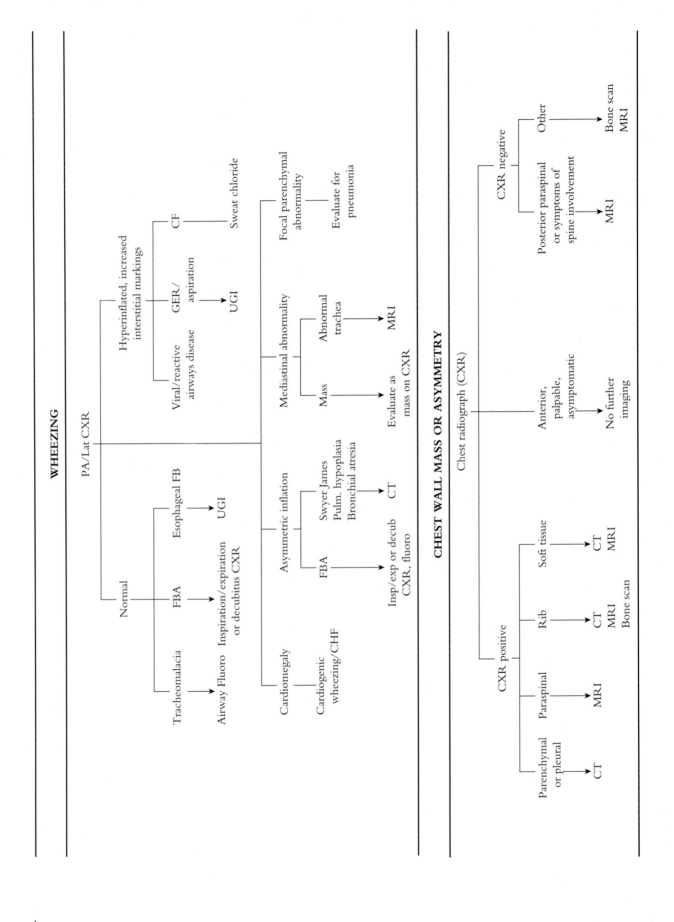

WHEEZING

PA/Lat CXR

Tracheomalacia — Airway Fluoro

Normal — FBA — Inspiration/expiration or decubitus CXR

Esophageal FB → UGI

Cardiomegaly — Cardiogenic wheezing/CHF

Asymmetric inflation

FBA → Insp/exp or decub CXR, fluoro

Swyer James
Pulm. hypoplasia
Bronchial atresia → CT

Viral/reactive airways disease

Hyperinflated, increased interstitial markings

GER/aspiration → UGI

CF — Sweat chloride

Mediastinal abnormality

Mass → Evaluate as mass on CXR

Abnormal trachea → MRI

Focal parenchymal abnormality — Evaluate for pneumonia

CHEST WALL MASS OR ASYMMETRY

Chest radiograph (CXR)

CXR positive

Parenchymal or pleural → CT

Paraspinal → MRI

Rib → CT
MRI
Bone scan

Soft tissue → CT
MRI

Anterior, palpable, asymptomatic → No further imaging

CXR negative

Posterior paraspinal or symptoms of spine involvement → MRI

Other → Bone scan
MRI

440

ABNORMALITY DETECTED ON CXR

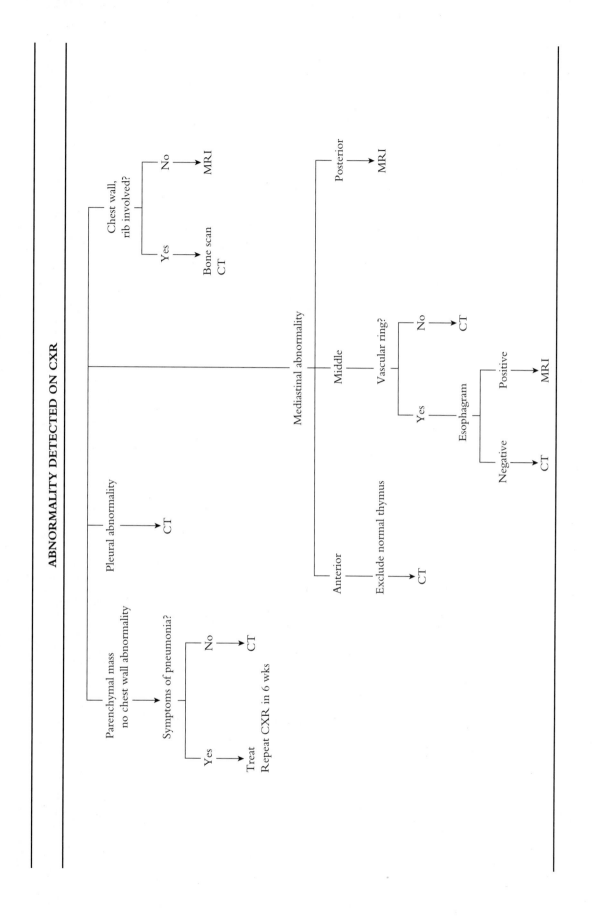

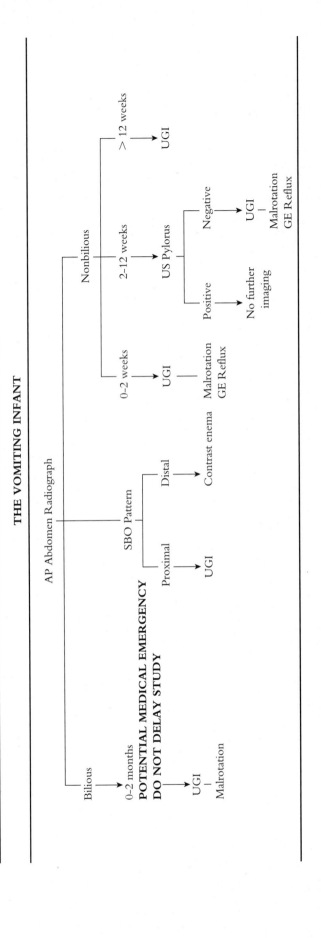

THE VOMITING INFANT

SMALL BOWEL OBSTRUCTION

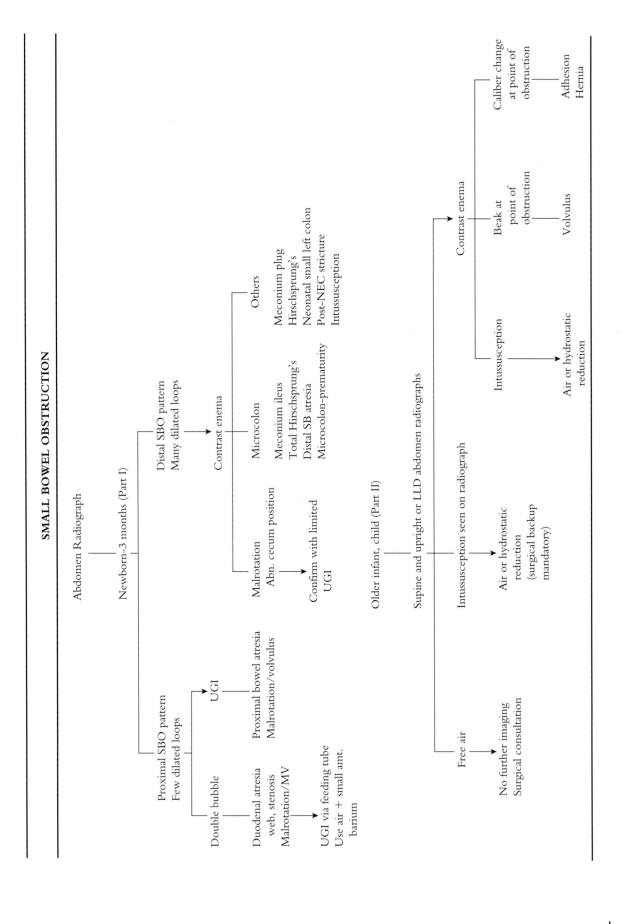

Abdomen Radiograph

Newborn–3 months (Part I)

Proximal SBO pattern
Few dilated loops

Double bubble
— Duodenal atresia web, stenosis Malrotation/MV

Proximal bowel atresia Malrotation/volvulus
— UGI
— UGI via feeding tube
Use air + small amt. barium

Distal SBO pattern
Many dilated loops
— Contrast enema

Malrotation
Abn. cecum position
— Confirm with limited UGI

Microcolon
Meconium ileus
Total Hirschsprung's
Distal SB atresia
Microcolon-prematurity

Others
Meconium plug
Hirschsprung's
Neonatal small left colon
Post-NEC stricture
Intussusception

Older infant, child (Part II)

Supine and upright or LLD abdomen radiographs

Free air
— No further imaging
Surgical consultation

Intussusception seen on radiograph
— Air or hydrostatic reduction (surgical backup mandatory)

Contrast enema

Intussusception
— Air or hydrostatic reduction

Beak at point of obstruction
— Volvulus

Caliber change at point of obstruction
Adhesion
Hernia

ABDOMINAL MASS

Abdomen and chest radiograph

Evaluate displacement of bowel loops, character of mass (calcified, air filled, etc.), location, possible paraspinal involvement

Evaluation of abdominal mass by cross-sectional imaging usually by US or CT. Outpatient study most often ordered for this indication is US because of lack of discomfort to the child (no IV or sedation required), comparative cost and radiation exposure considerations. Limitations of US include smaller field-of-view than CT or MRI, inability to image the lung for possible metastases, bowel gas, or body habitus restrictions. If mass incompletely evaluated by US or neoplastic, CT or MRI commonly obtained to define lesion more thoroughly.

US

Identify relation of mass to solid organs, involvement of solid organs by metastases, solid vs. cystic, homogeneous vs. heterogeneous, relation to vascular structures (displacement, encasement, or invasion)

CT

With oral but without IV contrast to identify calcification. Then with IV contrast to characterize mass, identify solid organ involvement, relationship to vascular structures

MRI

If paraspinal or intraspinal, multiplanar MRI without/ with gadolinium preferred to CT. Characterize, localize mass and its extension

Cystic Mass (Part I)

RUQ	Epigastric	Mesenteric	Renal	Adrenal	Hepatic	Variable	Spleen
Choledochal cyst	Pancreatic pseudocyst	Mesenteric cyst	Cystic kidney	Hemorrhage	Simple cyst	Ovarian cyst	2° trauma
Hepatic cyst	Duplication cyst	Cystic hygroma	MDK	"Cystic" NBL	Biliary ectasia	Meconium	Cystic
Duplication cyst		(lymphangioma)	Hydronephrosis		(Caroli's dis.)	pseudocyst	hygroma
Mesenchymal			Multilocular		"Cystic"	Pancreatic	"Cystic"
hamartoma			cystic nephroma		lymphoma	pseudocyst	lymphoma
			Tuberous sclerosis		Abscess	Duplication	
			"Cystic" lymphoma		Granulomas	cyst	
					Biloma		

444

ABDOMINAL MASS

Solid Mass (Part II)

Renal

< 1 year

Mesoblastic
nephroma
Wilms' tumor
Nephroblast-
omatosis
Angiomyo-
lipoma (TS)

> 1 year

Wilms' tumor
Nephroblast-
omatosis
Angiomyo-
lipoma (TS)
Leukemia/
lymphoma

> 10 year

Renal cell CA
Leukemia/
lymphoma
Angiomyo-
lipoma (TS)

Adrenal

Newborn

Hemorrhage
Neuroblastoma
(NBL)
→
Repeat US in
10–14 days

Hemorrhage will
liquefy

> 1 month

NBL
Pheochromo-
cytoma
Carcinoma
(precocious
puberty,
virilization)

Hepatic

Benign

Hemangioma
Adenoma
Focal nodular
hyperplasia
(FNH)

Malignant

Hepato-
blastoma (HBL)
Hepatocellular
carcinoma (HCC)
Fibrolamellar
hepatocellular
carcinoma
Leukemia/
lymphoma
Metastases

Obtain α fetoprotein level: elevated
in HBL and HCC, but not in
fibrolamellar HCC, nor in
benign liver tumors

Central scar: present in FNH
and fibrolamellar HCC

Calcified liver mass: HBL or
NBL, germ cell tumor, or
osteosarcoma mets

Spleen

Lymphoma
Metastases

**Diffuse,
peritoneal**

Leukemia
Lymphoma
Rhabdomyo-
sarcoma
Undifferentiated
sarcoma

Note: TS = Tuberous sclerosis.

445

ABDOMEN/PELVIC TRAUMA

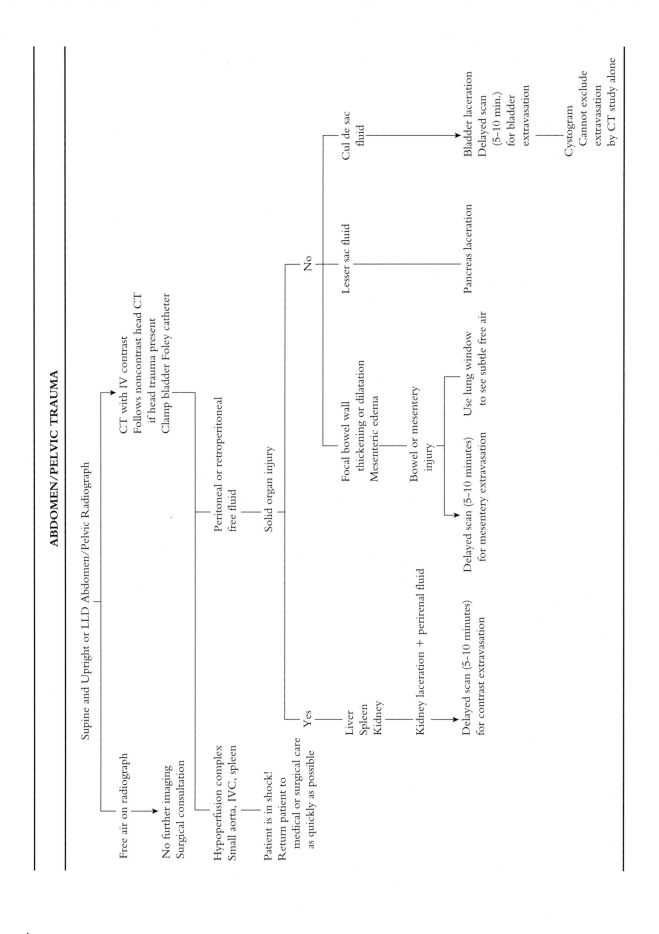

Supine and Upright or LLD Abdomen/Pelvic Radiograph

Free air on radiograph

No further imaging
Surgical consultation

CT with IV contrast
Follows noncontrast head CT
if head trauma present
Clamp bladder Foley catheter

Peritoneal or retroperitoneal
free fluid

Solid organ injury

Hypoperfusion complex
Small aorta, IVC, spleen

Patient is in shock!
Return patient to
medical or surgical care
as quickly as possible

Yes

No

Liver
Spleen
Kidney

Kidney laceration + perirenal fluid

Delayed scan (5–10 minutes)
for contrast extravasation

Focal bowel wall
thickening or dilatation
Mesenteric edema

Bowel or mesentery
injury

Delayed scan (5–10 minutes)
for mesentery extravasation

Use lung window
to see subtle free air

Lesser sac fluid

Pancreas laceration

Cul de sac
fluid

Bladder laceration
Delayed scan
(5–10 min.)
for bladder
extravasation

Cystogram
Cannot exclude
extravasation
by CT study alone

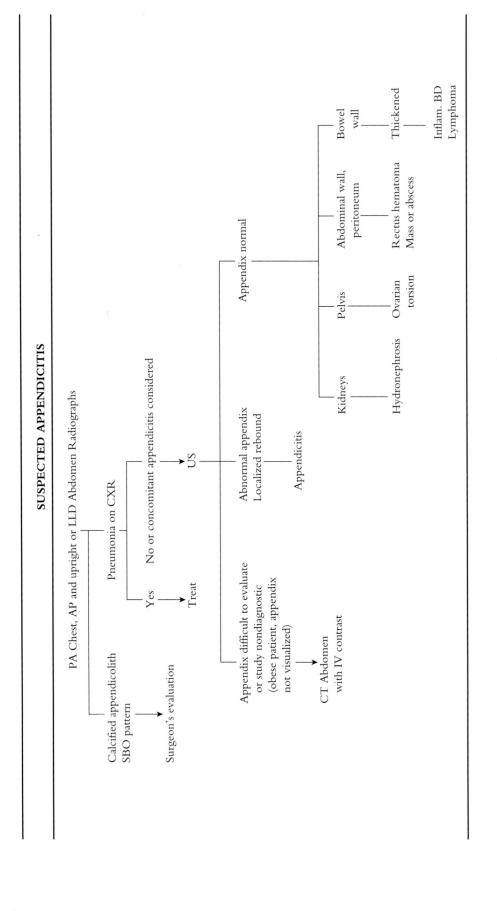

SUSPECTED APPENDICITIS

PA Chest, AP and upright or LLD Abdomen Radiographs

Calcified appendicolith
SBO pattern

Surgeon's evaluation

Pneumonia on CXR

No or concomitant appendicitis considered

Yes → Treat

US

Appendix difficult to evaluate
or study nondiagnostic
(obese patient, appendix
not visualized)

CT Abdomen
with IV contrast

Abnormal appendix
Localized rebound

Appendicitis

Appendix normal

Kidneys

Hydronephrosis

Pelvis

Ovarian
torsion

Abdominal wall,
peritoneum

Rectus hematoma
Mass or abscess

Bowel
wall

Thickened

Inflam. BD
Lymphoma

ACUTE ABDOMEN

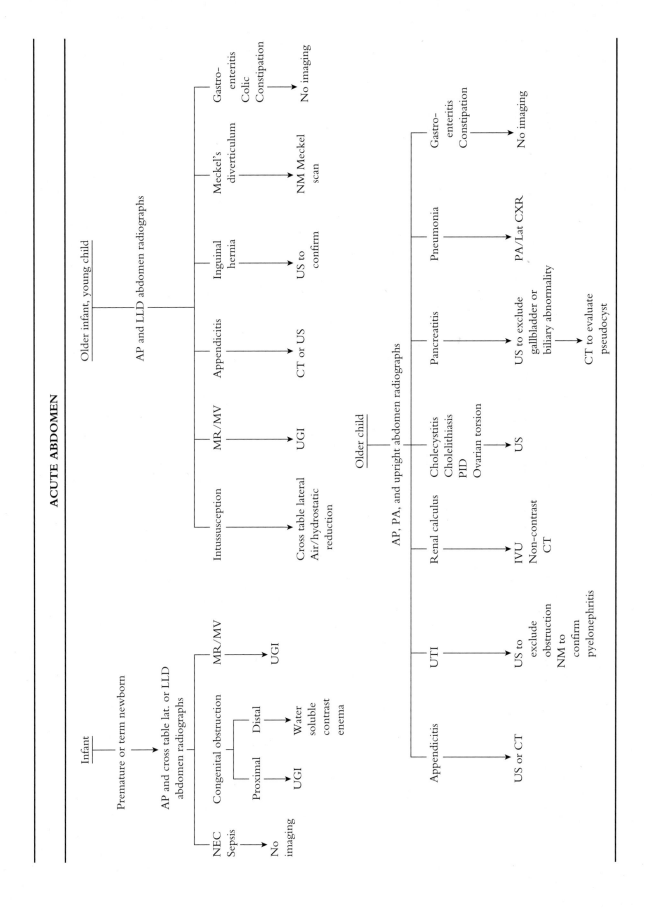

CHRONIC ABDOMINAL PAIN

Normal appetite
Normal physical exam
Normal laboratory studies
Periumbilical pain

Weight loss
Growth failure
Fever
Flank or pelvic pain
< 2 years of age

Yes → Functional abdominal pain → No imaging

No

No → Organic abdominal pain

Yes → Organic abdominal pain → AP or PA and upright or LLD abdomen radiographs

Urinary tract abnormality
Cholelithiasis
Choledochal cyst → US

Inflammatory bowel disease → UGI/SBFT

Lead intoxication → Knee radiographs to evaluate duration of exposure

Constipation
Lactose intol.
Giardiasis → No imaging

Unlike most functional disorders, functional abdominal pain may wake the child from sleep.

At most, 10% of childhood chronic abdominal pain is due to organic causes.

If an organic process exists, genitourinary and gastrointestinal causes are equally likely.

If no specific etiology is suggested by clinical evaluation, abdominal ultrasound is a reasonable examination. This may be followed by UGI/SBFT.

449

CONSTIPATION

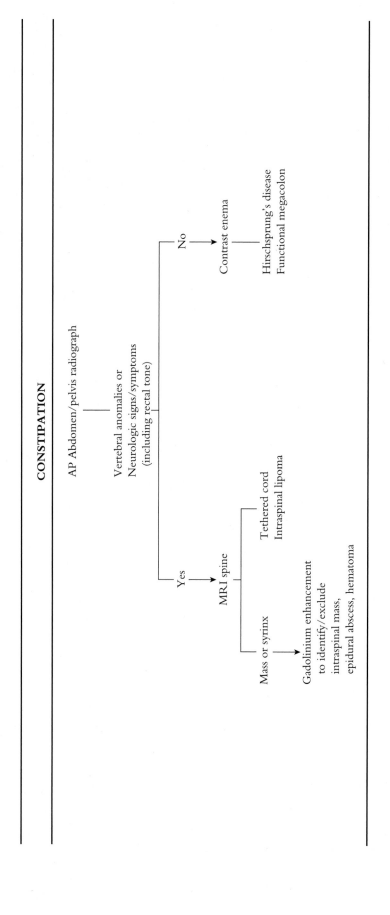

AP Abdomen/pelvis radiograph

Vertebral anomalies or
Neurologic signs/symptoms
(including rectal tone)

Yes → MRI spine

No → Contrast enema

Tethered cord
Intraspinal lipoma

Mass or syrinx → Gadolinium enhancement
to identify/exclude
intraspinal mass,
epidural abscess, hematoma

Hirschsprung's disease
Functional megacolon

DIARRHEA

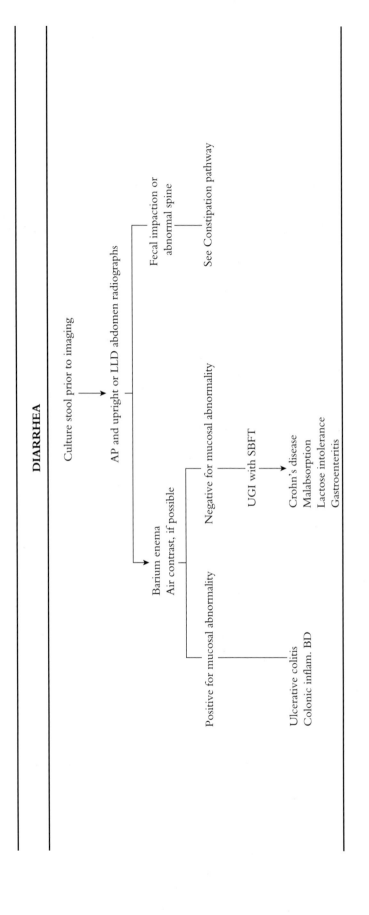

Culture stool prior to imaging

AP and upright or LLD abdomen radiographs

Barium enema
Air contrast, if possible

Negative for mucosal abnormality

UGI with SBFT

Crohn's disease
Malabsorption
Lactose intolerance
Gastroenteritis

Positive for mucosal abnormality

Ulcerative colitis
Colonic inflam. BD

Fecal impaction or
abnormal spine

See Constipation pathway

NEONATAL ABDOMINAL DISTENTION

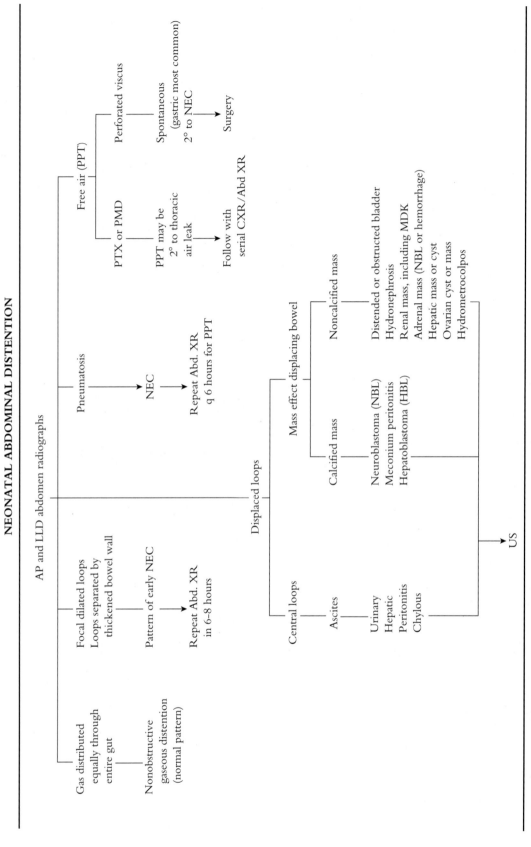

Note: PPT = Pneumoperitoneum; PTX = Pneumothorax; PMD = Pneumomediastinum; NEC = Necrotizing enterocolitis; MDK = Multicystic dysplastic kidney.

FIRST UTI

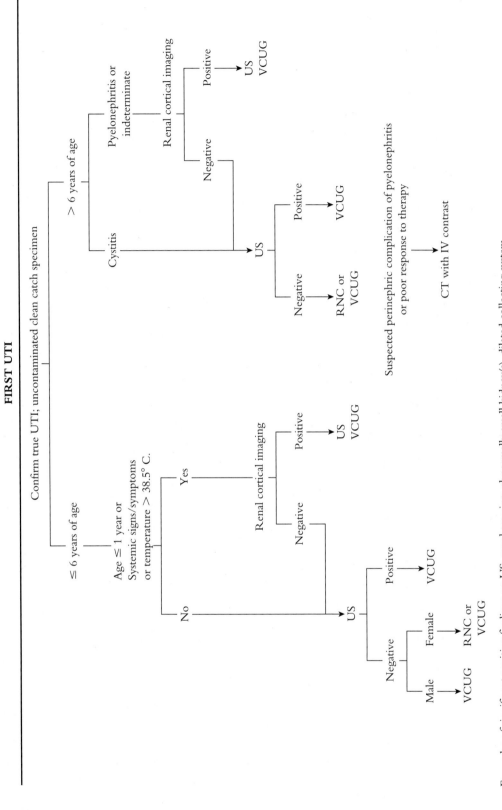

Confirm true UTI; uncontaminated clean catch specimen

≤ 6 years of age

Age ≤ 1 year or Systemic signs/symptoms or temperature > 38.5° C.

Yes

Renal cortical imaging

Positive → US VCUG

Negative

No

US

Positive → VCUG

Negative

Female → RNC or VCUG

Male → VCUG

> 6 years of age

Pyelonephritis or indeterminate

Renal cortical imaging

Positive → US VCUG

Negative

Cystitis

US

Positive → VCUG

Negative → RNC or VCUG

Suspected perinephric complication of pyelonephritis or poor response to therapy

CT with IV contrast

Examples of significant positive findings on US: renal scarring, abnormally small kidney(s), dilated collecting system.

Renal cortical imaging performed with 99mTc DMSA or glucoheptonate.

Radionuclide cystogram (RNC) requires 1/10 to 1/100 the dose of VCUG.

RNC is especially useful for follow-up studies and for children with a low likelihood of reflux.

TESTICULAR PAIN/SWELLING

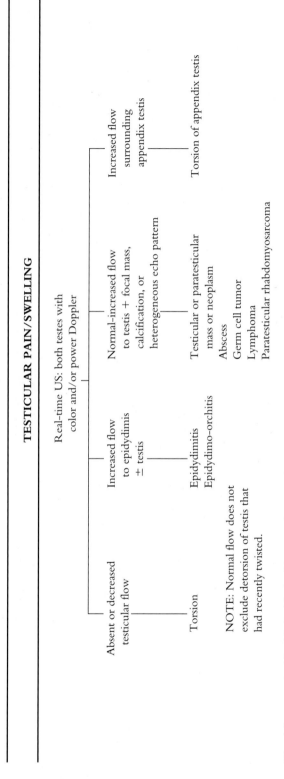

Real-time US: both testes with
color and/or power Doppler

Absent or decreased testicular flow

Torsion

NOTE: Normal flow does not
exclude detorsion of testis that
had recently twisted.

Increased flow to epydydimis ± testis

Epidydimitis
Epidydimo-orchitis

Normal-increased flow to testis + focal mass, calcification, or heterogeneous echo pattern

Testicular or paratesticular
mass or neoplasm

Abscess
Germ cell tumor
Lymphoma
Paratesticular rhabdomyosarcoma

Increased flow surrounding appendix testis

Torsion of appendix testis

Blood flow must be identified with confidence in the normal testis to ensure diagnostic examination for torsion in the symptomatic testis.
There is a limited grace period (usually 6 hours) for testicular viability following testicular torsion.
If US study is indeterminate, <u>immediate</u> urologic evaluation is mandatory.

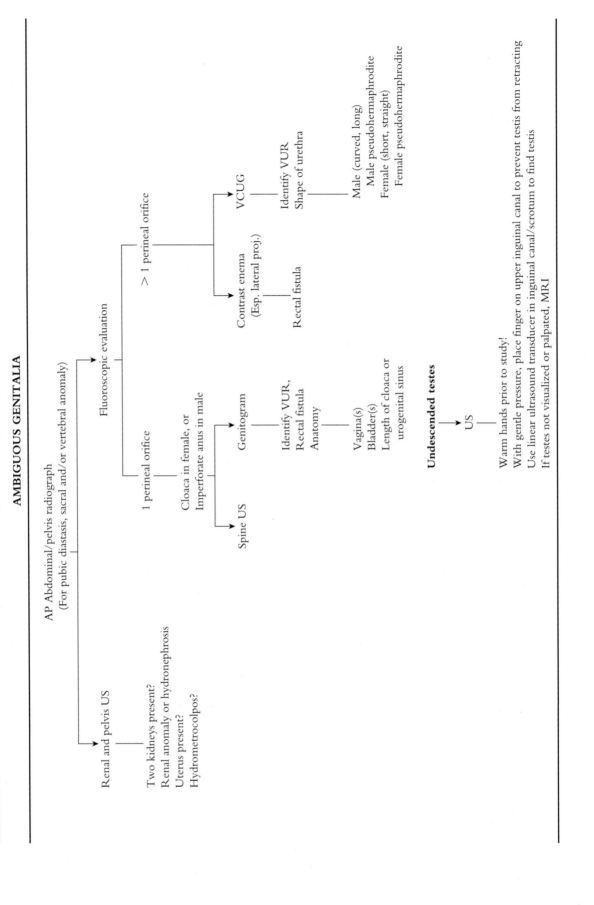

AMBIGUOUS GENITALIA

AP Abdominal/pelvis radiograph
(For pubic diastasis, sacral and/or vertebral anomaly)

Renal and pelvis US
- Two kidneys present?
- Renal anomaly or hydronephrosis
- Uterus present?
- Hydrometrocolpos?

Fluoroscopic evaluation

1 perineal orifice
- Cloaca in female, or Imperforate anus in male
- Spine US
- Genitogram
  - Identify VUR, Rectal fistula Anatomy
  - Vagina(s)
  - Bladder(s)
  - Length of cloaca or urogenital sinus

> 1 perineal orifice
- Contrast enema (Esp. lateral proj.)
  - Rectal fistula
- VCUG
  - Identify VUR
  - Shape of urethra
    - Male (curved, long) — Male pseudohermaphrodite
    - Female (short, straight) — Female pseudohermaphrodite

Undescended testes
- US
  - Warm hands prior to study!
  - With gentle pressure, place finger on upper inguinal canal to prevent testis from retracting
  - Use linear ultrasound transducer in inguinal canal/scrotum to find testis
  - If testes not visualized or palpated, MRI

APPENDIX 1: ROUTINE PROJECTIONS FOR CONVENTIONAL PEDIATRIC IMAGING

GENERAL NOTES

Use of gonad shields:

a. Whenever possible, the child's gonads should be shielded on all films where gonads are in the primary beam.

b. When a seated patient is having films taken of the upper extremity, it is very possible that the gonads are in the primary beam; therefore, the gonads should be covered with a glove or other protective device.

Trauma:

a. With the exception of films of the hips, comparison views are usually not necessary.

b. When a long-bone injury is suspected, the joints above and below the site of injury should be included on the radiograph.

c. Soft tissue radiography for a foreign body: A metallic marker should point to the site of injury on at least one view.

Detail films:

a. Whenever listed, detail film/screens should be used, except on follow-up orthopedic work, when plaster might obscure the image.

BODY

EXAM: Child Acute Abdomen

FILMS: AP SUPINE

AP UPRIGHT

PA ERECT CHEST★

The AP upright must include the pelvis to the symphysis. If the diaphragms are not seen, then Film #3 must be taken.★

EXAM: Infant Acute Abdomen

FILMS: AP SUPINE

LEFT LATERAL DECUBITUS (LEFT SIDE DOWN)

FOR EXAMPLE: Suspected NEC, Obstruction, or Intussusception.

EXAM: Routine Abdomen

FILM: AP SUPINE

FOR EXAMPLE: Tube placement evaluation.

EXAM: Trauma Abdomen

FILMS: AP SUPINE

CROSSTABLE LATERAL (if patient can't be moved)

If patient can tolerate positioning, then Film #2 may be AP UPRIGHT or LEFT LATERAL DECUBITUS.

EXAM: Routine Lumbosacral Spine
    FILMS: AP SUPINE
                LATERAL

EXAM: Lumbosacral Spine for Spondylolysis
    FILMS: AP SUPINE
                LATERAL
                RT OBLIQUE
                LT OBLIQUE

EXAM: Pelvis
    FILMS: AP SUPINE

EXAM: Chest for Possible Foreign Body
    FILMS: PA INSPIRATORY
                PA EXPIRATORY

If child is too young to cooperate, RT *and* LT LATERAL DECUBITUS Films can substitute for Film #2 (TOTAL OF 3 FILMS).

EXAM: Routine Chest
    FILMS: PA
                LATERAL

AP SUPINE and CROSSTABLE LATERAL films may be done if child is too young or too ill to stand. Films should be taken in Inspiration.

EXAM: Ribs
    FILMS: AP
                OBLIQUE (BUCKY)

NOTE: A third film for ribs seen below the diaphragm may be necessary.

EXAM: Sternum
    FILMS: CONED LATERAL

EXAM: Thoracic Spine
    FILMS: AP
                LATERAL

EXTREMITIES

EXAM: Ankle
    FILMS: AP
                LATERAL
                INTERNAL OBLIQUE 15 degree
                EXTERNAL OBLIQUE

DETAIL FILM/SCREEN COMBINATION.

EXAM: Calcaneus
    FILMS: LATERAL
                TANGENTIAL

SLOMAN VIEW (STANDING OBLIQUE)

EXAM: Clavicle

    FILMS: AP

                AP AXIAL 35 degree CEPHALAD ANGULATION

NOTE: Both clavicles may be included on newborn exam but it is not necessary to include both.

EXAM: Elbow

    FILMS: TRUE LATERAL 90 degree FLEXION

                AP

If elbow cannot be extended, AP projections of the distal humerus and proximal radius/ulna should be obtained using two exposures. Use detail film/screen combination. Lateral view must be a *true* lateral!

EXAM: Femur

    FILMS: AP

                LATERAL

EXAM: Finger

    FILMS: PA

                LATERAL

                OBLIQUE

NOTE: Detail film/screen combination.

EXAM: Foot for Club/Flat Foot

    FILMS: AP WEIGHT BEARING (OR SIMULATED WEIGHT BEARING)

                LATERAL WEIGHT BEARING (OR SIMULATED)

                LATERAL MAXIMUM DORSIFLEXION

NOTE: Weight bearing may be simulated by firmly pressing the foot against the cassette or a sponge.

EXAM: Routine Foot

    FILMS: AP

                LATERAL

                OBLIQUE

NOTE: Detail film/screen combination.

EXAM: Foot for Vertical Talus evaluation

    FILMS: AP WEIGHT BEARING (OR SIMULATED)

                LATERAL WEIGHT BEARING (OR SIMULATED) LATERAL MAXIMUM PLANTARFLEXION

EXAM: Forearm

    FILMS: AP

                LATERAL

NOTE: This is not an adequate examination for either the WRIST or the ELBOW. If pathology is suspected in either site, specific films for the wrist or elbow should be obtained. If an angulated fracture of the radius or ulna is found, images of the wrist and elbow *must* be included or obtained.

EXAM: Hand for Bone Age

    FILMS: PA of LEFT HAND AND WRIST

NOTE: Detail film/screen combination.

EXAM: Routine Hand

    FILMS: PA

                60 degree OBLIQUE

                LATERAL WITH FINGERS SPREAD

NOTE: Detail film/screen combination.

EXAM: Hip for Dysplasia

    FILMS: AP PELVIS

                FROGLEG LATERAL PELVIS

                VON ROSEN VIEW★

If the infant is in a harness, do Film #1 only. ★Film #3 should only be done on the initial exam.

EXAM: Routine Hip

    FILMS: AP PELVIS

                FROGLEG LATERAL

NOTE: FROGLEG LATERAL only on affected side. Shield gonads on LATERAL only.

EXAM: Humerus

    FILMS: AP

                LATERAL

EXAM: Knee for Osteochondritis

    FILMS: AP

                LATERAL 15 degree FLEXION

                TUNNEL (OR HUGHSTON) VIEW

EXAM: Routine Knee

    FILMS: AP

                LATERAL 15 degree FLEXION

EXAM: Knee for Trauma

    FILMS: AP

                LATERAL 15 degree FLEXION

                INTERNAL OBLIQUE

                EXTERNAL OBLIQUE

NOTE: Detail film/screen combination.

EXAM: Patella

    FILMS: PA

                TANGENTIAL

EXAM: Scapula

    FILMS: AP

                LATERAL

EXAM: Shoulder for Arthritis or Posterior Dislocation
    FILMS: AP
                POSTERIOR OBLIQUE

EXAM: Routine Shoulder
    FILMS: AP INTERNAL ROTATION
                AP EXTERNAL ROTATION
                ANTERIOR OBLIQUE ("Y"VIEW)

EXAM: Standing Feet for Orthopedic Evaluation (SEE CLUB/FLAT FOOT)
    FILMS: AP
                LATERAL in MAXIMUM DORSIFLEXION

EXAM: Thumb
    FILMS: AP
                LATERAL
                OBLIQUE

NOTE: Detail film/screen combination.

EXAM: Tibia
    FILMS: AP
                LATERAL

EXAM: Toe
    FILMS: AP
                OBLIQUE
                LATERAL

NOTE: Detail film/screen combination.

EXAM: Wrist
    FILMS: AP
                LATERAL
                NAVICULAR VIEW★

NOTE: Detail film/screen combination.
★Film #3 if Navicular fracture is suspected.

HEAD & NECK

EXAM: Adenoids
    FILMS: LATERAL FACE

NOTE: Soft Tissue Technique.

EXAM: Airway for Acute Symptoms
    FILMS: AP INSPIRATION
                LATERAL INSPIRATION

NOTE: Films should be taken while child is breathing in, not at the end of inspiration.

EXAM: Airway for Chronic Symptoms
FILMS: AP INSPIRATION
AP EXPIRATION
LATERAL INSPIRATION
LATERAL EXPIRATION

NOTE: This examination is performed to demonstrate upper respiratory tract obstruction, inflammation, or other disease. If the child is in serious or acute respiratory distress, only a SOFT TISSUE LATERAL NECK should be obtained.

EXAM: Cervical Spine
FILMS: LATERAL first
AP
ODONTOID (OPEN MOUTH)

NOTE: If the patient is in a collar for acute injury, show the LATERAL to an MD before removing the collar for further views.

EXAM: Facial Bones
FILMS: PA
WATERS
LATERAL
SUBMENTOVERTEX★

★NOTE: Film #4 only if zygomatic arch fracture suspected.
WATERS VIEW taken UPRIGHT if possible.

EXAM: Mandible
FILMS: TOWNES
PA
RT LATERAL OBLIQUE
LT LATERAL OBLIQUE

EXAM: Mastoids
FILMS: TOWNES
MODIFIED LAWS
STENVERS

NOTE: Show the request to a radiologist before performing exam. CT may be more appropriate study to evaluate fracture or mastoiditis.

EXAM: Nasal Bones for Trauma
FILMS: WATERS
LATERAL

NOTE: LATERAL on Detail film/screen.

EXAM: Orbits for Foreign Body
FILMS: CONED WATERS
LATERAL

NOTE: Detail film/screen combination.

EXAM: Routine Orbits
FILMS: PA
              WATERS

NOTE: Film #2 UPRIGHT if possible.

EXAM: Sella
FILMS: ` CONED LATERAL

EXAM: Sinuses
FILM: CALDWELL
           WATERS
           LATERAL

NOTE: All UPRIGHT if possible, but at least one film with HORIZONTAL BEAM. WATERS should be done with OPEN MOUTH if possible.

EXAM: Skull for Headaches or Short Stature
FILM: LATERAL

EXAM: Routine Skull
FILMS: PA
            LATERAL

NOTE: Film #1 can be AP if child is uncooperative. Film #2 should be done CROSSTABLE.

EXAM: Skull for Trauma
FILMS: PA
            LATERAL
            TOWNES

NOTE: Film #1 can be AP if child is uncooperative. Film #2 should be done CROSSTABLE.

EXAM: Soft Tissue Lateral Neck
FILM: LATERAL

NOTE: Do not force the child to lie down if he/she is in respiratory distress. This Film can be obtained CROSSTABLE LATERAL. Film should be taken DURING INSPIRATION WITH THE MOUTH OPEN.

EXAM: Temporomandibular Joint
FILMS: TOWNES
           RT OPEN MOUTH LATERAL OBLIQUE
           RT CLOSED MOUTH LATERAL OBLIQUE
           LT OPEN MOUTH LATERAL OBLIQUE
           LT CLOSED MOUTH LATERAL OBLIQUE

PROCEDURES

EXAM: Air Contrast Barium Enema for Rectal Bleeding, Suspected Colitis
FILMS: AP SUPINE ABDOMEN
           PA PRONE ABDOMEN

RT LATERAL DECUBITUS
LT LATERAL DECUBITUS
BOTH SUPINE OBLIQUES
CROSS TABLE LATERAL PRONE RECTUM.

NOTE: Total Films = 7. Consult with radiologist about Post-Evac Film.

EXAM: Air Contrast UGI for Suspected Ulcer, Bleeding
FILMS: AP STOMACH
PA STOMACH
RT LATERAL STOMACH
LPO STOMACH
UPRIGHT AP STOMACH

NOTE: Consult with radiologist before beginning this study

EXAM: IVP
FILMS: AP ABDOMEN/PELVIS (KUB) PRE-INJECTION
AP CONED KIDNEYS, 2 MINUTES
AP ABDOMEN/PELVIS (KUB), 7 MINUTES

NOTE: Show initial film to radiologist before injection. Show 2 and 7 minute films to radiologist before dismissing patient.

EXAM: Barium Enema for Constipation
FILMS: AP ABDOMEN PRE-STUDY
AP ABDOMEN FILLED
LATERAL RECTOSIGMOID FILLED
AP ABDOMEN POST-EVAC
LATERAL RECTOSIGMOID POST-EVAC

EXAM: Routine Barium Enema
FILMS: AP ABDOMEN PRE-STUDY
AP ABDOMEN FILLED
AP ABDOMEN POST-EVAC

EXAM: Routine UGI For Child
FILMS: AP ABDOMEN PRE-STUDY
AP ABDOMEN
RT LATERAL DECUBITUS STOMACH
LPO STOMACH

NOTE: INCLUDE FULL ABDOMEN ON AP

EXAM: Routine UGI for Infant
FILMS: AP ABDOMEN PRE-STUDY
AP ABDOMEN

NOTE: Include full abdomen on AP

EXAM: VCUG
FILM: AP ABDOMEN/PELVIS PRE-STUDY

SURVEYS

EXAM: Bone Age for infant <18 MOS
   FILMS: AP (TRUE) LEFT UPPER EXTREMITY INCLUDING SHOULDER AND HAND
              LATERAL LEFT KNEE, OBLIQUE LEFT FOOT AND ANKLE

EXAM: Bone Age for child ≥18 MOS
   FILMS: PA LEFT HAND AND WRIST

EXAM: Rickets Survey for premature infant
   FILMS: AP LEFT WRIST AND HAND

EXAM: Rickets Survey for infant or child
   FILMS: AP BOTH HANDS AND WRISTS
              AP BOTH KNEES

EXAM: Scoliosis Evaluation
   FILMS: UPRIGHT PA T-L SPINE
              LATERAL T-L SPINE

NOTE: 10 ft Tube-to-Film distance for PA. Include entire T-L spine on one film WITH PATIENT'S KNEES TOGETHER AND FULLY EXTENDED. LATERAL VIEW should be made WITH THE PATIENT'S ARMS EXTENDED STRAIGHT FORWARD, NOT OVER THE HEAD.

EXAM: Scoliosis Follow-up
   FILMS: UPRIGHT PA T-L SPINE

NOTE: 10 ft Tube-to-Film distance for PA. Include entire T-L spine on one film WITH PATIENT'S KNEES TOGETHER AND FULLY EXTENDED.

EXAM: Scoliosis Screening
   FILMS: UPRIGHT PA T-L SPINE

NOTE: 14 × 17 OR 14 × 36 10 ft PA WITH PATIENT'S KNEES TOGETHER AND FULLY EXTENDED. CONE TO THE T-L SPINE.

EXAM: Shunt Series to R/O Malfunction
   FILMS: AP CHEST
              AP SKULL
              LATERAL SKULL
              AP ABDOMEN

NOTE: Include Neck on CHEST and SKULL FILMS.

EXAM: Skeletal Survey for Non-Accidental Trauma
   FILMS: AP AND LATERAL SKULL
              AP AND LATERAL CHEST
              AP INDIVIDUAL LONG BONES
              AP PELVIS
              LATERAL COMPLETE SPINE

NOTE: A BABYGRAM is UNSATISFACTORY.

EXAM: Skeletal Survey for Dysplasia or Genetic Evaluation
FILMS: AP AND LATERAL SKULL

AP AND LATERAL COMPLETE SPINE

AP LONG BONES

AP PELVIS

AP CHEST

AP BOTH HANDS

APPENDIX 2   PEDIATRIC NUCLEAR IMAGING

Study	Isotope	Comment	Dose (μCi/kg)	Minimum (mCi)	Maximum (mCi)
Bone Scan	^{99m}Tc-MDP	Malignancy	285	0.600	20
		Others	175	0.600	15
Myocardial scan	^{201}Thallium-chloride		30		1.5
Right-to-left shunt	^{99m}Tc-MAA		100 to 400 μCi		
Gastric emptying	^{99m}Tc-SC	<2 yrs		200 μCi	
Gastric emptying	^{99m}Tc-SC	2–4 yrs		300 μCi	
Gastric emptying	^{99m}Tc-SC	≥4 yrs		400 μCi	
Liver-spleen scan	^{99m}Tc-SC		66	0.300	2
Hepatobiliary	^{99m}Tc-IDA		66	0.400	3
Meckel's	^{99m}Tc-pertechnetate		44	0.250	3
Gallium	^{67}Ga-citrate	Malignancy	110	0.250	7.5
		Others	33	0.150	2
Thyroid	^{99m}Tc-pertechnetate		66	0.015	3
Lung perfusion	^{99m}Tc-MAA		88	0.400	2
Renogram/GFR	^{99m}Tc-DTPA		55	0.250	3
	^{99m}Tc-MAG$_3$		80	0.300	3
Renal Cortical	^{99m}Tc-DMSA		33	0.250	3
	^{99m}Tc-Glucoheptonate		55	0.250	3
Transplant Renogram	^{99m}Tc-DTPA		285		12
Renal Flow	^{99m}Tc-DTPA		6.5		3
Cystogram	^{99m}Tc-SC	<2 yrs		300 μCi via bladder catheter	
Cystogram	^{99m}Tc-SC	>2 yrs		500 μCi via bladder catheter	
Scrotal	^{99m}Tc-pertechnetate		176	1.0	10

Key: MDP = methylene diphosphonate; MAA = macroaggregated albumin; DTPA = diethylenetriamine pentaacetic acid; DMSA = dimercaptosuccinate; MAG$_3$ = mercaptoacetyl triglycine; SC = sulfur colloid; IDA = iminodiacetic acid (HIDA, or dimethyl IDA; preferred agent is DISIDA, diisopropyl IDA)

INDEX

NOTE: *Italicized* page numbers represent images. Page numbers followed by Roman f and t refer to figures and tables respectively.

than ever. And he had. Mother simply hadn't understood business. Of course, Angelo had also promised not to tell his half brother they had the same father. That still tore at him.

He crossed the room and opened the door of the walnut curio cabinet, removing the small figure of a faerie resting on a shamrock. Mother had enjoyed these whimsical things. Worthless things. Still, he smiled, remembering.

From there, he glanced toward her small antique desk near the bay window. A light flashing on the phone drew his attention, and he crossed the room still clutching the figurine.

There was a message on her machine. An overwhelming need to hear her voice on the outgoing message gripped him, so he pushed that button first. Holding his breath, he waited.

He heard his mother's soft, lilting voice as she asked the caller to leave a message after the tone. *How can she be dead?*

Then he pushed the PLAY button to hear the new message left on her machine. As the electronic beep sounded, he reached for the STOP button, but a small voice made him freeze.

"Mamó, when are you coming for—"

Scowling, Angelo hit rewind and listened to the voice again. A child. Why would a child have called his mother?

Mamó. "Where have I heard that before?" He played the message again and again, struggling with memories better left buried—his disastrous marriage, their beautiful baby girl, her kidnapping and murder.

Why did the sound of some kid's voice on an answering machine make him remember that nightmare? The call was probably nothing more than a wrong number. Even so, he listened again, a cold sweat coating his forehead and his palms. His gut clenched and his throat tightened. It wasn't the child's voice that had triggered those memories.

Mamó. That one word. He looked at his mother's

teased her memory, and she had a sudden flash of those same eyes beneath the brim of her brother's cap when she'd tried to sneak her way onto the lads-only soccer team. "Irene Gilhooley, as I live and breathe!"

They hugged and chattered about childhood memories. Finally, Maggie asked, "Are you back for good then?"

"We'll see." Irene smiled, a dimple flashing in her cheek. "Aren't I part owner of Gilhooley's, after all?"

"Truly? You mean that ornery Kevin decided to let a mere lass join the business?"

Irene grinned again. "Da didn't give him any choice in the matter. I always have been half owner, but was too young and too busy seeing the world with Mum and Da to do anything about it."

Irene's parents had won the Irish Lottery during her sixth year of school. They'd immediately packed up their youngest child and moved to Crete. Maggie didn't remember seeing her since. Kevin, being much older, had stayed to take over his parents' pub. "So now you're back to help your aunt keep your brother in line?"

Irene laughed. "And to find myself. Let's get together over a bottle of wine and I'll tell you all about it."

"I'd like that." Maggie immediately recognized one of the things that had been missing in her life since returning to Ballybronagh. Friends. Most of the lasses she'd grown up with, including her best friend, had moved to Dublin, since jobs in small villages like Ballybronagh were hard to come by. Only a few were still in the area, and they were all married with children. In fact, some of their youngest ones would be Maggie's students. Her college roommate, Ailish, was her only truly close friend, and she missed her.

"Where are you off to now?"

Irene's words brought Maggie back to the present. "School. I'm the new teacher." Pride made her smile as she glanced at her watch. "And I'm late for a meeting. I'll come by Gilhooley's after."

Irene gave her another quick hug. "I'll be there, showing Kevin how to organize things better. 'Tis driving him off his nut, I am."

Irene's laughter as she walked away told Maggie that the woman enjoyed tormenting poor Kevin more than anything. Remembering all the times she and her brothers had bickered and teased each other made her smile and shake her head. As Mum often said, *some things never change.* Like Maggie's bad cooking . . .

Chuckling at herself, she walked across the schoolyard and climbed the steps to the back stoop. A soft breeze blew in from the sea, carrying with it the sound of voices raised in anger, almost in a sort of chant. She couldn't quite make out the words, but she couldn't deny the sudden panic that made her belly clench and her throat tighten. Even without looking, she knew there were no people arguing nearby, no one between her and the sea.

No one alive.

And isn't that the craziest notion?

Any crazier than cursed castles and reincarnation? Didn't she believe that Riley and Bridget had heard *Caisleán* Dubh's whispering? Aye, especially after they broke the curse.

She swallowed hard and glanced over her shoulder, toward the ruins. Odd that the voices she heard had nothing at all to do with *Caisleán* Dubh. A shiver skittered down her spine.

Or did they?

Five

Angelo Fazzini junior stood in his mother's suite rooms in the east wing of their Long Island home. He w all alone now. No wife, no children, no parents. No one carry on the Fazzini name or empire. He needed an h Maybe he should remarry.

Of course, that wouldn't bring Mother back. Still d astated from the shock of her sudden death, he wal around her sitting room, touching things that had longed to her. A curio cabinet filled with figurines f Ireland stood untouched against the far wall.

His breath snagged in his throat and he squeezed eyes shut for a few seconds, reeling in his emotions couldn't afford to spend weeks in mourning. He had ing business on hold already. He would finish his m ing today, then get back to work.

The news of his mother's private plane crashing the Atlantic had devastated him. She had always be strong, so proud, so disapproving. He smiled sad membering the last time she'd tried to convince l give up the business his father had worked so hard ate. Of course, Angelo couldn't do that. He'd pro his father that he would make them bigger and s rocker in the corner, remembering her sitting there singing Irish folk songs to her only grandchild. Mother had laughed at Angelo's comments about the baby not being able to understand her, but she had merely laughed and insisted on talking or singing to Erin all the time.

He released his breath in a long sigh, seeing his mother and daughter together again, right here in this room. Even more clearly, he heard his mother's words to her granddaughter.

"Talk to Mamó, wee one. Talk to Mamó."

None of this made sense. He had to know what *mamó* meant first. He would order Finn McAdam to track down where the call had originated, and once he had the facts, then he could make an informed decision, rather than the emotional one lurking just beneath the surface.

His own mother—

"Don't think. Talk to Finn and find a goddamned Irish dictionary."

He stalked toward the double doors separating his mother's suite from the rest of what now felt more like a mausoleum than a mansion. Pausing there, he glanced down at the figurine still clutched in his fist.

Without breathing, he drew back his arm and flung the fine porcelain against the wall, watching with a woeful lack of satisfaction as it splintered near his mother's desk.

And that damned answering machine.

Nick lurked in his room as long as possible, admiring his treasure. With the crucifix clean and tucked safely in his pocket, he joined his employer and her granddaughter in the kitchen. They were reading what appeared to be a newspaper.

"What's new?" He grabbed another cup of coffee and tried not to think about the now shiny crucifix.

"I'm thinking it's time for us to get out and about a bit more," Aunt Mo said. "Last night's party went well, don't you think?"

"Yep." Nick took a slug of coffee, eyeing the woman

over the cup's rim. With Erin in the room he couldn't remind his employer about the risks of appearing in public. Instead he said, "Ballybronagh seems quiet enough."

"That it does." Aunt Mo looked up and smiled, her eyes crinkling.

Half the time the woman was sly and calculating, and the other half he could almost forget she wasn't really his aunt. "So what do you have in mind?"

"Lunch at Gilhooley's."

Nick arched a brow. "Isn't that the local bar—I mean, pub?"

"It is."

He inclined his head toward the kid, who now watched them both with interest. "One of us is a minor," he said.

"This is Ireland." Aunt Mo turned her attention back to the newspaper.

"And your point would be . . . ?" He set the cup on the counter and folded his arms, waiting.

Aunt Mo pointed at an ad. "There it is. Today's special is fish and chips. Perfect."

"Is it all right for me to go?" Erin asked, her gaze shifting from Nick to her grandmother. "I'm only eleven, and Cousin Nick said—"

"Oh, aye." Aunt Mo laughed and hugged Erin to her side. "An Irish pub is both restaurant and pub—a family gathering place, and the center of any Irish village. Second to the church, of course."

Nick half expected the woman to cross herself after that blunder.

"Oh, good." Erin clapped her hands. "I'll go change to my pink jumper."

"You do that, lass." Aunt Mo turned her attention to Nick as soon as Erin had bounded up the stairs. "We need to get out in the community more. It's unnatural to be so isolated. For Erin."

Nick nodded. "She'll start school soon. Right?"

Aunt Mo sighed and stepped away from the table. "And doesn't that present a bigger problem?"

He started to ask what, but realized the answer before the words left his lips. "I don't think they'll let me enroll in school." He grinned to soften the words, recognizing his employer's concern. Hell, he shared it.

"I spoke with Brady Rearden last night about making a generous donation to the school."

"Oh, yeah—my cousin." Nick remembered the way the old man had come on to Aunt Mo. "I guess male charm runs in the family."

She laughed. "Well, you could take a few lessons from your cousin, lad."

"Lad?" Nick grimaced, but did it with a smile. Damned if the woman didn't seem more and more like his aunt than his employer. *Dumb, Desmond. Real dumb.*

Her expression sobered again. "I'm sure we're in agreement that Erin can't attend school without you along to— well, you know."

Nick nodded. "Go on. I'm listening."

"So I suggested to Mr. Rearden that you would make a good handyman."

"Handyman?" His voice sounded strained even to his own ears. Hell, it was all he could do not to growl. How frigging low could he sink? From detective to handyman? *Shit.* But it was a great plan. After all, he had a job to do, and this was a clever move. He had to hand it to the old woman.

"I realize you're overqualified, but this was the only excuse I could think of to justify you being at the school with Erin."

Nick released a long sigh. "I agree. Makes sense." He narrowed his eyes as he met his employer's gaze. "What about you? I thought you were half my job."

Maureen O'Shea set her lips in a thin line and squared her shoulders. "You can't be in two places at once, and I'm far more capable of taking care of myself than Erin is."

Suspicion niggled him. Despite this country's gun laws, he had to ask. "Do *you* have a gun?"

Aunt Mo's eyes widened and she glanced toward the stairs. Her expression shifted from shock to mischief by the time she blinked again. "I don't believe you want to know."

He studied her for several seconds. "You're right. If it's illegal, I don't want to know. What I *do* want to know is if you know how to use what I don't want to know about."

She lifted her chin a notch. "I do."

He should have known. He narrowed his eyes, refusing to let her out of this one.

She squirmed a little, but quickly recovered her usual dignity. "Have you changed your mind, then, about doing anything a bit . . . illegal?"

His gut clenched and so did his fists. He shoved them into his pockets, coming into immediate contact with the crucifix. A strange sensation washed through him—both protective and powerful.

"Maybe," he said. "No!" What had he been thinking? Breaking the law—even in Ireland—went against everything his father had taught him. He glanced upward, hoping Dad hadn't witnessed his near transgression. "No." His voice softened.

"I understand." She sighed and gave him a tight smile. "I understood from the start that you're an honorable man. Fair enough."

He pondered that a moment while gently rubbing the crucifix with his thumb. Would an honorable man keep this artifact to himself? "Thanks."

She cleared her throat. "Let's be hoping nothing like that will be needed."

"Yeah. Let's." He forcibly withdrew his hand from his pocket, feeling something like a hobbit after that frigging ring. *Bullshit.* He took a step toward his employer, determined to focus on business. "This is the former cop talking. Lots of people get killed with their own—"

"I won't."

He had to smile, despite the subject of their discussion. "I believe you."

The sound of Erin thundering down the stairs put an end to further conversation. So he would continue as an unarmed bodyguard and become a handyman. How would the school folks feel when they found out the only tools he'd ever owned were a simple hammer and a screwdriver?

Maggie would be at the school every day. Heat eased through him, chasing away thoughts of illegal weapons and mobsters and replacing that tension with another, far more pleasant kind.

"I thought you were changing into the *pink* jumper." Aunt Mo smiled at her granddaughter, who was now garbed in purple.

Erin smiled, a dimple flashing in her cheek. "I changed my mind."

Nick chuckled. "Women."

"Outnumber you in this house." Laughing, Aunt Mo grabbed her purse—a much smaller one than the one she'd carted from the States. "Let's go to lunch."

Out of habit Nick patted the spot where his holster *should* have been concealed beneath his denim shirt and leather vest. Erin ran to the front door and grabbed the handle.

"Wait, Erin!" Aunt Mo hurried to the girl's side.

Erin looked at her grandmother, obviously confused. "Aren't we going, Mamó?"

Of course, Nick knew exactly why Aunt Mo didn't want Erin dashing out the door. The poor kid was a prisoner in her own home. He felt silly doing it, but he managed an exaggerated bow and said, "A lady always waits for the gentleman to open the door."

She giggled and, as he straightened, he caught Aunt Mo's approving nod. He couldn't help himself, so he grinned in return and made a great show of swinging open the door, even as he discreetly surveyed what waited on the other side.

All clear. He held the door open and stepped outside, glancing up and down the road and across the treeless terrain. *Talk about nowhere to hide.* He wanted to think they were too worried, but he couldn't—not when the man they were hiding from was Fazzini.

"After you, miss. Madam." Nick bowed again, holding the position even as he kept his gaze aimed at the lane that passed by the cottage.

Erin kept giggling as she waited on the steps. Aunt Mo paused beside Nick with a wicked chuckle.

"Yikes!" He straightened and let the door slam.

His sweet little old aunt had goosed him.

Maggie had been home for months and this was the first time she'd been to Gilhooley's. Oh, and didn't it feel good to enter the pub with its dark wood and shining brass?

She stopped to greet old Séamus Doone, who spent most of his days rocking before the hearth at Gilhooley's or fishing. "'Tis about time you came to see me, lass," he teased.

Maggie laughed and tossed her hair over her shoulder. "And didn't I just see you at the *céilí* last night, Mr. Doone?" She bent to kiss his wrinkled cheek and he patted the hand she'd placed on his shoulder.

"So you're to be the new teacher," he said as she straightened. "The lads will not be learnin' a thin' with such a comely lass teachin' their lessons."

"I see you've kissed the Blarney stone again." Laughing, she thanked the dear charmer for his compliment and made her way to the bar. Gilhooley's was busy, as it often was at midday.

She looked around for Irene, but didn't spot her. Kevin finished building a Guinness and served it to Michael Kelly, at the end of the bar, then turned his attention to her. "What a pleasure 'tis to have the local teacher visit me humble establishment." He flashed her his best publican grin.

"Have all the men in Ballybronagh kissed the Blarney

stone today?" She laughed and leaned toward her brother's dearest friend. "I saw Irene earlier."

"Ah, me loving sister herself." He slapped his hand across his heart and staggered backward. "The bane of me bloody existence."

She couldn't help but laugh at his exaggerated reaction. "And hasn't Riley said the same thing about me a time or two?"

"No, of course not." Kevin grimaced and added, "As long as you don't try to cook, that is."

Maggie sighed. "Don't worry. I'll not be using either of you to test anything again."

He winced. "For that I'll be eternally grateful."

The expression on his face confirmed that he remembered the last time he'd tasted anything prepared by her incompetent hands. "I've learned my lesson, Kevin. I'm not a cook."

"Thank the Blessed Virgin."

"If you cross yourself, I'll be punching you in the nose, of course."

He clasped his hands together in front of him, the epitome of innocence.

Rolling her eyes, she asked, "Will Irene be about?"

"In the kitchen I fear."

"Is *she* a good cook?"

"To me knowledge, she's never cooked anything in her life," Aileen said as she placed a tray on the bar beside Maggie. "Kev, a pint of Harp and two Cidonas, please."

Maggie sensed that Aileen wasn't any more pleased than her nephew to have Irene underfoot. "Then what's she doing in the kit—"

A loud crash, followed by cursing, sounded from behind the swinging doors that led to the kitchen. Kevin darted through the doors, then staggered back a moment later, his expression haggard.

"What's she doing in the kitchen, you ask?" Aileen repeated. "Destroying it. What's she done this time?" She turned her attention to her nephew.

"Knocked down the whole bloody rack of pots." Kevin shook his head. "And isn't Mavis threatenin' to quit again already?"

"We can't be havin' that." Aileen took the tray from Kevin and balanced it on her shoulder. "Good cooks are hard to come by in Ballybronagh. Now if you'd just find a comely lass who can cook and get married, we wouldn't have to worry about your sister."

"Argh!" Kevin tossed a towel at his aunt as she walked away with her order, laughing all the way.

"That let's me off the hook," Maggie muttered under her breath.

"Come to eat at the competition, have you?" Kevin shoved the lunch menu in front of her with a grin.

"And doesn't it look as if business is doing well here despite the competition?"

"That it is. That it is." Kevin beamed. "Actually, once the B and B opens, I believe it will help our business even more."

"Good." The menu hadn't changed much over the years, and the prices were still reasonable. "I was hoping Irene could join me."

"Oh, and don't I wish she would at that?" Kevin sighed and added the final layer to a Guinness. Over his shoulder he added, "She's determined to earn her keep round here and will be—Jaysus save us—helpin' Mavis in the kitchen until one o'clock. I'll let her know you're here, though."

"Thanks."

Kevin disappeared through the double doors and Maggie felt a tug on her sleeve. She looked beside her and saw Erin O'Shea's smiling face.

"Hello, Erin," Maggie said. "Don't you look pretty in purple?"

"Thank you, Miss Mulligan." Erin leaned closer. "Mamó brought us here for lunch."

Mrs. O'Shea walked up behind Erin. "And we'd love for you to join us."

Maggie hesitated, then decided she would eat now and

simply chat with Irene after her shift. "I'd like that. Let's get a booth in the back corner, where it's quieter. I'll join you after I tell Kevin where I'm going."

After Kevin returned, she gave him a message for Irene and walked around the corner, where booths were filled with talkative diners. She spotted Mrs. O'Shea's snowy hair immediately in the last booth, and as she drew nearer her breath snagged. Seated with his back to the wall on the opposite side of the booth was Nick Desmond.

Her pulse sprinted forward like an eager thoroughbred, and her palms turned clammy. She wiped them on her jeans and slowed her pace, realizing with a mixture of joy and terror that she would have to sit beside Nick, since Erin was sharing the other seat with her grandmother.

Hip to hip. Thigh to thigh. With Nick. Heat flowed sweetly through her as she paused beside their table. His gaze met hers, surprise registering in his eyes.

"While you were outside talking to the *garda*," Mrs. O'Shea explained, "we invited Maggie to join us for lunch."

Nick smiled, unfolded himself from the booth, urged her to slide in first, then he joined her. He was a big man—tall, powerful, well muscled. Maggie sighed a little as the length of his thigh settled beside hers. His warmth seeped into her. It felt *good*. Simply good.

Oh, don't you mean better than good? All right, better than good. Stimulating. She felt as if a walking, living, breathing adventure had just sat beside her.

Aileen took their orders and winked when Maggie met her gaze. Was Maggie's attraction to Nick so obvious? She drew a shaky breath and met Mrs. O'Shea's knowing gaze. The twinkle in the older woman's eyes gave the answer. Aye, obvious to other women at least.

"Have you decided on the first day of school then, Maggie?" Mrs. O'Shea asked after Aileen had delivered their drinks.

"Three weeks from Monday."

Erin squeaked and clapped her hands. "I like school. I can't wait."

Maggie smiled at the child. "Where was your last school, Erin?"

"I went to the abbey school in—"

Mrs. O'Shea tipped over her water glass. Nick rose to gather all their napkins and sop up the mess. "Sorry about that. Clumsy of me," the older woman said.

"I'll get some more napkins." Nick walked away from the booth.

Maggie watched him until he turned the corner, deciding that the view from this side was every bit as nice as the other. There wasn't an unattractive millimeter on that man.

"Cousin Nick was *garda*—I mean police—in New York," Erin said, drawing Maggie's attention.

"Was he now?"

Erin nodded and took a sip of Cidona. "I really like the fizzies."

"Nick was a detective," Mrs. O'Shea said, her tone solemn. "One of the best."

"Then why—"

"Here we go." Nick passed the napkins around, a mischievous grin on his face. "No tipping the help."

Before Maggie drew her next breath he was beside her again. And was it her imagination, or had he scooted much closer this time? Now their shoulders, hips, and thighs touched. Heat spiraled through her and a tremor followed that had nothing to do with temperature. She was *hot*. And so was he.

'Tis in trouble you are, Mary Margaret.

Aileen brought plates heaping with crispy fish and chips. Erin's eyes grew round and Mrs. O'Shea actually moaned in anticipation. "Oh, it's been far too long," the older woman said on a sigh.

They all ate in silence for a few minutes, then Mrs. O'Shea asked, "What did the *garda* want?"

Nick cleared his throat and lifted a shoulder. "He was curious about the security system."

"Oh." Mrs. O'Shea's cheeks pinkened. "Was he now?"

"Security system?" Maggie chuckled and arched a brow. "In Ballybronagh? But why—"

"My fault," Nick said. "Too much time on the streets of New York, so I insisted. Overkill. Huh?"

She met his gaze and her heart skipped a beat. When he smiled at her like that she couldn't think or even breathe.

"Aye," Mrs. O'Shea said. "I can understand why the *garda* was curious. I'm sure no one else has one."

Maggie recovered herself enough to agree with Mrs. O'Shea. "The bank over in Kilmurray probably does, but no one here."

"Well, the officer—er, *garda*—was just curious," Nick said. "He seems decent enough."

"Guard Bailey is more than decent, though he's retiring next year," Maggie said. "He's been the *garda* here in Ballybronagh since I was about Erin's age, and his da before him. A family tradition, you might say."

She felt Nick stiffen at her side, and Mrs. O'Shea cleared her throat. "'Twas good of Guard Bailey to inquire. I must say the fish and chips are outstanding."

Maggie sensed the subject had been deliberately changed. Again she was struck with the certainty that Nick had secrets. It seemed every time she'd asked a question today, someone—usually Mrs. O'Shea—had changed the subject. There were definitely secrets at work here. Even so, Maggie was more than a little attracted to Nick Desmond, and wanted to know him better.

Much better.

For the first time in her life, she'd met a man who made her contemplate things she'd never experienced. It was like a powerful hunger pulsing through her with every beat of her heart. When he reached for his beer, she wanted to grab his arm and hold on tight.

"I like this." Erin forked a blob of coleslaw into her mouth and chewed.

"Everything tastes great." Nick turned sideways and met her gaze, his eyes intense. "How's yours?"

"D—delicious." Maggie licked her lips and reached for her water glass just as Irene came to the booth.

"There you are." She untied the soiled apron from around her waist. "Whew. What a mess."

"Mrs. O'Shea, this is Irene Gilhooley—a friend who's recently returned to Ballybronagh," Maggie said, remembering her manners. "Irene, this is Mrs. O'Shea, her granddaughter Erin, and nephew Nick Desmond."

Irene shook their hands and told Maggie she'd wash up and meet her at the bar in a few minutes.

"Maggie, we want to talk to you about the school. Will you be there later today?"

Maggie shook her head. "I'll be there for a few hours tomorrow afternoon, though."

"I'll send Nick by then."

"All right, Mrs. O'Shea." *Send Nick . . . ?*

They said their good-byes and Nick actually held her hand for a few seconds, as if he didn't want to let her go. She felt oddly bereft without his warmth at her side. Shaking herself, she made her way to the bar to wait.

Irene bounced out of the kitchen a moment later, a backpack slung over her shoulder. "Did the handsome Yank leave, then?" She leaned against the bar.

Illogical jealousy made Maggie feel uncomfortable and guilty. *Silliness.* "Aye."

"Pity." A crease furrowed Irene's normally smooth brow.

"What is it?" Maggie studied her friend's expression. "Is something wrong?"

"Not wrong, but . . ." Irene pursed her lips for a moment, then said, "I could swear I've seen Mrs. O'Shea somewhere before."

Six

Nick escorted Aunt Mo and Erin back to Donovan Cottage. Maureen O'Shea had put on an Oscar-winning performance, dodging questions, spilling water—the works.

The woman might not be exactly young, but she had more energy than half the New York City Police Department. "I think that went well," he said after they were safely inside their self-made prison again.

"We saw lots of people from last night," Erin said. "'Twas fun!"

"It was fun," Aunt Mo said. "We should do it more often."

"Suits me." Nick shrugged.

"Mamó?"

"What is it, Erin?" Aunt Mo asked.

"I'm so glad you brought me home to live with you. You're all I have." The girl shuffled her feet and smiled through crocodile tears. A moment later, she threw her arms around her grandma's shoulders.

For the next few minutes Nick stood helplessly by, watching the little girl pour her guts out. His heart wasn't as protected as he'd thought. He was too damned soft. Erin ought to know she was one lucky kid to have a grandmother who loved her enough to go through hell to protect her from her gangster old man. But that would mean telling the child the whole truth, and she sure as hell didn't deserve that. No one did. The less Erin knew about her heritage, the better.

"There." Aunt Mo gripped Erin's shoulders and held her up straight. "We all need a good cry now and then. Feel better now?"

"Aye." Erin sniffled and scrubbed her eyes with the backs of her hands. "I want us to be a family together forever. And Nick, too."

He cleared his throat, shifting his weight from foot to foot. The shit was getting deep, and he definitely didn't have the right kind of shovel for this touchy-feely kind.

"Well, now, your cousin is an awfully pretty young man for us to keep all to ourselves forever," Aunt Mo said, stroking Erin's hair. "Why, he might even get married someday and have children of his own."

"Then I'll have more cousins!"

Nick narrowed his eyes when his employer hugged her granddaughter and flashed him a sheepish look over the girl's shoulder. He mouthed the words *thanks a lot,* but he couldn't really be pissed at the old woman. Erin needed reassurance. Unfortunately, including him in their happy family picture was also a big fat lie.

How would Erin react when he headed back to the States next year? She believed they were cousins. Well, hell. He could write her letters and continue the pretense, but he wouldn't stay here and make more little cousins to entertain her. *Perish the frigging thought.* Hopefully, by the time Nick left, Erin would have so many friends here in Ballybronagh that she wouldn't even miss him.

If everything went as planned, he would return to New York, put Fazzini behind bars, and get on with his own life without Erin ever learning the truth. Hell, he could even send her Christmas and birthday gifts like a good cousin. She was a sweet kid. Her paternity wasn't her fault.

A soft knock sounded at the door, and Nick immediately tensed. He glanced through the window beside the door and saw Brady Rearden standing there, hat in one hand, flowers in the other. "Speaking of cousins, I hope you're up to company." He flashed his employer a grin and opened the door.

Aunt Mo rose and hugged her granddaughter. "Well now, don't I feel twenty years younger?"

"I'll bet," Nick muttered through a grin as Brady stepped into the cottage.

"Afternoon, Nick," the old man greeted. "Would your lovely aunt be about?"

"I would indeed, Brady Rearden," Aunt Mo said from behind them.

Nick watched his distant cousin hang his hat from a peg near the door, then turn to smile at Aunt Mo. *Yep, he's got it bad.*

"Don't you look lovely today, Mrs. O'Shea?"

Erin's eyes grew round when she saw the flowers. "Mamó has a beau!"

"Hey, you both rhymed." Nick grinned as both Aunt Mo and Brady blushed. "Want me to take Erin to the playground for a while?"

"I want to stay here, Mamó." Erin's smile hadn't waned.

"Of course you do, and you shall. I'll just put these beautiful flowers in water and put the kettle on for tea." Aunt Mo told the men to sit, then she took Erin and the flowers with her to the kitchen.

Nick sat and turned his attention to his *real* cousin. "So . . . have you lived here all your life?"

"Mostly, though I was in the States living with me daughter's family for eleven years." Brady sat in an overstuffed chair near the hearth. "And on me way home, wasn't I fortunate enough to meet Bridget Mulligan and her son Jacob?"

Aunt Mo and Erin returned with a tray bearing tea and

cookies—what they called biscuits here. Cookies were cookies as far as Nick was concerned.

"Tell me, Mr. Rearden, how is it that Bridget and Jacob were Mulligans before they settled here?" Aunt Mo asked as she poured tea and sat in her rocking chair.

"Oh, 'tis a sad tale, that one." Brady took a sip of his tea. "And I'd be proud if you'd use me given name, Mrs. O'Shea."

"Only if you call me Maureen." Aunt Mo smiled and Erin giggled.

Nick caught the kid's attention and winked, which made her giggle even more. Then a sobering thought barged into his brain. Had Aunt Mo figured out all the family genealogy in such a way that he could be cousin to both Brady *and* Erin without the old man getting suspicious? He made a mental note to grill his employer about that later.

"Now, about Bridget and young Jacob." Brady settled back into his chair—a sure sign that he would be staying a while. "Culley Mulligan was Riley's younger brother by two years, as I recall. Riley stayed home to run the farm and Culley went to university after getting his leaving certificate from me." Brady grinned, obviously proud of his many years of service as a teacher.

"Leaving certificate?" Nick echoed.

"Ah, you Yanks would call it a high school diploma." Brady set his teacup aside and folded his hands in his lap. "After graduating from university, Culley went to the States on holiday. He had a bit of wanderlust, that one did. Oh, but he was a fine lad. One of the best."

Brady fished a handkerchief from his pocket and dabbed his eyes. "'Tis sorry I am." After a moment, he drew a deep breath and continued. "Culley planned to tour the eastern half of the country by car. After leaving his uncle's house, he ended up in a small town in Tennessee, where he met and fell in love with our dear Bridget."

"It sounds very romantic," Aunt Mo said, her tone solemn.

"What happened then?" Erin asked, perched on the ottoman near her grandmother, her eager gaze fixed on their visitor.

The old man paused—for emphasis, Nick figured— then said, "Culley and Bridget eloped, but before he could even call home to tell his family the news, the dear lad was killed in an auto crash."

Erin gasped and Aunt Mo sighed. "Tragic," the older woman said. "Was Bridget hurt badly in the accident?"

"No, she wasn't in the car." Brady brightened somewhat. "And considering she was carrying our Jacob by then, 'tis a blessing, that."

"That's so sad." Erin's lower lip trembled. "Poor Bridget and Jacob."

"Aye, 'tis sad, Erin." Brady nodded. "The authorities didn't know about Culley's marriage, so his family here was notified of his death. Culley's mum learned about Bridget and her grandson years later and invited them here. That's when the curse was broken."

"Curse?" three of them asked in unison.

"Don't tell me you haven't heard about the curse of *Caisleán* Dubh?"

Nick saw the gleam in Brady Rearden's eyes and knew they were in for a juicy tale. In fact, watching the old man's expressions and use of his hands reminded him of his grandfather. *Genes will tell.* He grabbed a handful of cookies and settled on the couch to listen.

"In 1783, Aidan Mulligan fell in love with a peasant girl—a servant in the castle. However, his da had arranged a suitable marriage for Aidan, and forbade him to see dear Bronagh again." Brady's gaze shifted to Erin, then to Aunt Mo. "Some of this isn't suitable for young ears, I fear."

Erin groaned and rolled her eyes.

"I trust your judgment and discretion, Brady," Aunt Mo said and patted her granddaughter's shoulder. "Don't keep us in suspense. Go on."

"Well, the lass was brokenhearted, and she committed a

terrible sin." Brady bit his lower lip and Aunt Mo arched a brow. "Er, I'm meanin' she took her own life—a sin in the eyes of the Church."

"Of course. The poor dear." Aunt Mo gave an almost regal nod, reminding Nick of the day he'd first met her. She was a class act.

"Bronagh's aunt was furious with the Mulligans, and she placed a dark curse on the castle to punish them."

"Curse?" Nick raked his fingers through his hair. "You believe that sh—manure?"

"Nicholas." Aunt Mo aimed her disapproving eyebrow in his direction this time.

"Sorry."

"Not manure, lad." Brady glanced at Erin and Aunt Mo. "'Tis true. Bronagh's aunt was a powerful witch. I have the diary of the priest who attended her in her final days. She confessed it all to him—even the words to her spell."

"What happened?" Aunt Mo asked.

"Many generations of Mulligans were plagued with tragedies until the family sealed *Caisleán* Dubh and moved into the cottage where Maggie lives now." He leaned forward and grabbed a cookie. "After that, things calmed down a bit, though the curse killed Patrick Mulligan, too."

"Who was he?" Erin asked.

"Father to Riley, Culley, and Maggie." Brady sighed, sadness etched across his craggy features. "No one has ever known why he went into the sealed castle that day, but 'twas young Riley who found his da's body there. The lad dragged him outside all by himself."

"Terrible. Just terrible." Aunt Mo dabbed at her tears— real ones this time. "So how did Bridget coming here break the curse?"

"Fate. Nothing less than fate." Brady smiled a little sheepishly and added, "I have to tell you that while Riley and I were discovering all the facts about the curse, I spent a lot of time in confession. Tested me faith, it did, but me faith won."

"Of course it did." Aunt Mo leaned her chin in her hand. "Go on, please."

"What happened next?" Erin added.

"Young Culley had heard an odd whispering coming from the castle most of his life. No one else in the family heard it until after his death."

"That's weird." Nick's cop persona didn't buy all this magical woo-woo bull. He liked evidence. Facts. "Wonder why?"

"Even more weird, as you say, is the fact that after Culley's death, *Riley* began to hear the whispering."

"Whoa! That's creepy." Nick had to hand it to his cousin—the old fart could sure spin a tale.

"And after Bridget arrived, *she* heard it, too."

Aunt Mo pressed her hand over her heart. "Oh, because—may I guess?"

"Aye."

"Reincarnation? Soul mates."

"So we believe." Brady nodded. "Bridget and Riley fell in love and married. The last time either of them heard the whispering was at their wedding."

"Oooooooh, that's so sweet." Erin sniffled and pulled a tissue from the box on the table. "Isn't that sweet, Mamó?"

"Oh, aye," Aunt Mo said on a sigh. "Was Ballybronagh named for Bronagh, then?"

"Precisely." Brady nodded enthusiastically. "The priest's diary is filled with thoughts about how Aidan Mulligan changed the name of the village to assuage his own guilt. *Bronagh* means sorrowful."

"How sadly appropriate." Aunt Mo poured more tea into Brady's cup, then hers. "I'm glad the curse has been broken."

"Question?" Nick held up one finger and waited for their attention. "Do you all really believe this stuff?"

All three of them stared at Nick in shock. Aunt Mo said, "Of course we do. We're Irish."

"Well, so am I—by blood, that is—but I believe in facts."

"'Tis fact, Nick. Documented fact." Brady stiffened slightly. "Documented in the Church records, no less."

"All right. Sorry. It's just hard to swallow."

"Ah, he is a Yankee." Brady directed his comment toward Aunt Mo.

"True, true."

"Well, he'll come round in time." Brady's faded eyes twinkled when he shifted his gaze back to Nick. "Come by me cottage sometime and I'll share some of the diaries and records."

"I'll do that." Nick rose and walked to the window, shoving his hand in his pocket. The crucifix felt smooth and safe there. No one would take it from him.

"It belongs to me. A gift. Mine . . ."

Was the crucifix talking to him? This was getting weird. As he gazed out the window with his hand on the antique silver, he saw a flash of red hair on the road. It was late afternoon and Maggie was walking home. Nick's heart skipped a beat, as flames suddenly engulfed his view. He stepped back, blinking, actually feeling their heat. After a moment, he drew a shaky breath. The flames were his imagination, just like—

Oh, my God. Slowly he turned to face Brady again. "What happened to the witch?"

Brady pressed his lips into a thin line. "I'm afraid she was tried and . . . executed."

Nick swallowed hard. He didn't have to ask the method of execution used. A cold sweat coated his face and hands.

"Burn, witch, burn!"

Maggie paused at the edge of a cliff to watch the setting sun glitter across the sea. A gentle breeze blew her hair away from her face, and she inhaled deeply, savoring everything about this day. This place. This life.

She felt renewed—stronger than she ever had. Even the bewildering feelings she had for Nick Desmond made her feel more alive, more certain about the path she'd chosen. This was her home. Her life.

The air was cool. She hugged herself against a chill, but didn't turn to head home just yet. There was still plenty of light. Besides, she could find her way home in the darkest of nights.

In her peripheral vision, a shadow moved. She turned toward it, a shiver skittering along her spine. Two people stood gazing out at the sea, his arm around her, and the woman's head resting on his shoulder. *How sweet.*

She couldn't see them clearly, but they looked young. She blinked a few times to clear her vision . . . and they simply vanished. Confused, she took a step, knowing the drop-off to the sea below was steep. They couldn't have climbed down so quickly. Where had they gone?

She shook her head. It must have been her imagination—shadows from clouds skating across the sky between the earth and the setting sun. Or maybe wishful thinking? Nothing more.

Yet they'd seemed so real. . . .

You've gone daft, Maggie. She shoved thoughts of the imaginary couple aside and gazed out at the sea again, drawing several deep breaths to calm her nerves and soothe her soul.

The sound of footsteps made her heart stutter. Was it the couple? No. Somehow she knew who it was. Hadn't she seen him watching her from the cottage window only a few moments ago?

"Maggie?" he said softly.

She turned toward him, smiling. "Good evening, Nick." *Did you follow me here for a reason? Will you kiss me now, as I know you want? As I want . . . ?* "'Tis beautiful here—one of my favorite spots."

"Yeah." His voice sounded hoarse. He shoved his hand into his pocket and she saw him wince as if in pain.

"Are you ill?"

"No, not that." He released a shaky breath. "Brady just

finished telling us about the curse on your castle. Though I find it all hard to swallow, it's still creepy."

Maggie suppressed a shudder. "Creepy. True, but 'tis broken now. Everything's fine."

"That's good." He shook his head as if clearing his mind. "I needed air. Brady is staying for supper." He withdrew his hand from his pocket and reached toward her, pausing partway. "I had to come out here after I saw you through the window. You know, I've never met anyone like you." He stepped closer.

"Like me?" Her pulse put the speed of Michael Flatley's feet to shame. "I'm not sure what you mean by that."

His smile was quick and unguarded for a change. "Neither am I."

Maggie laughed again. "Your cousin is one of my favorite people, but he can outtalk anyone I know."

Nick chuckled, seeming to relax. "You can say that again." He turned his gaze toward the setting sun, appearing mesmerized by it. "I like it here."

"You mean here on this cliff, or here in Ballybronagh?" Maggie held her breath, uncertain why.

He paused, half turning to face her again. "Here on this cliff." His voice grew huskier, and he placed his large, strong hand on her upper arm. "With you."

She understood exactly what he meant. Didn't she feel the same sort of bewilderment about him? "I know."

He drew a deep breath and closed his eyes, then opened them as he released it. "It's almost as if I know you from . . . somewhere. I can't explain it."

A small gasp—her own—filled the lull between the rhythmic crash of the waves below. The warmth of his hand on her arm spread relentlessly throughout the rest of her body. Her breasts felt heavy beneath her jumper and her mouth went dry. The heat of her blood intensified and pooled low in her belly, augmenting her awareness of a powerful emptiness deep inside her.

And her awareness of *him.*

She blinked, waiting. Wanting.

"You're beautiful, you know," he whispered, leaning closer.

"So are you."

He chuckled again, bringing both hands up to cradle her face. His gaze captured and held hers as he lowered his lips to brush hers ever so lightly.

Jaysus, Mary, and Joseph. A shudder rippled through her and she leaned into his kiss. He teased her lips until they parted, allowing him to explore further, and sending her spiraling need into a fast and sure orbit.

His hands didn't leave her face to roam over her body, though she felt thoroughly pliant and well seduced in his arms. Like magic, he made her feel touched even where he hadn't. The intimacy of it made her sway, and, shamelessly, she eased her arms around his waist, loving the way his muscles bunched beneath her hands.

The sudden urge to touch him in ways and places she'd never touched a man exploded within her. Oh, and to be touched—aye, she wanted that, too.

She wanted more and pressed herself closer, feeling the hard pulsing maleness of him against her lower abdomen. Gasping, she broke their kiss and dropped her hands to her sides as shame washed through her. What had come over her? She'd gone a bit off her nut.

Their breathing sounding ragged in the ripening dusk, she looked up and met his gaze. What was it about this man? He made her want and yearn like no one she'd ever known.

He eased his hands from her cheeks to her shoulders. "I've wanted to do that since the minute I first saw you," he said. "I hope I didn't come on too strong."

Maggie had to laugh quietly. Hadn't she been the one to come on too strong, after all? "I'm glad you did. Kiss me, that is."

He smiled again and kissed her on the forehead this time. "Walk you home?"

"I'd like that." He took her hand in his and she glanced down to see their hands clasped together in the growing dusk. Something about the sight of their linked fingers and touching wrists, looked so very right. Intimate. *And doesn't it feel even better?*

Their pace slowed as they neared *Caisleán* Dubh. As always, Maggie tensed near the massive boulders around the foundation. Her breath caught and she reminded herself how silly it was to fear the castle. The curse was gone. There was no reason to be afraid.

"I thought I saw someone on the cliffs when I first left the cottage," Nick said, breaking the silence.

Maggie stopped in the shadow cast by the castle tower to stare at Nick. "A couple, was it?"

"Yeah." He glanced back from where they'd come. "Is that a hot spot for making out in Ballybronagh?"

"Making out?" She couldn't quite see his features in the shadows now.

"Uh . . . what we were doing a few minutes ago."

She saw the flash of his white teeth through the darkness and her face flooded with heat. "Oh, that. Um, nooooo. I think there's a spot up near Doolin for sparking."

"Sparking?" Nick chuckled again and surprised her by pulling her into a hug. Maggie savored the feel of being cuddled against his strong chest, his arms warm about her shoulders. He rested his cheek against her head and she sighed.

"I'm glad I went for a walk," he said, stroking her back, "and found you."

"So am I."

He kissed her again, very gently this time. When they parted he kept his hand on her face, gazing into her eyes. "I'd better take you home before I ruin the local teacher's reputation."

Maggie's face flooded with heat. "Aye, well . . ." Remembering her earlier plans, she said, "I need to stop here first to see my family."

"I'll walk you to the door." Nick took her hand again and started around the boulders.

"Wait, stop." A wave of dizziness washed through Maggie, driving her to her knees.

Nick was beside her before she drew her next breath. "What is it? Are you all right?" He gripped her shoulders gently as she rose, steadying her.

"I . . . I don't know." She drew several deep breaths and looked away from the castle. "I'm fine now. Thank you."

"Are my kisses *that* potent?" He stroked her cheek with the backs of his fingers, and she heard the smile in his voice.

"Maybe." She captured his hand in hers and pressed it to her lips. "I believe they are." She didn't dare tell him that she'd grown afraid of the very castle in which her family lived. "Would you like to come in?"

"I'd better get back. Supper with Brady. Remember?"

Maggie laughed and gave his hand a squeeze before dropping it. "He knows more about the curse than anyone. He's a historian."

"I noticed." Nick chuckled quietly. "I'd like to see you again," he said as they walked around the path that led to the massive front doors of *Caisleán* Dubh and the restaurant, Mulligan Stew.

"I . . . I'd like that, too." Maggie glanced through the windows at the well-lit dining room. "They've customers, so I'll go through the kitchen."

Near the side entrance he took her in his arms again and kissed her. Aye, his kisses were *that* potent.

"I'll come by the school tomorrow," he said, stepping away and into the shadows. "About one o'clock?"

"That's fine then."

He waved and jogged back toward the village.

Maggie waited there on the smooth stones of the patio, staring after him. She gripped the cold stone wall and leaned forward, peering into the darkness, hoping to catch another glimpse.

The moon peered above the horizon, bathing the landscape in silvery light with intermittent slices of evening fog. There was Nick's dark figure, running past the church now. A flash of bright light winked at her from his person. A reflection from silvery moonbeams, though she couldn't imagine what could have been so bright.

She kept staring until the dark figure vanished into the night. Then she shook her head and turned to go inside. He'd kissed her! She smiled and hugged herself.

And looked forward to tonight's dreams.

Seven

Thoughts of Maggie remained fresh in Nick's mind. Throughout dinner with Brady, he remembered Maggie— the sweetness of her lips, the softness of her body pressed so eagerly against his. Everything reminded him of her.

He shouldn't get involved with any woman right now, but she wasn't just any woman, and he couldn't seem to convince himself to leave her alone. *Impossible.* He couldn't wait to see her, to taste her again. Was she really as sweet as he remembered?

Damn. He didn't need this. He had a job to do, and his father's killer to put behind bars. If only he could have met Maggie at another time. Of course, this job was the only thing that had brought him to Ballybronagh. Without it, he never would have met or even heard of Maggie Mulligan.

The sound of Brady's voice as he bid them all good night jarred Nick back to the present just in time to watch the old man kiss Maureen O'Shea on the cheek. Nick told his womanizing cousin good night, then wandered back to stare out the window and into the darkness. He could barely make out the shape of the tower of *Caisleán* Dubh against the night sky. Maggie's cottage was inland some.

He'd seen it from a distance before, and the urge now to go knock on her door gnawed at him. He reached into his pocket and grabbed the crucifix, focusing on it and shoving thoughts of kissing Maggie Mulligan—and more—to the back of his mind.

Work. Fazzini.

"Duty."

That voice. Who was it and why was Nick hearing it? It seemed to mirror his thoughts at times. The other voice about burning witches was different. Evil. Terrifying.

And Nick really was going insane. When he returned to New York, he would see a doctor. A shrink.

More focused, he heard Aunt Mo and Erin putting things away in the kitchen and forced himself to walk in there to help. Still silent, he dried a couple of pans Erin had placed in the drainer and put them away.

"You've been distracted since your walk," Aunt Mo said. "Did something happen? Did you see . . . anyone?"

Realizing she was worried that he might have seen someone who could be a threat, Nick said, "Only Maggie Mulligan."

"Ooooh, so *that* would explain why you're so distracted." Aunt Mo sighed, obviously relieved. "That's nice then."

"She's pretty," Erin said as she drained the water from the sink and dried her hands. "Do you think she's pretty?"

Nick's face flooded with heat and his employer's knowing smile told him they saw right through him. "Gorgeous." No point in lying. "I walked her home."

"Did you now?" Aunt Mo's eyes twinkled and she started to hum as she wiped the counters and draped the rag over the edge of the sink to dry. "Isn't that nice?"

He didn't dare tell them how nice. He'd never hear the end of it. Sometimes he had to remind himself these people weren't *really* his family. His throat tightened. A few distant cousins like Brady were the only real family Nick Desmond had.

He had to concentrate on his job. On avenging his father. On clearing his own name. And, most of all, on putting Angelo Fazzini behind bars.

"Why don't you invite Maggie for dinner tomorrow evening?" Aunt Mo suggested. "We can talk about the school."

Nick wanted to have dinner with Maggie alone, but they barely knew each other. And he wanted to know her one hell of a lot better. Intimately.

His body tightened with longing and he nodded. "I'm supposed to meet her at the school tomorrow. I'll ask her then."

"Time for you to get to bed, Erin." Aunt Mo headed toward the staircase with her granddaughter. "I'll be back down in a minute, Nick. Will you still be up?"

"You bet."

"Good night, Nick." Erin stood on tiptoes to kiss his cheek, then scrambled toward the stairs.

"Night." She was a good kid, but playing nice all the time and knowing his plans to put her father behind bars made for a constant shitload of guilt. Still, it was for her own good as well as everybody else's.

Nick grabbed a beer from the refrigerator and sat at the table to wait. He took a long pull from the bottle and stared at the label. The dark red color of the letters reminded him of Maggie's hair.

He chuckled to himself and took another drink. When a guy started seeing a woman's hair color on his beer bottle label, that was a bad sign. If only things could be different. Maybe . . .

"Nah."

"Talking to yourself?" Aunt Mo asked as she emerged from the staircase and poured herself a cup of herbal tea. "No more caffeine for this old woman tonight." She pulled out a chair and sat across the table from him.

Nick had to grin. "You've taken to washing dishes like you were born to it."

Aunt Mo laughed quietly. "And wasn't I?"

He arched a brow. "For real?"

"My da was a poor farmer in County Cork."

"How . . ." He shouldn't ask, but curiosity nagged at him. "How did you meet . . . your husband?"

She pressed her lips in a thin line and was silent for some time. Finally, she said, "He was an American soldier, on his way home from Korea." She shrugged as if it meant nothing, but the expression in her eyes told the truth. "He and a friend came across the Channel on leave. He said he promised his Irish mother he'd visit her homeland if he ever got close enough."

"I see." Nick had trouble picturing Fazzini senior as having ever had a mother, let alone one from Ireland. "So that's how you met."

"Aye." She smiled sadly, obviously lost in her memories. "He was handsome and rich, and I was simple and poor." Her smile turned somewhat cynical. "I didn't know when he proposed that I was to be a souvenir for his mum."

"Ouch." Nick took another swig of beer. "Then there were more surprises."

"As you very well know." She rose and took her cup to the sink. "His mum took to me right away, and taught me to play hostess to important business associates. By the time she died, I knew my role well."

Nick stood and took his empty bottle to the bin. "Did she know . . . you know?"

"I don't think so." Aunt Mo stared into the distance at some memory only she could see. "I didn't learn myself until shortly before my husband's death."

"I'm sorry." What the hell else could he say? "I shouldn't have asked."

"No, it's all right. It helps keep things in perspective if I force myself to remember all the reasons I have for doing the things I've done."

He thought about that for a few minutes. "You're one hell of a woman, Mrs. O'Shea." He'd promised not to call her that F name again, and he wouldn't. Besides, to him, she wasn't that person.

"Thank you, Nick." She patted his cheek. "We make a good team. Don't you agree?"

"Yep—we put Walter Matthau and Jack Lemmon to shame."

She laughed openly now. "I can't imagine a finer nephew than you." She appeared suddenly uncomfortable and shook her head. "Funny, isn't it?"

"How real this seems, you mean?" He sighed and nodded. "Sometimes I have to stop and remind myself why I'm really here."

"Aye." She blinked several times. "Maggie seems sweet. Not that you need any encouragement there."

Nick couldn't deny her observation.

"There's nothing wrong with enjoying spending time with Maggie while you're here," she added.

He grinned. "If you insist."

"I'll not touch that one." She kept smiling.

Nick rubbed his chin, contemplating. "Of course, there's nothing wrong with you spending time with my cousin either."

"Ah, you've got me there, boyo." She patted his cheek again. "Brady Rearden is one of the most interesting men I've ever met."

"It's in the genes." Nick had never expected to have any family to make jokes like that about again. It felt strange and damned good, too. But it also made him remember Dad. "My father would've liked him, too. You could do worse."

"I'm not doing anything right now but making a new friend."

"Sure, lie to yourself if it makes you feel better."

"Ah, I think I'll turn in now." She laughed as she headed toward the staircase. "Sweet dreams, Nick."

He released a long, slow breath. "I hope so."

She yawned and waggled her fingers at him before she started up the stairs. Nick stood there for several minutes, alone in the kitchen. Finally, he checked all the locks, set the security system, and turned off the lights.

Alone in his room he pulled the crucifix out of his pocket and sat on the edge of the bed, turning it over in his palm, wondering about his obsession with it. He couldn't blame it on religion or greed. No, it was more than that. It belonged to him, as if it had been waiting here for him to find it.

"And if that isn't nuts, I dunno what is." Carefully he put it in his drawer and stripped off his clothes for bed.

In the dark he stared up at the ceiling, remembering Maggie. The way her softness had flowed against and around him during that kiss made him grow hard enough to tent the blankets. She had a lush, tight young body that would make any man want her.

However, Nick's feelings for this woman were a lot more powerful than mere lust. Why? That was what worried him most.

"Mine."

Both the crucifix *and* Maggie Mulligan . . . ?

Maggie helped her sister-in-law put away the last of the pots. Mulligan Stew was a great success. Tourists and locals went out of their way to taste the American chef's unique, Southern American cuisine—what Bridget called "comfort food"—served in a legendary castle. This evening an entire tour bus had scheduled a stop here.

"They wanted a tour of the tower," Bridget said on a sigh. "You should've heard your brother trying to explain to them that the renovations aren't complete and it isn't safe."

"Eejits." Riley stepped into the kitchen, his fists perched on his hips. "You'd think the lot of them had never heard of construction before."

"Well, the tower renovations were delayed a few years, Riley," Bridget reminded her husband. "With the Irish Trust paperwork snafu and such."

"They've probably read so much about the place, they were dying to see it," Maggie added. "Mulligan Stew has been reviewed in newspapers and on the telly."

Bridget beamed, her pride evident. "It's a real kick in the seat of the pants, too."

"I'm proud of you." Riley smiled at his wife.

"As if you haven't done as much work as I have." Bridget patted his cheek. "Did you get Jacob to bed?" She untied her apron and removed her chef's hat.

"I did, though I had to threaten him a bit."

Bridget merely laughed. "Sure you did."

Everyone knew Riley would never threaten or harm anyone, and especially not the lad who was both nephew and adopted son. Maggie smiled as her brother pulled his wife into his arms and gave her a quick kiss.

"Don't overdo." He rubbed his pregnant wife's back and shoulders. "And make sure you save enough energy for your husband."

Maggie blushed and grabbed her purse. "On that note, I'll bid you all good night." She headed for the door. "Tell Mum I'll stop by tomorrow on my way to the school."

"I will," Bridget said.

Riley kissed his wife's forehead and said, "I'll walk Maggie home. Wait up?"

"Of course." Bridget winked at him.

Maggie's face burned hotter. "And since when don't I know the way without my big brother's assistance?"

"It's late and you live alone now." He donned the old beret that hung near the kitchen door of the castle just as it had in the cottage all those years. " 'Tis my duty to protect the women of my family, and that includes you. Like it or not."

"Since when?" She sighed and hugged Bridget. "I'm not sure how you put up with the likes of him."

"He is a pain, but I can't think of anything I'd rather do."

" 'Tis me irresistible charm." Grinning, Riley opened the door. "After you, Mary Margaret?"

"Thanks for helping me clean up, Maggie," Bridget called after them.

"You're very welcome." Maggie didn't buy her brother's

story about needing to protect her for one minute. What was really on his mind?

Outside, Riley took her by the arm and whistled quietly as they strolled around the castle on the smooth path and up onto the road that wound its way across their land to the cottage. He was definitely up to something.

As they passed the stable, fog rolled in from the sea and shrouded everything, including them. Maggie pulled free of her brother's arm. "Enough of this silliness, boyo," she said. "Tell me the real reason for this sudden attack of chivalry."

In the darkness she couldn't see his face, but she sensed the tension thickening along with the fog. "Are you angry with me about something?" she prodded. "What—"

"I saw you." His words sounded clipped. Terse. "Kissing the Yank."

Oops. Maggie wavered for a moment between embarrassment and anger, but anger won. "And since when is it your job to spy on me, Riley Mulligan?"

"Jaysus, Mary, and Joseph—I wasn't spying. I was in the kitchen and there you were, right outside the window." He sighed and reached for her shoulder, giving it a squeeze. "It's just . . . we know nothing about the man. He's a stranger. And the way he was kissing you . . ."

She drew a deep breath of misty air and released it. "Riley, I love you. You're the best big brother any sister could ever have, but you haven't noticed that I'm grown now. A woman, Riley. Not a child."

"'Tis this woman thing that worries me," he muttered.

"Riley Francis Mulligan, I—"

He rested both his hands on her shoulders now. "Easy, lass. You're right in part." He sighed, his breath stirring the thickening fog between them. "But I love you, so I worry. 'Tis a big brother's right, I think. At least I resisted the urge to interrupt."

How could Maggie argue with that? "You're a big sweet oaf, but I'll forgive you. This time."

They started walking slowly toward the cottage. Her

cottage. *Home.* Some evening, maybe Nick would walk her home. They would be so thoroughly alone. Together.

With big old Riley watching over Maggie, that was unlikely. "Riley, give me the chance to make my own mistakes, please."

"You might as well ask me to sever my arm, lass." He chuckled low and gave her hand a squeeze as they reached the kitchen door. " 'Tis late and dark, so I'm going in just to make sure—"

"Riley!" She stomped her foot as her brother opened the kitchen door and walked through the cottage, flipping on every light in the place. He even went upstairs.

"Ow!" he bellowed from the stairs.

Maggie laughed. How many times in her life had she heard her tall brother smack his skull on that low beam? "Serves you right," she called.

She waited in the kitchen, tapping her foot until he returned with a sheepish expression on his dear face. "Satisfied that no one is lurking about, are you?"

"I am." He shoved his hands in his pockets and moved toward the door. As he reached for the knob, he turned to pin her with a solemn gaze. "Have a care, Maggie. You just met the Yank. Be careful. That's all I ask."

A few years ago, Maggie would've punched her brother for such overprotectiveness, but now she stood on tiptoes and kissed his cheek. "I promise to be careful. Good night."

"Fair enough." He left her standing alone in the kitchen, contemplating his words. She really didn't know Nick at all. If not for Mrs. O'Shea, she still wouldn't even know he'd been a police officer back in the States. And why had he tensed when she'd talked about Guard Bailey?

"Give the man time," she said to herself as she locked doors and turned off lights for the night. Though they hadn't talked enough to know much about their pasts, they had shared more than one breathtaking kiss.

The memory of his kisses made her feel warm and deliciously drowsy by the time she reached Mum's old room.

The large antique bed beckoned to Maggie. At first she'd resisted her mother's insistence that she should take the larger bedroom, since Maggie would be living alone in the cottage. But now it felt right. True, she had memories of visiting her mother in this room, but now it was hers. Mulligan Cottage was hers.

And, just maybe, she wouldn't *always* be alone here.

As she undressed for bed, she remembered her resistance to Mum's cajoling about her settling down and getting married. Nesting, she'd called it. Well, Maggie Mulligan wasn't nesting, but she had to admit that the thought of romance appealed to her just now.

She settled into bed with the covers pulled up to her chin and gazed into the darkness. Riley was right, and hadn't Maggie herself realized Nick Desmond was a man with secrets? She needed to learn more about Nick before she let him get closer.

Oh, and didn't having him closer sound appealing?

Maggie smiled when she opened the front door and saw Nick standing there. It was late and the fog swirled around him. He wore a dark jacket and his smile was tentative and guarded. "May I come in?" he asked.

She clutched the neckline of her simple cotton nightgown closer. Letting him into her cottage so late at night while she wasn't decently dressed was scandalous. Risky. But she swung the door open wide and shivered as he entered, brushing against her as he passed.

He seemed more mysterious now. More dangerous? "Don't be silly, Mary Margaret," she thought. She should get dressed, make tea, serve him something to eat. He was her first nonfamily guest in her cottage.

And the one she'd wanted most to invite.

She took his jacket and hung it on a hook near the door, her hands trembling slightly. An image flashed through her mind as if the scene before her eyes were changing. The freshly painted wall became dark wood. The metal hook where she reached out to hang Nick's jacket transformed into ornate brass, and his jacket suddenly felt heavier. For a fleeting moment, it looked like an old-fashioned wool cape.

She barely avoided dropping it and squeezed her eyes closed. He reached out to cover her hand and guide the jacket onto the hook. When she reopened her eyes, everything was perfectly normal, except the sight of his large hand covering hers. What had happened to her? How odd.

Nervously, she withdrew her hand and said, "I'll go get dressed. It won't take me a minute."

"Don't go." His voice sounded intense and husky. He stepped closer and reached out to wrap one of her wayward red curls around his finger. "You look perfect just as you are."

Maggie's mouth went dry and her heart danced a jig. Why was he here? What did he want? She shivered again, wondering. Nervously, she asked, "Would you care for some—"

He wrapped his arms around her waist and pulled her gently against him. His warmth seeped through her nightgown, warming her in more ways than one. "I only came for this. For you."

His lips covered hers before she drew her next breath. She searched for the courage to resist, to turn him away, to send him home where he belonged this late at night. Instead, she leaned into him, welcoming his kiss.

She wore nothing beneath the nightgown, and the feel of her bare breasts against the thin fabric and his warmth was delicious. He pulled her closer and tilted her slightly back against his strong arm, deepening their kiss.

His seeking tongue was silky smooth, hot, and

persistent. She moaned into his mouth, savoring the sensations swirling through her body. She wanted him closer; she wanted their clothes gone. Aye, gone.

They were so alone and she was vulnerable. Inexperienced. Riley had asked her to be careful, but right now that was the last thing she wanted to think about.

All she wanted was to feel Nick's flesh against her own, to be touched in ways and places she'd never been touched. She wanted this man to make her a woman in every way.

Dangerous. Aye, this was dangerous and exciting and powerful. Heat pooled low in her belly and her body clenched around the agonizing emptiness there.

He brought his hands around the sides of her rib cage, spreading his fingers possessively against her, so near her aching breasts she almost moaned again. It was all she could do not to beg him to touch her there—to touch her everywhere.

His thumbs brushed against her nipples and she broke the kiss, shock and joy mingling to boggle her mind even more. "I . . ." What could she say? What should she do? She should be afraid, and maybe she was just a little. But she wanted him more than she feared him.

He continued to brush his thumbs across her nipples and lowered his mouth toward hers again, but she remembered her promise to Riley and grabbed Nick's wrists to stop him. Gently but firmly she pushed his hands downward, away from her throbbing breasts. It was one of the hardest things she'd ever done.

"I want you," he said, his eyes intense.

"I want you, too, but . . ."

"We're both adults." He started to kiss her again, but she shook her head and stepped away.

"I don't know you well enough to . . . to . . ."
He walked to the door, slipped his jacket on and tied it at the waist. Without another word, he opened the door and walked out into the foggy night.
Maggie dropped to her knees, gasping for air. She ached with longing for the man. Why had he walked away, rather than allow her time to get to know him better? Why?
Nick Desmond was a man with secrets.

Maggie awoke with a start, wondering where she was. No longer in her bed, she was covered with a cold sweat and breathing heavily. A shiver rippled through her.

"Jaysus, Mary, and Joseph." She *remembered*. It *had* been a dream. Hadn't it? She turned on the lamp nearest the door where the strange visions had popped into her mind. Everything looked fine. Undisturbed.

This was all Riley's fault. If he hadn't reminded her how little she knew about Nick, she wouldn't have these nagging doubts. Nick wouldn't *really* be so secretive when she tried to get to know him better. Would he?

Swallowing hard, she walked toward the door, locked as it had been before she went to bed. Somewhat reassured, she turned to touch the hook that had transformed in her dream. She stepped closer, examining the smooth wall beside it that bore no resemblance to the dark wood she'd glimpsed briefly while hanging up Nick's jacket.

With a nervous laugh, she reminded herself that she hadn't really hung up Nick's damp jacket. She stepped nearer, her bare toes coming into contact with frigid water.

No. Impossible. She stooped down to examine the moisture, her heart thundering in her chest. A small puddle had formed beneath the coat hook, and a trail of droplets remained between there and the door.

Mother Mary, *had* it been a dream?

Eight

Nick had dreamed of kissing Maggie again last night, but at a more private location. He wanted her so much he ached—awake and asleep. Dreaming about Maggie hadn't been unusual or unexpected—definitely not unpleasant.

However . . . why, even in his dreams, didn't he press a little harder? Why was he holding back when she obviously wanted him as much as he wanted her? She was a grown woman—very nicely grown. He drew a shaky breath, still puzzled by his hesitation—as if she were made of glass or too precious to soil with his lust.

That didn't make sense. Remembering her response made his blood thicken and pool in his groin with a vengeance. She wanted him. He wanted her. They were both consenting adults. *Dammit.* Why hold back?

Was it because he'd always thought of Ireland as a place full of good, Catholic, virginal girls? But Maggie was no girl—she was every inch a woman. So why did he resist the urge to satisfy them both?

"Sense of duty . . ." The voice that answered in his mind wasn't his own. Again. "Sense of duty, my ass."

The only duty he had right now was to his employer and her granddaughter, and to his dead father. Also, if he screwed up by creating any kind of scandal in their new community, Aunt Mo would have his balls bronzed. "Ouch."

Focus, Desmond. Now *this* was more like it—his own guilty conscience. Other people's voices in his head was just too frigging weird. It had all started after arriving in Ballybronagh. Never before in his life had he heard or seen strange things. His grandmother had told him once that Ireland was a mystical place, and even the ever pragmatic Nick was starting to believe that.

"I'm not nuts." Resolved, he turned the crucifix over and over in his hand and stared at it. He'd also dreamed about another couple standing on the cliff, like the one he'd seen when he approached Maggie yesterday evening. Except this time fog and mist swirled around them. They'd stood with arms linked and their heads together, gazing out toward the sea.

In that dream he'd felt like a voyeur and realized that in reality he wouldn't have been able to see their faces, since only a bird would have been able to fly beyond the cliff to stare back at them. Even so, they remained unclear, as if deliberately blurred. Their clothing was dark and old-fashioned. The young man wore an odd hat—a tricorn? The woman's skirts were long and full, billowing in the breeze. She wore a bonnet tied beneath her chin.

They didn't appear wealthy. Though only characters in a dream, there was an intensity about them that was very real. At least to Nick . . .

He closed his fist around the crucifix and walked to the window. Why was he constantly drawn to the artifact, especially in light of this morning's lustful thoughts?

He gazed out the window where the tower of *Caisleán* Dubh dominated everything. Remembering the story about the curse, he shook his head to rid himself of dreams and thoughts of all things mystical or flat-out weird, then opened his palm to look at the crucifix again.

His chest tightened and his breath grew shallow. *Why?* Quickly, he shoved it into his pocket, his gaze drawn back to the castle. He swallowed the lump in his throat and turned deliberately away.

Now it was time for something far more pleasant. He drew a deep breath. *Maggie.* He was supposed to meet her at the school. His pulse quickened again, but for a good reason this time.

He left his room and made sure Aunt Mo and Erin knew he was leaving. He sure as hell hoped Erin wouldn't want to tag along today. Fortunately, they were busy baking a recipe Bridget Mulligan had given them. He said good-bye, locked the door behind him, and stared at the schoolhouse. Maggie was there.

"You got it bad, Desmond." What had come over him? He'd never reacted to anyone but Maggie this way before. It was exciting and scary as hell all at the same time.

And damned inconvenient. . . .

All the logic in the world couldn't dissuade him. Every time he considered his obsession with the crucifix, he realized his attraction to Maggie was just as powerful, just as disconcerting. Why? Did it matter why? Knowing why wouldn't change the fact that he had a serious case of the hots and something more.

The something more is what scared holy crap out of him. So much so, he had no intention of even trying to define it at the moment.

After a steadying breath, he reached the door to the schoolhouse. Right this minute the *why* definitely didn't matter. If all went well, his job here would be so easy he'd have plenty of free time to spend with her, and by the time it was finished, he'd know.

Know what? Nick hesitated with his hand on the doorknob. He'd written off his personal future along with his career a long time ago. He released a long, slow breath, afraid to consider that a gangster's widow was turning out to be his fairy godmother—god aunt? "Get a grip, dumbass." He shook himself and knocked as he turned the knob.

"Mag—" He froze, the acrid scent of something burning singeing his nostrils. Not just something. Something damned familiar to a former New York City vice cop, though if that bunch of smoldering weed she held was what it smelled like, it was the biggest joint he'd ever seen. "Maggie Mulligan, are you smoking pot in here?"

She stopped her walk around the classroom, the smoldering whatever-it-was clutched in her hand. "Nick . . . I didn't expect you so soon. I . . ."

"What is that stuff?" He walked inside, carefully closing the door shut behind him. It wouldn't do for the locals to get a whiff of this. "It smells like marijuana."

"First of all, I doubt most folks round here know what marijuana smells like." She stiffened and set her mouth in a thin line. "Secondly, 'tis sage. I'm smudging the school."

"Smudging?" He crossed the room, where chairs had been placed upside down on the tables, their legs jutting toward the ceiling like a line of soldiers at attention. "It stinks. Why are you stinking up the place?"

A blush bloomed in her cheeks and she gave him a look of utter impatience. Just now, she reminded him of his mother when he'd been about three and his favorite word was *why.*

"Well . . . 'tis supposed to . . ." She shook her head. "I'll explain after I've finished." She wrinkled her nose and circulated the room, waving her hand around as if painting the air with the odd bunch of smoldering weeds she had clutched in her fist. "It does stink, though."

He couldn't suppress his belly laugh, but he managed to resist the sudden urge to grab her and kiss her senseless. He noticed she seemed to pay particular attention to the corners of the room, and the windows and doors. She ducked into an alcove, then returned a moment later, coughing.

"There." She coughed again. "I think that should do it. You should've come earlier when I was burning cedar. Smelled much nicer."

Her smile made his breath hitch. She'd pulled her hair

back today, probably to keep from catching herself on fire while she "smudged."

The thought of Maggie and fire made him go cold all over—deep inside. In his soul.

In your what, Desmond? Get real.

"So . . ." He walked toward her, shoving aside the fear. "Are you going to put that thing out now?"

She laughed. "I've been reading up on cleansing rituals, but I must confess that I'm not sure of the proper way to extinguish it without offending . . . anyone."

"Offending?" Nick's eyes burned from the stench. "My nose and eyes are the only things around here to offend. Where's the bathroom?" The bough of smoldering sage was small enough now to flush without causing a clog. He reached for it, but she shook her head.

"No. I'll bury it on my way home later." She smothered the weeds in a bowl and set them aside.

A strange sensation crept over him. Was Maggie into magic? Was she Wiccan? And, if she was, why should that bother him? He'd always believed all religions took different paths to the same place. Still, something about this whole scenario made him uncomfortable, and knowing that made him pissed at himself.

He heard a sound and looked up to find her trying to light a match. The sight banished his earlier uneasiness and sent a surge of pure panic charging through him. One raspy slide across the narrow strip on the side of the box. Sharp. Anticipatory. A whiff of sulphur.

"No. Protect her. Save her." His blood turned to ice. His heart stopped. A cold sweat coated his flesh.

"What . . . are you doing?" he asked, walking slowly toward her, his gaze locked on her small hands striking the stubborn match against the side of the box.

She nodded toward a small white candle resting in a crystal dish on what he assumed was her desk. "Finishing the cleansing ritual. My book said to go through the building with a white candle." Her excitement charged the air around them.

He took the match from her and the box, battling against the image of fire he'd experienced several times since coming here. What the hell was happening to him? His hand trembled, but he managed to light the match anyway and touched the flame to the candlewick. A moment later the small candle flared to life. "Have you always been so superstitious?"

"Superstitious, is it?" She laughed and shrugged. "I suppose 'tis true. I am superstitious. I've always been fascinated with rituals, and what good Catholic isn't?"

"True."

She took the box of matches from him and unlocked a metal cabinet behind her desk and stashed them there. "Out of harm's way," she said, returning to the burning candle. "And won't Riley be surprised when he hears how many matches I've lit today? Or almost lit?"

She had a cute dimple in her left cheek when she smiled. *Damn, Desmond.* "I'm sorry, but why would Riley care about you lighting matches? I think you're old enough."

She laughed again. "Aye, but . . ." Her smile faded and she rubbed her hands together, her gaze seemingly drawn to the candle's flame. "For some reason, I've been afraid of fire all my life. I've managed to control it as an adult, but as a child I often woke in the middle of the night screaming. The nightmares were always about fire."

"I . . . I'm sorry." Nick could relate to her fear of fire in a big way these days. He shoved his fingers through his hair and cleared his throat. "I didn't mean to remind you of something unpleasant."

She waved her hand as if it meant nothing. "Well, now, shall we finish the cleansing?" Her smile returned and she picked up the crystal globe where the burning candle rested. Her hands trembled some and Riley took it from her.

"If you insist on doing this, *I'll* carry the candle."

She looked relieved and nodded. "Thank you."

"What are we supposed to do now?"

She took his free hand and led him around the room. "I imagine if I did some more research, I could find some words we could be saying, but this should do. 'Tisn't an evil place, after all."

"Not with you here," he said, staring straight ahead as he held the globe in the palm of his hand.

"What a sweet thing to say." She gave his hand a squeeze as they ducked into the small lavatory, and finally finished the circuit.

He placed the candle on the desk. "Blow it out now?"

She nodded and he did the deed, far too eager to get rid of any open flames than he should have been. "Let's go outside for some fresh air."

"We should open the windows first to let the negativity leave, and to welcome peace, health, and the nurturing of growing young minds."

"Let's send the stink out with the negativity. Especially if anyone else coming in here knows what pot smells like." He threw open all the windows on one side of the room, then helped her with the others.

She hesitated with both hands on the bottom of a window frame. "And how is it that Nick Desmond knows what marijuana smells like?"

He attempted a grin and shrugged, not ready for her to know how important a part of his life being a cop had been. Not that he'd ever be ready. "You know I used to be a cop. Vice. Knowing what it smells like came with the job."

"Ah, that's right." She walked with him to the back door, and they both stepped outside into the fresh air. "Mrs. O'Shea mentioned it yesterday at lunch. Being on the police force in New York must have been an exciting life."

"Yeah." He heard her unspoken question—why had he left his exciting career?—but he raked his fingers through his hair and stared out across the playground and cemetery. He tried not to let his gaze drift toward the old ruins where he'd found the crucifix. "Does it give any of the kids the creeps to play right next to the graveyard?" Even that was a safer topic than his former career.

Maggie appeared thoughtful, and he reached for her hand. They walked slowly toward the moss-covered stone wall separating the playground from the cemetery. "I remember being afraid once when I was a child. We were playing a game out here, and I thought I saw something over there." She pointed toward the ruins. "Something very strange."

Nick's heart stuttered. "Something shiny?"

"Oh, I've often seen something shiny over in the old ruins, but not that day." She looked in that direction again. "Come to think of it, I haven't seen that for a while now. That's odd."

Not a bit odd. He put his left hand in his pocket and draped his right arm across her shoulder, needing suddenly to touch her.

"Save her."

He squeezed his eyes closed, trying to ignore the voice, though he couldn't deny that was exactly how he felt right now. Protective. "What did you see? What frightened you?" He swallowed hard, feeling the metal in his pocket grow warm, almost pulsing with it.

With a gasp she turned toward him, her eyes wide. "Until now, I was never sure what I'd seen, but now I know. I remember! It explains why I've always been afraid. . . ." She bit her lower lip and pointed to the open area near the ruins. "A column of flame right there."

She trembled and he tightened his arm around her. He had to ask. "Was it real?"

"Only to me."

Angelo Fazzini paced the plush carpet in his office, waiting for Finn McAdam—the man he trusted above all others. Finn had called nearly half an hour ago. Where the hell was the man?

Finn's grandmother and later his mother had both worked for Angelo's family as housekeepers. He and Finn had grown up like brothers. Angelo had learned at his father's deathbed that they had the same father, though no one else knew the truth now that their old man was dead.

Angelo and Finn kept the Fazzini empire running together—just the way Father would have wanted. In fact, sometimes Angelo had to struggle against the urge to disregard his father's wish that Finn never know about his paternity. At least they didn't look alike, though both were blends of Irish and Italian.

Angelo paused beside his desk and picked up the copy of *Collins Gem Irish Dictionary* he'd purchased. Now he knew for certain that Mamó meant granny or grandma.

Who the hell had called his mother's private number and addressed her as *mamó*? And *why*? He slammed the book down on his desk just as a knock sounded at the door. "Come in," he barked.

"Testy today, are we?" Finn asked as he entered the office and closed the door behind him. "I thought for sure this one was a wild goose chase, boss, but I think we might have something now."

"What?" Angelo walked around the corner of his desk and slumped into the chair. "Sit. Talk." He slid the Irish dictionary closer to himself and let his hand rest on it. "Well?"

"Since the call was international and weeks old by the time I started trying to track it down, it was damned near impossible."

"But . . . ?" Angelo didn't have the patience for Finn's usual crap today. "Cut to it, McAdam."

"Was your mom religious?"

"You know as well as I do that she went to mass every week. Why?"

"The call came from a convent in Ireland."

"Convent?" Even more confused, Angelo shook his head. "That's *it*? Just a convent?"

Finn raked his fingers through his blond hair and glanced at the paper clutched in his hand. "There's a boarding school, too, run by the Sisters of—"

"School?" That nagging suspicion Angelo had been trying to deny shot through him like lightning and he lurched to his feet. "A *school?*"

"Yeah, a school." Finn narrowed his eyes. "Color me curious. What's the big deal?"

Angelo fell back into his chair with a plop and rubbed his forehead. His head ached. His gut ached. His physical hadn't gone well. He hadn't been sleeping worth a damn, and all because of a hunch that wasn't based on anything even remotely resembling fact. Why? He let his head fall back against the leather chair and sighed, then leveled his gaze on his most trusted assistant.

"Maybe nothing," he said. "Maybe everything. It may be crazy, but I can't let it go. I just *can't.*"

"Enlighten me, boss." Finn held his hands out to his sides, palms upward. "I can't help if I don't know what I'm looking for."

"Not what." Angelo released a long, slow breath. "Who."

"Okay. *Who?*"

He held his half brother's gaze for several moments, then said, "Erin."

Finn cleared his throat. "Have you been into the merchandise, boss?"

"Cute." Angelo drew a deep breath, determined to keep his cool. He rubbed his eyes and picked up the dictionary. "Look up the word *mamó.*"

"I already know what it means. That's what I called my grandmother. Why?"

Angelo pulled the small tape player from his desk drawer and pushed play. The sound of the child's voice made his breath hitch. He pushed stop after it ended and looked up at Finn. "Maybe it was just a wrong number, but I can't let it go."

"Angelo, think. How *could* it be Erin?"

"We never found her."

"That's not proof, and neither was that phone call."

Angelo rose and leaned on the desk's polished surface, locking his elbows. "There's more."

"What?"

One good thing about Finn—at least he knew when to cut the crap and get serious. "Mother was out of town."

Finn waved his hand over the top of his head. "Went right by me. When was she out of town, boss?"

So much for serious. Angelo mentally counted to ten. "When Erin was . . . kidnapped." He didn't want to remember that time. It hurt too much.

"Oh, yeah. That's right." Finn stood and started pacing. "I remember her flying home. She was still mourning T—" He paused and looked up at Angelo.

"You can say her name."

"Your wife."

"Teresa."

Finn's eyes widened in obvious surprise. "Right. Your mom flew home from wherever she went to mourn."

"And we searched for Erin. My child." Angelo had his emotions in check now, allowing the cold, calculating mind that had enabled him to build the organization his father had founded into something bigger and better. Impenetrable. Losing his only child to slimeball kidnappers had been Angelo's only failure. Teresa didn't count. Her life had been worthless and expendable.

But Erin mattered. She was his blood. "Do you know where my mother flew home *from* after Erin was kidnapped, Finn?"

He shook his head. "I don't have a clue, boss. Where?"

"I didn't remember either, so I asked *your* mother. She remembered."

"She remembers what I ate for breakfast when I was three." Finn stopped his pacing and stared at Angelo. "Holy shit. Ireland?"

"Got it in one."

"But when did she leave to go there?"

"Your mother isn't sure, and I haven't found anything in my mother's files about her using her private plane or a travel agent then either." Angelo cracked his knuckles, wishing he could smash a window or something instead. "It's almost . . . almost as if she wiped that trip clean. Covered it up."

"Do you realize what you're saying, boss?" Finn shook his head.

"Why do you think I put you on this instead of someone else?"

"You going to Ireland?"

Angelo held his breath for a few seconds. "Not yet," he finally said. "You go and do some preliminary work. See what you can learn at the convent."

"I'll get right on it."

"If you find . . . anything, then I'll join you there."

Finn touched his arm. "Remember, the kid won't know you if it's her."

"If it's her, she's alone now that Mother is gone." Angelo swallowed the bile rising to his throat at the thought that his own mother could have done anything so vile . . . to her own son. "Go find out for me. I trust you, Finn."

"I know you do, but I want a raise." He spun around and left the office.

"Anything you want," Angelo muttered as the door closed.

Alone with his tormenting thoughts, he listened to the tape again, wondering. How could he ever forget the day a few weeks before Erin's birth, when his mother had asked him to give up his "life of crime," as she'd called it? He'd laughed at her then.

He sure as hell wasn't laughing now.

Nine

After Maggie had accepted Mrs. O'Shea's invitation to dinner, she watched Nick walk away from the school. He hadn't kissed her this time, though she'd seen desire in his eyes. They'd been alone here in the schoolyard, and he'd seemed very tense about something.

Her story about the fire?

He probably thought she was one for the loony bin after catching her smudging the schoolhouse with sage, then hearing a bizarre tale of seeing fire that hadn't existed. "And isn't that the way to woo a man?"

Was that her intention? She paused to gaze across the graveyard. The wind shifted and a soft, soughing sound reached her ears.

The chanting. Fingers of ice drove themselves through her veins. She walked slowly toward the low stone wall separating the schoolyard from the cemetery and ruins, struggling merely to breathe.

Though unintelligible, the muffled sound grew stronger. Now she was almost certain the voices came from the ruins—if not from the fragments of her sanity. Her heart skipped a beat or more as she strained to discern words from the jumbled voices. More than one voice? Or was it the same voice repeating something in rounds?

"Rounds, is it now? You're bloody crazy." She shook her head as if to clear it, but couldn't bring herself to leave the wall.

"Rejoin the accurst . . ."

She held her breath and looked behind her, then back to the ruins. The murmuring stopped. Had she heard the words, or had it been her imagination running amok?

"And hasn't your imagination been doing just that lately?" she asked aloud, needing to hear the sound of her own voice to anchor herself in reality.

Enough nonsense. She'd heard nothing. 'Twas the wind and the sea—nothing more. She released her death grip on the wall and wiped her sweaty palms on her jeans.

Determined to forget the imagined words, she strode away from the wall and closed up the schoolhouse before heading home. At the curve in the road separating *Caisleán* Dubh from the fields and meadows of their farm, she paused.

What was happening to her? Why was she hearing voices and having bizarre dreams? Her face flamed. *Couldn't hormones have a wee bit to do with her dream?*

But it hadn't been only a sexy dream. Last night's dream had also frightened her—no sense in denying it. Even so, it had excited her even more, which probably explained her disappointment that Nick hadn't kissed her again today.

Of course . . . the day was still young. She hugged herself and glanced at the castle. She should stop and see Mum, and promised herself she would on her way back to town. Right now she couldn't bring herself to even enter *Caisleán* Dubh.

A shudder rippled through her at the thought, and she cut across the meadow where Oíche grazed contentedly on the summer grass. Riley's horse raised its head as she passed and gave a friendly nicker, but she didn't pause to stroke the lovely black beast as she normally would. "Tomorrow I'll bring you a treat. I promise. There's a good lad."

She quickened her pace, eager to call Ailish and tell her about the dream and the voices. Of course, she wouldn't give her friend *all* the details, but enough to make her point.

This morning Maggie had convinced herself that the puddle and droplets she'd discovered last night must have been left by Riley when he'd made his overly protective big-brother inspection of her cottage. And wasn't that possible? Well, at least it sounded more logical than a dream that left physical evidence in its wake. But how had she ended up downstairs? She'd never walked in her sleep before. . . .

Wasn't there a first time for everything? Perhaps if she kept reasoning with herself, the dreams and doubts would leave her in peace. She had a school to plan and more than enough work to keep her busy.

Despite Riley's urging, she rarely locked her doors. No one in Ballybronagh did, except for Maureen O'Shea, from what she'd heard. But the woman was a newcomer to their village. Soon enough she would realize there was no need here for locks and security systems.

The moment Maggie closed the door behind her, a sense of peace settled over her. She loved this cottage. Her home. Here she was safe.

"Safe from what?" She had to laugh at herself, albeit a bit nervously, as she made her way to the phone and dialed Ailish's number. Doubts eddied through her and she almost hung up, but a cheery *hello* foiled her plan.

"Hi, Ailish," she said into the receiver.

"Maggie, how are you? Did you get the new book I sent?"

"I did. Thank you." Maggie chewed her lower lip, searching for the words.

"What is it? What's wrong? I can tell something is wrong."

Maggie sighed and proceeded to tell her old roommate

about her dream—leaving out a few of the more delicious details. The most important points were that she'd found herself downstairs when she awakened, with water on what should have been a dry floor. The moment those words left her mouth, she added, "Of course, my brother was here just before I turned in, so he could have left wet footprints behind."

Several seconds of silence filled the line. "Did you see footprints, Maggie?"

She drew a shaky breath. "No. Only drops of water."

"That came from nowhere?"

"And when you put it that way, don't I really sound insane?"

"No," Ailish said in her calm, knowing way. "Is the cottage on a ley line?"

"A what?"

"Ley lines are paths of energy that run through the earth at sharp angles."

"Is there anything in the book you sent about—"

"A little." The sound of turning pages came through the phone line. "I'll read this to you. It's pretty basic. 'In 1921, Alfred Watkins noticed that ancient ruins seemed to fall in straight lines. He mapped several in England and also discovered that hilltops, churches, standing stones, castles, and burial mounds are connected by these lines.' And isn't Ireland a land filled with such things?"

"Connected?" Maggie's throat went dry as she remembered the voices. "We have ruins near the school."

"I'm going to take a holiday and come see this place for myself. I've been dying to see this castle of yours anyway. Are you up for some company?"

"I'd love to see you." Maggie released a long slow breath. "There's more."

"What is it?"

"I . . . I'm interested in someone."

"And wouldn't that be the man from your dream, of course?" Ailish laughed. "You didn't think you could hide that from me, did you, love?"

Maggie's face flamed and she cleared her throat. "He's an American—from New York. Former police."

"Rich? Handsome? Sexy?"

"Two out of three." Maggie laughed, pleased she'd called her dear friend. "I'm not so sure about rich, though his aunt seems well-to-do."

Ailish laughed as well. "And isn't handsome and sexy more important? Kind, good, spiritual?"

Maggie remembered how he hadn't pressured her to take their kiss further, even when she'd been eager enough. Was that why he'd been more aggressive in her dream? Because *she'd* wanted him to be so in real life? *Listen to yourself.*

She cleared her throat. "He's a gentleman, kind, good. I don't know about spiritual yet. If you mean does he go to mass, I have seen him there with his aunt and young cousin."

"I mean spiritual in a deeper way."

For some reason, the thought gave her pause. "I . . . I'm not sure I understand your meaning."

"Ah, Maggie, how could you room with me so long and not know what I mean?"

"Oh. That."

"*That.* Listen to you." Ailish laughed, but not mockingly. "Aren't *you* learning that you're spiritual in ways you never imagined?"

"I'm still not sure." Maggie glanced at the open book on her kitchen table. How would she ever explain her interest in Wicca and ley lines to Mum or Riley? "We'll see."

"Won't we now?"

Needing to change the subject, Maggie asked, "When will you arrive?" She stretched the phone cord as far as it would reach to allow her to grab a bottle of soda from the icebox. "I can't wait to see you."

"Friday. I'll ask directions in the village."

"Stop at the school first. That's probably where I'll be if you get here during the day." Maggie took a sip of cola.

"Or walking on the beach with your handsome, sexy Yank," Ailish said with a suggestive chuckle.

Maggie's soda bubbled in her throat and she coughed. "I've missed you."

"And I you. I'll see you Friday afternoon—I have to work the morning or Da will be furious. And I want to meet your Yank. I'll read his aura and let you know how spiritual he is."

Maggie ended the call and retrieved the most recent book Ailish had sent. She found mention of ley lines in the index, but there wasn't any more information there than what Ailish had already told her.

She sat at the kitchen table, allowing herself a few minutes to think before dressing for dinner. She'd been so focused on the mysterious drops of water that she'd nearly forgotten the way the wall and coat hook had transformed in her dream. And Nick's jacket had become a heavy, wool cloak.

A chill seeped through her and she shivered. She rose and went to the old books in what had been Da's study and later Riley's. All she knew about this cottage was that it had been built in 1900. What had been here before?

"Probably sheep or cows," she chided, unconvinced. She would ask Riley or Brady. They might know.

She hurried upstairs to change for dinner, but found herself drawn to her bedroom window. It faced the church and school in the distance, but nearer and to her far left she saw the tower of *Caisleán* Dubh.

A chill slid through her as she contemplated the sharp angles—ley lines?—that ran from the old church ruins to *Caisleán* Dubh . . .

And to this cottage.

Nick took a stack of plates from Aunt Mo and placed one at each place on the kitchen table. Donovan cottage didn't have a formal dining room—not that *he'd* ever had one before—but Angelo Fazzini's mother must have.

Not Fazzini. O'Shea. Maureen O'Shea. He cleared his throat. "This is one hell of a switch for you. Isn't it?"

Aunt Mo looked up from the pot she'd been stirring and smiled. "I'm enjoying myself."

"Playing house, huh?" Nick grinned when she rolled her eyes at him. "Five places for dinner? Let me guess . . ."

"Very funny." She put a lid on the pot and turned down the flame. "Your cousin is joining us."

"Hmm." Nick waggled his eyebrows. "Two nights in a row? Must be serious."

Aunt Mo's cheeks reddened, but her expression turned solemn. "'Tis glad I am that Maggie will come, too."

Nick swallowed the lump in his throat, hoping the old woman wouldn't notice. He'd been distracted by Maggie's odd behavior and her confession about having seen a column of fire.

Aunt Mo placed knives and forks beside all the plates. "Everything seems to be going well here," she said.

Nick paused. "So far."

Aunt Mo met his gaze from across the table. "So far."

"With any luck, the expense of me will turn out to be a big waste."

A smile curved the old woman's lips. "Not at all." She continued setting the table, then added, "Brady promised to bring up the notion of you working at the school this evening."

"Oh, yeah." Something else Nick had forgotten. It wasn't like him to let things slide this way. He was getting sloppy, and that could prove dangerous. "The new handyman or something?"

"Or something." Aunt Mo smiled again as someone knocked on the front door.

Erin stopped playing the piano in the front room and Nick accompanied his employer to the door. "All clear." He tried to sound flippant for Erin's sake.

"You're silly." She giggled.

"And you're giggly," he returned.

Aunt Mo laughed as she opened the door. "Brady, Maggie, come in. Welcome."

Brady removed his hat as he stepped inside, presenting his hostess with yet another bouquet of flowers. "These pale before your beauty."

Aunt Mo's cheeks glowed. "You're such a darling charmer. Thank you, Brady."

"I ran into Maggie out front, and brought her along." Brady winked and hung his hat on the peg where it had rested last night during his visit.

Cousin Brady was getting downright comfortable. Nick couldn't suppress a smile for his distant relative, but his attention swung very quickly to their other guest.

"Hi." Nick inhaled Maggie's scent. She smiled at him and his heart skipped a beat. The soft green sweater she wore clung to her curves in all the right places, and the crinkled-looking skirt fluttered to her ankles. His breath caught as his gaze traveled the length of her, settling at last on her lush, tempting lips. "You look gorgeous."

Erin giggled.

Maggie smiled. "I'm afraid I didn't bring you flowers."

Erin giggled louder and skipped away to torment Brady and her grandmother.

Damn, but this is weird. He hadn't realized it earlier, but this was like . . . a real date. And—even more strange—the idea pleased him. He'd get to walk her home later. His body warmed and tightened in anticipation of kissing Maggie good night again.

And more. Oh, yeah—he *definitely* wanted more. He deliberately dropped his gaze to her breasts again, and her soft gasp assured him that she'd noticed. So far, he'd treated her like something fragile, though what he really wanted was to taste every inch of her naked body, and to give them both what they obviously wanted.

Sex. Great sex. And plenty of it.

His blood supply pulled a U-turn that made him sway. He dragged in a shaky breath to steady himself, amazed at how powerful his urge was to throw her over his shoulder and carry her off to his bed.

Erin giggled again, reminding him that was the last thing in the world he could pull right now. Besides, that sort of Neanderthal behavior would frighten Maggie away, and he *definitely* had other things in mind for her. Delicious things.

Hoping no one would notice how thoroughly he filled out his jeans now, he took Maggie's small leather purse. "I'll just hang this here." He put it beside Brady's hat and took her arm.

"Thank you." Her voice sounded huskier than he remembered.

Make small talk, Desmond. "Gilhooley's is interesting. Is it family owned?"

"Aye. Gilhooley's has been here for centuries, passed from son to son."

"Not daughters?" He grinned.

Maggie laughed. "Well, now that you mention it, Irene is part owner with her brother."

"Did she go to college with you?"

"Oh, no." Maggie chuckled a little at that. "The Gilhooleys won the Irish Lottery years ago and moved away."

"I guess if I won the lottery, I'd move somewhere warm and sunny."

"I'd never live anyplace else," she said. "They moved to Crete."

"Sounds like a tough life." He rested his hand on the small of her back to guide her toward the bench before the front window.

Maggie sat and smoothed her skirt as Nick slid down beside her—as close as humanly possible. His heart skipped a beat and heat insinuated itself right where it counted.

Maggie chewed her lower lip and tilted her head at an angle, spilling her mane of red curls over one shoulder.

Enough small talk. Nick drew a deep, appreciative breath. Her hair smelled spicy, like cinnamon.

"Something in the kitchen smells good," Maggie said a bit breathlessly.

He'd like to make her a lot more breathless.

"I . . . I think maybe pride, more than anything, brought Irene back," she said.

Pride was something Nick could understand. He swallowed the sudden lump in his throat, unwilling and unable to consider what had once made him proud. And had nearly destroyed him . . .

"At least that's my guess." Maggie folded her hands in her lap, definitely nervous. "I should go help Mrs. O'Shea."

"Stay." Nick covered her hand with his own, acutely conscious of what lay beneath her primly folded hands and the silky folds of her skirt. "Brady and Erin are helping." His cousin laughed from the kitchen. *Great timing.* He couldn't suppress the grin that spread across his face. "We'd just be in the way."

"And wouldn't I do more harm than good in the kitchen anyway?" Maggie laughed, though it sounded nervous. "I'm a dreadful cook."

He gave her hand a squeeze, concentrating exclusively on the bright, vibrant woman sitting at his side instead. "A beautiful, dreadful cook."

"And aren't you and your cousin a pair of charmers?" She laughed and the sound trickled down his spine.

Nick's breath caught in his throat. A woman's laugh had never turned him on before, but Maggie's tiptoed inside him and did a little dance. He was in a bad way. Hoping he was being discreet, he adjusted his position enough to prevent his belt from pinching a very sensitive spot.

"If I'm charming, it's only because you're so beautiful." *You got it bad.*

A blush crept upward from the neckline of her sweater and bloomed in her cheeks. "Thank you," she whispered, her blue eyes darkening.

He turned her palm over and linked his fingers through

hers, wishing he could get closer to her now. Later, he would walk her home, and kiss her again. And again. "Just the truth." His voice sounded thick, hoarse.

"Well . . ." She gazed downward at their linked hands, her curls brushing against his arm. Maggie looked up and met his gaze. "How . . . how long are you planning to stay here with your aunt and cousin?" she asked.

Nick gnashed his teeth and inhaled slowly through his nose. He didn't want to alarm Maggie by reacting too dramatically, though her question was like a punch in the gut. He lifted a shoulder. "We'll see. I haven't thought too far beyond getting Aunt Mo and Erin settled here."

And getting revenge.

"Do you miss your home? Your parents?"

"They're dead." His gut was on fire. "There's nothing there to miss."

"Oh, Nick. I'm so sorry."

Her eyes glittered dangerously. The last thing he wanted was to make her cry. "It was a long time ago." He shrugged and leaned back, hoping he sounded more casual than he felt. "My aunt asked me to come to Ireland, so here I am."

" 'Tis glad I am you're here," she whispered, looking down at their linked hands.

Something in Nick's chest swelled and pressed upward against his throat. She made him want to feel things again—things that had died inside him along with his father.

"Are you interested in your Irish heritage?"

Yes, change the subject. Please. "I found Brady, didn't I?"

Maggie laughed, her eyes sparkling again. "There's no one who knows more about the clans of Ballybronagh and Clare itself than your own cousin."

"Trust me—I noticed." He winked. "My grandparents talked about Ireland a lot, so I figured this was my chance to see it for myself."

She seemed satisfied with his answer. Erin popped

around the corner from the kitchen, grinning as if she'd been hoping to catch them smooching. Nick fully intended to do just that, but not where the nosey kid could see them.

"Dinner's ready," Erin said.

Nick rose and kept Maggie's hand as they strolled into the kitchen. Erin raised her eyebrows as they passed and Nick couldn't resist winking at her. He was rewarded with another giggle—Erin's specialty, so he'd learned.

A roasted chicken with stuffing oozing from it sat on the table. Several steaming bowls surrounded it, filled with spuds, peas, white sauce, and a basket of brown bread. Nick pulled out a chair for Maggie and waited until she was seated. Aunt Mo and Brady occupied the other side of the oval table, with Erin on the end. That left him no choice but to take the chair right beside Maggie.

Smiling to himself, he sat. His employer invited Brady to say the blessing and Nick bowed his head, though he couldn't resist a side glance at Maggie through the veil of his lashes. After Brady's brief prayer, she crossed herself and he followed her example, remembering all the years of catechism he'd endured as a child.

His pulse quickened and he slipped his hand into his pocket to grasp the crucifix. It pulsed with heat and its warmth crept up his arm and across his chest. He muttered, "Spiritus Sancti"—something he'd probably learned a long time ago, but the meaning was lost to him now.

Maggie glanced up at him, obviously surprised. Liquid fire flooded his cheeks as he realized everyone at the table was staring at him as well. What had he said? And why?

"I didn't realize you were old enough to have learned Latin in catechism, Nick," Aunt Mo said.

"I'm not even sure what I said." He gave a nervous chuckle and pulled his hand from his pocket. The comforting warmth he'd experienced while touching the crucifix left him confused and embarrassed.

"You said 'Holy Spirit,'" Erin said. "I learned that at school."

"Of course you did." Aunt Mo passed the carving knife and a serving fork to Brady. "Would you do the honors, Brady?"

"Aye, a pleasure." Brady stood to carve the chicken, sniffing the steam wafting upward from the roasted bird. "And isn't that a heavenly aroma?"

Nick agreed and reached over to give Maggie's hand another squeeze. She blushed prettily and he suddenly wished they could skip dinner and take a walk. The need to have her alone unhinged him even more decidedly than touching the crucifix had.

"How are plans for the school coming along?" Aunt Mo asked as the various dishes made their way around the table.

"Well, I think." Maggie released his hand to spoon peas onto her plate and passed the bowl to Nick with a shy smile.

She seemed so young and innocent just now. Guilt knifed through Nick. He shouldn't have lustful thoughts about her, but he did. Confused by these new and contradictory values, he blinked as he took the bowl and served himself. She was a gorgeous woman, an adult, and he was a grown man with a serious craving. Why should that make him feel shame? The old Nick wouldn't have hesitated to pursue and even seduce a beautiful, willing woman if he wanted her. Oh, and he definitely wanted her. He held his breath for a long moment until Erin took the serving bowl from him.

"Maggie, how do you feel about having Nick work at the school?" Brady asked as he passed the platter of sliced chicken.

Obviously startled, Maggie looked up quickly. "Work?"

"Brady said there are some repairs that need doing," Aunt Mo said smoothly as she reached for her tea. "Nick needs to be busy, so Brady and I thought he might be the perfect person for the job."

" 'Tis true, but . . ." Maggie drew a slow, deep breath, riveting Nick's attention to her breasts again.

This new Nick wanted to seduce her, too. *Dammit.* That settled it. No more of this strange sense of honor and duty he'd been battling. Not that he would force anything— never that. Still, it was clear Maggie wanted him, too. He heard his name and dragged his attention back to the conversation.

"I'm not sure how we can afford to pay Nick or anyone else," Maggie said, her voice sounding strained. "We can barely afford to keep the school open as it is, and I've already donated most of my own salary back to the operating expenses."

Aunt Mo's eyes grew wide, and Nick wondered how she would get out of this one. She didn't want the villagers to know she was loaded, but it looked like she no longer had the luxury of keeping that particular secret.

"And hasn't Mrs. O'Shea—Maureen—come to our rescue?" Brady asked, beaming.

Maggie shook her head, obviously confused. "Our rescue?"

"I . . . well, let's just say money isn't a problem for me," Aunt Mo explained. "And it's high time it did some good. So I made a donation to the school—enough to cover this year's operating expenses, I think. Including Nick. I hope that's all right."

"Of course it's all right. It's wonderful! Thank you. I'm just surprised." Maggie looked at Nick. " 'Tis an old building. Are you good with tools then, Nick Desmond?"

A piece of chicken stuck in his throat and he washed it down with water. "Depends," he finally managed, trying not to think about tools of a more anatomical nature.

"My nephew is a man of many hidden talents," Aunt Mo said.

Erin clapped her hands together. "I'm so glad we came here."

Nick ate without really tasting a thing. All he wanted was to be alone with Maggie again. He'd walk her home, of course. Alone. In the dark. Maybe she would invite him into her cottage.

"Brady, do you know if another building ever sat where Mulligan Cottage is now?" Maggie asked.

"Aye." Brady stiffened somewhat and set his fork aside, obviously uncomfortable with her question. "No one has ever asked about it before."

Nick detected an unspoken *why* in his cousin's comment, which made him curious. "Is there something wrong with asking?"

Brady shook his head. "Not at all, though wouldn't I have rested easier if no one ever had?"

How un-Brady not to burst into an eager and long-winded explanation. Nick reached instinctively for Maggie's free hand in the folds of her skirt. It was cold and trembled slightly. Something weird was coming down. "Why?" Someone had to ask.

"And wasn't I merely curious?" Maggie managed to laugh, though it sounded forced.

"'Tis sorry I am for hesitatin'." Brady drew a deep breath and took a sip of tea. After setting his cup into its saucer again, he steepled his fingers beneath his chin and looked from Maggie to Nick, then back. "Me own uncertainty is the reason for not explainin' right away. You see, it appears Mulligan Cottage was built on the foundation of a smaller one once used by servants who worked in *Caisleán* Dubh."

Nick sensed that Maggie relaxed some, though she tightened her grip on his hand. "That isn't a bad thing, so why did you hesitate?" she asked.

"No, 'tisn't a bad thing at all." Brady reached for his fork again, obviously eager to move on to other topics. "'Tis the identity of the occupants that worries me."

Nick felt a shudder ripple through Maggie, though he couldn't imagine why. "Who was it?" He sensed she needed to hear the answer.

Even Aunt Mo and Erin seemed to hold their breath, waiting for Brady's answer.

The old man certainly had a gift for drama. Nick shoved a forkful of mashed potatoes into his mouth.

"The parish and Mulligan records indicate the original cottage was occupied by poor Bronagh and her lonely old aunt." Brady looked around the table. "The *cailleach*."

Ten

"*The* cailleach?" *Maggie* couldn't breathe for several seconds. Bronagh and her aunt had lived on the same ground where Mulligans had for over a century? How could her family have not known? And how could Maggie have felt safe and happy there?

"What's a *cailleach*?" Nick asked, his solemn tone reflecting her mood.

"A witch," Aunt Mo said, her expression passive.

Nick stiffened at Maggie's side, and she heard him grind his teeth. If hearing of a witch who'd died two centuries ago could unnerve him, how would he react to Ailish? For that matter, why did discussion of Bronagh's aunt disturb Maggie?

Because the witch's spell—the curse—had plagued Maggie's family for two hundred years. She closed her eyes and drew a steadying breath. "It seems odd that they—my ancestors—chose that site for the cottage." She reopened her eyes to meet Brady's gaze.

The old man smiled at her. "Ah, but the Mulligans didn't realize a spell had caused the curse until Riley and I read the old priest's diaries. Fascinating reading, though

I found myself going to confession more often." His cheeks blazed crimson and Mrs. O'Shea patted his hand.

"A real witch?" Erin asked, her eyes round. "A bad one?"

"Well, now, some thought so, though the priest insisted she was both pagan and Catholic," Brady said. "After all, she was only tryin' to avenge her niece. Her heart was broken, lass."

"My ancestors built the cottage and moved into it to *escape* the curse," Maggie whispered, as much to herself as to anyone, needing to make sense of nonsense. "On the same land where the witch responsible for the deed had lived?" The irony of this discovery made her voice rise a bit with every syllable.

Nick squeezed her hand and she glanced at his kind face. His tension had obviously passed. His gentle gaze held hers as she managed another deep breath. Odd that a man who excited her in so many ways soothed her now.

"Ah, but the curse only affected Mulligans *within* the castle walls." Brady took a sip of tea, obviously recovered from his uncharacteristic bout of reluctance. "And since, for whatever reasons, the Mulligans weren't aware of the *cailleach,* they had no reason to fear the land upon which her cottage once sat. Hasn't it been a safe haven for your family, Maggie?"

"It has." She managed, finally, to slow her racing heart.

"What an interesting history your family has," Mrs. O'Shea said evenly, her smile reassuring.

"You grew up in that cottage," Nick said, his tone neutral. "Were you ever afraid?"

Maggie released a sigh. "Never, and 'tis foolish I'm being now." She forced a smile and savored the warm, solid feel of his hand in hers. "I'm a bit tired is all."

"Been burning the midnight oil getting ready for the school to open?" His smile made her heart skip a beat.

"That I have." Maggie's cheeks warmed as she remembered *exactly* what—and who—had awakened her last night. That dream had started the string of questions in her mind about the cottage. That and Ailish's comment about ley lines . . .

Nonsense. Or was it? How could she discount the fact that the same witch who'd cast the spell had lived on the same soil where her cottage now stood? She forced herself to listen to the conversation.

"I made the afters," Erin said, accompanying her grandmother to the counter. "Chocolate *gateaux.*"

"What's that?"

"Cake," Maggie said.

"Yum. One of the first things I learned in Ireland is that *afters* means *dessert,*" Nick said. "Does it have gooey frosting?"

"Whipped cream and strawberries," Erin said.

Nick looked at Maggie again with that devastating grin of his. It never failed to make her heart flutter. She was more than ready to concentrate on other subjects—like the man at her side.

"A woman with taste." His voice lowered and his eyes smoldered as his grin transformed into something far more intense. More inviting.

More stimulating.

And isn't that a marvelous notion? Maggie smiled again. "I *do* have excellent taste."

His eyes widened, telling her he'd caught her double entendre. He inclined his chin a bit, as if in deference to the victor. "So do I."

The urge to crawl into his lap and plant a big wet kiss on his mouth made her squirm a bit. He held her hand, brushing small circles across the back of it with his thumb. Only when Erin placed plates heaping with chocolate and berries in front of them did he look away.

"You made this all by yourself?" Nick asked as he grabbed his fork and took a bite. "Mmm."

"Mamó showed me how." Erin took her seat again and forked a huge bite of cake into her mouth. "Oh, it *is* good!"

Brady nodded in agreement. "Perfect."

"You doubted it would be good?" Mrs. O'Shea arched a brow at her granddaughter. "Silly lass."

Erin wrinkled her nose and proceeded to eat in silence, as did the others. Maggie left only a few crumbs on her plate, amazed by how thoroughly the promise of chocolate could restore her appetite. *Temptation.*

And wasn't the man at her side more than a bit of temptation himself? Her heart pounded and her breath quickened. Nick Desmond was far more than merely a *bit* tempting. He made her want to be naughty. Very naughty.

He made her want to be kissed, touched, caressed. He made her want to toss caution aside and . . . and—

Oh. Shocked by the direction of her thoughts, a hot flush crept across her cheeks and she pulled her hand free and stood. "Let me help with the dishes."

Nick glanced up at her as if he knew exactly what had made her leap up from the table. His crooked grin insinuated itself into her heart and it was all she could do not to throw herself into his arms and invite him to have his way with her.

Aye.

"Nonsense. You're a guest and you've been working too hard as it is." Mrs. O'Shea rose and patted Brady's shoulder. "Besides, someone else offered first."

"So I did." Brady gathered dishes and carried them to the sink with Erin and Mrs. O'Shea. "And isn't it me pleasure?"

"I'll walk you home." Nick rose and took Maggie's arm.

"Thank you for dinner," she said, so nervous her mouth went dry. "Everything was delicious—especially the afters."

Erin directed a smile over her shoulder. "Thank you, Miss Mulligan."

They all bid their good nights, and Maggie finally found her purse draped over her shoulder and herself outside with Nick. Alone. She'd been so distracted earlier, she hadn't thought to bring a wrap, and hugged herself against the evening chill.

Nick slipped his denim jacket from his shoulders and settled it over hers. "Better?"

"Uh-huh, but now you'll get cold."

He cupped her chin in his hand and tilted it upward. Very briefly he brushed his lips against hers. Awareness sizzled through her veins, settling hot and deep in her center.

"Not a bit cold," he murmured.

With his arm draped across her shoulders, they walked slowly along the dirt road that wound its way toward the peninsula where the intimidating tower of *Caisleán* Dubh spiraled into the night sky. The top of the tower blended seamlessly with the darkness.

Was it her imagination, or did their pace slow more and more as they neared the curve that would lead toward Mulligan land? Maggie didn't mind the delay. In fact, she welcomed it, for it meant she could remain at his side that much longer.

As if in unspoken agreement, they paused near the cliff to gaze out at the sea. The moon cast a silver streak across its surface that seemed to point toward them. *Isn't that another silly notion?* Still, the thought remained.

Nick massaged her shoulder through the thickness of his jacket. The cool evening air and his nearness combined to make her nipples tighten beneath her jumper. Her thin cotton bra and the darkness were the only protection for her modesty.

Modest, however, didn't come close to describing her mood now. He half turned to face her, one hand on each of her upper arms. "I've been looking forward to this all evening," he whispered, the heat of his breath wafting across her face.

Her throat tightened, but she managed to murmur, "Me, too." Before she could draw her next breath, his mouth possessed hers.

There was nothing gentle, nothing subdued about this

kiss, and Maggie savored it, as if she'd been waiting a lifetime for this moment, this man. Desire unfurled through her veins, seeking each and every nerve ending along the way.

She threw her arms around his neck, and when his tongue parted her lips, she welcomed it. His arms slid around her waist and he pulled her snugly against him with a groan that rumbled through her bone marrow and settled unerringly in her womb.

Liquid heat swarmed through her as he explored her mouth. She returned his kiss, tentatively at first, then more boldly. That small step sent a thrill through her—a sort of feminine power, she supposed.

He massaged her hips and his jacket slipped unheeded from her shoulders. Maggie moaned, realizing she *couldn't* have stopped this even if she tried.

He cupped her bottom in his large hands and tugged her more firmly against his lower body. The hard resistance she encountered there made the fire low in her belly burn hotter, and she clenched agonizingly against an emptiness so powerful it made her groan.

"Maggie," he whispered, kissing his way across her cheek, down the side of her neck. "Maggie."

She captured the sides of his face with her hands and kissed him again. As he responded, she threaded her fingers through the soft dark curls at his nape, holding him to her.

Through some kind of haze, she became aware of him inching his hands forward until they rested against her rib cage, just beneath her aching breasts. Oh, she wanted him to touch her, to kiss her.

She simply *wanted.*

Gently, as if testing their weight, he cradled her breasts in his palms. A deep, throaty sound came from somewhere deep inside her, and he responded by brushing his thumbs across her nipples.

Maggie broke their kiss, gasping, her head lolling back and to the side as he traced tortuous circles around her erect nipples. "Jaysus, Mary, and Joseph," she muttered, unable and unwilling to pull away.

Nick eased one hand beneath the hem of her jumper, and the feel of him touching her bare flesh made her thrust her pelvis against his compelling hardness. A foggy thought about the shamelessness of her response tried to take root, but raw need obliterated it as he found her sensitive nipple through the thin cotton of her bra. Without the barriers between her tender flesh and his touch, the sensations escalated until she bit her lower lip to prevent the whimper that threatened.

They didn't speak. Maggie wasn't even sure they were breathing until she identified the ragged sounds stirring the air around them.

"I want you," he whispered against her ear, his voice trembling.

"I . . . I know." She licked her lips, desire battling uncertainty. "I know."

Cool air rushed across her abdomen as he nudged her jumper higher. Fog drifted in from the sea to transform the silvery moonlight into a surreal cocoon of privacy, as if no one else existed in this time, this place.

She should stop him, but she didn't. Couldn't. A combination of curiosity and need compelled her to watch his dark head dip as he drew her cloth-covered nipple deeply into his mouth.

The sweet-hot feel of him tugging against her sent her toward some unknown but strangely coveted place. She couldn't speak or even think as he arched her backward against his strong arm, enabling him to take her more thoroughly. She'd had no idea. . . .

A soft sound circled them, with an almost chanting rhythm. Maggie grew more aware of it and where they were. Common sense returned and she gently nudged Nick away and righted her sweater. His breathing rasped through the darkness as he straightened.

"I . . . I went too far," he whispered, remorse edging his voice.

"No." She stepped toward him, her heart thundering as she reached up to take his face between her hands. "No." She kissed him soundly as the chanting voices grew more insistent. If only she could blot them out or ignore them.

"No?" He held her in his arms, stroking her back as she rested her head on his shoulder.

"Not too far." She savored the feel of his nubby shirt against her cheek. "Just not yet."

"And not here."

Her knees trembled as he bent down to retrieve his jacket, then eased it around her shoulders. Nick's own spicy scent clung to the denim and his warmth eased through her. Slowly they walked toward her cottage. As they moved farther from the cliffs, the voices faded, though one echoed through her head just as they passed the base of *Caisleán* Dubh.

"The texture of his wool cape . . ."

Nick held Maggie's hand as they passed the castle. He'd never wanted a woman more in his life, nor had he lost control so completely. Once upon a time, he'd been considered cool with women. He'd had his share of dates while on the force, though the last couple of years he'd lived like a hermit.

One with a mission. He had people to protect, and promised revenge as his reward. Still, he couldn't help but want this woman. Spending time with her wouldn't keep him from his responsibilities. Besides, the thought of not seeing her, touching her, kissing her made his gut clench. He would find a balance between duty and . . . this. Passion? Romance? Lust?

All of the above? The thought made him smile and the chilly damp air gave him back enough self-control to think clearly. Oh, he was still horny as hell, but the more distance they put between themselves and that crazy-making acre of ground near the sea, the more at ease he felt.

The sudden urge to touch the crucifix slammed through him. His breath froze and a cold sweat coated his skin. He should have buried it back where he'd found it, but he couldn't. *"Mine!"*

His hand trembled with the need to touch the artifact right now, but he resisted by hooking the thumb of his free hand through his belt loop. *Damn it.* He was stronger than whatever force compelled him to keep the crucifix to himself. Wasn't he? Gradually he started to breathe again as they followed the bend in the road that would take them inland toward Maggie's cottage.

"During the day, I would cut across the meadow." Maggie dragged his thoughts back to the present. "But in the dark we might step in things we'd rather not have on our shoes."

Nick chuckled and gave her hand a squeeze, feeling himself relax. Remembering Brady's story about the witch, he glanced at Maggie through the silvery fog. Thank goodness she didn't know about one of the voices he kept hearing.

"Burn, witch, burn," it always said.

He was starting to feel as if he'd fallen into a bad horror movie. The voices, the crucifix burning a hole in his sanity, the formerly cursed castle, the witch, and—so Brady and Maggie claimed—reincarnation.

"Do you believe in the curse?" he asked. His voice seemed louder than normal, but that was in contrast to total silence. They'd walked inland far enough that he couldn't even hear the sea now. *"Really* believe it?"

"Aye, really." She paused and turned to face him. "Why do you ask again?"

He couldn't very well tell her about the voices, the vanishing couple, or—especially—about the crucifix. "You seemed a little freaked back there about the witch thing."

"Did I?"

She lowered her head and he reached out to cup her chin in his hand. Even through the foggy darkness, he could see her eyes widen. "Yeah, you did," he said gently. "I'm still not sure I buy into all this woo-woo crap, but you seem to."

"Woo-woo crap?" She laughed quietly. "Interesting choice of words."

He had to chuckle at that. "There are a lot of . . . weird things that happened here. Do you think any of them still happen?"

Maggie flinched and he felt her pull away, both physically and emotionally. He dropped his hand away from her chin. "I'm sorry." Nick realized he'd touched on something that upset her. Hell, it upset him, too. "I guess I'm starting to buy into this woo-woo stuff myself. It's kind of hard not to around here."

She seemed to relax at that and stepped closer. Her breasts brushed against his chest and he hardened between heartbeats. He wanted her and she wanted him. He'd felt her response earlier, and the need to follow through pulsed through him like an uncontrollable hunger.

A shiver rippled through her and he took that as an invitation to ease his arms around her again. He rested his chin on top of her head, inhaling the spicy scent of her hair. His heart swelled, pressing upward against his throat, making him wonder things he had no right to wonder.

Like what would it feel like to wake up beside her every morning? What would they talk about over breakfast? What would their children look like?

Whoa! He shoved those thoughts aside. Until he completed his assignment and had his father's killer behind bars, Nick Desmond couldn't have a life. Yes, he could enjoy a few stolen moments along the way, but he had no business contemplating a future with anyone. Anywhere.

No matter how much he wanted it.

She wiggled slightly and pressed herself more intimately against him. His erection throbbed as a reminder of his physical needs. Those were safer than emotions. He could handle sex—oh, could he *ever* handle sex right now. The touchy-feely crap was too much. His employer and Erin had already pushed him to the limit there with all this happy family pretense. Now there was Maggie . . .

He rubbed her back, stroked the long ripples of hair

flowing down to her waist, savored the feel of her soft curves against the hard angles of his body. "You feel good," he murmured against her hair.

"Mmm, so do you." She tilted her head back to look up at him. "Couldn't I stay here like this all night?"

The thought of staying all night with Maggie made him grow harder, if that was possible. "You're killing me," he whispered.

Maggie pulled back a little. "Did I hurt you?"

He chuckled and rested his forehead against hers. "It hurts so good."

"Oh."

He could imagine her blush, and that made him want her all the more for some reason. How innocent was she? He couldn't very well come right out and ask if she was a virgin. She was a college grad. How many gorgeous women made it through college as virgins?

But this was Ireland, and he'd already seen how different things were here. She responded to him as a woman who knew what she wanted, though.

He brought his hands up to frame her face and captured her lips with his. She melted against him and he ached to have her naked beneath him. Even better, he imagined her astride him, her pearly flesh bare and glistening, her wild red hair flowing about her like Lady Godiva.

Dangerous thoughts. His body ached and throbbed, reminding him how long he'd been without a woman in his life and in his bed. He wanted Maggie; she wanted him. Why shouldn't they indulge themselves?

She trembled as he deepened their kiss and pulled her tighter, nearly lifting her feet off the ground in his attempt to get close enough. There was only one way he'd ever be close enough to Maggie Mulligan. Only one way . . .

He pulled back to ask, "How far is it to your place?"

"Not far." She slipped her hand into his and started walking, as did he.

Nick could barely breathe, let alone think. Dad had told him not to think with his little head. *Well, Dad, it's not so little now.* All the more reason to keep his brain in gear. He had a couple of condoms in his wallet—a habit he'd learned years ago. Safe sex was logical, which meant he was using his brain. Right?

Every beat of his heart made him want and doubt and want again.

His reluctance still stymied him. Was it because she might still be a virgin? No. It was something more than that. Something he couldn't explain. In truth, the thought of another man ever touching Maggie made his gut twist into a knot.

"Mine. Protect her."

Why was he hearing the voice again now? They were far from the ruins.

"Burn, witch, burn."

And that other voice, too? Until a few days ago, he hadn't clearly identified the voices as two separate ones. Now he was sure. It seemed as if one was the good voice and one the evil.

Yep, a horror movie.

Next thing he knew, his head would do a three-sixty and he'd be flinging priests through windows. The thought made him stumble, though he didn't fall.

"Are you all right?" Maggie asked, dragging him back to the present. To reality.

"Nothing that can't be fixed." He tried to keep his tone light, though his thoughts were darkly frightening.

"Here we are," she said.

Nick hadn't realized they'd come so far already. She reached out to open the door, then stepped inside. After a moment light flooded the room and flowed through the doorway. He drew a shaky breath and took a step. Something stopped him there, right on the threshold. As if he'd walked into a brick wall, he stood frozen, unable to take a step.

"The parish and Mulligan records indicate the original cottage was occupied by poor Bronagh and her aunt, the *cailleach,*" Brady had said.

"Would you care for tea? I think I have some beer, too."
Maggie stood just inside the door. Light spilled around
her, setting her hair ablaze.

"Burn, witch, burn."

"Nick?" She reached toward him, took his hand in hers.
"Would you like to come inside?"

He'd like nothing better, so why didn't he? He squeezed
his eyes shut for a second and stepped into Maggie's
kitchen. Nothing weird happened. No voices. No fire. No
disasters.

"Are you all right?" she asked again.

"I am now." He managed a grin and pulled her against
him, kicking the door behind him shut with his foot. He
kissed her thoroughly, savoring the sweetness of her,
aching for more.

He felt a tremor ripple through her and broke the kiss.
Gazing down at her, he saw her wide, innocent eyes looking up at him. A potent blend of desire and uncertainty
swam in the blue pools.

She wasn't ready. Not yet.

"I'd better go." His voice broke. Walking away from
this beautiful, passionate woman would be among the
hardest things he'd ever done.

She bit her lower lip. "Have I done something wrong?"

"No, no." He rubbed her upper arms as he drew deep
breaths in a feeble attempt to ease the throbbing between
his legs. "I want this to be perfect. Rushing you wouldn't
be perfect."

Her cheeks flamed with color and she nodded very
quickly. "You're a good man, Nick Desmond." When she
met his gaze again, her eyes were moist. "I . . . I could be
persuaded to—"

"Don't." He pressed his finger to her lips and kissed her
forehead. "This may kill me yet, but I don't want to *per-
suade* you." Narrowing his eyes, he added, "I want you so
hot and bothered you'll strip off all your clothes and
spread yourself out on that table for me. I want to make a
several course meal of you. With dessert."

"Jaysus, Mary, and Joseph." She swayed and pressed the heel of her hand over her heart. "I . . ."

"When you're *really* ready." He kissed her very quickly, then opened the door and walked outside, pulling it firmly closed behind him. The chilly evening air washed over him and he gulped it into his lungs.

What he needed was a cold shower or a swim. He'd settle for the former.

The temperature had fallen in the few minutes he'd been inside. Of course, Maggie wasn't beside him now. She had a way of making him hot all over and under. "The shower for you, Desmond." He jogged out toward the road.

He'd forgotten his jacket, but he knew where to find it. Slowing his pace, a smile tugged at his lips as he shoved his hands into his pockets.

And touched that frigging crucifix . . .

"Protect her. Save her."

Eleven

The next morning Maggie decided to do what she should have done the moment she started hearing the voices. Determined, she marched over to *Caisleán* Dubh to ask Riley about the whispering he and Culley—and later Bridget—had heard from the castle.

The last thing she wanted was to worry her brother. Now that Bridget's morning sickness had passed and her pregnancy was advancing well, he seemed much calmer. However, Maggie needed information, and didn't it make sense to ask a man who had also heard voices from the past?

Maggie stopped halfway across the meadow. She had no way of knowing whether the voices were from the past or not. The ones Riley and Bridget had heard most certainly were. How did the chanting she heard relate to those whispers from the cursed castle?

Or did they?

Still, it made sense as much as any of this could. She shook herself and continued the short walk toward the imposing black tower and her family.

This time of day they would all be gathered in the kitchen for breakfast. Her dropping in wouldn't be considered unusual, and she could probably find out what her brother's schedule looked like today. She certainly couldn't discuss this in front of Mum or Bridget. They would worry that the curse had returned.

Maggie swallowed hard. And wasn't that really what she feared? Could there be ley lines connecting the old ruins, the castle, and Mulligan Cottage? Could those lines of energy have stored or carried the witch's spell to other places? To other people?

To Maggie?

A chill swept through her. No matter what, she had to ensure her family's safety first. Bridget's babe would come in October, and Jacob was only eleven. This new generation of Mulligan children would grow up without the shadow of a curse haunting them.

She stared up at the tower, then said, "Mother Mary, show me the way." After crossing herself, she walked around to the kitchen entrance. There was no reason for her to fear the castle—no reason for her to worry about the curse.

Yet worry she did.

A light mist filled the air, sending her already curly mane into a frenzy. She should've braided the mess, but was too eager to talk to Riley. The top half of the kitchen door stood ajar to the morning air. She peered inside and saw Mum dishing up eggs and spuds. Riley, Jacob, and Bridget all sat at the large wooden table in front of a sunny window.

Mum stood at the stove filling serving bowls. She looked up and smiled. "Top o' the mornin' to you, Mary Margaret. You're just in time for breakfast."

"One that's edible," Riley called.

Maggie rolled her eyes, grateful some things never changed. If only she could understand and explain all the strange feelings she'd been having, not to mention the voices . . .

"Don't mind your brother. Take this bowl and I'll grab

another plate and cup." Mum passed a bowl heaping with scrambled eggs to Maggie.

"How are you feeling this morning, Bridget?" she asked as she placed the bowl in the table's center. "You look well."

Bridget smiled. "I feel fantastic, though I'm eating everything in sight, and none of my clothes fit."

Maggie laughed. "And isn't it supposed to be that way?"

Riley reached over and rubbed his wife's round tummy. "You're sure there's only one, love?" he asked, his brow furrowed.

Bridget sighed and elbowed her husband. "You heard the doctor, Riley. I'm getting big as a barn, but there's only one baby."

Maggie sat across the table from her brother and sister-in-law, next to Jacob. "Are you ready for school to start?"

Jacob nodded. "I like school."

"You and Erin O'Shea will be the oldest students. There are five younger ones." Maggie poured herself a cup of tea. "I think you'll set a fine example for them."

Mum gave the blessing, then passed the steaming bowls around the table. A basket of Bridget's famous sourdough biscuits made Maggie's mouth water. She looked around the table for the gravy, which her brother was busy ladling onto his plate. To think they'd never eaten these American biscuits and gravy before Bridget came to them. Now they were a favorite at their table.

"We booked our first overnight guest for the B and B," Riley said between bites. "A Yank. He'll be here the end of next week."

"So soon?" Maggie swallowed a sudden lump in her throat at the thought. "The t—tower is ready then?"

"Yes." Bridget beamed as she sipped milk.

It was odd not to see Bridget without her customary glass of soda at breakfast, but Maggie's sister-in-law had given up caffeine until after the baby came. "The time will be over before you know it, then you'll have another baby to love." Maggie didn't want to talk about the tower, but it was necessary. "Are you excited that *Caisleán* Dubh will finally be open to guests?" The restaurant and bed and breakfast had been Bridget's brainchild from the start.

"Yes, and a little proud, too." Bridget turned her smile on her son. "I wish Granny was here to see this."

"She would have wanted the room at the very top," Jacob said. "Where she could look out at folks with her binoculars and holler at 'em."

Bridget cleared her throat and blushed a little. After the four years she and Riley had been married, hadn't they all grown accustomed to the wild stories of Bridget's late granny?

"And isn't your granny looking down on her grand-daughter right now, nodding her approval?" Mum asked in her calm, knowing way.

"And yelling 'Bingo!'" Bridget laughed and dabbed at her tears, then turned back to Maggie. "Anyway, back to Maggie's question. Yes, the rooms are ready. The furniture hasn't arrived for all of them yet. We finished the two rooms with a sea view first, but this guest requested one with a view of Ballybronagh."

"That's odd." Maggie couldn't imagine why anyone would rather look at the village than the sea. She lifted a shoulder. "A queer one, I guess."

"He sounds nice enough over the phone, but the request does seem odd." Bridget took a bite of scrambled eggs. "It's nice to eat something I didn't cook myself once in a while. Thank you, Fiona."

"'Tis me pleasure, lass, for you and the babe."

Riley cleared his throat.

"And for me big babe, too," Mum teased.

Riley growled, which merely made them all laugh louder. "Women. Will they ever stop pickin' on a man?" he asked young Jacob.

"Nope."

"There's Mamó's wise lad." Mum patted her grandson on the shoulder.

" 'Tis best to accept early in life that women truly run the world." Maggie played along, remembering all the times in the cottage when good-natured teasing was as important a part of a meal as the food. Bridget and Jacob hadn't wasted any time joining in the fun, and Riley accepted their ribbing with grace. At least, now he did. There'd been a time when he wore a perennial scowl. Didn't they all have Bridget and Jacob to thank for Riley's happiness?

"Granny taught me that women are always boss," Jacob said with an impish grin.

"She sure did." Bridget smiled sadly, obviously remembering the woman who'd been such an important part of their lives back in Tennessee. "If we have a girl, we've been thinking of naming her Sarah Jane, after Granny."

"I think that's a fine idea," Mum said. "Perfect."

"Thanks." Riley reached over to rub Bridget's belly again. "So do we."

"And if the babe is a lad . . . ?"

Riley stared at something only he could see, his expression solemn. "Patrick . . . Culley Mulligan."

Mum covered her face with her napkin, crying and laughing at the same time. "Oh, wouldn't your da and brother be proud?"

Riley cleared his throat and looked at his wife. "Neither of us even thought of any other name. It feels right."

"Then 'tis." Mum dried her eyes and they all ate in silence for a few minutes.

"Do you know much about your first guest?" Maggie asked. "Is he someone famous? A couple on their honeymoon?"

"He's a writer from New York. Said he wants some privacy to work and maybe do some research. He said he writes true-crime novels. Can't imagine why he'd want to do research in Ballybronagh."

"Well, he should find plenty of privacy here unless Brady gets wind of him," Riley said. They all laughed at that.

"Are you going to the school today, Maggie?" Riley pushed away from the table. "I have to pick up supplies, if you want to come along."

Relieved that her brother had given her the opportunity to talk with him alone, Maggie placed her napkin on the table and stood. "Shouldn't we help Mum with the dishes first?"

"Go on with you now," Mum said. "Haven't I been doin' dishes since I was younger than Jacob here?"

"And I'm not an invalid." Bridget stood, her condition more obvious than Maggie had realized. "I just look like I swallowed a bowling ball."

Laughing at her sister-in-law, she stepped outside. The air was thick with cool mist that seemed to hang there, rather than falling to the earth. It made Maggie's skin feel wonderful and her hair look dreadful. "It feels more like early winter than the end of August."

Riley headed across the road. "I'll need the lorry for the supplies."

They walked halfway across the meadow to where Riley's lorry was parked next to the tractor and the barn. Maggie climbed into the passenger side while her brother started the engine. It sputtered and coughed, then finally roared to life.

"I think it's time to buy a new one." He backed around, then drove forward across the rutted field until they reached the road. "With Bridget due in three months, I'll want a reliable one."

"Aye." Maggie watched her brother shift gears as he steered the lorry along the bumpy road. They passed *Caisleán* Dubh and made the turn back toward town. Directly ahead of them was the area near the cliffs where the church, the cemetery, and the schoolhouse rested. Beyond there were the crumbled ruins of the old church.

Now, Maggie. Ask him now.

She cleared her throat and shoved her stubborn hair back from her face. "Riley, tell me about the whispering you used to hear from *Caisleán* Dubh."

He shot her a curious look, then turned back to watch the road. "Don't you know as much as I do about it? Culley heard it all his life, and I after . . ."

Maggie would never forget the day they'd learned of Culley's death. "I know." She reached over and gave her brother's shoulder a pat. "And Bridget heard it, too."

Riley chuckled low in his throat. "Wasn't I shocked about that?"

" 'Twas fate."

He appeared solemn and nodded. "But I would have loved Bridget even without a curse or reincarnation. Never doubt that."

"Who could ever doubt that?" Maggie smiled and wrapped her arms across her abdomen. What her brother had with Bridget was what she wanted for herself someday.

With Nick Desmond?

Listen to yourself. She sighed and glanced at her brother's profile again as he eased the car to a stop beside the church.

He cut the engine and half turned to face her. "Why do you ask?"

"I . . ." She didn't want Riley to worry. If she told him about the voices, he would. She knew that with solid certainty. "Brady was telling the story of the curse to the O'Sheas, and I found myself wondering if you ever understood any actual words in the whispering. That's all." She lifted a shoulder, hoping she sounded more casual than she feared.

"Understood, is it?" He made a snorting sound. "It was like singing hovering around me every time I went outside or anywhere near the castle. I never understood a bloody word."

"Did Bridget?"

"She never said so and I never asked." Riley furrowed his brow and narrowed his eyes. "Why, Maggie?"

"I told you, I just wondered." She forced a smile, knowing she'd failed at not worrying her brother. "Hearing the story told again, and hearing their questions reminded me of all the details I never thought much about before. 'Tis only that."

"Hmm." Her brother sounded unconvinced. "Why is it, I wonder, that I think there's more to it?"

Maggie managed a laugh as she opened the door to escape Riley's questions. "Haven't you always been the suspicious one? Thanks for the lift." She scrambled out and slammed the truck door, but by the time she stood outside, she realized her brother had climbed out of the truck and stood by the open driver's side door. And didn't he look very unhappy for some reason?

"What might all this have to do with your Yank?" He arched a brow and waited, the mist swirling about his dark head and giving him an almost ethereal quality.

Her heart stuttered and her breath froze. "Nick. His name is Nick. And this isn't about him. 'Tis about my own, simple, foolish curiosity. I thought it odd that you never understood any words in all that whispering. Or singing, did you say?"

He lifted a shoulder. "'Tis how it seemed to us—like whispered singing."

Maggie forced herself to show no reaction, though she couldn't helped but wonder why Riley had presumed a connection between her question and Nick. "Well, now I have my answer. I'd best get to work."

"Maggie . . ."

She stopped partway up the steps and faced her brother again. "There's nothing to worry about, Riley. Honest." She started to turn, then remembered her news. "I almost forgot. Ailish is coming for a visit—arriving Friday afternoon sometime."

"Your roommate from university?" Riley seemed to relax. "The weird one?"

"Ailish isn't weird. Well, maybe a bit." Maggie laughed, remembering the weekend Bridget and Riley had visited her at school. Ailish had been doing some kind of ritual during the new moon. "Aye, she's coming for the weekend. I'd like to bring her round to see everyone."

"I'm sure Mum and Bridget will want her to come for lunch or dinner. We'll ring you up."

Riley was off the subject of the voices *and* Nick, thank the saints. Maggie waited until he'd returned to his lorry and driven away, then quickly crossed herself.

She hurried into the school, chilled through from the mist. The small stove in the corner beckoned, but there was no peat for a fire. She'd have to see if Riley had enough cut to spare some for the school, since chilly weather wasn't uncommon any time of the year in Ireland.

She arranged her lesson plans across her desk by grade and set about reviewing them all, but her thoughts drifted back to her conversation with Riley. He wouldn't let this drop—not her brother. He would remember and find another private time to confront her about it. Or, worse, he might ask Brady or Bridget. She had no choice but to talk to him again. Somehow, she had to ease his worry. She never should've said anything to him, knowing him as she did—ever the protector of Clan Mulligan.

She rubbed her eyes and shook her head, hoping to clear her thoughts so she could concentrate on her work. School would begin next week. Her dream of teaching would become reality.

"Concentrate, Maggie." She made a few notes about ideas for emerging readers, then turned her attention to a science project for the older students.

The temperature was dropping and she shivered. She glanced at her watch and realized almost two hours had passed. She should take her paperwork home to her nice warm kitchen.

The door squeaked open and she looked up to see Nick peering in to the school. "I was hoping I'd find you here," he said as he came inside and closed the door behind him.

The sound of Nick's warm voice banished the lonely silence. She smiled. "You found me."

"Brrrr. You planning to freeze your students?"

"So it would seem." Just seeing Nick made her warmer, but she felt a little embarrassed, remembering how he'd touched her and kissed her last night. Oh, the way he'd suckled at her breast . . . Her skin turned hot and prickly, but the chilly room made her shiver in contrast as she stood.

He walked toward her and placed his hands on her upper arms. "Hi." His lips brushed hers.

Maggie's knees trembled and her heart swelled with longing, but she resisted the urge to fling herself at him. He'd been a gentleman last night, and she would force herself to remember she was the local teacher with a reputation to protect. It wouldn't be easy.

"Lunch?" he asked, still holding her upper arms. "Aunt Mo is teaching Erin to make Irish stew, and they're going to knit something. Seemed like a real good time for a man to make an escape."

She laughed and nodded. Hadn't her brothers said the same thing often enough? " 'Tis a good day for making soup and knitting." Mum would call it a good day for nesting.

She almost gasped as she remembered her mother's comment about that when Maggie had announced her intention to move into the cottage. *Nesting.* Didn't Bridget have more than enough reasons for that? But not Maggie. Still, the thought didn't terrify her as it once had.

Nick flashed her his devilish grin. "How about lunch at Gilhooley's?" He glanced around the schoolhouse. "It's a lot warmer there."

Maggie laughed. "And I'll bet Mavis will have a pot of stew fit for angels simmering today." She wasn't really hungry after her huge breakfast, but a bit of warm stew and even warmer company sounded perfect.

"As long as it's fit for the likes of us, it'll do."

Nick waited near the door while she put away her lesson plans, then she joined him at the door. He opened it and they stepped onto the stoop. The soft chanting whirled around her again and she couldn't breathe. *Aye, it is chanting. Angry chanting.* It sounded like three syllables, repeated over and over again, but not loud or clear enough for her to actually understand.

Nick stiffened and she glanced sharply at his profile. A muscle in his jaw twitched as if his teeth were clenched, almost as if . . . as if he heard it, too.

No. That was impossible.

But hadn't Riley *and* Bridget heard the whisperings of *Caisleán* Dubh? Now she was really being nonsensical. *Change the subject, Maggie.*

"Lunch?" she asked.

She watched Nick's expression as he pivoted to face her. Confusion etched his features for several seconds, then he shook his head as if to clear it.

Had he heard the voices? The chanting?

Maggie's blood turned to ice and she reached for his arm, needing to feel his strength. Her touch seemed to snap him out of whatever thoughts—or voices—had gripped him.

"D—did you hear something?" she asked, her voice quivering.

He snapped his head around, his eyes wide. "Did you?"

"I thought so, but perhaps not." She forced a tight smile. Had she actually hoped someone else might share this madness with her? How unfair of her.

Or had she hoped for something like Bridget and Riley had shared . . . ? She squeezed her eyes closed, afraid to answer her own questions.

"Lunch," he said and took her hand.

They walked quickly away from the schoolhouse toward the village, but Maggie couldn't resist peering back over her shoulder before they rounded the bend in the road.

The dark silhouettes of a couple stood on the cliff, shrouded in the mist. She blinked and almost stumbled.

"Careful." Nick slowed his pace. "Am I walking too fast?"

"No." She released a long slow breath and faced forward. "Sorry."

As they passed Donovan Cottage, she looked back again.

The couple was gone.

Twelve

Nick forced himself to concentrate on the woman at his side, trying to forget those frigging voices. As soon as this job was over, he would find the best shrink in New York City. Why was he obsessed with a hunk of metal he'd found in some old ruins, and why were people—probably dead people, if they'd ever actually existed at all— talking in his head?

He had to hold on until his employer and her grand-daughter were safe and permanently established in Bally-bronagh. Then he could take the evidence, put Fazzini's ass in jail, and get help. For now, the thing to do was keep his mind off the voices. And the best way to do that was to turn all his attention on Maggie Mulligan.

Seduction. That's what he needed to think about. He wanted her and something kept stopping him from follow-ing through even when he had an invitation. Well, no more of that. He swallowed the lump in his throat, re-membering how sweetly she'd invited him into her cot-tage last night.

Tonight, he had to make sure history repeated itself. Or maybe some afternoon delight was in order. Oh, yes, he'd definitely enjoy making love to Maggie in the daylight.

This misty, crappy weather was perfect for cuddling up with a beautiful, sexy woman.

Maybe they could skip lunch. . . .

His stomach rumbled audibly and Maggie laughed. *Busted, Desmond.* Okay, so he needed to keep up his strength.

"Hungry, are we?" She slipped her arm through his as they neared Gilhooley's.

"Ravenous." He glanced down at her, deliberately keeping his expression as intense as his libido. He wanted her to know he meant business—that his hesitance had passed.

Her eyes widened and a blush bloomed in her cheeks. A slow, sexy smile spread across her face. "I . . . I'm hungry, too." Her voice sounded a little breathy.

"Mmm." He couldn't wait. "Do you mind if we have lunch somewhere more . . . private?"

She stopped midstep and turned to face him. The uncertainty he'd seen last night was still there, but not as strong as the naked desire shining in her beautiful blue eyes. He wouldn't push too hard—that wasn't his style—but he would definitely encourage her some.

"I want to make love to you, Maggie Mulligan."

She brought her fingertips to her lips and he heard her swallow. The urge to kiss her long and hard slammed into him, but even though the swirling mist gave the illusion of privacy, Nick reminded himself they were standing in the middle of Ballybronagh.

"I have some soup we can warm at my cottage," she whispered.

With a nod, he took her arm again and tucked it closer to his side, while his heart and other parts of his anatomy thundered in unison. "Sounds perfect."

They walked back the way they'd come, past Donovan Cottage, past the schoolhouse, past the church, and the cliffs where they'd kissed more than once. No voices called to Nick now, except the one from his body that no man could ignore regarding sexual matters.

And this was a supremely sexual matter.

Perhaps he could keep the voices away through sheer determination. The only other thing in his life he'd ever been as determined about as sleeping with Maggie was putting his father's killer behind bars.

He banished thoughts of his father and duty and turned his full attention to Maggie. The fog and mist blurred everything around them. Nothing seemed real or important now except this woman and his desire for her.

They quickened their pace as they rounded the curve that would take them beyond *Caislean* Dubh, which appeared as nothing but a dark mass in the mist, its tower completely invisible. They cut across the meadow, where he could see a pair of headlights near a shape that had to be the barn. The lights went out and Maggie froze.

"Riley," she breathed.

"Your brother can't see us in this soup," Nick whispered, steering Maggie out toward the road they'd followed last night. Riley Mulligan would undoubtedly take the shortcut across the meadow back to the castle. Nick's determination refused to consider any other option.

They didn't speak until they reached the kitchen door of Maggie's cottage. He felt her tremble slightly and gathered her closer. His kiss was thorough but gentle, and he hoped it would ease her mind. Even more important than his libido—which seemed more insistent with every beat of his heart—was his need to earn Maggie's trust. There was no room for fear now. Only trust and desire were allowed.

She melted against him and he felt her warm and soften in his embrace. "Mmm." He broke their kiss and remembered that her door had been unlocked last night. Without releasing her, he reached with one hand to open it.

Maggie walked inside and Nick allowed himself only a split second to muster his own courage. Whatever barrier had tried to stop him here last night was off duty now, thank God.

His blood burned, but he would take this slow. They

had all day. Aunt Mo didn't need him while she and Erin
stayed in the cottage to cook and knit. The security system
would protect them, and the whole village would come
running if it was triggered. He grinned to himself at the
thought.

"I'll heat some soup." Maggie's voice quivered slightly.
"I think we need a fire, too. It's grown chilly."

"Point me to wood and matches."

"Peat. Not wood." Maggie led him to the front room
and showed him the box of turf.

With her careful instructions, he finally had a warm but
rather smelly fire going. "Do you heat the whole place
from this one source?"

"There are small stoves in the bed . . . rooms."

They wouldn't need any additional heat in those rooms
today. He flashed her a grin as he straightened and she
smiled shyly in return. At the sight of that particular smile
of hers, his heart did something weird—sort of swelled
and pressed upward against his throat. He couldn't breathe
for a few, terrifying seconds.

This wasn't lust. This was something a whole lot
scarier.

He could deal with lust, with desire, and definitely with
a wild, hot affair. He drew a shaky breath at last and saw
her walking back into the kitchen. Had she always had
that nice little wiggle?

*Concentrate on the wiggle, Desmond. Wiggles are safe.
Emotions are not.*

He closed his eyes, remembering the first time he'd
seen Maggie, walking away from Donovan Cottage. Yes,
she'd always had that nice little wiggle. He blew out a
breath and adjusted his jeans, then followed that wiggle
back into the kitchen.

He stood in the doorway, just watching her. She opened
a can of tomato soup and dumped its contents into a pan,
added milk to it, and set it on the stove. After she turned
the knob, the flame flared up around the sides of the pan,
and she jumped back.

"Save her!"

Nick's blood turned to ice and he rushed over to turn off the stove. His heart hammered against his chest and his breath came in quick, rapid bursts. He finally focused on Maggie, who stood less than two feet away, her eyes wide and her chest rising and falling with her breathing.

He reached for her and she walked into his arms. The need to protect her was too powerful to ignore. Had the voice meant Maggie all along? He stroked her hair until she stopped trembling.

She'd admitted yesterday to a fear of fire, and he wasn't too crazy about it himself lately. He clenched and un-clenched his teeth until he felt control return. Besides the fact that he would make love with Maggie today, he knew one other thing for certain—he couldn't bear to see her cook. Not with her fire hang-up and his weird visions and voices. Not today. They could eat a cold lunch.

"Got any peanut butter?"

She burst out laughing and he found himself chuckling along with her. She stepped back, her eyes sparkling and her cheeks brighter. Damn, but he wanted her in a bad way. No, in a good way. The best way.

And he knew exactly how he wanted his peanut butter, but he didn't want to frighten her away. He'd eat peanut butter sandwiches the normal way now, then . . .

"Peanut butter it is. Have you ever had Nutella?"

"Nope."

"It's ambrosia—hazelnuts and chocolate the texture of warm honey. 'Tis good on toast or ice cream, or with peanut butter."

Strike the peanut butter. He knew exactly what to do with Nutella. "Sounds delicious."

She spun around and opened the icebox, which looked older than she was and then some, then bent over to re-trieve something.

The sight of her bent over that way made something snap. Nick's throat tightened and went dry; his blood hit the boiling point right between his legs. He stepped up behind her and cupped her butt, giving her cheeks a little squeeze. She went very still in front of him and he pulled her backward just enough to almost kill him. *Hell of a way to go, Desmond.*

The soft pressure of her jeans-clad curves against his insistent erection shattered what remained of his pitiful sense of decency. To hell with lunch. To hell with peanut butter.

He groaned and clasped her hips, pressing her back more firmly. The throbbing between his legs responded to the pressure with overt enthusiasm and he hissed a breath inward through his teeth.

She straightened slowly and he slid his arms around her waist, holding her against his chest without sacrificing a bit of the delicious contact below their waists. Her head fell back against his shoulder and he reached out with one hand to close the icebox.

"Lunch?" she asked, her voice quivering.

"Later." He kissed the side of her neck and felt a tremor ripple through her. He loved the feel of her nestled against him, but it wasn't enough.

He wanted skin.

Gently, he reached for the hem of her sweater and pulled it over her head. She raised her arms and helped him rid them of the barrier. He trailed his fingers across the smooth bare skin of her abdomen, right along the waistband of her jeans.

She trembled again but from desire, not fear. Definitely not fear. Not now. Somehow, he knew she was ready, and his heart soared, despite his determination to keep his heart disengaged.

Desperate to reveal more of her skin, he eased his hand between them and released the clasp on her simple white bra. It popped open and his anticipation went into orbit. With shaking hands, he eased the straps down her arms until it joined her sweater on the floor.

He'd worn a western-style shirt with snaps, and he yanked them free, baring his chest to her naked back. He could barely breathe as he eased the pale, luminous skin of her slender back against his chest.

"Oh, God. You feel so good." He nuzzled her neck again and found her breasts with his hands. A moan came from somewhere deep inside him and she answered with a small, sexy sound that nearly made him lose the shattered remnants of his self-control.

He had to take this slow, easy, and make it every bit as good for her as he knew it would be for him. He wanted his mouth on her—all of her—and to see her.

Slowly he turned her to face him, her nipples brushing against the hair on his chest. Her breasts were small and firm, nicely round, their nipples a coral several shades lighter than her russet hair.

He remembered the comment he'd made last night about spreading her out on the table, and he fought the urge to scoop her up and lay her there now. Not this first time. They would make love in bed today. Later, when she was more comfortable with him, on the table.

Gently he cradled her breasts in his hands, watching her eyes darken to a smoldering cobalt. She bit her lower lip and her lush curls fell across her bare shoulders.

He'd never seen a sexier image. "Where?" He brushed his thumbs across her nipples and she met his gaze. "Where?" he repeated, his voice breaking.

Her tongue swept out to moisten her lips. "Upstairs."

No hesitance remained in her eyes. She had the look of a woman who knew what she wanted and was determined to get it. *Thank God.*

Nick swung her into his arms and headed toward the *very* narrow staircase near the backdoor. "So much for drama," he said and she laughed. The sound made his heart do that peculiar swelling thing again.

A sudden lump formed in his throat and he allowed his gaze to drift from her face, down her silken throat, to her beautiful breasts. Oh, God. He couldn't wait. The table was looking better and better.

She squirmed and he set her feet back on the floor. Giggling, she dashed to the stairs and disappeared.

I'm dying and she's *laughing.*

Nick released a breath in a loud whoosh and staggered toward the stairs, so aroused he could barely walk, let alone think. He took the steps two at a time, eagerness spurring him upward.

Would she be naked by the time he found her? The thought stole what was left of his sense of reason and he ran up the last few steps.

And slammed his forehead into a low beam at the top of the stairs. "Ow!"

Maggie had just kicked off her shoes and squirmed out of her jeans when she heard Nick's cry. She winced. How many times had her brother smacked his noggin on that same beam? She peered into the hall and saw Nick rubbing his forehead, but her gaze quickly fell to his massive chest. *Jaysus, Mary, and Joseph, but he's beautiful.*

"Are you all right?" She gave him a sheepish grin. " 'Tis sorry I am. I should have warned you."

"Holy . . ." He stopped rubbing his forehead and his eyes widened. "You're . . . wow."

She'd almost forgotten that she wore nothing but her knickers. If she was going to do this—and she *definitely* was—she would do it right. Here she stood wearing maidenly white cotton when she felt more like black silk. She'd never realized before that she had this decadent, daring streak.

He took a step toward her.

She took a step back into the bedroom, hooking her thumbs through the elastic at her waist and tugging it lower. He stood framed in the doorway, all hers. He wanted her, and—*oh!*—didn't she want him more than anything? For today, at least, he would be hers.

Slowly she eased her knickers lower and he licked his lips. "What about you?" She could barely breathe. He was practically making love to her with his eyes. "Off with it now."

A crooked grin tugged at his full lips and a shock of black hair fell across his bruised forehead. She eased her knickers a bit lower and took another backward step. She should have been afraid, but the moment he'd filled his hands with her bare breasts downstairs, she'd known this was meant to be.

He was for her, and she for him.

"The only one," the old one said.

Her heart skipped a beat as he eased his shirt from his muscular shoulders and let it fall. He took another step, unbuckling his belt, then the buttons at the front of his fly.

"Oh." She took another backward step, her skin hot and prickly all over. She wanted him so much she couldn't bear another minute. "Nick?"

"Hmm?" He kicked off the runners he always wore and shoved his jeans downward.

She watched, breathless, as he pulled off one leg, then the other, and ridded himself of his socks as well. When he straightened again, he wore only a pair of dark blue briefs that barely covered the bulge there.

Maggie swallowed hard, her belly tightening in fear and anticipation. She'd grown up on a farm—knew the technicalities, so to speak. Mum had told her some things, too. However, Mum had left out the glorious, bold, wonder of what led up to the loving.

"I want you naked," she whispered brazenly, even as she backed another step toward the bed.

"Turning my words back at me?" He wasn't smiling now, and the intensity of his perusal made her sway.

"Aye." She dropped her knickers to the floor and kicked them aside. A sense of vulnerability washed over her and she wished she'd kept them on a bit longer. For several seconds she stared at his feet, then slowly allowed her gaze to drift upward, lingering where his thumbs remained near the waistband of his briefs.

Fear and uncertainty shot through her—not about going

through with this. She couldn't imagine *not* making love with Nick now. What she feared was being unable to please him. She didn't know what to do next. She didn't know *how.*

All she knew was she desperately wanted to have him inside her. A small gasp came from her throat and her vagina clenched against the unbearable emptiness. Perhaps *she* didn't know what to do, but her body obviously knew what it wanted. Needed.

His expression gentled somewhat and he walked slowly toward her, his briefs still in place. He paused in front of her and simply stared at her. Finally, he put his arms around her and pulled her against him.

The feel of his bulging briefs against her belly made her burn for him. She whimpered slightly when his mouth covered hers in a kiss that stole her breath. She wanted this so much—wanted him. He explored her mouth with his tongue and she returned his explorations fully, allowing her passion and need to flow through them both.

He broke their kiss, panting, and stared intently into her eyes. "Be very sure," he whispered, his nostrils flaring slightly.

She wanted this more than food or water or virtue. She wanted Nick Desmond to teach her the meaning of love, and to fill her so full she would never want again. "I . . . I'm sure."

He scooped her into his arms and carried her the last few steps to the bed and laid her carefully upon the quilt. He stood beside the bed, devouring her with his eyes.

Heat crept from her face, down her throat, across her breasts, to settle low and hot and deep.

She returned his scrutiny, feasting on the sight of the dark hair covering his chest, and allowed her gaze to follow it down to the V, where it disappeared in his briefs. She watched as he slowly inched the fabric down his slim hips.

The part of him her body craved sprang free. She

gasped and bit her lower lip. He was so very large. Would he fit inside her? Her body clenched again in anticipation.

Her gaze shot to his face and she saw a question in his eyes. Swallowing her doubts, she rose onto her knees and covered his hands with hers.

Together, they eased the fabric downward until it fell to the floor. Maggie looked between them, where the length and breadth of him seemed to expand right before her eyes.

The urge to touch him stemmed from curiosity almost as much as desire. Tentatively, she wrapped both hands around his shaft. He flinched and a bead of moisture appeared at his swollen tip. She looked back up and met his gaze. His eyes were glazed with passion, and he took her shoulders to press her down to the mattress, leaving her no choice but to release her prize.

And, despite the fact that she had no one with whom to compare Nick Desmond, she had no doubt that he was quite a prize. He covered her, and everywhere the hot length of him brushed against her was a molten kiss—her hip, her belly, her upper thigh.

He kissed her again hungrily and she threaded her fingers through his hair. So this was what it felt like to lie naked with a man. No longer afraid, a thrill shot through her unlike anything she'd ever known.

"I will not let him go."

She shoved the old one's voice aside and concentrated on the way he trailed kisses down the side of her throat, to the curve of her shoulder, to the valley between her breasts. He cupped her breasts in his large hands and they swelled, eager for his touch.

He flicked his tongue against her nipple and she moaned. Then he traced circles around it before finally claiming it with his mouth.

"I will make him mine."

Yes, he was hers. This felt so good. She arched toward him, offering her breast to his hot mouth. He drew deeply and she linked her fingers behind his neck, holding him against her, never wanting him to leave.

She drew a deep breath, focusing on his hungry feasting of her breasts—first one, then the other. A low growl rumbled from inside her and she reached downward, wanting to touch him again, but unable to reach him.

A moment later he kissed his way down her abdomen, lingering to swirl his tongue in circles around her navel, then going lower still. His kisses left a trail of fire in their wake.

Maggie didn't know what to expect next. All she knew was she didn't possess enough power to even think of stopping him. More importantly, she didn't *want* to stop him. This was right. Destined. She'd known it in her heart the first moment she saw Nick Desmond. He was hers. She ached and throbbed and wanted. Oh, the wanting!

"Love me. I give me heart."

He pressed the heel of his hand against her and her insides convulsed again around that emptiness. Would he end their suffering now? She knew he wanted her as much as she wanted him, and she was eager to experience it all.

He stroked her moist folds with his fingers and she groaned shamelessly. Gently, he parted her and slid his fingers inside. Her breath escaped in a loud whoosh and he shifted until he was between her knees.

She opened her eyes, confused. Would he come back up here to take her now? Would he show her the meaning of all this? Would he give her what she wanted so much she nearly wept?

He stroked her with his tongue. Shocked, Maggie reached down to push him away, but he covered a particularly sensitive nub with his mouth and drew gently. Shock waves of raw need echoed through her, and rather than shove him away, she wove her fingers through his hair and let her knees fall apart. *Jaysus, Mary, and Joseph!* She'd had no idea—none at all.

"I know the feel of him. The taste of him."

No. She didn't know yet, but she wanted to know. Her

blood turned molten, and everything converged where his mouth and fingers drove her rapidly insane. Her pelvis angled toward him, her insides clenching around his fingers. Something was happening. She remained poised on the brink of something she craved—something she had to find or go mad.

Then everything happened at once. Her body contorted, her toes curled, her lungs froze, as a wash of liquid fire scorched through her in an explosion of sensation unlike anything she'd ever imagined.

He kissed her inner thighs, eased his way back up the curve of her hip, gently stroking and petting her. "That was . . . amazing," she whispered, stretching languidly as he looked up at her through hooded eyes.

Then she remembered that this wasn't finished, and the knot of heat in her womb unfurled again, spreading its flame through her blood. She reached down and cupped his face as he nuzzled her breasts.

His erection brushed against her slick folds and her breath caught. Now he would take her. Now he would finish this.

"'Tis only beginning. I will not let him go."

She couldn't even fathom letting him go right now. She whimpered when he kissed her again, and she reached down between them to brush her fingers against his hot, moist tip.

A low rumble started from his chest and reached his lips as a growl. Maggie swallowed it with her kiss, feeling it reverberate through her body.

He pressed himself against her and she opened for him. Somehow knowing what to do, she guided him inside her. She was hot and wet and he slid partway in and stopped, his breathing labored.

"Does it hurt?" she asked softly, stroking his hair away from his face.

"I . . . forgot something." He withdrew and left the bed. She watched the play of muscles on his butt as he dug through the pockets of his jeans and tore something open with his teeth. When he returned to her, she realized what he'd forgotten.

"Oh." Heat flooded her cheeks as he covered her again, his erection now sheathed in a condom. The thought hadn't occurred to her. Of course, contraception wasn't commonly taught in Catholic homes.

Again he pressed himself inside her and she opened, desperate now to have him fill her. She clenched around him, drawing him inward, eager for more. Why did he hold back?

"Now," she whispered, pressing her knees against his hips in encouragement. "Love me."

Nick froze. *Love me.* Her words slammed into him with all the finesse of a wrecking ball. He couldn't think about love—not now. They were both so turned on they'd probably die if he didn't finish this. Imagine the scandal if they were both found dead in this position.

A smile tugged at his lips until she wrapped her long, slender legs around his waist and drew him inward. "Oh, God." He couldn't hold back much longer. They were both well past the point of no return.

He eased himself deeper into her tightness, holding his breath as she compressed around him. She was incredibly tight. He should stop. He shouldn't go through with this.

"Protect her."

He'd put on the frigging condom. They were protected. The damned voice had followed him here. He shoved it away and inched toward heaven.

"She is forbidden. You have committed yourself to duty."

He wouldn't listen.

"Nick, please?" She looked up at him with pleading eyes. "Don't stop." She locked her ankles behind him and angled her pelvis more fully against him.

Nick tried to hold back, but she was too powerful, too tempting. "Oh, God, Maggie." She wiggled her hips. "You're killing me."

"And what are you doing to me, Nick Desmond?" she whispered and bit the lobe of his ear. "Now."

Surrendering, Nick thrust himself inside her. She opened to him after a brief resistance, and the heat of her nearly killed him. "A virgin." He shouldn't have. He shouldn't have. He was pond scum.

"Save her."

You're a little late with that advice, pal. He pushed up on his elbows and met her gaze. He saw pain . . . and something more. The something more was the most dangerous of all. He saw her heart, her vulnerability.

She wiggled her hips again, then contracted around him like a vise—a velvet fist of heat and sensation. "It doesn't hurt now," she murmured, tickling his ear with her tongue.

"Wanna bet?"

She giggled, and he kissed her again, but her laughter was contagious and he chuckled along with her. Never in his life had he laughed with a woman in bed. "This is serious, Maggie," he teased.

Her expression sobered. "Show me serious, Nick Desmond."

He always did love a challenge. He withdrew almost completely and she tried to follow. "Let me," he said. He stroked the length of her again, watching her eyes for any sign of pain.

What he saw was beauty, passion, more. He couldn't deal with more. *Too late.* She moaned and caught his rhythm, meeting him thrust for thrust as if she'd done this a thousand times.

She demanded every inch he had and gave more than she took. Maggie Mulligan's passion was even more powerful than he'd imagined, and he'd imagined—hoped for—plenty. She angled her hips to take him deeper. Every stroke drove him closer.

He quickened his pace, thrusting harder and deeper. Her muscles gripped him with mounting intensity until he could barely breathe. Sweat trickled between them as they created heat and more heat.

He felt as if he could leap tall buildings and then some. He wanted to watch her. The veins in her neck showed through her fair, almost translucent skin as she soared with him, meeting his thrusts with a hunger that left him breathless.

She tightened again in a relentless vise, and he saw her eyes roll backward, and her back arched off the bed. "Now," he said, and drove himself into her, answering her need and his own.

The explosion shook him. It had been a long time, but he hadn't expected *this*. Maggie took him with a sweet-hot passion that brought everything he had converging to that place where she pulsed around him. The heat of it scorched him. Branded him. Nuked his sorry ass.

He looked down at her, their breathing raspy in the small room. The window was fogged over both inside and out. "You're amazing. I . . ." He swallowed hard, suddenly recognizing the words he hadn't consciously thought, but had been about to say.

She slid her feet along the backs of his legs and twined her ankles with his calves. "Amazing," she echoed. "Like burning up on the inside."

Her words made his heart skip a beat, then race forward.

"Burn, witch, burn."

Thirteen

Maggie opened her eyes to sunlight spilling through the lace curtains her mum had made. Every muscle in her body ached, but in a good way. She smiled, remembering everything. They'd never eaten lunch, and had settled for grilled cheese sandwiches—which Nick had insisted on cooking—as a light dinner before coming back upstairs.

She gradually became aware of the warm body pressed against her back. Nick had fallen asleep. If anyone learned he'd spent the night here, the village would never let her teach a single class.

"Nick?" She shook him gently and he groaned. "'Tis morning."

"Uh-oh." He sat upright in bed, his hair tousled and morning stubble covering his jaw.

He looked delicious.

As if he sensed her gaze on him, he looked at her through sleepy eyes. "Good morning." Then he kissed her gently. "Sorry. I should've gone home, but you wore me out." His sheepish grin stole her heart.

She blinked back the stinging sensation in her eyes and swallowed the lump in her throat. There'd been no promises or declarations of love between them, nor had she expected them. Still . . .

Listen to yourself, Mary Margaret. She drew a shaky breath and reached out to touch his cheek. "You need a shave." She smiled. "Are you wanting breakfast?"

"I'd love it, but—"

The phone rang and Maggie's heart stopped. *Don't let it be Mum or Riley.* She climbed out of bed, acutely aware of her nakedness, and answered the phone on the third ring.

"Hello," she said, facing Nick as she spoke, and recognizing the worry etched across his face.

"Good morning, Maggie," the woman said. "It's Maureen O'Shea. This is awkward, but Nick—"

"Mrs. O'Shea. He's here. Just a moment." Maggie squeezed her eyes closed as Nick came to her side and took the phone.

"Aunt Mo, I'm sorry. I—"

His eyes widened and crimson bloomed in his cheeks. Whatever his aunt had said must have embarrassed him.

"I'll be home in fifteen minutes," he said. The color in his cheeks brightened even more and he cleared his throat. "I . . . well, if you insist. Thanks. Bye."

After he hung up the phone he looked at her with a bewildered expression. She touched his forearm. "I'm sorry, Nick. Did I cause any trouble for you?"

He chuckled and blinked. "She told me to make sure I call before I stay out all night again so she won't worry." Shaking his head, he added, "Imagine that."

"Why shouldn't she worry? She's your aunt." Maggie bit her lower lip. "What else did she say?"

He arched a brow. "She said, 'Tell Maggie no one will hear of this from me.'"

The breath she'd been holding rushed out of her lungs. "Well, thank the saints for that. 'Tis rather exciting. I've never done anything . . . scandalous before."

"You're very good at it." His eyes smoldered as he held her gaze.

She gave him a peck on the cheek and he wrapped his arms around her, pressing his erection against her hip. Nick Desmond was proving himself to be what her friends at university had called *randy*. Her cheeks warmed, but she remembered her responsibilities and said, "I'll get dressed and—"

"Don't do that." He nuzzled her neck. "Aunt Mo said to take my time, and I intend to do just that."

"Mmm." Warmth flowed through Maggie. "I'd like that, but I have to go to the school and finish the work you kept me from yesterday. Ailish is coming for a visit."

"Who?"

"Ailish was my roommate at university and my dearest friend," Maggie said. "She's coming for holiday."

"Staying here?" Nick pulled back a little, a mischievous twinkle in his heavily lashed eyes.

"Aye."

"Then that will put a cramp in our love life, so we'd better make the best of this morning."

Love life? Awareness sizzled through Maggie. "Give me a minute to myself, then I . . . I'll meet you in the shower. We'll save time that way."

His eyes widened and his hot erection pulsed against her. A surge of wickedness swept through her and she glanced down at it. "Promises, promises."

He burst out laughing and she broke free and raced to the bathroom to turn on the water. It always took forever for the water to get warm upstairs, so she turned on the hot and took care of other pressing matters.

How would she face Mrs. O'Shea? Well, she simply would. She and Nick were adults, after all. Before she climbed into the shower, she glanced at herself in the half fogged mirror.

She looked different. Like a woman. Her nipples appeared swollen, and there was a red mark on her neck from Nick's whiskers. She touched the spot with her fingertips, remembering, and the truth struck like a bolt of lightning.

She was in love.

The realization stole her breath. Tears welled in her eyes and she blindly reached into the shower to turn on some cold water to run with the hot, until the temperature was right. She climbed in and allowed her scalding tears to wash away in the warm spray.

Aye, she loved him. Dare she hope he might love her, too?

"His love of piety and traditions is stronger."

The old one's voice angered her and she lathered shampoo into her hair and scrubbed. Nick Desmond wasn't interested in piety or traditions. What rot.

And where was Nick? He should have joined her by now. She peered around the shower curtain and saw him slipping through the door, his muscles rippling from the simple effort of bolting the door. Ever the Yank to lock even this door.

He spotted her and smiled, but she saw worry in his eyes as well. "Is something wrong?" she asked as he climbed into the shower.

He placed both his hands on her upper arms. "First, don't worry. He didn't see me."

Maggie's face went numb. "Riley?"

Nick nodded. "He was pounding on the kitchen door. I looked out the upstairs window and saw him stomping away when no one answered."

"Stomping. That would be himself all right."

"He probably figured you were at the school."

Maggie shook her head. "And wouldn't it be just like him to go see for himself?"

"Mary Margaret," Nick said, ducking until his nose was level with hers. "You're an adult and you never would've heard him from the shower anyway. Don't worry about this."

Then he kissed her so tenderly she wept again. He kissed away her tears, rinsed her hair for her. Then he soaped the washcloth with her favorite cinnamon-scented bar and bathed every inch of her.

He played her like a master musician with a finely tuned instrument. Her body hummed with desire. Nick was slow, deliberate, patient.

Last night had been an earth-shattering, desperate type of passion—the kind Maggie had read about in those yummy romance novels. This was different but every bit as wondrous. She felt worshipped, adored, cherished.

"I took him within me and made him mine to keep."

He lifted her and braced her back against the warm shower wall—she wrapped her legs around his waist. Warm water flowed around his back and down their bodies. He nipped at her wet breasts, teased them with his tongue, and she clung to him, ached for him.

He trembled with his own passion and she angled herself to take him, riding him as he supported her weight with both arms and body. Her explosion came in a charge of heat that brought more tears to her eyes. He tensed and released himself into her. She couldn't get close enough and her body swallowed him with greed.

As he eased her feet to the shower floor, the water had begun to cool. They rinsed quickly and she turned off the water. They dried each other and she wanted him all over again.

"I'll never get tired of this. Of you," she whispered, and the look in his eyes made her sway. Was that love burning there? Would he say the words? Should *she*?

"I gave him me heart. Me trust."

Nick would never hurt her, but something—perhaps the old one's words—made Maggie keep her declaration to herself. For now.

After he was dressed, he kissed her. "I'll circle around the back way to town so no one at the castle will see me. Okay?"

She smiled as she tied her robe. "Thank you. For *everything*."

"Mmm." He kissed her and slipped his hands inside her robe. "Maybe—"

She laughed. "Go on with you, Nick Desmond. I've work to do."

He kissed her again and brushed his thumbs against her nipples. She was tempted. So tempted. "I've work," she repeated against his lips, and he backed away.

"All right. I'm going." He snapped his shirt closed and buckled his belt, then stuck his hands in his pockets. The expression on his face was one of pure horror.

"Nick?" She rushed to his side and touched his arm. "What is it?"

He pulled his hand out of his pocket and gulped several deep breaths. "I . . ." He swallowed so hard she saw his Adam's apple travel the length of his throat and back. "That last time. We shouldn't have."

Confused, she shook her head. "What was different about—"

Then she remembered the thrilling, molten rush of his seed.

"I took his seed into me. . . ."

Nick kicked himself all the way back to Donovan Cottage. He'd taken her virginity, and he'd failed to protect her. Horny old Nick had to have her one more time. One more for the road.

No, it hadn't been like that—never could be with Maggie. She was . . .

Terrifying.

He drew a shaky breath as he found the lane that curved around to enter Ballybronagh from the east, and he quickened his pace. The road was muddy and rutted, but once he found the paved one that served as the village's main street, he broke into a jog.

The minute he'd put his hand in his pocket and touched that crucifix, he realized how he'd failed her.

"Protect her," the voice had said.

Yet he'd failed her.

The odds were against her becoming pregnant from one unprotected encounter, and she'd insisted it was the wrong time of her cycle for that to be likely. Still, he would worry. At least he had been tested for HIV, so that wasn't an issue. That didn't excuse him—he was the older, more experienced one, and he *knew* better.

"'Tis your duty."

"Go to hell," he muttered, slowing his jog to a brisk walk as he entered the village. He didn't need any supernatural or imaginary voices telling him about duty. True, he'd stayed out all night when he should have been with his employer and her granddaughter doing his *job,* but . . .

No buts. He'd screwed up royally. He'd placed Maggie's reputation at risk, and shirked his duty to the woman paying him more per month than he'd earned in the last few years combined. He should have slipped away as soon as it was dark enough, but he hadn't wanted to leave Maggie's side. The rest was easy. He'd fallen asleep after the greatest sex of his life and hadn't stirred until this morning, when he'd had the best shower of his life.

A smile tugged at his lips as he opened the squeaky garden gate of Donovan Cottage and strolled up the walk to the front stoop. He punched in the password on the control panel and let himself in the front door.

Aunt Mo stood in the kitchen doorway, eyebrows arched. "Well? . . ."

Nick's face heated and he closed and locked the door behind him. "Well . . . I blew it. I should have come home last night."

"But? . . ."

She wasn't going to make this easy, even though she'd seemed pretty damned nice about it on the phone earlier. "Where's Erin?" The last thing he needed was the kid with the bionic hearing and eyesight to witness this.

"Taking a nice, long bubble bath." Aunt Mo turned and walked back into the kitchen. "I saved some oatmeal."

"Oh, goodie," he muttered.

She whirled around with a wooden spoon in hand and he held his hands up in surrender. "Just kidding."

She made a slight grunting sound and dished oatmeal into a bowl and set it on the table. "I made coffee."

"Thanks." Nick couldn't figure out why she seemed pissed at him now when she hadn't been earlier. He drizzled honey on the oatmeal and picked up his spoon. She set the cup of coffee on the table and positioned herself in the chair across the table from him. To stare.

He took a bite of the warm, sweet cereal, but felt her gaze on him and dropped the spoon back into the bowl. "I told you I'm sorry about not calling or coming home." He felt like a teenaged boy explaining himself to his mother.

"What about Maggie Mulligan? What about her family? What about her reputation? Couldn't you have found someone in a neighboring village to . . . to . . . ."

"To *what*?" Nick narrowed his eyes, waiting for the inevitable. "I think you need a verb there."

"Sully?" She leaned back in her chair and folded her arms across her chest. "She's the local teacher. Such a dear, sweet lass."

The sweetest. Guilt made his throat tighten and his gut twist. "I've been kicking myself about it enough, but I give you my word that I won't hurt her." *Unless I already have.* He reached for his coffee cup and took a gulp, surprised his hands weren't shaking.

"Do you plan to marry her then?"

He spewed coffee and grabbed his napkin. "I . . . don't have to answer that."

She stiffened. "Indeed, you do not."

He took another sip of coffee and set the cup aside. "We . . . it just happened. We've been attracted to each other since day one. This wasn't one-sided either. We're grown-ups. Remember?"

Aunt Mo drew a deep breath and released it very slowly. "I apologize. It *is* your business, and you *are* both adults."

"Thank you for that." He took another bite of lukewarm oatmeal.

"Of course, I *will* hold you to your promise about not

hurting her." Aunt Mo stood and carried her cup to the sink. "Furthermore, I'm confident Riley Mulligan will see to that."

"And I'll offer to help him kick my sorry ass, but it won't be necessary. I won't hurt her."

"She came to me a virgin and I coveted her."

Nick shuddered against the voice—the same one that always told him to "protect" and "save" her. Now the voice was getting way too personal.

"I'm not sure men and women understand hurt the same way, but I'm going to trust you on this one."

She wasn't his real aunt, though he felt like a properly chastised nephew right now. He managed a tight smile just as the phone rang. Aunt Mo—way too much like an aunt—answered it, leaving him to sulk in his oatmeal.

He hadn't thought of anything but putting Fazzini behind bars since Dad's death. Marriage? A family? Those things sounded too normal, too happily-ever-after for the likes of Nick Desmond.

Happily-ever-after was as make-believe as the voices in his head—voices that now seemed to be talking *to* him, rather than just filling his head with noise—as fey, leprechauns, and ghosts or goblins. Ireland seemed to be crawling with make-believe. Even so, that idyllic life would never be part of Nick's future.

But with Maggie . . . ?

That tight fist around his heart triggered the alarm to his personal danger zone again. *Don't think about it. Just don't.*

He finished the oatmeal and stood to carry his bowl to the sink just as Aunt Mo hung up the phone.

"That was Bridget Mulligan."

Oh, shit. Riley saw me.

"They're having an impromptu dinner party this evening for a friend of Maggie's who's arriving today."

Relief rippled through Nick. "Oh?"

"We're all invited to dine at Mulligan Stew at seven."

"Seven. Got it."

Aunt Mo patted him on the shoulder as she passed. "Don't look so forlorn, lad. Your guilty conscience doesn't show. Much."

I wouldn't count on it.

It took every bit of courage Maggie could muster to stop by *Caisleán* Dubh on her way to the school. Facing her mother and brother after her night of decadence was terrifying. Would they be able to see the difference in her?

"No, of course not." She drew a deep breath of the bright morning air. The rain and fog had cleared, leaving everything fresh and clean.

The top half of the kitchen door stood open, and Maggie opened the bottom one. "Hello?"

Mum came bustling in from the dining room. Fiona Mulligan ushered her youngest child into the kitchen. "We're havin' a dinner party this evenin'."

"Did Riley tell you about Ailish?" Maggie asked.

"Aye, 'tis why we're havin' a dinner party, silly lass."

"Party?"

"I sent Riley to tell you this morning, but he said you weren't home."

"I must have been in the shower." Maggie's cheeks warmed and she looked down at the slate floor. It was safer. "'Tis nice of you to have a dinner for Ailish. Thank you."

"Layabout this morn', Maggie?" Riley asked from the doorway.

She looked up sharply and met her brother's gaze. He arched a brow, folded his arms across his broad chest, and leaned against the doorjamb. "A bit, I suppose," she finally said.

"I just want to make sure you're safe and happy alone in the cottage. There's room for you here." Riley shoved himself away from the doorjamb and grabbed an apple from a bowl on the counter. "'Tis a man's duty to *protect* his family." He stared at Maggie as he took a bite of the apple.

Mum leafed through a recipe book Bridget favored. "And haven't we already discussed Maggie livin' at the cottage, Riley? 'Tis settled."

Maggie resisted the impulse to stick her tongue out at her brother. "Thank you, Mum," she said instead.

"I've chores." Riley took several more bites of the apple, then dropped the core in the garbage bin labeled for the chickens. He paused near the door and his gaze settled on his sister again. "Mum told you about the party then?"

"She did." Maggie rose and told herself she was imagining the questions in Riley's eyes. "I need to get some work done at school, and that's where Ailish is coming to meet me."

"We'll expect you both to come round before seven," Mum said. "Don't we have plenty to keep us busy gettin' ready for the party? Oh, and Bridget invited Brady and the O'Sheas."

And Nick? "That's fine then." Maggie's pulse quickened and she deliberately avoided her brother's gaze as she walked past him and stepped outside. "We'll be here early, Mum, to help."

"Thank ye, lass."

"As long as you don't cook anything," Riley added, following her outside.

" 'Tis a beautiful day," she said.

Riley kept pace with her as they walked around the castle. Near the boulders, where the uneasiness always struck her, Maggie held her breath, waiting for the voices, but they didn't come this time. At least *that* was a relief, even if having her brother hovering over her was not.

"Well, I'm off to work then." She pivoted toward Ballybronagh, but Riley grasped her elbow to stop her.

"Wait, lass," he said, his tone gentle.

Maggie swallowed and turned to face her brother. "What is it?"

He looked upward for a moment, then pinned her with his gaze. "I *saw* you."

All the air rushed out of her lungs and she swayed. A

second later, she remembered that she was a woman grown and had a right to privacy. "What do you mean you *saw* me?"

"Yesterday, walking home."

Maggie pulled her elbow free of her brother's grip. "So you saw me. I've work to do."

"With Desmond."

She chewed her lower lip, then summoned her pride and lifted her chin a notch. "Aye."

"Is draggin' it out of you what it takes to get the truth, lass?"

Angry now, she folded her arms across her rib cage and narrowed her gaze. "I don't lie and you know it."

He nodded. "'Tis secrets you're keepin', lass. You don't know him well e—"

"And why would a brother object to his *grown* sister inviting a friend to lunch?" *Understatement isn't a lie. Exactly.*

"Friend, is it?" Riley pressed his lips into a thin line. "I'm thinkin' there's more to it. Friends don't kiss the way you two were the other evening."

"'Tis making a habit of spying on me, you are." She turned toward the schoolhouse again. Her heart thundered in her chest and her eyes burned. She didn't like having harsh words with Riley, but this was none of his business. He pushed too far.

The crunch of gravel beneath his big feet alerted her that he followed. Exasperated, she stopped and whirled around. "Give it a rest, boyo."

"One more thing—because you're my baby sister and I love you," he hastened to add.

She heaved a sigh and asked, "And how could I be arguing with that? You fight dirty, Riley Mulligan."

"Only when it matters, lass."

Her anger dissipated and she took his hands in hers. "I love you, too, Riley, but I'm entitled to my privacy."

He appeared to ponder that, then gave a curt nod. "Fair

enough, but . . ." He raked his fingers through his long, dark hair.

"But what?"

His eyes were pleading. "Can you not see the man has secrets, Maggie?"

She blinked, unable to answer. Hadn't the same thought passed through her own mind at least a hundred times?

"Just . . . be careful. That's all I ask."

She nodded and her brother pulled her into a big hug. He kissed the top of her head, then released her. " 'Tis late I'll be if I don't hurry along now."

"Drive safely." Maggie watched him stride across the meadow and climb into his lorry. She stood staring until he'd driven out of sight, waving to her as he passed.

"Hold your love. Keep him. Don't let him go."

Fourteen

Angelo answered his cell phone on the first ring. The digital display told him the call was from Finn. "Talk," he said into the receiver.

"Friendly, aren't we?" Finn sighed into the receiver. "I can see the look on your face from an ocean away, boss."

Angelo popped two antacids into his mouth and chewed furiously. He'd practically been living on the damned things. "Talk, damn it."

"Okay. I went to the convent and talked to the Reverend Mother. When I asked her about any little girls there named Erin, she got real uptight."

Erin. The skin around Angelo's mouth tingled. He grabbed a tissue and mopped perspiration from his forehead. "Did you see the kid?"

"Nope. This is where it gets interesting."

"Keep talking." Static filled the line. "Finn. Can you hear me? Talk, damn you!"

"Just a sec." *Crackle.* "Lemme move over by the window. That better?"

"Yeah."

"When I told the nun that I was searching for a missing child, she stopped hedging and came clean." The sound of papers being shuffled came through the line. "The girl was checked outta the school on the *same day* the call went to your mother's private line."

Angelo released a long, slow breath. "Who the hell checked her out?" Was it his Erin? After all this time?

"Are you sittin' down, boss?"

"Tell me who the fuck checked her out!"

"Easy, Angelo. Easy. It was the kid's grandma. Her *mamó.*"

Mamó? "She's dead. That's im—"

"Boss, the girl asked for Mamó when she called. Right?"

"Yeah."

"That doesn't mean she wanted Maureen Fazzini. It was probably a wrong number and the wrong Erin."

"Maybe. I still want you to follow up. Find them. See them with your own two eyes."

Finn chuckled into the receiver. "Like I knew you'd say that, so I got friendly with this cute chick who records real estate transactions in this part of Ireland. I figure if the woman was taking her granddaughter home to live, she might move or something."

"And?"

"Someone with the same last name as the kid closed on a cottage the same week she was sprung."

Angelo swallowed the lump in his throat. "What . . . last name, Finn?"

"Well, it sure as hell ain't Fazzini."

"Finn."

"O'Shea, man. Doesn't ring any bells."

Angelo picked up a pencil and bounced the eraser end on his desk. "I've heard it, but I'm not sure where."

"Like I said earlier, this is all probably nothin' but coincidence. A kid named Erin dialed the wrong number. End of story."

"So when will you pay a call on this Mrs. O'Shea and her granddaughter?" Angelo let his head fall back against his chair.

"Knowin' you like I do, I made a reservation at the only hotel in that village." Finn made a snorting sound over the phone. "A bed and breakfast of all things. It's in a cursed castle. Can you believe it?"

"I don't give a shit where you're staying." Sometimes Angelo wished his father had never told him Finn was his half brother. Then he could fire his ass without guilt. "When do you check in and how far is it from this cottage the bitch bought?"

"Wednesday, and from what I can tell on the map, I'll probably be able to see it from my room. I'll take binoculars."

"Sooner. Call and change your reservation. And take a damn camera. You can e-mail pictures." Angelo grabbed a pen and paper. "On second thought, give me the particulars. I'll be joining you."

"I kinda thought so."

Angelo jotted down the name and phone number of the hotel and the village.

"Anything else?" he asked Finn. "Are you staying sober?"

"Yeah, yeah."

"Call me after you get to Ballybronagh."

"Sure thing," Finn said.

"I'll meet you there. Book me a room under the usual alias." Angelo disconnected the call and staggered over to the bar, sloshed scotch into a glass, then drained it.

His health was in the toilet, but from what the doc had told him, all the drinks in the world wouldn't make any difference now. Pancreatic cancer. He'd lost a lot of weight without trying, and the tinge of yellow in his eyes was undeniable now. Well, hell, everybody had to go sometime.

He had to find out about the girl first. Erin. If she was *his* Erin, then he would bring her home and leave the family business to her as it should be. The real money came from the drugs of course, but she really never needed to know about that. There were enough legitimate businesses used as a front to keep her busy. Finn would run the more profitable but less public portion of Fazzini Enterprises.

Of course, Erin—*if* this was Erin—would need a guardian for several more years. Finn or his mother would do it. If the girl wasn't his daughter—he sighed—then he had no choice but to tell Finn about his paternity and leave everything to him.

Angelo poured another drink.

Maggie actually squealed with delight when she saw Ailish walk through the schoolhouse door. She dropped her paperwork and ran across the room to throw her arms around the woman who had been her roommate for four years.

"*Céide Milé Fáilte.*" Maggie pulled back to look at her friend. Ailish's perfectly straight, glossy black hair still hung to her slender waist, and her bright green eyes were as bewitching as ever. She giggled, realizing how appropriate that was. "You look wonderful."

"And you." Ailish gave her a peck on the cheek, then tilted her head and narrowed her eyes. "Something is different. It will come to me."

Liquid fire filled Maggie's cheeks.

"Ah, so it's like that, is it?"

Maggie cleared her throat and walked back to her desk, fidgeting with her paperwork. "Like what?"

"The man from your dream," Ailish said. She placed her hand on Maggie's shoulder. "Or a dream come true?"

Maggie bit her lower lip and faced her friend. Until this moment she hadn't realized how desperately she needed someone who might understand. "Aye."

"Ah, Maggie." Ailish smiled and hugged her again. "My Maggie is in love."

Maggie squeezed her eyes closed until Ailish released her. "Aye."

Ailish pursed her lips. "And why wouldn't you be

dancing with joy about that?" She stroked Maggie's hair.
" 'Tis sad you are."

"Not sad. Not exactly."

Ailish frowned and took Maggie's hand, turning her
palm over and staring at it for several moments. When she
looked up, her expression was solemn. "Ah. I see."

"See what?"

"You've slept with him."

Maggie laughed. "Not even *you* can tell that from looking at my palm."

Ailish flashed a sheepish grin. "No, but can't I tell by
your reaction? Talk to me."

Maggie nodded. "I'm finished here. Let's go back to
my cottage and get ready for the party."

"Party, is it?" Ailish nodded approvingly. " 'Tis a lovely
thought, but unnecessary. I do hope your young man will
be there."

Maggie smiled this time. "I think so."

"Good. I can't wait to meet your Yank."

My Yank. More and more, Maggie hoped it proved true.
She lifted a shoulder at Ailish's knowing gaze. "I really
care about him. It's . . . frightening."

"Sounds wonderful to me." Ailish walked slowly to the
window and stared out toward the graveyard. " 'Tis a
quaint village, Ballybronagh."

"That's one way of putting it." Maggie couldn't help
but laugh. "Compared to Dublin, it must seem like the end
of the earth to you."

When Ailish turned to face her again, Maggie saw great
sadness in her friend's eyes. Something was wrong.
"What is it, Ailish?"

Her friend drew a deep breath and smiled, though it
didn't reach her eyes. " 'Tis nothing a holiday won't
cure." She pointed toward the window. "Are those the
ruins you mentioned?"

Maggie sighed. "Aye."

"What are we waiting for?"

Ailish's mischievous smile and twinkling eyes told

Maggie she had no choice but to give her friend the grand
tour. "What, indeed?" *Except my sanity, that is.*

Maggie put away her paperwork and made sure the
schoolhouse was in good order. She pulled on her jumper
and headed toward the backdoor. "I assume you have your
car."

"I do." Ailish opened the door. "First, this. It beckons to
me."

Me, too. Maggie suppressed a shudder and followed her
dear friend outside. " 'Tis a beautiful day."

"Obviously." Ailish glanced over her shoulder, her eyes
dancing with mischief. "Come along, Maggie Mulligan.
Hiding won't change fate."

"Fate, is it now?" Maggie laughed, but it sounded
forced even to her ears. *Was Nick her fate?* Her heart
pressed against her throat. *I hope so.*

*"I gave him me love, me innocence, and he turned
away."*

"Fate," Maggie repeated. Nick wouldn't turn away
from her.

"Aye, fate." Ailish rolled her eyes. "You're in a bad
way here. But won't we be dealin' with that later? Now,
let's see these ruins of yours."

Not mine. Definitely not mine.

They walked across the graveyard, and Maggie pointed
to her da's grave and various other Mulligan ancestors.
Ailish remained very quiet until they passed through the
gate and neared the ruins. Of course, that was a point
Maggie never passed. Something always warned her away
from the ruins, though she had no idea what.

Ailish pressed her hand to her heart and dropped to her
knees in the grass. "Oh, Maggie," she said, her eyes
closed, "do you feel it?"

Maggie blinked, staring at her friend, who knelt on the
ground as if in prayer. "Feel what?" *All I feel is the fear.*

"The *power.*"

"Danger lies here," the old one said.

"Is it . . . ?" Maggie cleared her throat and watched as

Ailish closed her eyes and swayed rhythmically. "A ley line?" She had to tell Ailish about the old one and the chanting.

Her friend's eyes opened and she stood, though she grabbed Maggie's arm for support. "'Tis sorry I am. This place obviously confuses you. We'll visit again later."

"If you insist."

Ailish laughed and took Maggie's hands. "Ah, I've missed you so, dear friend."

"Enough of this. We have to get beautiful for the party."

"I'm looking forward to it." Ailish stood a full head taller, and she looped her arm over Maggie's shoulders. "So tell me his name."

"Nick." Maggie drew a deep breath and closed her eyes again. "Nick Desmond."

"The only man I ever loved."

A ripple of light appeared, despite her closed eyes.

"Look, Maggie." Ailish's tone was intense. "Now."

Maggie opened her eyes, confused. What was it? The ripples appeared again, like heat waves wafting off the earth's surface. "What . . . ?" Maggie took a step backward, toward the gate.

Ailish took her hand and followed her. "There, now. 'Tis enough for today, lass. Let us go to your cottage now."

"What was that?" Maggie's throat went dry, and she dragged in a shaky breath.

"Power." Ailish led her steadily through the gate without stopping. "Yours, I think."

"Nonsense. I have no power." Maggie glanced back over her shoulder and gasped. The mysterious couple stood near the stones that might have been a hearth a couple of centuries ago. They appeared fuzzy even this close—almost transparent. "Are they ghosts?"

Ailish tightened her grip on her hand. "Perhaps." She drew Maggie through the gate and let it close behind them. "'Tis one of the questions we'll ask later. Not now."

"If they aren't ghosts, then—"

"Shh." Ailish kept Maggie's hand in hers until they'd left the ruins and the graveyard behind and were almost to her tiny car. "There's time," she said as she opened the door and urged Maggie into the passenger seat.

Maggie stared across the schoolyard, the graveyard, and toward the ruins. She no longer saw the couple, though she felt them somehow. The power Ailish had mentioned?

A shudder spiked through her at the thought. The ley line theory made more and more sense, especially since she'd started hearing the chanting at the cottage, too. Here. The castle. The cottage. Didn't the locations form a perfect triangle butting up against the sea?

Ailish climbed into the car and started the engine. She backed up and pointed the car toward the road. "Which way?"

Maggie pointed toward the daunting black tower of *Caisleán* Dubh. "You have to ask?"

"Ah."

Maggie reached over and grabbed Ailish's arm before they pulled onto the dirt road that curved toward the sea and the castle. "What is the power?" she asked, almost as afraid to know than to wonder.

Ailish met her gaze, her green eyes wide and sincere. "Make no mistake, Maggie. There's magic here."

Maggie's throat constricted and she drew a shaky breath. "Wasn't the curse enough magic to last us a thousand lifetimes?"

A knowing smile spread across her friend's face. "Aye. You're getting warmer, I think. Let's go party."

"'Tis glad I am you've come," Maggie said as Ailish steered her car onto the dirt lane.

Ailish glanced over and nodded. "As am I."

Maggie leaned her head against the back of her seat and glanced toward the cliffs where Nick had first kissed her. The couple were there again. By the saints, she was going mad. No. She wasn't going mad. Ailish had seen them, too. They were real.

"I must keep him. Hold him. I will not lose him again in this life."

Maggie remained silent. Since yesterday while she was in Nick's arms, the old one had started speaking directly to *her*. She should be terrified, but she sensed that the voice—definitely an old woman—meant her no harm. She seemed almost to be advising her.

And now haven't you gone totally off your nut, Maggie?

The image of the couple slowly faded as Ailish steered her car around the curve. Had Ailish seen them again? Maggie didn't ask, deciding to wait until they were at the cottage to discuss the weird happenings further.

"The castle is magnificent." Ailish slowed her car almost to a stop as they passed the massive boulders around the foundation. "I'd like to hear more about this curse."

"At the cottage." For some reason, Maggie needed the comfort of her own home right now. Despite the fear of ley lines, of power, of voices and vanishing couples, Mulligan Cottage was home. It always had been.

"Aye, always."

Why are you talking to me? Maggie thought. *Who are you?*

She closed her eyes again as Ailish increased the car's speed. Home. She simply wanted to go home, and to enjoy her friend's visit. And she would see Nick again tonight. Today was a time for happiness—not for brooding.

"I'm assuming that darling cottage is yours." Ailish pointed across the meadow.

"Aye." Maggie's smile widened as she looked at her home again as if for the first time. "It is darling, isn't it?"

Ailish nodded as she turned into the long lane. The lone shade tree before the cottage made it look like something from a storybook.

"Are you lonely here by yourself?" Ailish asked as she parked the car in the worn place beneath the tree.

"No, never." Maggie opened her door and climbed out as her friend did. *How could I be lonely with voices in my head?* She sighed and almost laughed at herself. And she certainly hadn't been lonely yesterday, or last night, or this morning.

Remembering the shower, her face flooded with heat. Nick's lovemaking was more amazing than Maggie could ever have imagined. After he'd left this morning, she'd counted the days since her last period, just to make sure. She was toward the end of her cycle, thank the saints.

Ailish popped her trunk and pulled out a large satchel. "This is it. I pack light."

"You do." Maggie walked up the steps and opened the front door, which she rarely used. The long porch was unusual for an Irish cottage, and no one ever used it much. Looking at it now with the flowering vines and rails, she wondered why. It spoke to her. Maybe she'd put some chairs and a table out here to use in fair weather.

" 'Tis a feel-good place," Ailish said.

Maggie smiled and nodded. "Welcome to Mulligan Cottage, Ailish Delaney."

Ailish stepped through the open door and stopped near the coat hooks where Maggie's dream had occurred. " 'Tis an old place. Older than it appears."

Maggie cleared her throat. "I . . . I've just learned that a servant's cottage was on this foundation before the Mulligans built this one in 1900."

Ailish walked farther into the front room, slowly turning. Her gaze swept the place, and she nodded. "Someone important lived here." She frowned and bit her lower lip. "There was tragedy. Loss. But there was love, too."

"Oh, Ailish." Maggie closed the door and leaned against it. "Aye. Tragedy. Terrible tragedy."

"Tell me."

She nodded and pushed away from the door. "The dream I told you about?" At her friend's nod, Maggie con-

tinued, "It took place in this room. The water was there."
She pointed at the floor beneath the coat hooks.

Ailish dropped her satchel and purse and walked to that
place. She pressed her open hands against the wall and
closed her eyes. After a moment, she rested her cheek
there as well.

"What . . . what is it?" Maggie asked, her throat tight
and dry.

Ailish didn't answer for several seconds. Finally, she
pushed away from the wall and wiped her palms against
her jeans. "Do you know if any of the original cottage was
here when they built yours? Did they add on to a portion
of it, perhaps?"

Maggie sighed. "I don't know, but after I told you
about my dream on the phone, I remembered something I
forgot to tell you."

"What?" Ailish approached Maggie.

"In the dream, when I hung up Nick's denim jacket, it
seemed to change into a long wool cape—a very heavy
one. I think it was . . ."

"Wet." Ailish nodded. "That would explain the water
on the floor."

"It was a *dream*, Ailish."

Ailish retrieved her satchel and purse from the floor. "Is
there anything else about your dream that you haven't
mentioned?"

"The wall." Maggie's voice was barely audible. "The
one you were touching just now."

Ailish's eyes widened. " 'Tis old."

"In my dream it . . . transformed from the clean, white
it is now to old dark wood."

"Ah." Ailish nodded, seeming satisfied. "We'll find the
truth, love. I am sure of one thing, though."

Maggie wasn't sure of *anything* except her love for
Nick, for her family, and her desire to teach. Everything
else was confusing. "What?"

"She means you no harm."

An icy chill washed through Maggie and she swayed. "She?"

"Aye." Ailish slung the strap of her purse over her shoulder. "The old woman who once lived here."

"There were two."

"So you *do* know."

"Aye." Maggie released a long, slow breath. "'Tis *very* glad I am that you've come. I have much to tell you."

"And don't I have the feeling this will be interesting?"

"I want tea before we get ready for the party."

"Aye, tea. And talk." Ailish followed Maggie into the kitchen. "This is the newer part of the cottage. It has always been a loving, happy place."

"True." Maggie plugged in the electric kettle Riley had bought her to use at university. Now she used it to avoid having to light the stove so often. She spooned tea leaves into a sunny yellow pot and set out matching cups and saucers. The tray was bright and cheery. Just looking at it and knowing Ailish was here made everything seem better.

The only thing missing was Nick. The man she loved.

"The only man I ever took within me loins. The only man I ever gave me heart."

Aye, Maggie had taken Nick within her loins and given him her heart. Though she hadn't told him her feelings, she suspected he knew. Somehow, she doubted she could truly hide her feelings. Even grouchy old Riley suspected. She smiled to herself again.

"You really love him." Ailish touched Maggie's arm. "It shows."

"I was just thinking the same thing." Maggie unplugged the kettle and wet the leaves. The fragrant steam wafted upward and she drew a deep, appreciative sniff. "This is what I needed. Tea and friendship."

"And wine for later. I smuggled some from da's cellar before I left."

"You always do." Maggie flashed her friend a grin, remembering all the weekends at university when they'd sipped wine from Mr. Delaney's expansive collection.

They sat at the large wooden table, where Maggie had eaten meals all her life. Ailish was like the sister she'd never had.

She took a sip of tea and watched Ailish sweeten hers as she always did. They knew each other so well now—their habits, their fears, their dreams.

"So tell me about the women who lived here before," Ailish said, then took a sip of tea. "Ah, 'tis perfect."

"Aye." Maggie took another sip before answering. "I didn't learn about this until after my dream when I asked Brady Rearden what had been here before Mulligan Cottage."

"The dream made you wonder then?"

Maggie nodded and refilled both their cups. "The wall and coat hooks changing, though it *was* just a dream."

"A dream that left water on the floor?"

"There is that." Maggie drew a cleansing breath. "I asked and Brady told me that Bronagh and her aunt lived here when they worked for the Mulligans in *Caisleán Dubh*."

"Ah, I remember the story about her." Ailish nodded and reached for the sugar. "Bronagh was the lass who fell in love with your ancestor, and who ended her life when he married another."

"The same." Maggie glanced out the window at the tower now. "The Mulligans never even knew her name until Brady's research turned up the diaries kept by the parish priest during and after the *cailleach*'s trial."

An impish grin appeared on Ailish's face. "A witch, is it? Don't I resemble that remark?"

Maggie's cheeks warmed. "Sorry. But in those days . . ."

"I know. 'Tis fine. Go on with your story."

"Ballybronagh is named after Bronagh. Aidan Mulligan changed the name of the village to honor her, as he spent most of his life mourning her. In fact, his wife died after giving him one son, so he had much to mourn. As near as we can determine, Mulligans who came after Aidan never spoke Bronagh's name, and eventually forgot, though the story was handed down from generation to generation."

" 'Tis so sad." Ailish sighed and took another sip of tea. "What about the aunt? The witch?"

"Well, you know about the curse."

"Aye." Ailish rolled her eyes. "We spent hours talking about it at university. Remember?"

"How could I forget?" Their fascination with the tragic love story and the legendary curse had been a favorite topic for late night discussions. "Didn't I tell you how the curse came to pass? I'm not remembering now."

Ailish furrowed her brow. "Ah, I do remember. The aunt cast a spell. Your brother Riley and Bridget broke that spell, and fulfilled Bronagh and Aidan's destiny."

"Exactly."

Ailish's expression grew very solemn. "Your ancestors built their cottage to escape the curse placed on *Caisleán Dubh*."

"You remember as well as I do." Maggie gave a nervous laugh and twisted her empty cup in its saucer.

"They built this cottage on the same soil where Bronagh and her aunt—the *cailleach*—had once lived."

" 'Tis bizarre." Maggie shook her head, wondering again why they had done such a thing. "Of course, the Mulligans had omitted the part of the story dealing with the witch's spell until four years ago when Brady and Riley pored over the old priest's diaries."

"So they may not have realized who once lived here."

" 'Tis the only logical explanation." Maggie reached across the table and gave Ailish's hand a quick squeeze. "About the ley lines . . ."

"The power." Ailish nodded, the expression in her eyes seeming far wiser than her years. " 'Tis here as well."

"And at *Caisleán* Dubh." Maggie swallowed the lump in her throat. "I've felt . . . whatever it is there, too."

"Won't I be seeing that for myself soon enough?" Ailish smiled gently. "Show me my room and we'll make ourselves gorgeous for the party."

"I'm eager for you to meet Nick and give me your thoughts." Maggie couldn't help remembering the doubts Riley had instilled in her heart about Nick's secrets.

"Me, too. Your Yank is one lucky man, Maggie Mulligan. Don't be forgetting that."

"Why did he forsake me love for his duty?"

Fifteen

Nick dropped the crucifix into his pocket. Damn it, he wanted to leave it here. He'd tried three times to leave his room without it, but he couldn't. Finally, he surrendered and walked into the kitchen where his employer and Erin waited.

He wore a gray tweed sport coat—the only thing he owned that resembled a suit—with a blue-gray sweater and navy Dockers. Of course, everyone in Ballybronagh had seen him wear the same jacket to mass every Sunday. The only shoes he had besides his running shoes were the leather hiking boots he wore now.

Aunt Mo was gussied up in a fancy purple dress, and Erin looked like one of those dolls he'd seen in shop windows back in New York. "Well, don't you two look spiffy?"

"Thank you, sir." Erin curtsied and giggled.

Aunt Mo gave him the once-over. "We should have bought you a new wardrobe before leaving New York."

Nick shrugged. "Sorry—" He bit the inside of his lip. He'd been about to call her "boss" in front of Erin. Forgetting she was his employer made it easier to play his role, but it also made him uncomfortable as hell. Still, it was safer than accidentally calling her boss in front of the kid.

But she wasn't his aunt. Erin wasn't his cousin. The reminder made his gut twist. He was going soft. Since Dad's murder, Nick had worked hard to keep himself isolated from other people who might care about him and expect caring in return. Damn it, now he *cared* about them both.

And he cared even more about Maggie.

Erin walked over and took his hand in hers. "Escort me to the ball, handsome prince."

"Heh." Nick grinned down at her. "Careful. I might turn into a frog."

"Ribid," Aunt Mo said as she pulled a fancy shawl around her shoulders. A knock sounded at the door. "Brady was invited, too. He's stopping by for us."

Nick followed her to the door, knowing she was starting to forget all the reasons they had for being careful. As was he. This job was too easy, and that worried him. If Junior tracked them down after they'd stopped worrying . . .

He peered through the window. "Me charming cousin himself," he said in an exaggerated Irish brogue. Nick was still getting used to the fact that he had a *real* cousin here, and that there were more Reardens here and in the States he hadn't met. More people to care about. *Shit.*

So why did the notion give him a warm fuzzy? *Warm fuzzy, Desmond? Now you're really losing it.*

Aunt Mo opened the door and Brady removed his hat and bowed. Dressed in a dark suit, he looked every bit the country gentleman. From another century. Nick had to grin, though. The old fart was a flirt and a half.

"Well, if it isn't my handsome prince come to escort me to the ball." Aunt Mo winked at Erin.

"Ribid." Nick tried to appear innocent in response to his cousin's questioning look, but Erin's giggling made that tough.

Brady's face reddened, but he didn't miss a beat. "Shall

we?" He crooked his arm and Aunt Mo slipped hers through his and batted her lashes back at Nick and Erin.

"This is pretty lame," he muttered.

"What does that mean?" Erin asked as he set the security system and they hurried outside.

He took her hand and joined Brady and Aunt Mo on the walk. "In this case it means something is silly." *Not enough.* "And old-fashioned. Sort of."

"I think old-fashioned is charming," Aunt Mo said and patted Brady's arm.

"Indeed." Brady put his hat on and walked toward the gate.

It was early enough that he couldn't even call it twilight yet. He looked around as usual and saw no one skulking about. As usual. *Don't get lazy or careless, Desmond. Just don't.*

He watched Aunt Mo and Brady strolling ahead of him and Erin. They made a nice couple—both sort of old-world. Old-fashioned. He'd seen the looks they exchanged. Maggie made Nick feel like being old-fashioned. Hell, he wanted to play white knight and all that, too.

"Protect her. Save her."

Hush. Knock it off for a while. Whoever the hell you are . . .

The voice's timing was uncanny—almost as if it read his mind. That was rich. It was *in* his mind. Nick sighed and tried to shove it all aside.

He was going to *Caisleán* Dubh. To Maggie. The thought of seeing her again made that swelling in his chest start again, and he knew more and more that he'd failed at keeping his heart disengaged.

"Do you plan to marry her then?" Aunt Mo had asked.

A gentleman would've married her. After all, she'd been a virgin. He was her first lover.

And he wanted to be her only lover.

Damn. The danger signals were failing him again.

He had no business thinking about anything except finishing his job, and that included returning to New York with the evidence his employer had promised.

So why had he seduced Maggie Mulligan?

Because he'd wanted her more than any woman he'd ever met. Because her smile warmed him through. Because he'd needed to feel her goodness surround him and drive away the demons that haunted him. Because . . .

Don't go there, Desmond.

Her family would be there tonight, and that meant Riley. *Himself,* as Maggie called him. Her brother and protector. Would anyone notice how things had changed between them? Well, they would find out soon enough.

Lights flowed from the black castle, including from some of the tower rooms. Nick was more than a little curious about the place after all the stories he'd heard.

Enough of this. He glanced down at Erin. "Ready to party, kid?"

"Aye." Erin grinned. "Jacob will be there."

Aha! "That's right. Isn't he about your age?"

"Eleven like me." Erin giggled again. "Oh, we're almost to the castle."

Nick looked toward Maggie's cottage. Was she still there or already at the castle? A soft light burned toward the front of the cottage, near the front door if he remembered correctly.

Maggie. He drew a deep breath, remembering how she'd felt, tasted, responded. He'd replenished the supply of condoms in his wallet, hoping he would need every last one of them and more.

And buying condoms in Ballybronagh was *not* an easy task. He'd had to go to the chemist—what they called a pharmacist here—and *ask.* Talk about embarrassing. Back in the States a guy just picked them up with the bread and milk and dropped them in the shopping cart. At least no one else had been in the shop at the time.

If Maggie didn't have company tonight, he'd sneak over for a visit after seeing Aunt Mo and Erin safely locked in their bubble. He hardened in anticipation. But she *did* have company.

This would be a *very* long weekend.

They walked along the path that led past the big boulders surrounding the back and sides of the castle. A movement at the top of one boulder snared his attention. It looked like a woman in a long skirt with her hands stretched toward the sky.

"Stop this madness!"

A cold sweat popped from every pore on Nick's body, and his gut twisted and burned.

"What have ye done? Stop this!"

The urge to scramble over the boulders and drag the woman away from the castle slammed into Nick. He even took a step in that direction, but Erin tugged gently on his hand and looked up at him curiously. He blinked at her and looked back at the boulders.

The figure was gone.

"What have ye done?" the tormenting voice repeated.

Nick drew deep gulps of air and kept following Aunt Mo and Brady with Erin's hand still clutched in his. He had to keep himself anchored in reality here. Keep his head screwed on straight. Banish that frigging voice.

It must have been a shadow on the boulders. Nothing more. But what about the old man's voice in his head? The odd comments?

Knock it off, Desmond. He drew a deep breath and tried to concentrate on anything *but* the weird images and voices.

At the front entrance of *Caisleán* Dubh, Brady turned an ornate handle, and they heard the chimes all the way outside.

"Too cool," Nick said, earning him another of Erin's smiles. She was a good kid, and she obviously took after her mother and grandmother. He found it hard to believe she had a drop of Fazzini blood in her veins.

Riley Mulligan appeared at the huge glass doors and

swung them wide. *"Céide Milé Fáilte,"* he said and ushered them into the main hall of the castle.

At least now Nick knew that meant he was welcome here, and not that he was pond scum and deserved to be gelded. If Riley ever learned what had happened between Nick and his sister, castration was a likely fate.

Nick winced and shoved the thought aside when it was his turn to greet Riley. He offered his hand and noted the hesitation in the other man's eyes. Finally, Riley shook it, but he didn't smile as he had while greeting the others.

"Let me take your wraps," Riley said as he walked away from Nick.

Maggie's brother knew something.

"Mulligan Stew is closed for this private party tonight. You're all in for a treat. Haven't my beautiful wife and mum been toiling away in the kitchen?"

"Not Maggie, I hope," Brady said, smiling.

"You know better, dear friend." Riley laughed and took their hats and coats to an alcove.

Nick felt Maggie before he saw her. He tingled all over, and warmth filled his chest. He turned toward the staircase that wound its way into the tower. There she was, standing at the top of the stairs with Bridget and another woman he guessed was Ailish.

They started down the stairs and Nick couldn't look away. Erin had skipped off to the kitchen with Aunt Mo to find Fiona Mulligan and Jacob.

Maggie wore a soft lavender dress that fluttered with some kind of uneven skirt around her ankles. It clung to her hips and waist, accentuated her breasts—oh, her so tempting breasts—and left her arms and shoulders completely bare.

He ached to kiss her bare shoulders, the gentle slope of her long, slender neck, and her breasts. His heart thundered and his throat tightened. As she neared the bottom step, he noticed her hair was pulled high on her head, where it fell in soft curls down her back.

A hand clamped down on his shoulder, and he froze. He

knew without looking who it was, but he forced his gaze away from the woman he wanted far more than he should, and faced her brother's fierce expression.

Riley Mulligan stood very near Nick's height. They were both big men, though Riley's physique had more bulk, and it was all muscle. Nick was in good shape and a few years younger. Theirs would be an even match, though he hoped it wouldn't come to that for Maggie's sake.

"I'd like to know your intentions toward my sister," he said quietly. Menacingly. "Soon. Meanwhile, you'll be minding your manners where she's concerned, if you get my meaning." His smile was deadly. "And I think you do."

Riley moved away before Nick could respond. How could he blame the man for wanting to protect his sister? Nick didn't have any sisters, but if he did, he would have kicked someone like him out the door. No problem.

Then Maggie was beside him. He swung around to face her, and seeing her this close again was like a punch in the solar plexus. He couldn't breathe. He couldn't think. All he could do was stare and want and ache.

"Your duty. Protect her. Forbidden . . ."

"Nick," she said. "I'd like you to meet Ailish Delaney from Dublin. She was my roommate at university and is here on holiday."

A short one, I hope. "Pleased to meet you." Nick took the woman's hand and felt her gaze as if she had X-ray vision. She stared at him as she shook his hand, probing. He sensed questions, but had no idea what they were, let alone how to answer.

Riley and Ailish were trying to protect Maggie, yet he was the one hearing voices in his head about protecting her. Weird and more weird.

"Nick came to Ireland with his aunt and young cousin," Maggie explained.

Bridget joined them, her belly twice as big as the last time he'd seen her. "Make way for the fat lady," she said in her smooth, Tennessee drawl. "Nick, it's good to see you here again."

"You look glowing," he said, and she did.

"Another charmer. I swear, Ireland is crawlin' with them, and this one's not even from here."

"The truth."

"Honest to a fault, Nick? I heard you were a policeman back in New York," Bridget said. "I know Jacob would love to hear more about that. He loves movies and TV shows about American cops."

Nick stiffened and felt Maggie's hand on his arm. Somehow, she'd figured out that his former career wasn't something he enjoyed talking about. "Boys Jacob's age usually do," he finally said.

"I'd best poke my head in the kitchen to see how Fiona is doing with the final touches. We let the staff have the night off." She laughed as she waddled toward the kitchen. "One extra pair of hands isn't much of a staff."

With Maggie's hand still on Nick's arm, the urge to kiss her was so compelling that he half turned and placed his hand on the small of her back. "I've missed you," he heard himself say.

"And I you."

"So this is your Yank," Ailish said.

Stunned that he'd forgotten others were present, Nick blinked but kept his hand resting on the small of Maggie's back. He couldn't bear to be so close to her without touching.

"Nick, I . . ." Maggie bit her lower lip and blushed. "I told Ailish that we're . . . seeing each other."

He blinked. Of course she would have told her best friend. "Good." He met Ailish's gaze and still felt as if he were being subjected to a Vulcan mind meld or something.

"Well, he's handsome enough." Ailish grinned and turned to Maggie. "Two out of three, you said?"

Nick frowned. "Two out of three *what*?" He kept his

voice low. Had Maggie told Ailish that he hadn't used a condom that last time?

Maggie blushed again and Ailish laughed. "'Tisn't anything bad, boyo," Ailish said. "I asked Maggie if you were handsome, rich, and sexy. She said two out of three."

He relaxed somewhat and found himself massaging Maggie's back and inching closer. She smelled like the cinnamon soap they'd used this morning. He would never smell cinnamon again without thinking of her. And remembering . . .

"Aye, and isn't he the smitten one?" Ailish teased.

Nick swallowed hard and dragged his gaze away from Maggie and looked at Ailish again. She didn't seem as suspicious now, though there were still questions in her eyes. Somehow, he sensed them.

"The feeling is mutual," Maggie said as Nick moved his hand from her back to link his fingers with hers.

The truth was he didn't want to keep this a secret. Ailish and Aunt Mo knew, and Riley suspected. Couldn't he and Maggie simply *date*—or whatever they called it in Ireland—without anyone getting all uptight about it? Hell, what was the proper protocol for something like this in Ireland?

"Question." He glanced around the room and saw Brady and Riley huddled over some books on the far side of the hall. The others must be in the kitchen. "Is there some reason why we need to keep it a secret that we're, uh, seeing each other?"

Maggie blinked, appearing surprised. "I . . ." She laughed and shook her head. "For some reason, I guess I thought so, but well, no."

Ailish laughed, too. "So why is it a secret?" Her gaze became probing again. "And is it the only secret you're keeping?"

Nick stiffened and tugged at the neckband of his sweater. "The only one worth discussing." He hoped he sounded more flippant than he felt.

Ailish narrowed her eyes for a moment, then turned toward Maggie. "At dinner, I'll let it slip that you two are walking out. That should take care of it."

Maggie chewed her lower lip. That was an adorable habit of hers. Nick had to fight against the urge to help her. Realizing where his thoughts were headed again, he cleared his throat.

"I guess that would work, but . . ." Maggie sighed. "Maybe Nick should talk to Riley first."

Nick coughed. "What about your mom? Shouldn't she be the one I ask? Do adults still ask *permission* to come courting around here?"

"Some do." Maggie laughed openly now. "And Mum will be dancing a jig. Trust me."

"Then I'd much rather talk to her." Nick grinned again, but realized Riley was the one he had to convince. The guy was already suspicious, so coming clean—to a certain extent—was the right thing to do. "Can I have witnesses, just in case?"

"Look at it this way, Nick," Ailish said, her voice lowering to a sultry whisper. "You won't have to stop yourself from holding her hand or kissing her hello and good-bye in polite company then."

"Point taken." Nick drew a deep breath. "Now is as good a time as any, and my cousin can be my witness."

Maggie gave a nervous laugh and Ailish winked. "Go for it, boyo."

"'Tis your secret to carry to your grave. Your shame. Your sin."

And that was bull. Nick squared his shoulders and strode across the room to the men, who had their heads bent over some old books spread out on a massive table. They looked up when he stopped beside them.

"Cousin Nick, I was just showin' Riley here some of the records I've been translating about the old priest and the *cailleach.*"

Nick had heard enough of the stories to know what priest Brady meant, and that the *cailleach* was the witch

who had cast the spell that started the curse. "Interesting."
He wondered how to change the subject.

"Aye, 'tis fascinating." Brady turned his attention to a
page and pointed at an entry. "There, Riley. This is where
the *cailleach* was sentenced. Father Brennan was sick
about it. He encouraged leniency, as did the Mulligans. In
the end, she refused to reverse her spell, though she did
regret wishing ill to the Mulligans. So she was burned by
order of the landlord and self-appointed magistrate.
British, of course." Brady sighed.

"Burn, witch, burn."

Shut up. Go away.

Nick drew a deep breath to clear his mind—he hoped.

Then Riley looked up at him expectantly, as if he knew
that Nick had something to say.

"I wanted to . . ." Nick tugged at the neckline of his
sweater again, wishing he'd worn a T-shirt under his
jacket instead. "Uh, I wanted to ask your . . . blessing to
call on Maggie," he blurted, refusing to use the word *permission.*

Riley arched a brow, but the unmistakable flicker of respect appeared in his blue eyes. Nick should have known
that a man like Riley Mulligan could only appreciate
courage and honesty. He wouldn't underestimate this man
again.

"I'm fond of her and the feeling is mutual," he added.
"We'd like to see each other." He left out the fact that they
already *were* seeing each other.

"You're wanting to walk out with my sister?" Riley's
expression grew solemn. "I appreciate the asking, man to
man. Maggie's a smart, independent lass, and I'm a stubborn big brother. Ornery when I'm crossed, if you get my
meaning."

Oh, Nick definitely understood his meaning. However,
he and Maggie were entitled to their privacy, and Riley
didn't need to know the details of their relationship. Aunt
Mo knowing was bad enough.

"I do." Nick thrust out his hand and Riley shook it firmly. "Thank you."

"I trust you'll be a gentleman, of course," Brady added, his eyes twinkling.

A surge of mischief niggled at Nick. Unable to resist, he said, "I'll be every bit the gentleman you were with your Bridget before you were married."

Brady cleared his throat and damned if Riley didn't blush. Nick couldn't suppress his grin. He'd definitely touched on something.

"I'll just leave you two to your research then," Nick said, then made his way back toward Maggie and Ailish, who stood there smiling at him. His ego swelled. This was nuts. Why did he feel like a conquering hero just for talking to Riley? He smiled to himself again as he reached Maggie's side and took her hand, kissed her cheek.

The reward had definitely been worth the risk.

"Well, now, isn't that a sight for these old eyes?" Fiona Mulligan asked with a wink.

They would expect Nick to stay and . . . and . . .

Guilt made his throat clench. *Damn.* He'd taken things this far. Now he had no choice but to play along. "Thanks, Mrs. Mulligan."

The older woman smiled, then made her way around the hall with a tray filled with champagne flutes. "*Sláinte,* one and all," she called, making certain everyone had a glass. "Dinner will be served in ten minutes."

"Nick," Ailish said after Fiona had left them. "Let me see your palm."

Maggie laughed and Nick shrugged as he released Maggie's hand and gave it to Ailish. "You read palms?"

Ailish grinned. "No."

He pulled back, but she held fast. "Then what—"

"I read people," she said, narrowing her eyes as she looked into his instead of at his palm.

"She does, Nick," Maggie said. "I lived with her for four years."

Nick swallowed hard and watched Ailish. He didn't believe in this stuff. She wouldn't be able to tell why he was really here just by staring at his frigging palm.

"You're a man with secrets." She glanced first at Maggie, then at him. "Also a man of honor with a strong sense of duty." She nodded approvingly.

Nothing incriminating. Nick kept his expression bland; she wouldn't feel his racing pulse in his hand.

"Though . . ." She frowned.

"What?" he asked, hoping she was faking all this.

"You're a bit obsessive." She looked from his eyes to his palm again.

Nick's face warmed and he took a sip of champagne, hoping he looked a hell of a lot cooler than he felt.

"Oh, this is interesting." Ailish's dark brows swept upward.

"What?" Maggie asked.

Ailish looked up at Nick, her expression open and sincere. "You've been here before."

Nick's heart skipped a beat, though he had no idea why her comment should disturb him. "We attended a party here earlier in the summer," he said. "So, yes, I've been here before."

"No." Ailish caught and held his gaze. "You don't understand."

"I guess not." He took another sip of champagne, sensing Maggie's gaze on him.

"You've been to Ireland—*here*—in an earlier life."

Sixteen

Maggie was so happy that Nick had spoken to Riley she could have danced a jig. It was all she could do not to shout to them all that she was a woman in love, and a woman in every way.

Of course, she resisted, but didn't hesitate to sit beside Nick at dinner. They no longer had to hide the fact that they were interested in each other. Not that anyone needed to know just *how* interested.

What had Ailish meant about Nick having been here in an earlier life? Perhaps she meant his ancestors. Maggie thought of Riley and Bridget, who'd been brought together again in this life.

Was she being a silly, romantic fool to think that, maybe, she and Nick were destined to be together? Or was it the old one's words that had planted the seeds for Maggie's newest fantasy?

Maggie helped her mum serve the meal. That was considered safe even for Maggie. Oh, she could cook a few things, thanks to Bridget and Mum's patience, but 'twas safer if she avoided it as much as possible. They were all in agreement there. They had allowed Maggie to prepare the only dish she seemed capable of not ruining—the wonderful Mississippi mud pie Bridget had taught her to make. In fact, it appeared on the menu now as "Maggie's Mississippi Mud Pie."

After hot vinegary salads Bridget called "kilt lettuce," they had the dish for which the restaurant was named as the main course—Bridget's Bodacious Mulligan Stew. Warm sourdough bread dripping with butter made the rounds, and everyone ate until they swore they couldn't take another bite.

"Y'all *will* eat dessert," Bridget announced. "Maggie made it."

Riley groaned, but Maggie simply smiled. The old Maggie would've thrown something at him. In fact, she suspected if they didn't have company, she would have anyway. The thought made her smile widen.

"Don't worry, boyo," she said sweetly. "Didn't young Jacob help his Aunt Maggie dig the very freshest mud just for you?"

Mrs. O'Shea and Erin's eyes grew wide, and Bridget laughed.

"Mud?" Nick echoed from her side, and Maggie had to squeeze his hand, just because.

"Ah, 'tis relieved I am that the mud is fresh." Riley crossed himself and Nick laughed.

As Maggie served Nick his slice of pie, she whispered, "I think Riley likes you, Mr. Desmond. You learn fast."

His eyes smoldered. "So do you, Miss Mulligan."

Jaysus, Mary, and Joseph. She returned to her chair with her heart running a fifty-meter dash.

"I think Jacob was right." Nick held Maggie's hand under the table. "His mom is the world's best cook, and his aunt Maggie's mud pie is heavenly."

"I'll drink to that." Riley raised his mug and smiled. "But don't let the mud pie fool you, lad. Maggie's cooking is not a thing of beauty."

This time Maggie very calmly tore off a piece of biscuit, set it in her spoon, and shot it at her brother. It landed right in the middle of his pie. He arched a brow and

sighed, flipped the biscuit away with his thumb, and re-
sumed eating.

Mrs. O'Shea and Erin laughed along with Brady, and
Mum merely heaved a weary sigh and muttered something about the Virgin.

All was well at the Mulligan table.

They all toasted the chefs with either champagne or
beer, except for Bridget and the children, who had milk.

"Brady, what are you researching now?" Mum asked.

"Now, what makes you think I'm researchin' anything?" Brady winked. "As I was tellin' Riley before this
fine meal, I'm workin' on the sequel to my first book."

"First book?" Mum echoed. "By the saints, does that
mean you sold it, Brady?"

Brady puffed up with undeniable pride. "That I did.
The story of Aidan and Bronagh and *Caisleán* Dubh.
We're still working on a title. I thought of *Mulligan Stew,*
since it certainly was a stew, but . . ."

"Congratulations!" Riley raised his mug again. "And I
think *Mulligan Stew* is a perfect title."

"So do I," Bridget said.

"When were you going to tell us, man?"

"I just did."

They all laughed and drank to Brady's success.

"'Tis wonderful news," Maggie said. "What will the
new book be about?"

"This research is even more fascinatin' than for the first
book, lass." He squirmed with delight as he warmed to his
subject. "I've continued readin' Father Brennan's diaries
beyond the point where the poor *cailleach* was executed."

"Executed?" Ailish echoed, her green eyes snapping.
"Simply for being a witch?"

"For causin' the curse," Brady corrected. "The Mulligans and Father Brennan opposed her sentence and
begged for leniency. Alas, they failed and the landlord ordered the old one burned to death."

Ailish winced as did Maggie. Something cold trickled

down Maggie's spine and spread through her. Fear. No, terror. Brady had called the *cailleach* the "old one." Why?

"'Tis glad I am the Mulligans opposed that," Mum said. "Even though she caused years of misery for the family, takin' her life for doin' something while she was beside herself with grief was . . . terrible."

"I agree." Riley set his mug aside. "From what we've learned—rather from what Brady has learned—Bronagh's aunt cast her spell to give her niece a second chance at love."

"And life." Brady drank from his mug. "Isn't it all in the first book?"

"I'll drink to that," Bridget said, toasting with milk. They all laughed.

Except Maggie. She could barely breathe, let alone laugh.

"And I." Riley leaned over and kissed his wife.

Maggie didn't want to hear the tale about the old witch being burned again. Maybe his new book would steer the discussion in a new direction. "So what is the second book about?"

"'Tis about Father Brennan," Brady said. "The man and the priest—who he was and why he defended the old one." He chuckled and added, "Though from what I can tell, the priest was a few years older than the *cailleach*."

"What happened to the priest afterward that could be of enough interest for a book?"

"Well, 'twas actually what happened *before* that interests me, if I can find it," Brady explained. "However, the information wasn't revealed in his early diaries. Later, as he grieved over Sinéad's death—"

"Sinéad?" Nick interrupted.

Maggie tightened her grip on Nick's hand as the cold inside her intensified. *Sinéad.* The name reverberated through her. She shivered, and he moved the hand holding hers onto her lap. What had come over her? Why did this story terrify her so?

"Aye, that was the *cailleach*'s name, lad." Brady

paused for a drink, then continued, "As I was saying, 'tis clear from the priest's diaries that he'd known Sinéad all his life, and that she meant a great deal to him."

"You speak of a priest, Brady," Mum said, her tone solemn. "Are you suggestin' they were—he was . . ."

"In love with Sinéad?" Brady shrugged. " 'Tisn't clear as yet, but I must let the research tell the tale, wherever it leads."

"Sounds like it'd make a great movie," Nick said. *The Witch and the Priest.* Definitely a blockbuster."

Bridget laughed. "Maybe a movie of the week or a miniseries. I still remember how Granny loved *Roots* and *Rich Man, Poor Man.* She didn't miss a single second of those programs."

"Who knows?" Brady shrugged. "We'll see after I've finished translating all the diaries."

"Let me know when you do." Mrs. O'Shea elbowed him gently. "I'm dying of curiosity."

Why did the stories about Sinéad's execution make Maggie feel like she could lose her dinner? A shudder rippled through her and Nick rubbed her thigh with the backs of his knuckles.

" 'Tis interestin'," Mum said. "I'll grant you that, though I hope you find the priest was true to his vows."

"Aye." Brady appeared thoughtful. "Remember that the Penal laws banned Catholicism—and even being Irish, for that matter—from the end of the seventeenth century until the middle of the eighteenth. 'Tis possible that Father Brennan postponed his decision a bit."

"Perhaps he struggled with his decision *because* of her," Mrs. O'Shea suggested. "If it's true, her heart must have been broken. Then to lose her niece so tragically . . ."

"His love of piety and traditions was stronger than the love he professed for me."

Maggie swallowed the lump of chocolate in her throat, then reached for her champagne and drained it. Nick retrieved the bottle from the ice bucket and refilled her flute.

Why did Brady's new research frighten her so? What was it about the *cailleach*'s tragedy that felt as if it were her own? A shiver raced down her spine. More and more, she felt certain she knew whose voice spoke to her. Hearing her name here tonight made her suspicion even stronger.

Why was Sinéad speaking to Maggie? *Why?*

Again she had to wonder—did the old one's voice and the chanting have anything to do with the curse? If so, she had to make sure her family was safe.

And she had to know *why* Sinéad had chosen her.

Nick remembered Ailish's words: *"You've been to Ireland—here—in an earlier life."*

What the hell did that mean?

And why did this corner of Ireland have more than its share of curses, spells, witches, and reincarnated people? Nick was losing count of how many times he'd been asked to suspend disbelief since his arrival here.

After dessert he managed to find Aunt Mo alone long enough to let her know he was going to walk Maggie and Ailish back to the cottage. Aunt Mo gave him an approving nod, and he knew she and Erin would be safe here with Riley and Brady until he returned. Fortunately, Brady was enjoying telling stories too much to question why he wasn't trusted to escort them back to Donovan Cottage himself.

Along the way to the cottage beneath a star-studded sky—which both Ailish and Maggie told him western Ireland was famed for—Nick held Maggie's hand and Ailish walked off to one side. He looked warily at the dark outline of the cottage.

"When we walked over earlier, there was a light on in your cottage, and you two were already at the castle," he said. "Maybe the bulb burned out."

"We didn't leave any lights on," Maggie said. "Did we, Ailish?"

"I don't remember any. Where was the light, Nick, and what did it look like?"

What did it look *like?* Nick had to think about that one for a moment, and once he did, he realized it hadn't seemed quite . . . right. "More of a glow, I guess—like a candle? Near the front door, as I recall."

But why would Maggie, who was afraid of fire, leave a candle burning? It didn't make sense. "Maybe it was the sun reflecting off a window." Of course, that would have been much brighter. Maybe he'd just imagined the light, though he couldn't quite convince himself of that.

They walked along in silence, and clouds gathered rapidly to block out the moon and the stars as they neared the cottage. So much for stargazing.

"Looks like we're in for a fast-moving storm," Nick said. He hadn't seen much in the way of violent weather since his arrival.

Ailish sniffed at the air. "Aye." She looked up at the sky. "Wind, driving rain, lightning." She turned her head toward Nick in the darkness. "Perhaps you should stay the night."

Maggie gasped and Nick damned near died. He'd like nothing better.

"Thanks, but I have to see my aunt and cousin safely home." He gave Maggie's hand a squeeze and his breath caught and held. He grew hard enough to make him know what he wanted and to want it *now*. But he wasn't going to get it—not tonight.

Maggie opened the kitchen door and flipped on the lights. Nick went inside and insisted on looking around, since he'd seen what could have been a light earlier.

"Don't you sound just like Riley now?" Maggie laughed.

The champagne had loosened her inhibitions a bit, and he wished desperately for the opportunity to find out how much. He'd like to try the Nutella she'd mentioned. Warm. Spreadable.

Oh, God.

He took several deep breaths and made the mistake of glancing at Ailish, whose green eyes flashed as if she knew exactly what he was thinking. Oddly, she also seemed to approve. He no longer felt as if she were probing for answers to unknown questions, and realizing that made him more curious than about why she'd questioned him earlier. That had been obvious, since she was Maggie's friend.

Ailish walked across Maggie's kitchen in her flowing dress. She looked . . . otherworldly. *Get with the program, Desmond.*

Then again, maybe he was, finally. All this talk of curses and witches and priests who might have been in love was enough to make any man question what was real, normal, or halfway in between. At least, any American male. Irishmen probably had an advantage where paranormal stuff was concerned.

Something compelled him to meet Ailish's gaze again. The expression in her green eyes was approval and encouragement.

What the hell had changed?

Ailish laughed and spun in a circle, her black hair and silky dress floating around her. " 'Tis going to read the cards, I am. To see what's past and what is yet to be. Good night, darlings."

"Sleep well, Ailish," Maggie said. "Bridget loved the attic rooms before she and Riley married. I hope you do, too." She released Nick and hugged her friend.

"Night," Nick called as Ailish seemed to float out of the kitchen and up the stairs.

Weird. He arched a brow at Maggie, who whispered, "She's a witch, of course."

"Of course?" Well, he'd actually known men and women back in New York who were Wiccan—a few who were on the force. He was cool with this, as long as no one cast any more evil spells on families or castles. Even so, there seemed to be a *lot* more magic involved with

witches here—at least, to his knowledge. "All right."
What else could he say?

Maggie smiled up at him, her eyes filled with trust and
that something more he didn't want to think about.

"*'Tis forbidden. Ye tasted carnal pleasure once, but
must forsake it now for duty.*"

That voice was becoming more and more annoying.
And making Nick more and more uncomfortable.

"I want you, Nick," Maggie whispered.

This was more than champagne talking. He remembered her passion and swayed as his blood supply redirected itself. *Lightheaded—that's you, Desmond.*

He dragged Maggie against him with a single, powerful
tug. He wanted her desperately—possibly even more than
he had last night, and that was saying a hell of a lot.

She came up on tiptoes to reach his mouth with hers
and the heat rushed through him relentlessly. Ruthlessly.
He shuddered in her arms, barely preventing himself from
taking her to the table now.

Reluctantly he broke their kiss. "I wish I didn't have to
go," he said between gulps of air.

"Me, too." She pouted and reached up to brush his hair
away from his eyes, which made his heart do that funny,
flip-flop thing again.

He couldn't look away from her Mulligan-blue eyes.
She held him prisoner, and he couldn't think of any place
he'd rather be.

He was in deep shit.

Damn it. He wasn't supposed to fall in love—not now.
But he had.

I love you, Maggie Mulligan. He swallowed the lump
in his throat and simply drowned in the blue depths of her
beautiful eyes. *Sap.* No, this was more important than his
ego, than the career he'd lost.

And more important than revenge?

He tensed and held her at arm's length, trying not to remember the sight of his father dying on the sidewalk.
Closing his eyes, he told himself that after he'd done his

duty, he could come back to her. For her. To her. For her. Whatever. As long as it was Maggie.

"Ye vowed your life to service."

Shut up.

His blood roared through his head, pounded through his veins, nearly blinded him. This wasn't simple lust. There was nothing simple about it.

He was in love. Madly, passionately, deeply in love.

Nuked. Fried. Buried.

In love.

"I'll dream about you," he whispered, touching his fingertip to the tip of her nose.

"Aye." Maggie's voice had a breathy, ever-so-sexy quality. "Ring me up tomorrow?"

"I promise."

"Remember your duty. Protect her. Save her."

Yeah, I remember, damn it. Shut the hell up already.

He should leave. Now. Instead, he just stood there with Maggie in his arms, wanting to say the words. "Dinner was great," he said. "I like your family."

"I think they like you, too. Even Riley." She trailed the tip of her tongue along the side of his neck.

Damn. He didn't want to leave.

"I guess you'd better go," she said sadly and kissed him again.

He poured all his love into the kiss, hoping it would suffice until he was free to come to her without the burden of duty hovering over him. God, she felt so good. He wanted her so much. Needed her.

Finally, he pulled back and drew several deep breaths to bring himself under control. "I'd better go while I can still walk."

She laughed—a low, sexy sound. "Remember to dream."

"And you." He kissed her forehead, knowing he had to make his escape now. Otherwise, he would take her to the table and search her kitchen for Nutella and similar contraband.

With a sigh, he opened the door and dashed out into the threatening storm.

Lightning flashed, and Maggie realized she was no longer in her bed. She blinked and waited for her eyes to adjust to the darkness. Wind blew her nightgown against her and the lightning illuminated her surroundings.

She stood outside on her own front porch. She must have walked in her sleep again, though she didn't remember having a dream this time. Strange.

With trembling fingers she reached up to pull at the neckline of her gown. Stiff lace met her fingers. She distinctly remembered putting on a light summer cotton gown without a hint of lace.

She was still asleep and this was a dream. Of course, that was the only explanation. So why didn't she turn around and go back to her warm bed, instead of standing here on the porch in a storm?

"He will come to me now."

"Who?" Maggie whispered, her heart hammering. "Who will come? Who are you?"

"Ye know. In yer heart, ye know."

A violent shudder ripped through her. For a few, terrifying seconds she couldn't breathe. "Sinéad." In her heart she knew who, but the why of it had her confused.

"'Tis back to my bed I'm going now," she said. "To sleep. Go away. Leave me alone."

Maggie turned to reach for the door, but couldn't find it. Something was different. Where was she? What was happening?

Thunder rumbled and lightning flashed across the sky again. The wall of her cottage was dark wood rather than the fresh whitewash it should've been. "Jaysus, Mary, and Joseph." Like the dream. It was happening again.

She heard a step creak behind her, and she spun

around, frightened. The sky quieted, the wind died. Everything seemed surreal. Even her. "Who . . . ?"

A large, dark figure stood a few feet away. She swallowed hard, but her fear slowly dissipated. "'Tis you," she said, and took a step toward him. "I knew you would come back."

He pulled her against his chest. She tilted her lips up to his, drank from him, melted against him. The air about them seemed to come alive as he untied the ribbon holding her strange nightgown closed and eased the garment from her shoulders. It fell to the porch floor with a whisper. He looked down at her nakedness for several seconds, then groaned as he removed his wool cape and spread it on the porch floor and placed her gown atop it.

She urged him to remove his clothing, and soon they stood wrapped in each other's arms, flesh against flesh, heart against heart.

Desperation charged the air between them, as if they had waited their entire lives for this moment. He worshipped her with his lips, tongue, teeth, and she clung to him, took him within her body.

"Give yerself to me and no other," she murmured.

He didn't answer with words, though he took her body with a passion that left them both straining and breathless. They shuddered together in completion, bound by love yet torn apart by duty.

"I give ye me heart. Me body," she breathed. "Pledge yourself to me."

They clung together in the odd stillness of the night. Finally, he raised up on his elbow and cradled her face in his palm.

He said something, but the words were unclear. She wanted—needed—to hear him.

"I took ye within me and made ye mine," she whispered.

After a moment she felt his tears dampen her

cheek. Silently he pulled her to her feet and they dressed.

"I love ye, and ye are mine," she repeated.

Again he cradled her face in both hands. She felt his sadness—his regret.

"Ye cannot walk away from our love. Do not do this."

She reached into her pocket and withdrew a small bag when she saw that he would leave—that, at least in his heart, he had no choice.

"Me gift to you," she said, her heart broken beyond repair. "Carry it with ye always. Remember . . ."

Then he was gone.

Maggie bolted upright in her bed. She was alone. She groped at her nightgown—the same, simple cotton one she'd worn to bed. She'd dreamed again. None of it had happened.

"He came to me only once."

"Why are you telling me this?"

The old one didn't answer. The woman in her dream had been no older than Maggie. A young Sinéad? Or had it been Bronagh and Aidan Mulligan? That didn't make sense. Of course, none of this made sense.

Maggie threw back the covers and walked to the window. Lightning still flashed in the distance, behind the dark tower of *Caisleán* Dubh.

She went to the bathroom and drank cool water while looking at herself in the mirror. What had happened? Whose voice was she hearing? Whose life was she seeing in her dreams?

And *why*?

More importantly, why did her life and her dreams seem intertwined? This was the most terrifying thought of all. Why? Why? Why?

Too anxious now to sleep, she walked into the hall and looked up the narrow staircase that led to the attic room. Was Ailish awake? She walked up two steps and saw a

light under her door. Relieved, she knocked on Ailish's
door.

"Come in, Maggie," her friend called.

Maggie opened the door and saw Ailish with a purple
cloth spread upon the small night table. A single candle
burned in its center, and a deck of tarot cards sat beside it.

"I was expecting you," Ailish stated, her expression
solemn. "Come. Sit."

Maggie knew Ailish's ways enough not to feel uncomfortable with them. Still, tonight she was wary for some
reason.

"Come." Ailish smiled and pointed to the chair on the
other side of the table. "If I'm to read your cards, you
need to shuffle."

It wasn't as if Ailish had never read the cards before for
Maggie. Far from it. Maggie drew a deep breath and
crossed to the chair and sat. She reached for the deck, and
her fingertips brushed against Ailish's hand.

A bluish light glowed there for a moment, startling her.
She pulled back, but Ailish reached out and took her hand
firmly in her own. Something pulsed from Ailish and into
Maggie.

"Do you feel it, Maggie?" she whispered. "'Tis the
power."

"What power?" Maggie shook her head and swallowed
hard. "Yours?"

"Aye. And yours." Ailish turned Maggie's hand over
and placed the cards in her palm. "'Tis a new deck given
to me by a friend who said I would soon have a reason to
use them. She was right. They're for tonight."

"I have no power." Maggie shuffled the cards slowly,
wanting to talk about the dream. "I don't."

Ailish's eyes twinkled in the candlelight and she pointed
at the cards. "Once more. Cut them if it feels right, and
ask your question."

Maggie did have a question. More than one, actually.
She cut the deck once. "I . . . I've been hearing voices.
One clear one, and others raised in . . . some sort of

chant." She drew a shaky breath. "Whose voice is it? That is my question." She dropped her hands to her lap and waited.

"Only one question?" Ailish asked in her knowing way.

"For now."

Ailish turned over the top card of the deck, then met Maggie's gaze over the flickering candle. " 'Tis your own voice you hear."

Maggie shook her head. "No."

Ailish drew another card. " 'Tis from the past."

"Who is it?"

"I told you, darling." Ailish met and held her gaze. " 'Tis your own."

Maggie shook her head. She couldn't accept that.

Ailish drew another card, and her brow furrowed. "I didn't expect this. Heed the old one's words, Maggie. There's danger."

How did Ailish know that she'd grown to think of the voice as the "old one?" Maggie swallowed hard. "Danger?"

"Aye." Ailish's expression grew intense. "She means to protect you from suffering her fate."

Brady had referred to Sinéad as the "old one," and now Ailish used the same phrase. "Who is the 'old one?' " she asked carefully.

Ailish turned over the Queen of Wands. "You. This is you and this is the old one. Heed her words, for they are yours."

Maggie shook her head again. "That makes no sense." She stood and started toward the door. "I—I'm too nervous for this. I can't think."

"You had another vision."

"Another dream." Maggie whirled around to face Ailish again. "But how did you—"

"I just know." Ailish stood and went to Maggie and patted her shoulder. "You've never doubted me before."

"I—I don't want to, but I'm so confused." Maggie tried to blink back the tears, but they slipped from her eyes anyway. "I've fallen in love, yet I think I may be losing my mind as well."

"School starts Monday." Ailish gave Maggie's hand a squeeze. "For now, be busy, be happy, and enjoy your Yank."

"You said there's danger." Maggie narrowed her eyes. "How will I know?"

"You have a protector." Ailish's voice was gentle, encouraging, but the look she gave Maggie was filled with magic and promise.

"More than one, it seems."

Seventeen

Dreams—no, nightmares—filled Nick's sleep. He awakened tense, exhausted and desperate. Afraid.

He sat up in bed, realizing he had something clutched in his fist. The crucifix. He blinked. When had he gone to the dresser and taken it from the drawer?

Then his dreams came flooding back to him. Fire. Storms. Running. More fire. Always the fire. Always the fear. His visit to Ireland was starting to resemble Dante's frigging *Inferno.*

He opened his palm and stared down at the crucifix. Was it making him crazy? No, that was silly. But . . . *Think, Desmond.* When had the voices started? *Think!*

The day he'd found the crucifix. He'd heard the evil voice first, then he'd stumbled and fallen. Church bells, too. Almost immediately after he'd found the crucifix, the other voice started, and it seemed to talk directly *to* him.

He climbed out of bed, aching from the tension. After a hot shower, two aspirin, and fresh clothes, he felt marginally better and went out to have breakfast with Aunt Mo and Erin.

He poured coffee and carried it to the table, his mind drifting back to his discovery about the crucifix and the voices. Maybe if he stopped carrying it . . . ? As if he could. Thinking about it increased the pounding in his head to the nuclear level.

"What do you make of Brady's research, Nick?" Aunt Mo's question dragged his attention back to the breakfast conversation. "I think it's fascinating."

"Yeah." Nick took a sip of coffee, then another. The caffeine jolt was just what he needed right now. "Weird, too."

"Imagine a witch casting a spell that lasted centuries. Bridget and Riley's story is very romantic." Aunt Mo poured juice into a glass and slid it toward Nick. "Didn't you sleep well?"

"What? Oh, yeah. I had a nightmare." Fire. Always fire. Why?

"Too much mulligan stew and mud pie?"

"Something." He cleared his throat. "Or all the talk about . . . burning people."

"Burn, witch, burn."

Oh, my God. Numbness tingled around Nick's mouth. Brady. He had to talk to Brady. The crucifix. The priest. The fire. The voice. "Holy . . ."

"What is it, Nick?" Erin asked. "You look like you have a tummy ache."

"No. I'm . . . fine. Just tired." Nick drank more coffee and drained the juice, too. Get his blood sugar up. Get his head on straight. Go talk to Brady.

"If you don't need me for anything, I'm going to visit Brady for a while," Nick said, planning his strategy as he spoke. "He wants to show me some photo albums of all my cousins."

"That's a fine idea," Aunt Mo said. "I know he's been eager to get to know you better. He's also lonely since his son's family moved to the States."

"If you don't need me for anything, I'll walk over there now."

"Of course. Take some scones along, since you didn't eat. They're fresh."

"You're getting downright domestic." Nick managed a smile.

Aunt Mo arched a brow. "Erin's teaching me."

They all laughed, and Nick made his exit. The security system was armed, and they were staying in to finish readying Erin's clothes for her first day of school.

Nick walked through the village to Rearden Cottage and knocked on the door. His cousin answered and Nick held up the napkin-wrapped scones. "I come bearing gifts," he said, trying to sound cheerful.

"Nick, lad. Come in." Brady removed his spectacles and swung the door wide. "I was just finishing up another of Father Brennan's diaries. The man was very prolific in his later years. After Sinéad's execution, he became something of a recluse."

Nick didn't have to worry about dragging information out of Brady. He had to grin about that as he followed his cousin into a cluttered kitchen that screamed *bachelor.*

The crucifix was burning his thigh through the fabric of his pocket. He usually reached in and removed it when that happened, but now he resisted the impulse. It was nuts to believe a hunk of metal was manipulating him, but right now his whole world was kooky.

"The kettle is on." Brady eyed the bundle in Nick's hand. "What have you there, lad?"

"Scones. Aunt Mo sent them."

"Ah, a fine woman. Fine." Brady put plates on the table, poured tea, and they both sat down to nibble. " 'Tis glad I am you've come to visit."

Nick took a swig of tea and managed not to grimace. He really couldn't develop a taste for the stuff, but he could fake it for a while if he considered it merely a vehicle for the delivery of caffeine. "I—I'm curious about the story you told last night about that priest and the witch being burned."

"Burn, witch, burn," the evil voice said again.

Nick swallowed hard and reached into his pocket.

" 'Tis an amazing tale, Nick." Brady rested his ankle

across his knee and leaned back in his chair. "I'm more and more convinced that there were secrets between Sinéad and Father Brennan."

Nick's fingertips brushed against the crucifix and they tingled at the contact. Slowly he pulled it from his pocket, afraid.

"Mine."

He had to do this. He had to learn the truth. "Do . . . do you know if he ever owned anything like this?" Nick forced himself to hold his open palm out on the table.

Brady adjusted his glasses and reached for the crucifix.

Nick gritted his teeth. His hand trembled.

His cousin looked up at his face. "Are you all right, lad?"

Nick released a breath in a loud whoosh. "No. I'm not all right. Take it. Take it away."

"No!"

"Please, just take it." Nick closed his eyes until he felt his cousin remove the hot metal from his palm. He felt as if a part of himself had been amputated.

"Mine. Ye lost what was given. Her gift to me . . . Gone!"

Nick gritted his teeth and forced himself to look across the table and meet Brady's worried frown.

"Your hand." His cousin's expression was gentle, questioning. "'Tis burned, lad."

Nick looked. The shape of a cross was burned into his palm where the crucifix had lain just a moment ago. That hadn't happened before. His throat tightened as his cousin took his hand and looked from it to the crucifix, then back.

"Mother Mary," Brady whispered.

"Do—do you know anything about that thing?"

"Where did you find it?" Brady turned it over in his hand, examining it closely. "'Tis very old."

"The ruins. I saw it sparkle from far away, and finally went to look." He dragged his gaze from the crucifix and back to his cousin's eyes. "I think it . . . wanted me to find it."

Both of Brady's brows rose. "Interesting."

"It's nuts, but that's not all." This part would be harder. "I—I'm hearing voices. Two different ones. One keeps telling me the crucifix is 'mine,' and that I must 'protect' someone. 'Save her.' I've come to think of it as the 'good voice.'"

"Wait. I'm gettin' more o' me notes." Brady left the crucifix on the table and shuffled into a room off the kitchen.

Nick reached slowly across the table for the crucifix.

"Keep it safe. 'Tis mine."

Brady headed back toward the table with a wooden box. Nick withdrew his hand, but his gaze lingered on the crucifix. His cousin slid it toward the center of the table and pulled a small book off the top of the stack in the box, along with a steno pad.

"Father Brennan sketched a crucifix in one of his later journals. He'd lost it and was very upset, as it had been a gift." Brady flipped through the aged pages very carefully. "Here 'tis. His diaries are written in old Gaelic and some Latin, which is why reading them has taken me so many years. I've translated the important things to English in me notes."

Nick stood and walked around the table. His cousin picked up the crucifix again and laid it on the page beside the faded drawing. "All crucifixes are pretty similar," Nick said.

"Aye, but some are very ornate. This one is simple and made of silver, as was Father Brennan's. Furthermore, you found it in what would have been *his* church." Brady translated the words beneath the drawing. "He wrote this in 1792—almost ten years after Sinéad's execution. *'I lost her gift to me today. I have searched everywhere and cannot find it. I failed her in life, and have truly lost her now.'*"

"What does it mean?" Nick asked, a strange sense of despair clawing at him.

"Tell me more about the voices, lad." Brady looked up at Nick. "You said there were two. What does the other one say to you?"

Nick squeezed his eyes shut, his gut twisting. Finally, he opened them and met Brady's worried but curious stare. "It's shouting—always the same words."

"What are they, lad?"

Nick swallowed hard. "Burn, witch . . . burn."

Finn McAdam found the castle easily. Hell, he could see the black tower from miles away. Ballybronagh and *Caisleán* Dubh sat on a spit of land thrusting out into the sea.

And, for some damned reason, it gave him the creeps.

He parked his rental car in the lot overlooking the sea, and removed a silver flask from his jacket pocket. He took a swig, knowing he'd have to replenish his stash soon. After retrieving his bag from the backseat, he climbed out of his car and entered the castle through the front doors.

A gigantic Irishman saw him struggling with the door and his bag and came over to take it from him. "You'll be Mr. Mac Finn, then," he said. "I'm Riley Mulligan. *Céide Milé Fáilte.*"

"A hundred thousand welcomes, as I recall. Thanks for letting me move up my reservation." This place was a hell of a long way from New York. "Interesting place you got here."

"Thanks. Come sign our guest book and I'll show you your room."

This man was no bellboy—definitely the manager or even the owner. Finn followed Mulligan across the expansive lobby or whatever they called it. He scribbled his name in the guest book. "I'll need a room for my, uh, agent, too. He'll be arriving sometime late tonight or tomorrow morning."

Mulligan scratched his head. "Well, we're not quite ready for more guests, but I think we can make do." He pulled out a pad of paper. "What's your agent's name?"

"Angel. Frank Angel."

"Interesting name." Mulligan scribbled it down. "You'll be paying by credit card?"

"I'm strictly the cash type." He pulled out his wallet. "How much deposit do you need?"

Mulligan blinked, grinned, shrugged. "You're our first guest."

Finn rolled his eyes. "Great. Just great." He withdrew a few bills. "Here's five hundred. We'll settle up when I check out, or I'll bring you more if I go over that amount. Deal?"

Mulligan narrowed his eyes and a muscle flinched in his jaw. Finn had no desire to piss off the giant. He just wanted to get to his room and start unraveling this mess before Angelo arrived.

"Sorry. I'm beat," he said.

"'Tis fine then." Mulligan wrote out a receipt and locked the money in a drawer. "I'll show you your room then, Mr. Finn."

As they climbed up the curving staircase that led into the tower, Finn felt the place closing in on him—almost as if he were being watched.

"This floor is family quarters," Mulligan explained as they started up yet another flight. "Guest rooms will all be from the third floor up, and eventually we hope to install an elevator for those in wheelchairs."

As if I give a shit. However, once they moved up to the fourth floor where Finn's room was, the feeling of being watched passed. *Creepy.* The room was filled with antiques, like something out of a travelogue. Mulligan crossed and opened heavy drapes and light streamed through.

"It'll do." He held out a few bucks but Mulligan shook his head. "Suit yourself." Finn shoved the bills into his pocket and walked over to the French doors. "I can see the village from here. Good."

Mulligan opened the doors that led to the balcony. "Aye. To your left there are the church, cemetery, and schoolhouse. Inland from there is the village proper. Gilhooley's Pub is one of the finest in Clare."

Finn pointed at the cottage directly across the meadow. "Whose place is that?"

" 'Tis Mulligan Cottage, where we lived before the castle renovation."

"Anybody live there now?" He turned and met Mulligan's gaze and wished he hadn't asked.

"Aye, but 'tis family only—private."

Save me from this bull. "Someone told me there might be a cottage for sale here. That's why I asked."

Mulligan furrowed his brow for a few seconds and said, "Aye, Donovan Cottage was for sale, but 'tis sold now."

"Donovan. Just curious, but where might it be?" He looked back out the open doors and the giant pointed at the cottage that sat between the schoolhouse and the village. "It's just as well it sold. I'd rather have a view of the sea."

"But . . ." Mulligan shook his head and muttered something, then said, "Enjoy your stay."

After the Irishman left, Finn removed his binoculars and walked out onto the small balcony. He aimed the lenses directly at the cottage Mulligan had said recently sold, assuming it was the one Mrs. O'Shea had purchased. Not wanting to make his host suspicious with too many questions all at once, Finn hadn't asked the buyer's name. Later would do.

As long as he had the information before Angelo arrived.

Maggie watched as Ailish gathered dill, fennel, marjoram, yarrow, and mint. She tied bundles of the herbs with red thread and placed them on the kitchen table. A white candle burned in the center.

Ailish had explained that protection spells were best performed the third hour after sunset and during the waxing moon. The moon was waning now, but they would do one anyway since Maggie was anxious. She made Maggie promise to repeat the steps right after the new moon in the third hour after sunset.

"Also, this is very important to remember. Promise me."

"I promise."

"What's *not* spoken during a spell—emotionally—can be as important and powerful as what is." Ailish drew a deep breath. "Don't let yourself be distracted, darling. Promise."

"I promise."

"Close your eyes now. Breathe deeply, exhale, center yourself." Ailish did the things she'd instructed Maggie. "You remember well."

She touched the bundles with her ritual knife and said, "I charge thee, protective herbs, on this day and in this hour, to be a protection and safeguard against all adversity and evil. Protect well this house and all who dwell within. As I will, so mote it be!"

"So mote it be."

Maggie tingled all over, but waited quietly until Ailish turned to face her.

"We'll hang one bundle of herbs in each room." Ailish handed her the words of the spell, with one slight correction in the wording for when Maggie performed it during the third hour after sunset—the hour of Mars.

After they finished hanging the herbs in every room, Ailish carefully put away her tools. It was late morning on Saturday and Maggie still had lessons to plan for the first day of school on Monday.

"I love being here, and I'll visit again," Ailish said when they returned to the kitchen. "But I think you should have some privacy now."

Maggie swallowed hard. She wasn't afraid to be alone.

Not really. "I'm glad you've come, and I'll hold you to your promise to come again."

"I'd like to go visit the ruins again before I go." She smiled. "With you."

Maggie drew a deep breath and nodded. "'Tis time I faced all the things that have been happening. I think that is where I begin."

Ailish gave Maggie's hand a squeeze. "I think your local historian could have answers, too. Didn't you say Brady was the one who helped Riley unravel the curse?"

The bottom seemed to fall out of Maggie's stomach. "Aye." She swallowed hard and drew a shaky breath. "I'll visit him after the ruins."

"I'll take my bag along and leave from there, if you're sure you don't mind."

"I'll be fine. Thank you for coming, and for the protection spell." Maggie hugged her friend. "Let's go explore some ruins."

"I suspect a certain Yank could be convinced to visit with you this evening," Ailish said as they carried her things to her car.

Maggie's cheeks warmed, but she didn't even pretend to deny her heart. "I love him."

Ailish looked across the roof of her car and held Maggie's gaze. "I know." She laughed and climbed behind the wheel.

Maggie laughed as well as she slid into the passenger side. "You're a good friend, Ailish Delaney."

"The best, and don't be forgetting it." With a grin Ailish started her little car and they drove back around the meadow, past the castle, and rolled to a stop beside the school. "I can see why you always walk."

"Not even time to warm the engine," Maggie said.

"What are some of the specific words you've understood from the voices, Maggie?" Ailish asked as they walked through the graveyard toward the ruins.

"Mostly things that sound like a woman who lost the man she loved. Old-fashioned words about . . . her loins and such." Maggie grinned when Ailish laughed. "Well, 'tis true. I—I call her the 'old one.'"

"Ah. Where have I heard that before?"

"It must be a terrible burden to always be right," Maggie teased.

"Aye, but someone has to do it." Ailish gave her a quick hug. "Jokes aside, I'm *not* always right, love. I make mistakes. But I have to tell you something else I read in your cards."

Maggie didn't speak. She simply waited for Ailish to continue. Her palms turned sweaty and she closed her eyes.

"I couldn't tell if the cards were meant for you, or your protector. The old one."

Maggie narrowed her eyes. "I'm starting to have trouble telling the difference between her words and my thoughts, too. It's . . . scary."

"I told you that she means you no harm."

"You also told me you saw danger."

Ailish nodded. "Two things seemed wrong with the cards I drew—the warning of danger and . . ."

Maggie grabbed Ailish's forearm. "And *what?*"

Her friend sighed and pinned Maggie with her gaze. "Are you and Nick using contraception?"

Maggie's face flamed. "All but once."

Ailish nodded. "Still, I can't shake the feeling that the card wasn't meant for you, and it was definitely not meant for me unless we're talking immaculate conception."

Maggie managed a smile. "'Twas late in my cycle."

"And aren't there millions of little Catholics running round whose mums said, 'But 'twas late in my cycle?'"

Maggie laughed and hugged her friend again, then pulled back to look into her eyes. "Let's go back to your thoughts about the reading, and I'll let you know when I know about . . ."

"Any new little Catholics?" Ailish grinned. "'Tis teasing I am, love. Sorry."

"In my second dream—the one you called a vision—
they made love on the porch."

Ailish's eyes widened. "Truly? So this could follow the
fertility message in my reading."

"Aye." Maggie sighed and they started walking again,
slowly. "The problem is, I don't know who *they* are."

"I think, somehow, you do." Ailish's expression was
filled with certainty. "The porch and front wall of the cottage are older than the rest."

"And that's where both my weird, sexual dreams have
occurred."

"You've only had two? Ever?" Ailish laughed when
Maggie punched her in the arm.

"Now, seriously, have you understood any other things
the old one has said to you?"

"Once. Here." Dizziness swept through Maggie and she
stopped halfway across the graveyard. "She said, 'Rejoin
the accurst.' Does that make sense?"

Ailish stopped and grabbed Maggie's forearm. "Are
you sure? Be very sure."

"I . . . I think so. Why?"

"Since we first met, I've felt you're an old soul." Ailish
gave her a sheepish grin. "Bear with me. I know you're
still learning to believe some of what I accept as truth."

"That's one way of putting it." And wasn't Maggie be-
lieving more and more these days? "An old soul?"

"Aye. Wise beyond your years, as you've lived many
lives and retained some of that wisdom from each of your
past lives."

"Then why can't I cook?" Maggie gave a nervous
laugh, but Ailish wasn't laughing.

"I'm afraid of water, because I drowned in an earlier
life. Some are afraid of heights because they fell to their
deaths in earlier lives. Obviously you weren't a good cook
in at least one of yours."

"I guess that makes sense. I've always wondered if it's
because of my fear of fire." She thought back to the read-

ing again, and she asked the question she had to ask. "You said the voice I hear is my own. What did you mean?"

That I am Sinéad?

"That's the part I think you know in your heart," Ailish said very gently.

Maggie squeezed her eyes shut and nodded. "Aye. But how can I accept that in another life I may have . . . cursed my own family?"

Ailish took Maggie's hand. "No one is perfect in any life, darling."

"True." Maggie drew a deep breath. "I don't think Sinéad ever married or had children."

"Be sure. I think she did, based on my reading," Ailish said while chewing her lower lip. "Ask Mr. Rearden."

"I will." She pointed toward the open area between the ruins and the cemetery. "Once when I was a lass attending school here, I looked over there and saw something no one else could see."

"What was it?"

Maggie's throat constricted, and the panic threatened. She drew several deep breaths until she felt some control return. "A column of fire."

Ailish remained silent for several seconds. When she met Maggie's gaze, her expression was grim. "'Tis very likely that the old one was executed at the church."

"I know." More and more, Maggie knew and didn't like it.

"You're starting to understand, I think," Ailish said gently.

Maggie sighed. "I wonder if Sinéad could cook."

Ailish laughed. "Let's go play on a ley line."

Maggie froze. "I—I think I'm afraid."

"Don't be." They passed through the gate to the ruins and Ailish again seemed transfixed, as if some great power flowed here.

Maggie paused beside her friend and looked toward the stone area where she'd seen the couple during her last visit. She felt older now. Wiser? Certainly more weary.

"Close your eyes, Maggie," Ailish whispered. "Feel the pulsing of the earth beneath our feet. Allow it to flow through your body, to your center. Breathe deep. Don't fear it—welcome it."

Maggie closed her eyes and she *did* feel something. It reverberated through her body—a pulsing cadence that seemed to climb from the earth, through the soles of her shoes, to flow with her blood.

"What is it?" she whispered.

"We don't need a divining rod here." Ailish laughed. "I felt it at the castle, and also at your cottage." She looked up quickly and met Maggie's gaze. "Don't let it frighten you. 'Tisn't evil."

Maggie wasn't so certain. "Something is."

"People can be evil, Maggie." Ailish walked toward the crumbled stones. "And sometimes those evil souls live again and are just as evil. Or worse."

"Do not let him go. Love him. Keep him."

Maggie didn't struggle against the voice this time. "She's talking to me again."

"Good. Listen. Tell me what she's saying." Ailish led Maggie into the center of the crumbled stones, where they'd seen the couple yesterday. "What do you feel here?"

Maggie's heart stumbled, and she swayed. "Anger."

"She said, 'I gave ye me love and ye betrayed me for piety.'" Maggie looked around, half expecting—even hoping—to see the woman whose voice filled her head. "I've heard her use the word *piety* more than once."

"Interesting." Ailish led Maggie across the stones and back onto the grass. "It looks like this may have been a doorway."

Maggie froze, listening, then repeated the words for Ailish. "'I do not care how many lives I suffer for this, if indeed I do.'"

"Oh, that's *good.*" Ailish led Maggie a few steps farther. "Anything else?"

Maggie couldn't breathe. Her throat burned; her eyes

stung. She nodded. "'Ye took me virginity when it was offered . . .'"

"Definitely a woman scorned," Ailish whispered.

"'Now leave me with me dignity in the end. 'Tis done. Let it be.'"

Maggie fell to her knees as a great sadness welled within her. "My God," she whispered. "Is she talking about . . . Nick?"

Ailish stooped beside her. "No, Maggie." She took Maggie's hand and pulled her to her feet again. "'Tis about Sinéad and her lover."

"Why am I hearing it *now*?" Tears seared Maggie's eyes, nose, throat. "I've lived here all my life and never heard her or the angry chanting until I came home from university. Why?"

"Angry chanting?"

"It sounds like many voices raised in anger. They chant the same three words over and over, though I can't understand them."

"Interesting." Ailish appeared thoughtful and led Maggie back through the gate and the graveyard until they stood together outside the schoolhouse. "I *think* 'tis because your life has reached a point where it parallels hers to a certain extent, if that makes sense."

Maggie chewed her lower lip and drew slow, deep breaths. "It does. What she's said to me seems to relate, somehow, to . . . Nick. And me. Even to . . . to . . ."

"Sex?"

Maggie managed a laugh and mopped her tears with her sleeve. "Thank you, Ailish. You've helped me." She hugged her friend. "'Tis sad I am to see you go."

"I know, but I sense you need your Yank more than you need me right now." Ailish pulled back and patted Maggie's cheek. "Don't fear this. I don't feel evil."

"What about . . . the curse, Ailish?" Maggie felt weak from having finally said the words aloud. "Does what's happening to me have anything to do with the curse?"

"I can't say it doesn't," Ailish said in her practical way.

"Ask Brady for the words to the spell and e-mail them to me. Let me know if anything else disturbs you."

At Ailish's car, they said their good-byes and Maggie watched her dearest friend drive away. Exhausted, she went into the school and washed her face. That restored her some, and she decided to walk to Brady's now, then return to her paperwork.

Brady's cottage wasn't far, but she had to pass Donovan Cottage along the way. The need to see Nick stole through her, but she kept walking. She would ring him up later and invite him to dinner this evening. Ailish was right. Maggie needed her Yank right now.

The thought of lying in his arms again warmed her, and she walked faster and felt more alive than she had all day. By the time she knocked on Brady's front door, she felt happy and more like herself.

Of course, she realized, she was also much farther from the ley lines. The thought gave her pause, but she had heard the old one's voice in various places. At least the chanting had yet to follow her this far from the ruins. She drew a deep breath and squared her shoulders as the door opened.

The man who stood there was much taller and younger than Brady Rearden. "Nick?"

"Maggie?"

"I think you two know each other," Brady teased from behind Nick. "Come in, Maggie. Come in."

"I just answered while Brady was getting some more notes," Nick explained as they walked through to the kitchen.

The men had obviously been busy. "What's all this?" she asked, indicating the books and papers strewn across the table.

"Research," Brady said, obviously doing what he loved most. "Sit, lass. Have a cup. 'Tis still warm." He pushed the pot toward her and she grabbed a cup and saucer from the cupboard before sitting as close to Nick as possible without crawling into his lap.

The memory of having her legs wrapped around him in the shower made her cheeks burn. Her hand trembled as she poured *very* strong tea into her cup. She wanted Nick again. Inside her. Beside her. Tonight.

Always.

Her heart stuttered and she felt him reach for her hand. Eagerly, she linked her fingers with his and met his gaze. *I love you.* Tonight, she would tell him and pray the truth wouldn't frighten him away.

She used her free hand to add lots of milk to the inky tea and took a sip. Brady made dreadful tea.

"Awful, isn't it?" Nick whispered in her ear.

"Where's your friend from university?" Brady asked, peering over the rim of his reading glasses.

"Ailish had to go home today." She gave Nick's hand a squeeze and leaned over to whisper in his ear, "Dinner?"

"Mmm."

Brady was busy leafing through pages. Nick leaned down and whispered, "Dessert."

"Ah, here's the part I was lookin' for." Brady slid the diary toward Nick along with a page of notes. "Not all of this is legible, but what I *was* able to translate is enough to make me wonder if Father Brennan was in love before he joined the priesthood. Read it, lad. Tell me if it has anything to do with what—"

Nick cleared his throat loudly. Brady looked up and blushed to his ears. "Sorry, lad." He flashed his cousin a sheepish grin.

Confused, Maggie sensed secrets were being kept. More secrets. Her gaze fell on something silver on the tabletop. She reached toward it, her hand trembling. "What's this?"

She barely touched it with her fingertip and a flash of reclamation soared through her.

"A pledge of me love and devotion. Me promise to love him always. And something more . . ."

Eighteen

Nick's vision blurred as he watched Maggie reach for the crucifix.

"'Twas a gift."

He shook his head and focused. She pulled her hand away from the silver crucifix after barely touching it and closed her fist around air. She met his gaze, and he saw great sadness there; it echoed through his own heart. He couldn't breathe, and his throat burned.

Brady rose, oblivious to the undercurrents swirling between Nick and Maggie. "I just thought of somethin' else. I'll be right back." He disappeared again into the room he called his office.

Nick placed his hands on both sides of Maggie's face and kissed her, breathed in her spicy scent, savored the taste and feel of her. "Invite me to dinner again," he murmured against her mouth. "Say yes."

"Yes. Aye." She kissed him, tracing the line of his lips with her tongue, driving him wild. "I'll kill you if you don't come to see me."

Nick grinned, concentrating on this woman rather than that hunk of silver on the table. "I think Ailish figured out we want to be alone."

Maggie nodded. "Didn't she say as much as she was leaving?"

"She's a good friend."

"The best."

They kissed again, tongues mating, giving and taking. Heat unfurled through Nick, setting every inch of him into expectant mode. "I'm not sure I can wait," he whispered and kissed her again.

Brady cleared his throat from across the room. Nick and Maggie both looked and saw a red-faced Brady hesitating. Obviously, he'd seen them.

"So . . . 'tis that way between you," he said with a smile as he returned to the table. "A handsome couple if ever I saw one."

"Thanks." Nick took Maggie's hand again beneath the table. He saw them as a couple now. A few days ago he couldn't have imagined feeling this way, and now he couldn't imagine it *not* being this way.

He still had a job to do. Would she wait for him? He remembered how she'd given herself to him, and he prayed she would wait. A future with Maggie? The thought terrified him even as it gave him hope.

This beaten failure of a cop might actually have a life after death—so to speak. He shook himself and dragged his attention back to the present. "I should get back to Aunt Mo and Erin for now." He stared at the crucifix.

"I'll keep lookin' for more information about your discovery, young Nick." Brady picked up the hunk of silver and looked at it, then directed his gaze at Nick. "I'll let you know if I find anythin'. I will say that my instincts about Father Brennan have been pretty accurate until now. My gut says this belonged to him, that he lost it, and that Sinéad gave it to him."

"Why . . . would a witch give someone a crucifix?" Nick asked. "Or am I being ignorant?"

"You are being ignorant." Brady chuckled quietly. "Many pagans are also Christians, and vice versa, I might add. This was particularly true in times past, though often the pagan part was kept secret from the Church."

Nick nodded, not wanting Maggie to know the whole story just yet. Maybe someday he'd tell her about his momentary insanity—or whatever it was—but not now.

He reached toward the crucifix and took it from his cousin's outstretched hand. It pulsed in his grasp.

"Mine. Do not lose it again. 'Tis mine."

He rose and put it into his pocket. A sigh of relief rippled through him. He'd missed the feel of it.

Bilbo Baggins, move over.

He looked at Maggie then, saw concern in her eyes. She obviously sensed something. The light in her eyes changed from blue to orange to red, and suddenly all Nick saw were flames.

He didn't scream. He couldn't. But he knew what he had to do. He looked away from the woman he loved, shoved his hand into his pocket and pulled the damned crucifix from his pocket. He held it out toward Brady.

"You keep this for me, please," he said, his voice sounding strained. "Until we figure out where it came from."

Brady stood, his eyes wide and filled with questions. "As you wish, lad." The old man placed it in the wooden box where he kept the diaries. "'Twill be safe here."

Turning away from it was pure torture, but Nick had to do it. He was stronger than that hunk of metal. He looked down at Maggie and forced a smile. "What time is dinner?"

"Six?"

"How about five?" he asked.

Brady chuckled. "Don't you two make me feel young again? I think I'll call on Maureen again this evening."

"She'd like that," Nick said. He bent down and kissed Maggie on the cheek. "I'll see you at five."

He left Brady's cottage and the crucifix as fast as he possibly could. Outside, he paced in the yard, feeling the absence of the crucifix as if it had been cut from his heart. He almost went back inside to retrieve it. Almost.

Instead, he ran all the way to Donovan Cottage.

Maggie waited until she heard the front door close. "Brady?"

"Aye, lass?"

"M—may I see the crucifix again, please?"

A curious expression crossed the old man's face, but he reached into the box and withdrew it, then placed it gently in her open palm.

"'Tis me gift to him. Me pledge. Me trust."

"So you believe this belonged to Father Brennan?" She met the old man's gaze. "Why?"

"He mentioned it in his diaries, and Nick found it in the ruins of the old church." Brady adjusted his glasses on the bridge of his nose and looked through the pages until he found the passage. "Ah, here 'tis. He lamented the loss of his crucifix. 'My silver crucifix is gone. 'Twas a gift from someone I loved and who loved me as no one else ever has.' "

"Me gift to him."

Maggie swallowed hard. "Do you . . . know who gave it to him? Who loved him?"

Brady set his mouth in a thin line. "I don't want your mum angry at me, but you heard what I said last night about Father Brennan's feelings for Sinéad."

Ailish had spoken of power, of past lives, of wisdom. Sinéad. That was the truth Maggie had skirted around all these weeks.

"He loved piety and tradition more than me."

Aye, Sinéad had loved Father Fergus Brennan. Maggie turned the crucifix over in her hand, afraid to ask, but knowing she had to. "Could you read the curse to me, Brady? Riley told me you have it."

"Aye." Brady enthusiastically placed the diary he'd been reading into the box and withdrew another. "Here 'tis, all nicely translated."

Maggie closed her hand around the crucifix and listened, determined to keep her mind and heart open to the truth. Whatever it was.

> *A darksome curse on them that walke these halls*
> *May they finde only death and miserie.*
> *No joying be withstood within these walls*
> *Much daunted by sore sad despaire they be!*
> *Until that cruell, disdayned destinie*
> *Beguile them torne asunder with her power,*
> *Rejoin the accurst for all eternity with*
> *her so fierce bewronged within this*
> *tower and ende this spelle, forever, in*
> *that blessed hour!*

The words reverberated through Maggie. She knew them. *Mother Mary help me.* She knew those wretched words.

She spoke softly after Brady finished. "Sinéad stood on the boulders at the base of *Caisleán* Dubh, round back, I think." Maggie closed her eyes, knowing Brady listened intently. "Sinéad felt the cold wind against her face. Rain pelted her yet she climbed higher. She'd written the spell carefully so she wouldn't forget a word. 'Twas night—"

"Lass . . . ?" Brady reached over and touched her hand. "Tell me how you know this. How you see it."

Maggie blinked and met his worried expression. "I— I'm not sure."

"Is there more?"

She reached upward. "Sinéad reached toward the sky. Lightning flashed and thunder shook the earth. She spoke the words of her spell, then . . ." Maggie opened her palm and stared at the crucifix. "Then *he* came and dragged her from the boulders."

"Father Brennan?" Brady was taking notes now.

Maggie smiled at the dear man. "I . . . think so." Now only one thing frightened her. "Brady, is my family safe? Is the curse really broken?"

"Of course. Bridget and Riley fulfilled what Sinéad sought to accomplish." Brady shook his head and sighed. "I know she did what she did out of love for her niece, but 'twas still wrong. Many Mulligans suffered because of it."

Maggie nodded, her chest tight and her eyes burning. "Bronagh and Aidan were reunited through reincarnation."

"Aye." Brady crossed himself and gave her a sheepish smile. "I'm feelin' the need to go to confession again, lass."

Maggie had to laugh. "You're not the only one, Brady." She drew a steadying breath. "Sinéad did what she thought she had to do. Father Brennan tried to stop her, but he was too late." She thought of the ley lines and wished, suddenly, that Ailish were here so she could ask her.

"Do you know what ley lines are, Brady?"

"Aye." He removed his glasses. "I've studied things of that nature since discovering the origins of the curse. You might say I've broadened my mind a great deal." He smiled again.

"Ailish believes the old church ruins, *Caisleán* Dubh, and my cottage are connected by ley lines."

Brady shrugged. " 'Tis possible. Why?"

"I've . . . been hearing voices."

Brady's eyes widened. "You, too?"

"Not like the ones Riley and Bridget heard," Maggie said quickly, still holding the crucifix. "Well, I hear one set of voices that sounds like angry chanting. The other voice belongs to an old woman, and I think she's speaking directly *to* me."

Obviously taken aback, Brady straightened. "Lass, do you think . . . ?"

"Sinéad." She squeezed her eyes shut for a few seconds, then met Brady's solemn gaze. "I have to make certain my family is safe. Could Sinéad's spell have traveled along the ley lines? Could it have spread to others? Perhaps even . . . ." Maggie turned the crucifix over in her palm.

"Even what, lass?"

"To herself?"

Brady sighed. "I'm not an expert on these matters, lass. I'm merely an old teacher turned historian and writer." He shrugged and shook his head. "Tell me this: Do *you* believe the voice speakin' to you belongs to Sinéad?"

Tears spilled from the corners of Maggie's eyes and she nodded. "I do." She held the crucifix up to the light shining through the back window. "God help me."

"Me gift to him. Me love . . ."

"Ask yourself another question. Do you think she means you harm, lass?"

Maggie remembered Ailish's words about the old one wanting to help Maggie—to save her from a "similar fate." Sinéad had lived her life alone: her niece dead, her lover—if Brady was right—married to his church.

Maggie didn't want to be alone.

"Jaysus, Mary, and Joseph."

"What is it, lass?"

"I . . ." She shook her head, trying to gather her thoughts. "She wants to protect me. She means me no harm."

"There you have it then." Brady steepled his fingers beneath his chin. "Her dream of giving Bronagh a second chance to wed Aidan has come to pass, after a fashion, so her mission was fulfilled. Her goal met."

"Aye."

"So why would she mean anyone harm? Not that we should forget all the Mulligans who perished because of her spell, of course." Brady crossed himself again.

"Of course."

He smiled sadly. "The British landlord was a zealot who felt it his duty to see Sinéad burn."

Maggie cringed and swallowed hard. "Why is she talking to *me*, Brady?" She shook her head, totally baffled. "*I'm* a Mulligan!"

"I wish I knew the answer, Maggie." He reached over and patted her hand, touching the crucifix. " 'Twas very sad," Brady continued, watching her very closely. "Are you thinkin' what I am about this?"

Maggie smiled. "That Sinéad gave the crucifix to Father Brennan, and that was why it was so important to him?"

"Do me a favor, lass?"

"Return this when you see Nick for dinner." Brady looked down for a moment, then met her gaze. She saw uncertainty and hope shining there. " 'Tis important, I think."

"Me gift to him. Me pledge. And something more . . ."

"I will. I—I need to get some work done this afternoon. Thanks for your time, Brady."

He stood and accompanied her to the front door. "Do let me know if you learn anythin' more," he said. "I'll do the same."

"Aye. Thank you." She walked out and closed the door behind her. It was time for Maggie to face all her demons.

Sinéad was speaking to her for a reason. Was it merely because Maggie lived in her home? Ailish had said the voice Maggie heard was her own.

Mother Mary . . . am I Sinéad?

Brady watched her walk away and shook his head. He rushed back to the notes left on his kitchen table and remembered the day he and Riley determined that he had been Aidan Mulligan in an earlier life, and that dear Bridget had been Bronagh. That had worked out well. Very well.

Riley had heard the whispering of *Caisleán* Dubh.

Bridget had heard the whispering of *Caisleán* Dubh.

They'd fallen in love before they recognized their past lives.

And now . . . He crossed himself again and shook his head. " 'Tis madness. More madness."

Nick had heard a voice about duty, and fate led him to Father Brennan's lost crucifix. Brady already suspected there had been more between the priest and the *cailleach* than anyone realized.

And sweet Maggie was hearing a voice that made Brady wonder if Ballybronagh was due another miracle.

He put away his diaries and notes, donned his jacket and cap, then did what any good Irish Catholic should do under such circumstances.

He went to confession.

Nick spent the afternoon trying *not* to reach into his pocket in search of his prize. He'd lost it. No, he'd given it to Brady. He shook himself and focused on the evening ahead.

After ensuring that Aunt Mo wouldn't need him this evening, he made her promise to arm the security system even while Brady was there, and not to open the door to him without looking first. She laughed and told him to go to Maggie and have a wonderful time.

He intended to do just that.

He stopped at the market and bought a bottle of wine, a jar of Nutella, and flowers. No fancy roses for his Maggie. He bought her a mix of wildflowers—fresh, bright, happy flowers. Then he walked back past Donovan Cottage and the schoolhouse, amazed that he heard no voices, saw no vanishing couples on the cliff. All he saw was the tower of *Caisleán* Dubh spiraling upward into a partly cloudy sky.

Yes, leaving the crucifix with Brady had been the right thing. So why did he feel so lost without it? With a sigh he focused on the road ahead of him and kept walking.

As he passed the castle, he decided not finding Riley there guarding the way was a good omen. Since it was only late afternoon, Nick cut across the meadow where a huge black horse grazed.

"Nice horsy," he said, just in case.

The beast glanced up at him, snorted once, then returned to his dinner.

Nick kept walking. It wasn't like the horse was a bull

that would charge or anything. He glanced back over his shoulder. Was it? Besides, he was wearing blue—not red.

He looked ahead and saw Maggie's cottage. His heart broke into a sprint. *Maggie.* "You are in deep shit, Desmond." The thought made him smile. "Bring on the shit," he muttered.

As he neared Maggie's kitchen door, he remembered two things. First of all, she couldn't cook. That made him grin again. Secondly, he'd stopped thinking about the damned crucifix.

Okay, so maybe thinking *damned* before *crucifix* was a sin. He glanced upward. "Sorry." He didn't want to offend anyone. Not God. Not Riley Mulligan. And not anyone who might have lived before them.

He drew a deep breath and kept walking. Tonight, he would hear no voices. A beautiful woman waited just a dozen or so feet ahead, and the sun shone on his back.

What could be better?

He stopped. Confused. He turned and stared back toward the castle. What the hell had happened to him? He had a job, a mission, revenge to seek. What was with this happy-go-lucky bullshit?

"Desmond, get a grip," he muttered. The horse nickered way too close to his shoulder. He glanced warily back at the huge beast. "You following me?"

The horse nodded. Really, it did. "Why?"

It snorted and pawed the ground, nodding again. "Nice horsy."

Nick jogged the rest of the way, proud of himself for only glancing back twice to see how close the big black horse really was. It had stopped to graze again. *Smart horse.* He grinned and bounded up onto the stoop at Maggie's back door.

Still grinning like a fool, he knocked. He heard footsteps heading toward the door. He drew a deep breath as they neared. The door swung open quickly.

And he stared into the grinning face of Riley Mulligan. "Shit."

Nineteen

Maggie hadn't planned on walking into her cottage to find a flood on her kitchen floor, but at least that had redirected her thoughts to practical matters instead of voices and curses and . . . other unexplained phenomena.

She found the leak under the sink and tried to fix it herself, but realized she didn't have the proper tools or the expertise. Reluctantly, she surrendered and did the only thing she could do under the circumstances. It galled her to admit defeat—and hadn't she managed to at least turn off the water by herself?—but she called her nearest male relative.

Now the leak was fixed and her brother seemed to tarry as he collected his tools and prepared to go home. "Well, I know you're eager to get home to Bridget." She urged Riley to leave. Nick would arrive at any moment.

"Aye." Riley wiped off a wrench and placed it in the wooden box he always kept handy. It held most things needed for emergency repairs. "That should hold you for a while. If it starts to leak again, give a yell."

A knock sounded on the kitchen door. She glanced at the clock. It had to be Nick. She wasn't expecting anyone else and it was two minutes before five. She sighed.

Brothers were placed on this earth for the express purpose of fixing leaky faucets and torturing their sisters. What other reasons could there be, since she rushed to the back door, but he beat her there? She covered her face as he swung it open with a nasty smile on his face. She hadn't even had time to get prettied up for Nick.

Not that Riley would appreciate that argument, if she'd expressed it. For that matter, how had Riley known it was Nick at the door? Big brother's intuition?

There stood Nick—handsome, sweet, smiling Nick—a bouquet of flowers in one hand and a shopping bag in the other.

And her big, sweet, hulk of a brother to greet him.

Maggie groaned.

Nick sighed.

Riley guffawed.

"Nick." She ducked under Riley's arm. "'Twas good of you to come for dinner." She took the flowers he extended, though his gaze shot questioningly to the human mountain standing behind her. "I had a leak under the sink. Wasn't Riley good enough to come fix it for me?"

"That's nice," Nick said on another sigh.

"Thank you, Riley." She placed the wooden toolbox in her brother's paw. "Do give Bridget and Mum my love."

He nodded, then turned his usual scowl on poor Nick. "Desmond," he said.

"Mulligan," Nick returned, his eyes questioning as he met Maggie's gaze.

Helplessly, she did nothing but shrug. What was a woman to do with dueling testosterone thrashing about?

"Tell Mum I'll come by tomorrow." Maggie barely resisted the urge to give her brother a nice, swift kick in the seat of his breeches.

Riley glanced back over his shoulder, his eyes hooded, brows drawn together. "Aye." He took a step out the door, all but filling it. Maggie shifted to the side to give him room. "Have a care," he said to Nick as he finally—thank the Virgin—walked out the door and across the meadow.

"Sheesh." Nick glanced back over his shoulder at Riley's departing backside. "Stubborn cuss."

"Aye, but he's a good, loving brother."

Nick flashed her a sheepish grin. "I can't argue with that. I like the idea of you having someone else looking after you when I'm not around."

Maggie didn't like the sound of him not being around. "You're here now." She forced a smile. "I'm afraid the leaky faucet and Riley's interminable presence have delayed dinner."

"My appetite is on other things." Nick stepped inside and kicked the door closed behind him. "I brought wine and . . . dessert."

Her eyes widened and her face suffused with heat, remembering his reference earlier today about dessert. "Oh," she squeaked and locked the back door—something she never did. In fact, she'd already locked the front. A smile curved her lips.

"I planned to cook." She folded her arms and released a sigh.

"Oh." He sounded underenthusiastic at best. "Why don't *I* cook instead?"

Maggie smiled and stepped closer to him, pressing herself wantonly against him. "I think you cook quite nicely, Nick Desmond."

He actually blushed, and the realization that she—Maggie Mulligan—had made this gorgeous man blush made her laugh with delight.

"You put the flowers in water, and I'll make omelets." He placed his grocery bag on the table and pulled out a bottle of red wine. "I think this needs to breathe or something. My experience is mostly with Budweiser."

Maggie smiled. "Omelets sound nice," she said. "I'll open this and . . ." She felt her cheeks warm. "And I'll slip into something more comfortable."

Nick looked over his shoulder and said, "Okay." His voice sounded a bit high-pitched as his gaze drifted down the length of her.

Maggie smiled self-consciously and dashed up the stairs. She'd planned, after all, to make herself beautiful before he arrived. Fate had other plans. Well, wouldn't she just make up for that now?

She took a quick shower and put on lotion and the scented oil Ailish had given her. It smelled exotic and sexy—everything Maggie wasn't. She brushed her hair until it shone, billowing in deep russet waves that fell to her waist. She applied powder and lipstick, and slipped on the deep bronze silk wraparound shift Ailish had given her.

The silk slid across her skin. She'd never felt anything quite like it, especially since she wore nothing beneath it. She glanced in the mirror and drew a deep breath, her nipples clearly outlined beneath the tissue-thin fabric.

Decadent. Nick would love it. Confident of that, she walked back downstairs to the aroma of onions and peppers. A man who cooked for a woman definitely had his merits.

She peered around the corner. The table was set with the flowers, the wine, and plates heaped with omelets dripping with cheese. All served by a sexy hunk of man.

Life could be worse.

Maggie needed this total abandonment. Later, she would think about the voices and Sinéad. Father Brennan. The crucifix she would return to Nick. All those things could wait. *She* could not.

Her body vibrated with her need for this man who cooked and cared for her. He cast her an adorable grin as she approached the table.

His eyes grew wide and his mouth fell open. "Wow," he said. "You look . . ."

Maggie swallowed hard. "What?"

"Gorgeous." He took three long steps and slid his hands around her waist. "I like this slippery stuff." He eased his hands along her hips and back up to the sides of her breasts. "I'm a dead man."

She frowned. "Have I done something wrong?"

"You're naked under there."

Heat and shame washed through Maggie. "Aye." She lowered her guilty gaze and turned away. "I'll go dress."

Nick grabbed her hand and pulled her against him, her breasts flattening against his chest. "Don't you dare." He covered her mouth with his, pulling her up and against him. He cupped her bottom with his hands and moaned into the kiss.

She buried her trembling fingers in his hair and pressed her hips against the growing, throbbing heat of him. She wanted him inside her again so much she could barely stand it.

"I had him once before he betrayed me heart."

No, she wouldn't listen. Nick would never betray her. She pulled back slightly, breaking their kiss. "Food?"

He kept his forehead against hers as he slowly allowed her silk-clad body to slide until her bare feet were on the floor again. "Food." He kissed her quickly, then escorted her to a chair, seated her, and placed the napkin on her lap.

His hand brushed against her nipple as he withdrew. A delicious shiver shimmered through her and she looked up into his eyes. Her love for him swelled within her and she almost blurted out the words, but kept them within her heart for now. Later tonight, she *would* tell him.

He took the chair next to hers and took a bite of his omelet. She liked watching him eat. A dark curl fell across his forehead, making her itch to push it back and so much more.

She glanced at the clock on the wall. Six o'clock. They had hours together before he would have to leave. The thought of her brother watching through a tower window for her lover to pass by on his way home made her grin.

"What is it?" Nick asked.

"I was just thinking about Riley watching for you to walk home later."

"He will. Won't he?" Nick's expression grew solemn.

"Since I intend to be very busy this evening, and very distracted, I'll set the alarm on my watch for eleven, just in case. I want to make sure Riley sees me walking home."

Maggie laughed as she watched him push a few buttons on his watch. "Thank you," she murmured, deciding not to mention that she had already set the alarm clock in her room as well.

He looked up and smiled. "Eat." His voice sounded rough and his eyes darkened. "You'll need your strength."

She drew a deep breath and tried to think of intelligent conversation. Her brain seemed to have disengaged itself in lieu of her libido. *Come on, Mary Margaret.* "School starts Monday. I guess we should stop there tomorrow and make sure nothing needs to be repaired before classes begin."

"Good idea." His eyes twinkled as if he understood that she was trying to stall. "I've never actually done handyman work, you know."

"Really?" Maggie laughed. "I guess your aunt wants to keep you busy."

He looked away long enough to make her realize he was being secretive again. She took another sip of wine, determined not to be nosey.

"Your brother and most of the villagers probably think I'm a bum."

His words surprised her, but didn't she have enough experience with brothers to recognize wounded male pride when she saw it? "Have you . . ." She bit her lower lip, remembering how he'd tensed up when they discussed Guard Bailey at Gilhooley's. Still, she wanted Nick to be happy here in Ballybronagh, and that meant doing something that made him feel worthwhile. Right? "Maybe you should talk to Guard Bailey."

He looked up sharply, his eyes narrowed. "I thought that was a *family* business."

Now she'd made him defensive. She reached over and covered his hand. "So it has been, but Guard Bailey and his wife never had any children." When he looked up, she added, "He's the last."

Nick's Adam's apple traveled the length of his throat, and the emotions playing through his eyes showed a deep sadness. Loss. And longing.

Someday he would tell her what had hurt him so. Someday he would share all his secrets.

"Dinner is delicious. Perfect." She drank deeply from her glass. "Everything . . ."

"Delicious." The expression in Nick's eyes was deadly.

A hot rush shot through her, settling relentlessly low. She resisted the urge to squirm in her chair as she took a bite, then another, barely tasting the food. Her mind, her body, and her heart were more concerned with other matters.

Her breasts felt heavy and swollen, her nipples stimulated by the slippery silk. She was so ready for Nick she could barely swallow the last few bites. Finally, she looked up and saw him watching her, his plate empty. He took a sip of the dark red wine, his eyes hooded as he stared at her over the rim of his glass.

"Mmm." Nick stood and collected their dishes. She started to push away to help, but he said, "Sit."

Maggie smiled and obeyed, enjoying the play of his muscles beneath his lightweight shirt as he worked. Soon, only their wineglasses sat on the long, scarred table.

Nick closed the curtains on the window beside the back door, and the one over the sink. She looked at him curiously and drained her glass, which he immediately took to the counter along with his. He reached into the grocery bag he'd brought along and pulled out a jar of Nutella.

"Oh, I have some ice cream for that." She pushed away from the table and stood.

He slid his hand around behind her and set the jar on the table, along with a handful of square, cellophane packets. Condoms. Before she drew her next breath, she found her body flush against his. The look in his eyes made her dizzy.

"What?" Her voice was little more than a strangled whisper as desire spiraled through her.

He reached down and untied her sash and the slippery silk slid down her back and to the floor. "I've dreamed about doing this."

She licked her lips and unbuttoned his shirt. "You mean the k—kitchen?" As she exposed his chest, she rubbed her hands against it, loving the roughness of the curling hair.

"About having *you* in the kitchen." He kissed her mouth, her cheek, her jaw, nuzzled the lobe of her ear. "About having you for dessert."

Maggie giggled. His hot breath against her ear tickled in delicious, decadent ways. A tremor rippled through her as she eased his shirt from his powerful shoulders and reached down to unbuckle his belt.

He stroked her bare back with long, sensuous strokes while she unbuttoned the snug fly of his jeans. Soon, she had it open and pressed her hands against his heat.

He growled and kicked off his runners, then shoved his jeans down and away. He dipped his head and drew her nipple into his mouth.

"Ah." Maggie linked her hands behind his neck. It hadn't been a dream. This felt every bit as good as she remembered. "Nick."

"Mmm." He scooped her up into his arms, but instead of heading for the too-narrow stairs, he sat her bare bottom on the table.

"Wha—"

He smothered her question with a kiss and eased himself between her thighs. This was an interesting position. She wrapped her legs around him and pulled him closer, then remembered his briefs were still in the way. She pushed them downward until he impatiently finished the job for her.

When he stepped between her open legs again, the heat of him made her clench around the void he would soon fill. He reached behind her, his chest hairs rubbing against her sensitive nipples.

"I took him within me once, and carried the memory with me always."

Maggie squeezed her eyes shut. She had already taken Nick within her more than once, and she intended to keep doing it. The wicked thought made her smile as she felt him fumbling with something behind her back. He was probably opening the condom now. Soon he would fill her again. Her body wept in anticipation.

She heard a pop and an odd vacuumlike sound. A moment later, Nick's hands were on her breasts, but something felt . . . different. She looked down and found him spreading the sweet, sticky Nutella across her bare skin.

Her eyes widened as she realized what he had in mind. Before she could draw another breath, he pressed her back onto the table and slowly, torturously, savored his dessert with enough enthusiasm to almost kill her.

"Mmm." He moaned and drew her nipple deeply into his mouth, then the other.

"I want you," she whispered, her hips leaving the surface of the table in search of what her body craved. Him. Only him. Always him.

Through a haze of desire, she watched him scoop another handful of gooey, hazelnut-flavored chocolate, but instead of covering her breasts, he deposited it between her legs. Maggie's eyes widened. "What—"

He looked at her through hooded eyes, his expression intense. Carefully, deliberately, he sat in a chair and draped her legs over his shoulders, then feasted on her.

This was . . . obscene. She'd never . . . Oh, that felt good. Her shock gave way immediately to pleasure so profound she couldn't breathe. She twined her fingers through his thick, wavy hair as he devoured her—licking, laving, loving.

"Nick." She whimpered and moaned until the sweet-hot rush of completion rocketed through her. And again. He stood then and moved the jar off the table and tore a condom open with his teeth. She pushed up onto her elbows to watch him roll it down his impressive length. He took a step toward her, and she realized his intent.

He cupped her bottom with his large hands and lifted her up and toward him. She wrapped her legs around his waist and laid back, unable to support her weight any longer. He slid into her in one, smooth stroke.

Instant joy erupted through, rippling to a crescendo of bright star bursts behind her closed eyes. Her body contracted and swallowed his with a voraciousness that left her shuddering and begging for more. Always more. He thrust into her, guiding her fully against him, leaving no room for her to settle back to earth before she soared again.

He gave and gave, and she took hungrily. Through veiled lashes she looked down to where his body entered hers. The intimacy of it was so incredibly *right* with this man. She knew in her heart that no other man would ever take this one's place in her heart or in her body. This was the man she loved—would always love.

With one final thrust he pulsed inside her and the sweetness of completion shimmered through her yet again. She stretched, supremely sated. Gradually she grew aware of the hard table beneath her and looked up at him. The expression in his eyes was everything she'd ever hoped and more.

He loved her. She saw it there as clearly as if he'd spoken the words aloud. Her heart smiled as she sat up slowly to rest her arms across his shoulders. She looked up into his eyes, their noses almost touching.

"I love you, Nick Desmond."

She heard him swallow and he kissed her gently, cupping his Nutella-sticky hands around her face. "I don't deserve you," he whispered. "God help me, but I love you, Maggie Mulligan."

She kissed him and tears of joy trickled down her cheeks. He kissed them away and said, "Shower."

"I love you so much, Nick," she said. "So very much."

"I love you more than anything or anyone ever." He smiled and she knew he spoke the truth. "No matter what happens, please know that."

No matter what happens?

Icy fingers of fear shot through her.

"His love of piety and traditions was stronger than the love he professed for me."

Finn waited until dark, then made his way to Ballynowhere. Endoftheworldville. Boringcity. He didn't take his car so no one would hear him leave or return.

At the outskirts of the village he stopped across the road from Donovan Cottage and watched the windows with his binoculars for several minutes. A few shadows moved past the front window, but no one stood still long enough for him to get a good look.

After tonight Angelo would be here, and Finn needed a drink. His flask was empty. He remembered the pub on the far side of town and shoved his binoculars into his backpack before heading that direction. He'd get ripped tonight, then dry up again starting tomorrow. Angelo would kick his ass if he found out Finn was drinking again.

Thinking about that made him need a drink even more. He'd sit in a quiet corner where no one would notice him. Who the hell would recognize him in a place like Ballybronagh anyway? And, just maybe, he'd find someone willing to talk about the O'Sheas.

He shoved through the door into the smoky, noisy pub and made his way to a table in the main part of the bar, away from any direct lighting. With his back to the wall, he waited until a cute blonde came over to take his order.

"I'm Irene," she said. "What can I get you?"

How about you for starters? She was young, but old enough. "Jameson's," he said. "Double."

He watched her stroll over to the bar and place his order, then she drifted into the back room for a few minutes before collecting his whiskey and returning to his table. "Will you be wanting a tab or pay as you go?"

He handed her some bills. "I'll pay as I go." Just in case he needed to leave in a hurry. "When you get a break, come join me? I'm an author visiting Ballybronagh on a research trip. Maybe you could answer a few questions?"

"An author?" She lifted a shoulder. "Well, why not then? 'Tis the least I can do for a visiting Yank."

Confident he'd found someone willing to talk—hopefully someone who knew something he could actually use—he leaned back to sip his drink. His hand trembled and he drained the whole glass before he returned it to the tabletop.

Irene made rounds again and he ordered another double. She didn't have any reaction at all to his thirst and he smiled. Ireland definitely had its high points. She returned with his drink and he smiled up at her. "Due for that break yet?"

She sat in the empty chair across the table from him. "I can take a few. What do you want to know about Ballybronagh?"

He stuck out his hand. "I'm Mac Finn."

"Pleased to meet you, Mac Finn." She shook his hand. "I'm Irene Gilhooley."

"Ah, you own the place?" He sipped his drink much more slowly this time.

"My brother and I do." She rolled her eyes. "I'm about ready to go back to our parents' villa in Crete, though. Driving me off my nut, my brother is."

"Nice place, Crete." Enough small talk. Finn leaned forward. "I'm looking for a family named O'Shea. Do you know them?"

"Aye." Irene's eyes brightened. "Mrs. O'Shea, her granddaughter, and her good-looking nephew bought Donovan Cottage."

"A nephew?" That part probably blew Angelo's crazy theory out of the water. "How old?"

"Older than me but younger than you." She grinned and glanced over her shoulder at the bartender. "My brother is giving me the eye. I should get back to work."

Finn put his hand on her wrist, but released it very quickly. He didn't want to frighten her. "Just a little more information, so I can try to figure out if they're the O'Sheas involved in this missing child case I'm writing about."

"Missing . . ." Irene pulled her chair in closer. "What missing child?"

"A baby kidnapped over ten years ago from Long Island. Her father is very wealthy. Problem is, though, no one ever asked for a ransom and no trace of the kid was ever found." Finn liked the way the blonde's eyes glowed while he talked. "I have newspaper articles I've been saving, and . . . an anonymous tip brought me here."

" 'Tis incredible." She chewed a fingernail, then aimed it at him. "What do the O'Sheas have to do with this?"

"Nothing possibly. I can't tell you everything about my anonymous tip, of course, but I will show you some of the articles, if you think you might be able to help find the little girl."

"Girl?" Irene sat up straighter. "And you said she was a baby ten years ago?"

Finn nodded. "I'd rather you not mention the case I'm working on for my book to anyone. They might scoop me."

"Ah, I understand."

"What do you know about the family?" He tried to sound casual.

"They seem to have a lot of money, if that means anything. Oh! I do remember something odd. They installed a security system. Can you imagine anyone doing that in Ballybronagh?" She laughed.

"No. I can't." Finn filed that information to give Angelo. "Seems sort of . . . suspicious, really."

She nodded and rested her chin on her fist. "When I first met Mrs. O'Shea—the grandmother—I thought she

Angelo Fazzini had arrived at *Caisleán* Dubh late last night, and he was in a shitty mood. In his archaic room he stared at the small computer screen displaying the digital photos Finn had taken as the villagers left mass that morning.

"There." Finn pointed at the monitor. "He look familiar, boss?"

"Yeah. Why?" Angelo looked for the zoom control in the software and enlarged the photo. "Goddamn cop!" He looked up at Finn, who nodded. "The one who had to be taught a lesson."

"The same. Looks like he forgot what he learned." Finn stood beside the small table in Angelo's room at *Caisleán* Dubh. "He was warned."

"I remember the details." Angelo pulled a roll of antacids out of his pocket and popped two into his mouth.

"You sure are eatin' a lot of those, boss."

Angelo didn't respond. "Desmond. That was it. What the hell is he doing here?"

"I figure someone hired him."

"For what?"

"He's pretending to be O'Shea's nephew, but I figure he's her bodyguard." Finn reached down and opened the next photo. "Tada! Your dear, departed mother."

Angelo couldn't breathe. The top of his head damned near blew off. He tugged viciously at his collar and sent a button flying. "God damn her soul to hell." He stood and paced the room. "Why did she do this?"

She'd asked him to give up his "life of crime" before Erin was born. He hadn't realized how serious she was.

"The old broad was a lot smarter than any of us thought," Finn said. "She must've been planning this for years."

Angelo swallowed the bile rising to his throat and trudged back to the computer. "I want to see Erin." His own mother had *stolen* his child.

"Sure, boss."

looked familiar. I realized later why that was, but I'm sur
it was just coincidence."

"Familiar?"

"My parents subscribe to the Sunday *New York Times*
It's always late since it comes across an ocean to them
but I enjoyed reading the society pages and such."

New York. Finn's interest went into overdrive. "Wha
about the *Times*?"

She gave a nervous laugh. "Just before I left Crete
there was a big article about a wealthy woman who wa:
killed in a private plane crash. The picture looked lik
Mrs. O'Shea—white hair, very polished, dignified." Irene
stood and shrugged. "Don't they say we all have a double
somewhere?"

"So I've heard." Finn pulled a folder out of his backpack and leafed through the clippings in the dim ligh
until he found the one he sought. "Bearing in mind tha
this was more than ten years ago, does this woman look
familiar at all?"

Irene squinted down at the page. "Maybe, but it's hard
to be sure. You know who you should ask?"

"Who?"

"Maggie Mulligan. She's the local teacher and is walking out with Mrs. O'Shea's nephew."

Finn replaced the article and offered her his hand.
"Thank you, Miss Gilhooley. You've been very helpful."

"Can I get you another drink, Mr. Finn?"

He shook his head. "No thanks." He gave her a bill
much larger than necessary. "Keep the change."

Finn had his cell phone in his hand before the pub door
closed behind him. He punched in Angelo's private number. The voice-mail message popped up almost immediately. He was probably either out of range or in flight.

Finn kept walking until he came to Donovan Cottage
again. *Security system. Granddaughter. Last name
O'Shea. Grandmother died in private plane crash.*

Or didn't . . .

• • •

Angelo plopped into the chair again as the next photo came into focus. His breath caught.

Finn said, "She looks like . . ."

"Teresa." Even the sound of his late wife's name left a bad taste in his mouth.

"Not a bit like you."

"But she *is* mine. And *nobody* takes what's mine." *Not even my own mother.* Women couldn't be trusted. He'd known Teresa was weak and would betray him. Getting rid of her had been easy.

And now the only woman he'd ever trusted had committed the worst betrayal of all. Dear old Mother had kidnapped Angelo's only child. Even worse—kept Erin hidden for more than ten years while she planned their new life.

Without him.

Maureen Fazzini deserved to suffer. He gnashed his teeth. She would die at the hands of the son she'd betrayed.

But how? It had to be painful and prolonged. And he would be her executioner.

"Boss, you okay?" Finn waved a hand in front of him.

"Yeah." He mopped perspiration from his face and focused on the screen. "It's hot as hell in here."

"You're kidding? I've been freezing my ass off—"

"Turn on the air."

"Boss, we're lucky they even have electricity in this dump."

"Figures." Angelo closed his eyes and drew a deep breath. "Revenge. Justice." He turned his attention back to the monitor. "Who's the redhead?"

"Schoolteacher. I've been doing my homework. Lots of talkative types in this place. Guess where Desmond spends most of his time when he isn't playing nephew?"

"Can't say I blame him." Angelo popped another antacid. "You think the redhead is our ticket to get him out of the way?"

"Yep, and I figure we can't move in on your mom and the kid until we do."

"Did you say tomorrow's the first day of school?" Angelo looked away from the screen to stare at his half brother.

"Yep. The proprietors of this place like to talk." Finn rolled his eyes. "The chef is a hillbilly. Great grub, though."

Angelo didn't give a shit about food. "If you were a teacher and tomorrow was the first day of school, where would you be today?"

"At school?"

Angelo crossed his arms. "Go watch. Desmond might visit his woman at the school. If he does, call my cell phone."

"What do you have in mind, boss?"

Angelo met Finn's questioning gaze. "Just going to visit my *mother.*" He clenched his fists. "Then take my daughter home."

"Gotcha." Finn grabbed his backpack. "Once Desmond is at the school, we move." He reached over to turn off the computer.

"Leave it." Angelo stared at the photo of his daughter again, then at the redhead.

Fury whipped through him. He saw flames. His anger at his mother was understandable and justified, but why did the schoolteacher make his palms sweat? She was a looker, but the urge that swept through him was to wrap his hands around her pretty neck.

"Shut it down." His hands shook as he watched the screen go black. He stood and walked to the window. "Binoculars." *Take care of business, Angelo. The teacher means nothing except a way to distract Desmond.*

Angelo aimed the binoculars toward the village. "I see the church. What's that building next to it?"

"School."

"Figures. It's Ireland." Angelo looked beyond there. "And that pile of rocks?"

"Ruins of the old church. I walked over there this morning. Kinda creepy."

Angelo trained the binoculars on the ruins again. An odd trickle of excitement raced through him. He heard angry shouting in his head, saw a column of flame near the ruins. *Yes!*

"Burn, witch, burn!"

Twenty

Fire. Flames. Greedy, all consuming, murderous.

Nick's dreams were filled with nothing but the screaming and the horror of watching a human being—an old woman—being burned to death.

Why had Brady sent the crucifix back to Nick? *Why?* Maggie had presented it to him as he was leaving her cottage last night. Her expression had been as intense as his dreams that followed.

"A gift," she'd said.

His answer after he'd taken it into his hands had been one word: "Mine."

After hours in Maggie's arms, he should have dreamed of her. Instead, there was the fire. Always the fire. The burning.

"Burn, witch, burn," the grating, evil voice said.

"Protect her. Save her," the voice of good argued.

A shower and breakfast had revived him enough to accompany Aunt Mo and Erin to mass. The busier he kept his mind, the less room there was for the voices.

And Maggie was there. Sweet Maggie. She'd reminded him about coming over to the school later today to discuss any last minute repairs. He could hardly wait.

After mass he escorted Aunt Mo and Erin home. As they all headed for their own rooms to change into more casual clothes, Aunt Mo asked Nick to meet her in the front room before he left for the school. She went to help Erin start her catechism lesson in her room, which alerted Nick that this was to be a private conversation.

When Aunt Mo came downstairs, she did something she'd never done before. She closed the sliding door between the small parlor and the kitchen. Something important was cooking.

Nick met her gaze. "What is it?"

"It's time. I—I don't think we need a bodyguard anymore." She smiled. "Do you?"

Heaviness settled over him. "I haven't seen anything here to make me believe you and Erin are in danger." He swallowed hard and avoided her gaze.

"School will begin tomorrow, and Erin will make friends. She'll want to go places and do things with other children." Aunt Mo drew a shaky breath and folded her hands in front of her. "I don't want her to feel like a prisoner in her own home. Especially not after living in a convent all these years."

He nodded. "When do you want me to leave?"

"I don't." She smiled again. "And what about your evidence?"

Nick's heart skipped a beat. He'd been so distraught about losing his make-believe family, he'd almost forgotten. "Thanks. Yes, of course, I'll need that."

"There's a safe-deposit box in your name. I'll give you the key when you're ready to go back. Everything you need is in there. Everything." She sighed and pressed her lips into a thin line. "So you're still planning to leave?"

He met her gaze then and saw sadness there. He could relate to that like a kick in the gut. This news should make him *happy*. She was going to reward him with the evidence that would put his father's killer behind bars, clear his name, and shut down the Fazzini drug empire forever. A dream come true.

Except . . . now he had new dreams.

"I . . ." He sighed. "I'm confused. This pretend life feels too real."

"Then let's keep pretending."

He blinked. "What?"

"There's no reason in the world why you can't continue to be my nephew."

Fullness clogged his throat. "It would be best if I keep in touch with Erin. No need for her to know the truth, and if I just drop out of her life . . ."

"She would grieve. As would I." Aunt Mo crossed the room and put her hand on his sleeve. "I have to say this, Nick Desmond. You're more like a son to me than a nephew. I want to be a part of your life, if you'll let me."

He blinked, took a step. "Aunt Mo." He could no longer think of her any other way. "I'd like that."

She smiled, seeming satisfied with his answer. "I'm glad that's settled. And you're welcome to live here with us as long as you wish."

Relief eased through him. He hadn't lost his new family. "Thanks. I'll make arrangements to go back and put the evidence in the right hands, then . . ."

"What about Maggie?"

He smiled. "I think you know how I feel about her."

"Of course. You're in love." Aunt Mo's smile widened. "So you'll come back."

"If she'll have me."

She laughed at that. "Oh, she'll have you. Make no mistake."

Yes, he believed she might. Remembering last night warmed him in more ways than one. No one had ever insinuated herself into his heart this way. It was both exciting and frightening as hell—like the roller coaster at Coney Island.

"I'll make arrangements to head back to New York later in the week," he said, thinking out loud. "After I finish there," he drew a deep breath, "I'm coming back to look for a job."

"Handyman work not to your liking then?"

He lifted a shoulder, almost as afraid to say this as he had been to admit his love for Maggie. "I'm going to ask Guard Bailey about residency requirements for being a cop in Ireland. If he's willing to give me a chance."

Aunt Mo clapped her hands together. "You didn't let the bastards win," she whispered.

"Neither did you." He squeezed his eyes shut. "But *I* almost did."

She looked up at him, her eyes shining. "You're strong and brave and *good.*"

Nick hugged her. "Thank you." He had to blink several times to clear his vision. "That's all I . . . ever wanted to be. Like my dad."

She pulled away and met his gaze. "Never forget that your father is *very* proud of his son."

"Yeah." Nick forced air into his lungs. "I believe he is."

"Starting today, you're my nephew—not my bodyguard."

"Suits me." He grinned and added, "Does that make the five grand my allowance?"

She punched him in the arm. "Get on with you. Didn't you say you have work at the school?"

He kissed her on the cheek. "Thanks, Aunt Mo." Then he headed for the door, amazed that he was even more eager to see Maggie than the evidence against Fazzini. "I'll be back later."

"Take your time. Bridget is coming for tea."

He grinned as he walked the short distance between Donovan Cottage and the schoolhouse. They didn't need a bodyguard, but they still wanted him. Family. He'd found a real cousin and an adopted family that were more important than blood ties.

And Maggie. He broke into a run as he neared the school, eager to see her smile, hear her voice, hold her in his arms. He opened the door and strode inside.

Irene Gilhooley stood beside Maggie's desk. Whispering. A chill forged its way through him.

"Protect her. Save her."

He had to get rid of this crucifix. Throw it into the ocean or something. Dragging a deep breath, he quelled the sudden terror and the urge to take the hunk of silver out of his pocket.

Suddenly he realized Brady hadn't returned the crucifix to *Nick.* He'd returned it to Father Brennan.

Nick couldn't breathe for a few minutes. Was he possessed? Why did he hear both the priest's voice and the other, evil one?

Get a grip, Desmond. "Hello," he called.

Irene spun around, her mouth forming a perfect circle. She looked guilty. Nervous. "I—I was just going." She looked back at Maggie, then swept past Nick without a word.

He heard the door close and turned his attention back to Maggie. "What's with her?"

"I . . ."

Maggie looked very pale and her hands trembled as she sorted through the papers on her desk. Nick crossed the room and reached down to capture her trembling hand in his, but she pulled it away and looked up at him. Her eyes flashed.

"Don't touch me," she whispered. "Not now."

Something had upset her. "What is it? What's wrong?"

She stared down at her desk while he tried to understand her mood. No, anger. She was pissed and he had no idea why. She'd been smiling and laughing at church.

"Maggie, please." He reached for her hand again, but she snatched it back before he could touch it. "What the hell is going on?"

She stood and paced the room. He waited helplessly beside her desk until she finally returned and stood there, staring at him. Her hands were clenched in front of her. A tear spilled from her eye, and he reached toward her again, but she glowered.

Nick grabbed her shoulders and said, "Look at me."

Slowly she lifted her gaze, and he saw betrayal and accusation there. "You lied to me." The words were barely loud enough to hear. "You lied. You and your bloody secrets."

The chill returned with a vengeance. A roaring sound thundered through his head, much like the flames in his nightmare. "Why do you think I lied, Maggie?" he asked gently. "Tell me."

"Irene told me . . ." She drew a shaky breath and her lower lip trembled. "There's a man here looking for a missing child."

Panic shot through Nick like a dull blade. "What man? What child?"

She narrowed her eyes. "Why do I get the feeling you already know?"

"What child, Maggie?" he repeated, knowing he sounded guilty of whatever nefarious activity Irene had insinuated.

"A babe stolen from her parents more than ten years ago in New York." Her voice rose a little with every syllable. "The man is looking for a family named O'Shea. Erin is eleven. I can add, Nick, and 'tis clear you've kept secrets. If I wasn't so certain about that, I wouldn't have listened. 'Tis time to tell the truth now. Until you do, I have nothing more to . . . to say." Her lower lip quivered and tears trickled down her cheeks.

My God. He gave Maggie a little shake. "Listen to me."

She shook her head. " 'Tis only truth I'll listen to now."

"Aunt Mo and Erin are in danger." He grabbed her chin and forced her to look at him. *"Danger.* Do you hear me? I'll explain everything later. I promise. I have to get to them."

"Burn, witch, burn."

He bolted out the door.

Danger? Maggie's eyes widened. "Ailish . . ." She'd said, *"Heed the old one's words, Maggie. There's danger."*

Maggie had seen terror in Nick's eyes when he'd raced out the door. "Heed the old one's words," she repeated with her own voice.

"I cannot let him go. The babe in me womb . . ."

Maggie swayed and gripped the edge of her desk for support. Her period had started this morning. She wasn't pregnant. But Sinéad had conceived a child that night on the porch when her lover came to her. Maggie swallowed hard as realization grew. "Bronagh."

She brought her knuckles to her mouth and bit down hard. The pain helped anchor her, and enabled her to see the truth she'd denied since the old one had started speaking to her.

Sinéad had been Bronagh's mother—not her aunt. Her *mother.* The grief the *cailleach* had felt then swept through Maggie now. No wonder she'd named her babe Bronagh—the Irish word for sorrowful.

"His love of piety and traditions was stronger than the love he professed for me."

"Father Brennan. Fergus." Maggie moaned as tears streamed down her face. Sinéad had conceived his child. Brady was right. They'd fallen in love. Maggie saw it all clearly now. The young Sinéad must have gone away to deliver her child in secret, then returned claiming Bronagh was her orphaned niece.

"Sorrowful." Maggie dried her tears and realized another truth. Rather than trying to prevent Father Brennan from entering the priesthood, Sinéad had loved him enough to bear the burden of raising their child in secret.

Father Fergus Brennan never knew.

"Danger." Maggie shook herself and remembered the look of terror in Nick's eyes. The man she loved.

"The only man I ever loved. Enough to let him go . . ."

"No." Maggie left the papers strewn across her desk and ran out the door. She had to find Nick.

Sinéad had let Fergus go, but Maggie wasn't Sinéad. This was a different lifetime.

"Bronagh."

Maggie stumbled.

"Bronagh," the old one repeated.

Confused and terrified, Maggie dashed toward Dono-van Cottage.

Nick saw the car parked on the road and his heart slammed against his chest.

"We don't need a bodyguard," Aunt Mo had said.

They needed a miracle now. He imagined Aunt Mo hadn't set the security system after he left. She'd believed they were safe.

Nick went to the back door and peered through a window. The kitchen was empty. Carefully he opened the door and slipped inside, wishing again that he had his gun. He listened. Waited.

"My own mother!" a man shouted from the front room.

Nick's blood turned frigid. Fazzini. Their worst nightmare.

"I don't know who y'all are, but you'd best hightail yourselves right on out of here."

"Shut up, bitch."

Bridget was here. *Damn.* A creak on the steps sounded louder than gunfire. Nick's heart stopped when he saw Erin tiptoeing down the steps. When she reached the bottom, he grabbed her hand and stooped low enough to look directly into her eyes.

The shouting from the next room would keep Fazzini from overhearing. "Run to *Caisleán* Dubh," he whispered. "Tell Riley we need help. Stay there. I'll come for you."

Eyes wide, Erin nodded. Nick opened the door just enough to let the child squeeze through. He watched her run until she rounded the curve and was out of sight. And safe.

"Why?" Fazzini asked.

"Yeah, why?" another man asked.

"Shut up, Finn."

Fazzini's henchman, too. *Shit.* Nick took a few steps toward the drawer where Aunt Mo kept some tools. He eased it open and grabbed a hammer.

The sliding door stood open just enough for Nick to

peer into the front room. He saw Bridget Mulligan in the rocking chair, her hand resting protectively across her belly. He could only see one side of the room, where McAdam stood near the entryway. Fazzini was somewhere to the right where Nick couldn't see him.

"I asked you why you stole my daughter," Fazzini said.

Based on the proximity of the man's voice, Nick guessed he stood with his back near the partially closed sliding door.

"To protect her from the life you chose for yourself," Aunt Mo said.

The sound of his aunt's voice gave Nick hope.

"Where's Erin?" Fazzini's voice broke. "Where's my daughter?"

"She's not here," Aunt Mo answered.

"Bullshit," McAdam said.

Wanna bet, asshole? Nick needed a plan. If only he had his damned gun.

"You don't look well, Angelo," Aunt Mo said. "Are you ill?"

"As if you give a shit," Junior hissed. "Finn, go upstairs and find Erin. Bring *my* daughter to me."

Nick barely had time to flatten himself against the wall before the door slid open and his old nemesis stepped through. Nick clobbered him with the hammer and caught him before he fell. He dragged the scumbag into his room off the kitchen.

Then he remembered the duct tape in his closet. Dad had always said a man should never be without a roll. Nick almost grinned. With a hammer and duct tape as his only weapons, maybe he was a handyman after all.

He searched his prisoner and found another useful tool. Didn't it figure that the good guys couldn't have guns in Ireland, but the bad guys had found a way? Disgusted, Nick evened the odds.

Once McAdam was secure, Nick crept back into the kitchen. With the sliding door open now, he could see Fazzini's back.

The man who'd ordered Dad's murder.

He raised the gun and took aim. He wasn't a killer. Still, the urge to pull the trigger thundered through him. He broke into a cold sweat and he couldn't breathe.

No, Nick Desmond wasn't a killer.

"Protect her. Save her."

The voice of Father Brennan? Nick drew a deep breath and inched toward the door. Bridget's eyes widened, and he knew she'd seen him. He held a finger to his lips, and she looked away.

"My granny always said men like you get what's coming to them in this life," Bridget said.

Junior's laughter was maniacal. "I'm taking my daughter home where she belongs. That's what's coming to me."

"Angelo, leave her be," Aunt Mo said. "Erin doesn't know you. She's safe here from your world. If you love her, turn around and leave."

"Y'all don't want her to see her daddy like that, do you? Holding a gun on her granny?"

"Shut up!"

The drug lord had lost his cool. He shifted his weight to his other foot, enabling Nick to see the angle of his right arm. The bastard had a gun, too.

"Erin is mine. She belongs with me."

"Not anymore," Aunt Mo said. "You chose crime over fatherhood."

"You self-righteous witch!" Fazzini roared in a familiar voice.

"Burn, witch, burn!"

My God.

"Let Bridget leave now," Aunt Mo said calmly, obviously recognizing her son's near hysteria. "Let her go home and I'll tell you where Erin is."

"You expect me to believe *you*?" Fazzini took a menacing step. "Finn, where the fuck *are you*?"

Nick crept closer. He turned the gun around to use the

butt on the back of Junior's skull, but the front door burst open.

And Fazzini fired.

Maggie threw open the door without knocking and bolted into the cottage.

A gun exploded. Bridget screamed. Mrs. O'Shea fell. The blood . . . Nick lunged through a doorway for the stranger holding the gun. Maggie ran toward Mrs. O'Shea.

The bad man dodged Nick and grabbed Maggie, his arm like a snake whipping out to wrap around her throat. Nick froze in a half crouched position, his eyes murderous. He also had a gun.

Maggie couldn't breathe. She clawed at the man's arm. He backed toward the door. "Drop it, Desmond," he ordered.

Nick stooped lower and laid the gun on the floor.

"Kick it over here and put your hands up."

Nick obeyed, his gaze locked on Maggie's. She hadn't trusted him enough.

"His duty came before love."

"Nick," she croaked, which made the man's arm tighten even more.

"Didn't you learn the first time, pig?" the man taunted. "Wasn't your old man's blood enough?"

Maggie watched the flash of pain in Nick's eyes.

"You hurt her and you're a dead man, Fazzini."

The man called Fazzini kicked the gun out the open door and dragged Maggie closer. "I don't know what you did with Finn and Erin, but you better listen this time."

Nick made no sound, but she saw his heavy breathing, and now she saw fear blended with his rage. Fear for her. If only she'd trusted him . . .

But he hadn't trusted her enough to tell *her* the truth. They were both at fault. It didn't matter now. She still loved him, and Mrs. O'Shea needed a doctor.

Bridget stood slowly. "You two go on and argue all day if you want. I'm going to tend Mrs. O'Shea now."

"Fazzini. Her name is Maureen Fazzini." He spat on the ground. "My *mother.*"

"Then I reckon I'll go tend Maureen." Bridget lifted her chin a notch. "Riley and Jacob will be stopping here to fetch me on their way back from Doolin soon enough, so I reckon you'd best leave us be."

"Riley isn't home?" Nick asked, his tone wretched.

"Shut up!" the man bellowed.

"Bronagh," the old one said.

Bridget *was* Bronagh. Maggie felt Sinéad's love for her daughter flowing through her. Bridget was one of the bravest women Maggie had ever known. She loved her like a sister.

Mother Mary, keep Bridget and her babe safe, Maggie prayed.

Fazzini kept his gun on Nick even when Bridget lowered her pregnant self to her knees and turned Maureen onto her back. The old woman moaned and Maggie felt her captor flinch.

"She's alive," Bridget said. "She needs a doctor."

"Let the bitch bleed." He swung his attention back to Nick. "Listen well, Desmond."

"I'm listening." He stood straight and tall, his expression masked. "Talk."

"I'm taking your woman to the ruins," he said.

"There's danger," Ailish had said.

"Why—"

"Shut up and listen." Fazzini waved his weapon again. "You send Erin to me there within twenty minutes. Alone."

Nick didn't even blink. "Or . . . ?"

"I will carry out my duty."

Nick's eyes widened as if he understood the man's cryptic words. "And *I* will do *mine.*"

"Twenty minutes, Desmond."

Fazzini dragged Maggie through the door and kicked the extra gun into the shrubs. Panting and sweating, he released his grip on her neck and shoved her ahead of him.

"Walk," he ordered, and she felt the gun barrel against her back. She willed herself not to cry.

"Faster," he barked.

She ran and heard his heavy steps behind her. "Stop!" he shouted as they neared the school. "You know where your fate awaits." His tone changed and Maggie froze.

"Me executioner has come for me."

Maggie blinked, trying to understand Sinéad's words. This was the danger Ailish had warned her about. *Jaysus, Mary, and Joseph.* Now Maggie understood why Ailish hadn't been sure who was in danger.

Fazzini gave her a shove between the shoulder blades and Maggie turned into the schoolyard. She walked through the cemetery, past her da's grave. Tears stung her eyes.

"Fergus cannot save me now. 'Tis too late. Too late."

Fazzini gave her another shove as they neared the gate that led to the ruins. Maggie staggered forward, breaking her fall against the low stone wall. She gasped for air while the man opened the gate. He grabbed her arm and flung her through it. She fell and her shoulder struck a rock. Pain shot through her, but she bit her lip to hold her silence.

"I will not let him see the fear in me heart."

"Get up, witch," Fazzini kicked her in the ribs. *"Get up."*

Maggie pushed to her feet. Her arm wasn't broken at least. He gave her another shove toward the ruins and she turned around to keep from falling over anything else.

Fear clawed through her. Someone had laid wood for a fire in front of the old church.

"Fergus cannot help me now. No one can."

The moment they left, Nick called Guard Bailey and stooped beside Bridget and Aunt Mo. The old woman's eyes fluttered open, and alarm instantly registered.

"Erin," she said, her voice weak. "Where's Erin?"

"Safe." The bullet had entered her shoulder. "Junior has Maggie. I have to go."

Bridget grabbed his arm. "Nick, wait—"

"I *have* to do this."

She nodded. "I'll wait here for Guard Bailey and Riley. Be careful."

"Call Fiona," he said. "Tell her to keep Erin there no matter what."

"Good," Aunt Mo whispered. "Good."

Nick grabbed the phone on the table and set it near Bridget on the floor. She started dialing, and he ran out onto the stoop. Where was the gun? Fazzini couldn't have bent over to pick it up while holding Maggie.

Maggie. He had to save her.

"I must save Sinéad. The landlord means to carry out her sentence."

Nick didn't have time to search for the gun. He ran as far as the school, then cut across the side farthest from the cemetery and ruins. At the back of the school he saw two figures, but from this distance he couldn't be sure what they were doing.

At least there were a few trees between the school and the ruins. He ran to one and flattened his back against it. Fazzini looked busy, but Nick was still too far away to see them clearly. He dashed to the next tree and saw Maggie's red hair blowing in the wind. She stood very straight, as if tied to—

"The landlord has tied Sinéad to a cross. Not only will he burn her, but he will desecrate the church with his hatred."

Terror shot through Nick. He no longer heard the evil voice to counter Father Brennan's, and he knew why.

Because the evil voice had found a new home.

Nick's heart thundered and his breath came in raspy gasps. He bolted for the tree nearest the ruins and waited for his breathing to quiet. Sweat poured into his eyes. He reached up and wiped it away and checked his watch. Nine minutes of the twenty remained.

"The landlord fears the Mulligans will try to stop him."

Nick dropped to the ground and crawled to the stone wall. Now he could hear as well as see.

"Burn, witch, burn," Fazzini chanted. "Burn, witch, burn. Burn, witch, burn."

Maggie's eyes were wide but dry. She was tied, to a post—not a cross—but it was bad enough. At her feet, wood had been laid for a fire. Nick spotted the gasoline can nearby.

The bastard had staged this nightmare before ever going to Donovan Cottage.

"Burn, witch, burn," Fazzini continued as he sprinkled gasoline on the wood. He still had the gun clutched in his other hand, and the expression on his face was one of consummate evil.

He set the can aside and looked at his watch. Then he shaded his eyes and gazed into the distance. Nick ducked lower, which meant he had to take his eyes off the monster for a few precious seconds.

"Damn you, Desmond."

Nick pulled Father Brennan's crucifix from his pocket and stared at it. *Help us.* After a moment he shoved it back into his pocket and held his breath, waiting and hoping for some sound that would tell him it was safe to look again. He couldn't risk the crazy bastard hurting Maggie. Though it was clear he had planned the fire—*God help me*—the fact remained that he still had a gun as well.

Nick wasn't sure who was more dangerous—the "landlord" or Junior. Then he remembered his father's murder and the countless lives that had been destroyed or lost because of Fazzini's drugs.

"This was supposed to be for Mother," Fazzini muttered. "But a burned witch is a burned witch."

Maggie made no response. Worried, Nick eased upward and peered over the wall. Flames leapt up behind Maggie.

"Save her now. Save her!"

With a roar Nick flew over the wall and tackled Fazzini. The bastard reeked of gasoline. His gun clattered across the stones out of reach, and Fazzini's insanity seemed to strengthen him. They rolled several times and Nick made sure it was toward the fire.

Toward Maggie.

With one final burst of power, Nick flung his father's murderer into the flames. Junior's scream echoed through the cemetery, and church bells rang—the same distant, surreal ones Nick had heard before.

The bastard's clothes were ablaze. Fazzini ran toward the sea and disappeared with another scream over the cliffs.

The flames had just reached Maggie's skirt. Nick lunged for her and fumbled with the ropes. Too much time. Hurry. Hurry.

"Save her."

"I'm trying, damn it." Nick finally dragged the post and Maggie away from the burning wood. He lowered her to the ground and threw himself onto her burning skirt. He was terrified he might fan the flames instead of smothering them.

The sound of men shouting broke through the roaring of the fire. Nick lifted his head and looked down at Maggie. Black soot streaked her face, but she appeared unharmed.

"You saved me," she said, her voice hoarse. "And Sinéad."

Nick nodded, not trusting his voice just now, then looked to make sure her skirt was no longer burning. "Are you hurt?" he asked.

"No."

"Thank God." With trembling hands he released the ropes and helped her stand just as Riley, Brady, Guard Bailey, and half the village came racing through the graveyard. They carried an odd collection of clubs and knives. Riley hefted a broadsword that must have belonged to a medieval ancestor.

"Where is he?" Brady demanded, murder in his faded eyes. He had an antique short sword clutched in his fist.

"Dead, I think." Nick kept his arm around Maggie. "He was on fire and ran off the cliff."

Several men broke away to investigate.

"Is Aunt Mo all right?" Nick asked.

"Aye." Brady lowered the sword. "When I saw what he'd done, I was ready to draw blood."

"I can see that." A halfhearted smile tugged at Nick's lips, and he pulled Maggie even closer. "They're both okay and the man who tried to hurt them is dead."

Guard Bailey stepped forward. "I've taken the one you left bound at the cottage into custody. Good work, Desmond."

Riley reached out to touch the backs of his fingers to his sister's cheeks. "Ah, lass. He tried to *burn* you?"

Nick released her to go to her brother. It wasn't easy, but it was necessary. He watched her hug Riley. A moment later she was back at his side, linking her fingers with his.

"Nick saved my life," she said. "He fought that madman with his bare hands and saved me. Only my skirt was burned."

A tear appeared in the corner of Riley's eye. He cleared his throat and clapped Nick on the shoulder. "You're a good man, Nick Desmond."

"Thanks." Riley Mulligan's approval meant more to Nick than he could have imagined.

"But . . ." Riley shook a finger in Nick's face. "Keeping secrets for whatever reason is what brought evil men with guns to Ballybronagh. No more secrets."

"No more secrets." Nick swallowed hard, his eyes burning.

"Your word is enough for me." Riley nodded.

"Thank you."

Guard Bailey and Brady went to the cliffs, and Nick gave Maggie's hand a squeeze as he met Riley's gaze. "I want to marry your sister." He turned to look at her. "If she'll have me."

"Maggie?" Riley asked.

"He is for me and I for him," she said emphatically. "I will marry you, Nick Desmond. Right after you explain all your secrets, that is."

"I will. But I'll need Aunt Mo's blessing for part of it."

Maggie smiled. "Then my answer is *aye*."

Nick kissed her and Riley cleared his throat. "In that case, you have my blessing," the Irishman said. "Mrs. O'Shea and Erin are at the castle, where they'll stay until she's well enough to go home. 'Tis I who'll need the doctor if I don't get back to tell Bridget and Mum that all is well."

Nick and Maggie gave their statements to Guard Bailey, and she made sure he knew where to find the extra gun so it wouldn't fall into innocent hands. After Fazzini's burned and broken—and very dead—body was recovered, Gilhooley's opened despite it being Sunday, so the villagers could gather to discuss the day's events. By the time Nick and Maggie were able to head toward *Caisleán* Dubh, it was dusk. They stopped at the curve in the road that would take them to Mulligan land. There, they gazed out toward the sea and saw them.

Except this time the man and woman standing arm in arm on the cliffs weren't young and innocent. They were old and wise. He wore a long wool cape, and she a shawl. Nick tightened his hold on Maggie's hand as the couple turned to face them.

"Sinéad and Fergus," Maggie whispered, her tone filled with awe.

Nick inclined his head toward the man whose words had filled his mind these past weeks. The man did the same.

Nick reached into his pocket and withdrew the crucifix. Together, he and Maggie approached them. Knowing what he had to do, Nick opened his palm and extended the crucifix toward Fergus.

Sinéad smiled and said, "Me gift to you."

Fergus reached out and took it from Nick's palm and said, "I thought it lost forever. Thank ye."

Sinéad and Fergus took a few steps backward, their hands joined. The years slipped away and they were young again. Slowly the couple faded, and Nick knew that he and Maggie would hear no more voices.

He turned to face Maggie, cupping her lovely face in his hands. "Together at last."

Maggie's eyes shone with love. "Now and always."

Epilogue

The Clare Champion: Caisleán Dubh, Ballybronagh.

The first week of October was an eventful one for the citizens of this small village when Mary Margaret Mulligan married American Nicholas Desmond in a ceremony held at the legendary *Caisleán* Dubh. Ailish Delaney of Dublin served as maid of honor, and the groom's cousin, Mr. Brady Rearden of Ballybronagh, as best man. Father Thomas O'Malley officiated.

The surprising event of the day was the birth of Patrick Culley Mulligan to parents Riley Francis and Bridget Colleen Mulligan—brother and sister-in-law of the bride. The lad was in such a hurry that the grandmother and the groom—a former New York City police officer who once assisted in a birth on the subway—delivered him in the tower of *Caisleán* Dubh. Young Patrick Culley is the first child to be born in the castle since it was sealed in 1899.

The newlyweds will honeymoon in Connemara. Patrick Culley and his mother are doing well, and the proud new da is expected to make a full recovery.

DEB STOVER has received, since her debut in 1995, the 1999 and 1997 Pikes Peak Romance Writers' Author of the Year Award, the 1999 Dorothy Parker Award of Excellence, a 1998 Heart of Romance Readers' Choice Award, two Colorado Book Award nominations, and seven *Romantic Times* nominations, including two for Career Achievement. Deb has received more than a dozen other Readers' Choice Awards, including Romance Novel of the Year from *Affaire de Coeur.*